1998
YEAR BOOK OF
PATHOLOGY
AND LABORATORY
MEDICINE®

Statement of Purpose

The YEAR BOOK Service

The YEAR BOOK series was devised in 1901 by practicing health professionals who observed that the literature of medicine and related disciplines had become so voluminous that no one individual could read and place in perspective every potential advance in a major specialty. In the final decade of the 20th century, this recognition is more acutely true than it was in 1901.

More than merely a series of books, YEAR BOOK volumes are the tangible results of a unique service designed to accomplish the following:

- to *survey* a wide range of journals of proven value
- to *select* from those journals papers representing significant advances and statements of important clinical principles
- to provide *abstracts* of those articles that are readable, convenient summaries of their key points
- to provide *commentary* about those articles to place them in perspective

These publications grow out of a unique process that calls on the talents of outstanding authorities in clinical and fundamental disciplines, trained literature specialists, and professional writers, all supported by the resources of Mosby, the world's preeminent publisher for the health professions.

The Literature Base

Mosby and its Editors survey more than 1,000 journals published worldwide, covering the full range of the health professions. On an annual basis, the publisher examines usage patterns and polls its expert authorities to add new journals to the literature base and to delete journals that are no longer useful as potential YEAR BOOK sources.

The Literature Survey

The publisher's team of literature specialists, all of whom are trained and experienced health professionals, examines every original, peer-reviewed article in each journal issue. More than 250,000 articles per year are scanned systematically, including title, text, illustrations, tables, and references. Each scan is compared, article by article, to the search strategies that the publisher has developed in consultation with the 270 outside experts who form the pool of YEAR BOOK editors. A given article may be reviewed by any number of editors, from one to a dozen or more, regardless of the discipline for which the paper was originally published. In turn, each editor who receives the article reviews it to determine whether the article should be included in the YEAR BOOK. This decision is based on the article's inherent quality, its probable usefulness to readers of that YEAR BOOK, and the editor's goal to represent a balanced picture of a given field in each volume of the YEAR BOOK. In addition, the editor indicates when to include figures and tables from the article to help the YEAR BOOK reader better understand the information.

Of the quarter million articles scanned each year, only 5% are selected for detailed analysis within the YEAR BOOK series, thereby assuring readers of the high value of every selection.

The Abstract

The publisher's abstracting staff is headed by a seasoned medical professional and includes individuals with training in the life sciences, medicine, and other areas, plus extensive experience in writing for the health professions and related industries. Each selected article is assigned to a specific writer on this abstracting staff. The abstracter, guided in many cases by notations supplied by the expert editor, writes a structured, condensed summary designed so that the reader can rapidly acquire the essential information contained in the article.

The Commentary

The YEAR BOOK editorial boards, sometimes assisted by guest commentators, write comments that place each article in perspective for the reader. This provides the reader with the equivalent of a personal consultation with a leading international authority—an opportunity to better understand the value of the article and to benefit from the authority's thought processes in assessing the article.

Additional Editorial Features

The editorial boards of each YEAR BOOK organize the abstracts and comments to provide a logical and satisfying sequence of information. To enhance the organization, editors also provide introductions to sections or individual chapters, comments linking a number of abstracts, citations to additional literature, and other features.

The published YEAR BOOK contains enhanced bibliographic citations for each selected article, including extended listings of multiple authors and identification of author affiliations. Each YEAR BOOK contains a Table of Contents specific to that year's volume. From year to year, the Table of Contents for a given YEAR BOOK will vary depending on developments within the field.

Every YEAR BOOK contains a list of the journals from which papers have been selected. This list represents a subset of the more than 1,000 journals surveyed by the publisher and occasionally reflects a particularly pertinent article from a journal that is not surveyed on a routine basis.

Finally, each volume contains a comprehensive subject index and an index to authors of each selected paper.

The 1998 Year Book Series

Year Book of Allergy, Asthma, and Clinical Immunology: Drs. Rosenwasser, Borish, Gelfand, Leung, Nelson, and Szefler

Year Book of Anesthesiology and Pain Management®: Drs. Tinker, Abram, Chestnut, Roizen, Rothenberg, and Wood

Year Book of Cardiology®: Drs. Schlant, Collins, Gersh, Graham, Kaplan, and Waldo

Year Book of Chiropractic®: Dr. Lawrence

Year Book of Critical Care Medicine®: Drs. Parrillo, Balk, Calvin, Franklin, and Shapiro

Year Book of Dentistry®: Drs. Meskin, Berry, Jeffcoat, Leinfelder, Roser, Summitt, and Zakariasen

Year Book of Dermatologic Surgery®: Drs. Greenway, Papadopoulos, Whitaker, and Barrett

Year Book of Dermatology®: Dr. Thiers

Year Book of Diagnostic Radiology®: Drs. Osborn, Groskin, Dalinka, Maynard, Pentecost, Rebner, Ros, Smirniotopoulos, and Young

Year Book of Drug Therapy®: Drs. Lasagna and Weintraub

Year Book of Emergency Medicine®: Drs. Wagner, Dronen, Davidson, King, Niemann, and Roberts

Year Book of Endocrinology®: Drs. Bagdade, Braverman, Horton, Kannan, Landsberg, Molitch, Morley, Nathan, Odell, Poehlman, Rogol, and Ryan

Year Book of Family Practice®: Drs. Berg, Bowman, Davidson, Dexter, and Scherger

Year Book of Gastroenterology®: Drs. Aliperti and Fleshman

Year Book of Geriatrics and Gerontology®: Drs. Beck, Burton, Ostwald, Rabins, Reuben, Roth, Shapiro, and Whitehouse

Year Book of Hand Surgery®: Drs. Amadio and Hentz

Year Book of Hematology®: Drs. Spivak, Bell, Ness, Quesenberry, Wiernik, and Horowitz

Year Book of Infectious Diseases: Drs. Keusch, Barza, Bennish, Poutsiaka, Skolnik, and Snydman

Year Book of Medicine®: Drs. Klahr, Cline, McCallum, Frishman, Utiger, Malawista, Mandell, and Jett

Year Book of Neonatal and Perinatal Medicine®: Drs. Fanaroff, Maisels, and Stevenson

Year Book of Nephrology, Hypertension, and Mineral Metabolism: Drs. Schwab, Bennett, Emmett, Hostetter, Kuman, and Toto

Year Book of Neurology and Neurosurgery®: Drs. Bradley and Gibbs

Year Book of Nuclear Medicine®: Drs. Gottschalk, Blaufox, Neumann, Strauss, and Zubal

Year Book of Obstetrics, Gynecology, and Women's Health: Drs. Mishell, Herbst, and Kirschbaum

Year Book of Occupational and Environmental Medicine®: Drs. Emmett, Frank, Gochfeld, and Hessl

Year Book of Oncology®: Drs. Ozols, Eisenberg, Glatstein, Loehrer, Tallman, and Wiersma

Year Book of Ophthalmology®: Drs. Wilson, Augsburger, Cohen, Eagle, Grossman, Laibson, Maguire, Nelson, Penne, Rapuano, Sergott, Spaeth, Tipperman, Ms. Gosfield, and Ms. Salmon

Year Book of Orthopedics®: Drs. Morrey, Beauchamp, Currier, Tolo, Trigg, Swiontkowski

Year Book of Otolaryngology–Head and Neck Surgery®: Drs. Paparella and Holt

Year Book of Pathology and Laboratory Medicine®: Drs. Raab, Cohen, Olson, Sirgi, and Stanley

Year Book of Pediatrics®: Dr. Stockman

Year Book of Plastic, Reconstructive, and Aesthetic Surgery®: Drs. Miller, Bartlett, Garner, McKinney, Ruberg, Salisbury, and Smith

Year Book of Psychiatry and Applied Mental Health®: Drs. Talbott, Ballanger, Frances, Lydiard, Meltzer, Schowalter, and Tasman

Year Book of Pulmonary Disease®: Drs. Jett, Maurer, Ryu, Strollo, and Wenzel

Year Book of Rheumatology®: Drs. Panush, Hadler, LeRoy, Liang, Reichlin, Simon, and Weinblatt

Year Book of Sports Medicine®: Drs. Shephard, Drinkwater, Eichner, Torg, Alexander, and Mr. George

Year Book of Surgery®: Drs. Copeland, Bland, Deitch, Eberlein, Howard, Luce, Seeger, Souba, and Sugarbaker

Year Book of Thoracic and Cardiovascular Surgery®: Drs. Ginsberg, Wechsler, and Williams

Year Book of Urology®: Drs. Andriole and Coplen

Year Book of Vascular Surgery®: Dr. Porter

1998

The Year Book of PATHOLOGY AND LABORATORY MEDICINE®

Editor-in-Chief

Stephen Raab, M.D.

Associate Professor, University of Iowa, University of Iowa Hospitals and Clinics, Iowa City, Iowa

Editors

Michael B. Cohen, M.D.

Professor, Departments of Pathology/Urology, University of Iowa; Director, Division of Cytopathology, University of Iowa Hospitals and Clinics, Iowa City, Iowa

John D. Olson, M.D., Ph.D.

Professor, University of Iowa; Director of Clinical Laboratories, University of Iowa Hospitals and Clinics, Iowa City, Iowa

Karim E. Sirgi, M.D.

Denver-Aurora Pathology Associates, P.C., Chairman, Pathology Laboratory, Columbia Presbyterian/St. Luke's Hospital, Denver, Colorado

Michael W. Stanley, M.D.

Professor of Pathology, University of Minnesota Hospitals and Clinics; Chair, Department of Pathology, Hennepin County Medical Center, Minneapolis, Minnesota

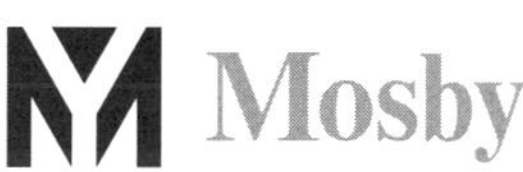

St. Louis Baltimore Boston Carlsbad Naples New York Philadelphia Portland London
Madrid Mexico City Singapore Sydney Tokyo Toronto Wiesbaden

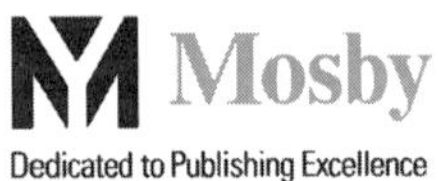

Mosby

Dedicated to Publishing Excellence

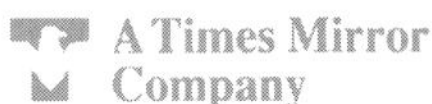

A Times Mirror Company

Acquisitions Editor: Gina G. Byrd
Developmental Editor: Kelly J. Poirier
Manuscript Editor: Stephanie M. Geels
Production Assistant: Laura Bayless
Manager, Literature Services: Idelle L. Winer
Illustrations and Permissions Specialist: Steve Ramay

1998 EDITION
Copyright © 1998 by Mosby, Inc.

Printed in the United States of America
Composition by Reed Technology and Information Services, Inc.
Printing/binding by Maple-Vail

Editorial Office:
Mosby, Inc.
11830 Westline Industrial Drive
St. Louis, MO 63146

International Standard Serial Number: 1077–9108
International Standard Book Number: 0–8151–9722–5

Contributing Editors

Ronald Feld, Ph.D.
Associate Professor of Pathology, Department of Pathology, University of Iowa College of Medicine; Laboratory Director of Chemistry, University of Iowa Hospitals and Clinics, Iowa City, Iowa

Dana Grzybicki, M.D., Ph.D.
Assistant Professor, Duquesne University School of Health Sciences, Pittsburgh, Pennsylvania

A.S. Knisely, M.D.
Denver-Aurora Pathology Associates, Denver, Colorado

Michael A. Pfaller, M.D.
Professor, Department of Pathology, University of Iowa College of Medicine; Co-Director, Microbiology Laboratory, University of Iowa Hospitals and Clinics, Iowa City, Iowa

Annette J. Schlueter, M.D., Ph.D.
Fellow Associate, University of Iowa, University of Iowa Hospitals and Clinics, Iowa City, Iowa

John F. Turner, Jr., M.D.
Assistant Professor of Pathology, University of Iowa; Hematopathologist, Department of Pathology, University of Iowa Hospitals and Clinics, Iowa City, Iowa

Table of Contents

Journals Represented

Mosby and its editors survey more than 1,000 journals for its abstract and commentary publications. From these journals, the editors select the articles to be abstracted. Journals represented in this YEAR BOOK are listed below.

Acta Cytologica
Acta Paediatrica
American Family Physician
American Journal of Clinical Pathology
American Journal of Dermatopathology
American Journal of Gastroenterology
American Journal of Hematology
American Journal of Medicine
American Journal of Nephrology
American Journal of Obstetrics and Gynecology
American Journal of Pathology
American Journal of Respiratory and Critical Care Medicine
American Journal of Roentgenology
American Journal of Surgical Pathology
Annals of Surgery
Annals of Surgical Oncology
Annals of Thoracic Surgery
Annals of Vascular Surgery
Archives of Neurology
Archives of Otolaryngology-Head and Neck Surgery
Archives of Pathology and Laboratory Medicine
Archives of Pediatrics and Adolescent Medicine
Blood
Breast Journal
British Journal of Cancer
British Journal of Obstetrics and Gynaecology
British Journal of Surgery
Cancer
Cell
Chest
Clinical Chemistry
Critical Care Medicine
Diabetes Care
Diabetic Medicine
Diagnostic Cytopathology
European Journal of Cancer
Hepatology
Human Pathology
International Journal of Cancer
International Journal of Gynecological Pathology
Journal of Clinical Microbiology
Journal of Clinical Oncology
Journal of Clinical Pathology
Journal of Cutaneous Pathology
Journal of Heart and Lung Transplantation
Journal of Infectious Diseases
Journal of Neurology, Neurosurgery and Psychiatry

Journal of Neuropathology and Experimental Neurology
Journal of Neurosurgery
Journal of Pathology
Journal of Pediatric Hematology/Oncology
Journal of Pediatrics
Journal of Urology
Journal of the American Academy of Dermatology
Journal of the American Medical Association
Leukemia
Medicine
Modern Pathology
Neurology
New England Journal of Medicine
Obstetrics and Gynecology
Pediatric Pathology & Laboratory Medicine
Prenatal Diagnosis
Prostate
Seminars in Oncology
Surgical Neurology
Thrombosis and Haemostatis
Transfusion
Urology

STANDARD ABBREVIATIONS

The following terms are abbreviated in this edition: acquired immunodeficiency syndrome (AIDS), cardiopulmonary resuscitation (CPR), central nervous system (CNS), cerebrospinal fluid (CSF), computed tomography (CT), deoxyribonucleic acid (DNA), electrocardiography (ECG), health maintenance organization (HMO), human immunodeficiency virus (HIV), intensive care unit (ICU), intramuscular (IM), intravenous (IV), magnetic resonance (MR) imaging (MRI), and ribonucleic acid (RNA).

NOTE

The YEAR BOOK OF PATHOLOGY AND LABORATORY MEDICINE® is a literature survey service providing abstracts of articles published in the professional literature. Every effort is made to assure the accuracy of the information presented in these pages. Neither the editors nor the publisher of the YEAR BOOK OF PATHOLOGY AND LABORATORY MEDICINE® can be responsible for errors in the original materials. The editors' comments are their own opinions. Mention of specific products within this publication does not constitute endorsement.

To facilitate the use of the YEAR BOOK OF PATHOLOGY AND LABORATORY MEDICINE® as a reference tool, all illustrations and tables included in this publication are now identified as they appear in the original article. This change is meant to help the reader recognize that any illustration or table appearing in the YEAR BOOK OF PATHOLOGY AND LABORATORY MEDICINE® may be only one of many in the original article. For this reason, figure and table numbers will often appear to be out of sequence within the YEAR BOOK OF PATHOLOGY AND LABORATORY MEDICINE.®

Publisher's Preface

Please join us in welcoming Stephen Raab, M.D. as the new editor-in-chief to the YEAR BOOK OF PATHOLOGY AND LABORATORY MEDICINE. He has assembled an outstanding group of individuals—Michael Cohen, M.D.; John Olson, M.D., Ph.D.; Karim Sirgi, M.D.; and Michael Stanley, M.D.—to complete the editorial board. We know you'll agree they've done an excellent job on this, their first edition of the YEAR BOOK.

Introduction

Welcome to the 1998 edition of the YEAR BOOK OF PATHOLOGY AND LABORATORY MEDICINE! For those who routinely read the YEAR BOOK, you will note that there is an entirely new editorial board composed of both academic and private practice pathologists. These individuals were chosen in part because I view them as friends, and also because I believe that these individuals have novel insights in specific fields of pathology. As the new editor-in-chief, my explicit instructions to them were to "write whatever," and if you knew me you would know that, despite the tongue-in-cheek, this is exactly what I did say. But knowing the other members of the editorial board you would know that for every article chosen there will be a stimulating, thought-provoking, and hopefully controversial comment. The more controversy the better.

As you are aware, there is so much that is published in pathology and related medical fields that it is difficult to keep abreast, let alone to determine what is useful. Our job was to do this for you. The format of the this year's YEAR BOOK is similar to previous ones, although we have added chapters on anatomic pathology outcomes and anatomic pathology techniques. I would appreciate your comments and suggestions regarding the YEAR BOOK, so please e-mail me or the other editors. Happy reading, or whatever!

Stephen Raab, M.D.

PART I

ANATOMICAL PATHOLOGY

———

1 Respiratory System and Mediastinum

Postmortem Findings in Lung Transplant Recipients
Husain AN, Siddiqui MT, Reddy VB, et al (Loyola Univ, Maywood, Ill)
Mod Pathol 7:752–761, 1996

1–1

Background.—Lung transplantation is now an accepted treatment for patients with end-stage lung disease. To further understand the factors that limit survival of such patients, autopsy findings in 1 series of lung transplant recipients were reviewed.

Methods.—Data from 37 patients were analyzed. These patients represented 77% of 48 patients dying after lung transplantation performed at 1 center between 1986 and 1995. The overall mortality for the 131 patients undergoing lung transplantation in that period was 36.6%.

Findings.—Among the 12 patients dying within 30 days of transplantation, intraoperative and postoperative complications caused the deaths of 6, and bacterial infection with pneumonia in the transplanted lung caused the deaths of 6 others. Eleven of the 18 patients dying 1 month to 1 year after transplantation died of infection, including cytomegalovirus infections (in 5), nonviral infections of the transplanted lung (in 5), and encephalomyelitis (in 1). Another 3 patients in this group died of posttransplantation lymphoproliferative disorder; 3, of chronic airway rejection; and 1, of unrelated causes. Of the 7 patients dying after 1 year posttransplantation, 4 died of chronic airway rejection, 2 of unrelated causes, and 1 of bacterial infection. In 23 patients undergoing native lung examination, 5 had bacterial pneumonia in addition to primary disease; 3, posttransplantation lymphoproliferative disorder; 2, cytomegalovirus; and 1, aspergillosis. Overall chronic rejection was the cause of death in 7 patients and was seen concomitant with the primary disease in 3.

Conclusions.—The most common cause of death in this series of lung transplant recipients undergoing autopsy was infection, responsible for 48% of the deaths, followed by chronic rejection in 19%, surgical complications in 19%, and posttransplantation lymphoproliferative disorder in 7%. In another 7%, the cause of death was unrelated to transplantation. Rejection was not a major cause of death in the early and intermediate posttransplantation periods. Thirty percent of native lungs had significant

"

pathologic findings in addition to the primary disease. In the intermediate posttransplantation period, significant left ventricular hypertrophy was observed; this may have been caused by cyclosporine-induced hypertension.

▶ Although most of us probably do not see many specimens from patients with lung transplants, lung transplantation, as Husain et al. suggest, is now an accepted modality for treating end-stage pulmonary disease.[1-3] More and more of these patients, after transplantation, will eventually be seen in hospitals where their original transplantation was not performed, and thus academic and community pathologists will see more of these specimens.

Husain et al. did a good job in documenting the causes of death in 37 patients with lung transplants. Like most pathologists, when I see a specimen from a patient with a lung transplant, I look for rejection or infection, and it was interesting to note how the proportion of patients who died of rejection or infection changed as length of survival posttransplant increased. Those who died within 30 days of transplant did not die of rejection, and their fatal infections were bacterial or fungal and not viral. Those who died from 30 days to 1 year after transplantation died of rejection, infection (including cytomegalovirus), or posttransplant lymphoproliferative disease. Deaths resulting from chronic airway rejection may occur as early as 6 months posttransplantation. Those who died 1 year after transplantation died of rejection and, less frequently, infection. Of course, these data depended on a number of factors, such as the aggressiveness of treatment for rejection and primary lung disease. This means know how your pulmonologist bases his treatment on your diagnosis.

S. Raab, M.D.

References

1. Billingham ME: The pathologic changes in long-term heart and lung transplant survivors. *J Heart Transplant* 11:252S, 1992.
2. Yousem SA, Burke C, Billingham M: Pathologic pulmonary alterations in long-term human heart-lung transplantation. *Hum Pathol* 16:911, 1985.
3. Tamm M, Sharples M, Dennis C, et al: Obliterative bronchiolitis (OB) in 120 consecutive heart-lung transplants (HLT). *Am Rev Respir Dis* 147:197A, 1993.

Clinical-Pathologic Analysis of 40 Patients With Large Cell Neuroendocrine Carcinoma of the Lung
Dresler CM, Ritter JH, Patterson GA, et al (Washington Univ, St Louis)
Ann Thorac Surg 63:180–185, 1997

1–2

Background.—Large cell carcinoma of the lung with neuroendocrine differentiation is still not well understood. Pathologic guidelines for classifying these tumors is needed to help determine prognosis and to guide treatment.

Methods.—The records of all patients undergoing lung cancer resection at 1 university since 1986 were reviewed, and all patients with large cell neuroendocrine carcinomas were identified. There were 40 patients, 32 with high-grade disease and 8 with intermediate-grade disease. Twenty-five patients had stage I disease; 6, stage II; 6, stage III; and 3, stage IV. The mean follow-up was 19.8 months.

Findings.—At the time of the study, 15 patients were alive with no evidence of disease, 6 were alive with disease, and 15 had died of disease. Patients with stage I disease had a 5-year survival of 18%. All-stage 5-year survival was 13%. Eighty percent of the patients with stage I or II disease died of disease. Postoperative chemotherapy, radiation therapy, or both were given to 9 of 26 patients with stage I disease, of whom 67% died. Thirty-five percent of the 17 patients with stage I disease died after no postoperative treatment.

Conclusions.—The prognosis for large cell neuroendocrine carcinomas identified histologically is remarkably bad, even in patients with very early stage disease. Survival is not improved with adjuvant treatment.

▶ This is an interesting work in which Dresler et al. described their classification scheme of neuroendocrine carcinomas of the lung and presented their survival data of patients with large cell neuroendocrine carcinoma. I agree with the authors that the concept of neuroendocrine tumors is confusing and appreciate their attempt to simplify the situation. The proposal to rename as neuroendocrine carcinomas all tumors with light microscopic neuroendocrine features is appealing and does away with the terms of *carcinoid, atypical carcinoid, large cell anaplastic carcinoma,* and *small-cell carcinoma.* Dresler et al. proposed to grade these neuroendocrine carcinomas (grades 1 to 3) on the presence of geographic necrosis, cell size, mitoses, nuclear molding, and nucleoli. This classification scheme probably does not add much to simplify the understanding of carcinoids (grade 1 neuroendocrine carcinoma in their system) and small-cell carcinomas (grade 3 neuroendocrine carcinoma, small-cell type), but it does help with the terms of *atypical carcinoid* (grade 2 neuroendocrine carcinoma) and *large cell neuroendocrine carcinoma* (grade 3 neuroendocrine carcinoma, large cell type).[1, 2]

I particularly agree with doing away with the term *atypical carcinoid,* which I find annoying and noncontributory. A grade 2 neuroendocrine carcinoma falls between the spectrum of carcinoid and small-cell carcinoma, but has smaller nuclei, fewer mitoses, less nuclear molding, and general absence of nucleoli compared with grade 3 neuroendocrine carcinoma. Following the assumption that a grade 2 neuroendocrine carcinoma is an atypical carcinoid, others would say that these tumors look like carcinoids but have focal necrosis and more mitoses and nuclear atypia. Prognostically, patients with grade 2 neuroendocrine carcinoma do worse than patients with carcinoids and better than patients with small-cell carcinoma. This study had so few of these grade 2 tumors, and the data would have been more convincing if more of these tumors had been presented.

A grade 3 neuroendocrine carcinoma, large cell type, has features of small-cell carcinoma but has larger cells, less molding, and more prominent nucleoli. The data from this study showed that patients with grade 3 neuroendocrine carcinoma, large cell type, do terribly, regardless of treatment.

Do we need a new classification scheme? I think the answer is yes, and this is a good one, although given the conservatism in medicine, it may take a great deal of difficulty to change from our current system. It may be difficult for pathologists and clinicians to completely do away with the terms *carcinoid* and *small-cell carcinoma*.

S. Raab, M.D.

References

1. Travis WD, Linnoila RI, Tsokos MG, et al: Neuroendocrine tumors of the lung with proposed criteria for large-cell neuroendocrine carcinoma: An ultrastructural, immunohistochemical and flow cytometric study of 35 cases. *Am J Surg Pathol* 15:529–553, 1991.
2. Wick MR, Berg LC, Maj MC, et al: Large cell carcinoma of the lung with neuroendocrine differentiation. *Am J Clin Pathol* 97:796–805, 1992.

The Prognosis of Resected Lung Carcinoma Associated With Atypical Adenomatous Hyperplasia: A Comparison of the Prognosis of Well-differentiated Adenocarcinoma Associated With Atypical Adenomatous Hyperplasia and Intrapulmonary Metastasis

Suzuki K, Nagai K, Yoshida J, et al (Natl Cancer Ctr Hosp East, Kashiwa, Chiba, Japan; Natl Cancer Ctr Research Inst East, Kashiwa, Chiba, Japan)

Cancer 79:1521–1526, 1997

1–3

Introduction.—It can be difficult to determine morphologically whether radiologically undetected intrapulmonary solitary nodules found in the resected lung are atypical adenomatous hyperplasia (AAH) or intrapulmonary metastasis (PM) from the primary lesion. Resected specimens of lung carcinoma with concomitant AAH or PM were reviewed retrospectively for the prognostic importance of these findings.

Methods.—Between 1972 and 1996, 1,360 patients underwent resection of lung carcinoma at the study institution. Atypical adenomatous hyperplasia was present in 137 patients, and PM, in 106. Primary lung neoplasms and nodules were examined microscopically by conventional hematoxylin-eosin stain. A histologic diagnosis of AAH was based on 3 criteria: a lesion with well-defined boundaries with proliferation of single layered atypical epithelial cells; abundant cytoplasm and a rounded or domed appearance of the cells; and hyperchromatic nuclei and prominent nucleoli. Only isolated AAH, a solitary nodule separate from the main tumor, was included in the study. Intrapulmonary metastasis was defined as a mass independent from the primary tumor but with identical histopathologic features (Fig 1, C and F).

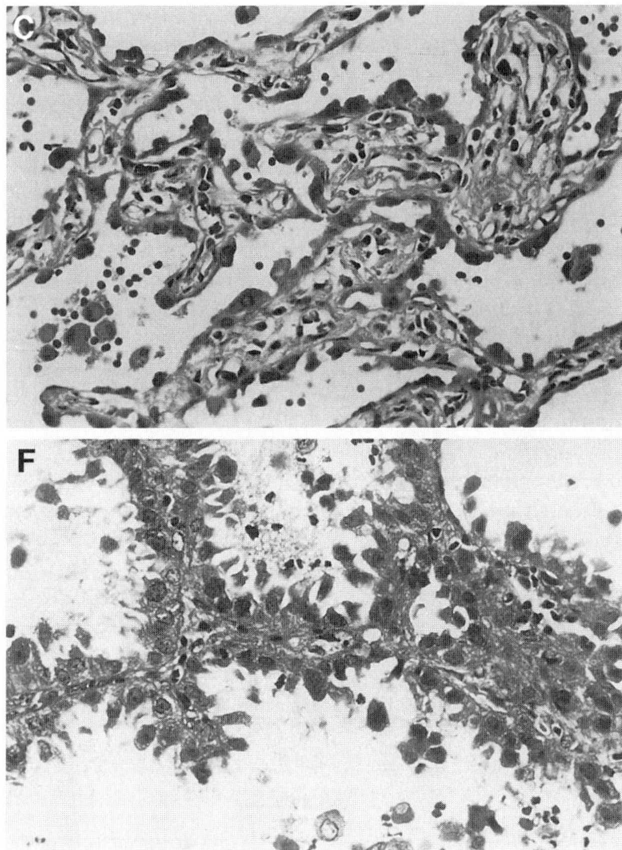

FIGURE 1.—Histopathologic findings of atypical adenomatous hyperplasia and intrapulmonary metastasis with hematoxylin-eosin stain. C, atypical adenomatous hyperplasia from a patient with well-differentiated adenocarcinoma; original magnification, ×100. F, intrapulmonary metastasis from a patient with well-differentiated adenocarcinoma; original magnification, ×100. (Courtesy of Suzuki K, Nagai K, Yoshida J, et al: The prognosis of resected lung carcinoma associated with atypical adenomatous hyperplasia: A comparison of the prognosis of well-differentiated adenocarcinoma associated with atypical adenomatous hyperplasia and intrapulmonary metastasis. *Cancer* 79:1521–1526. ©1997 American Cancer Society. Reprinted by permission of Wiley-Liss, Inc., a subsidiary of John Wiley & Sons, Inc.)

Results.—The 5-year survival rates of patients with AAH were 72.9% in stage I, 60.6% in stage II, 27.1% in stage IIIA, 0% in stage IIIB, and 0% in stage IV. These rates did not differ significantly from the overall survival rates for all patients with lung carcinoma; thus, prognosis was not affected by the concomitance of AAH. The most common histologic type of resected lung carcinoma in patients with AAH was well-differentiated (w/d) adenocarcinoma; fewer patients with PM had w/d adenocarcinoma. Overall, the 5-year survival rate was significantly better for patients with AAH (64.6%) than for those with PM (35.5%). And among cases of pT1-2, NO w/d adenocarcinoma, most of which were bronchioalveolar carcinoma, survival was significantly better for concomitant AAH than for PM.

Conclusions.—A finding of AAH does not in itself affect the prognosis of resected lung carcinoma. The significant difference in survival in these patients with AAH or PM and w/d adenocarcinoma, especially bronchio-alveolar carcinoma, suggests that conventional pathologic examination was generally able to distinguish morphologically between these lesions.

▶ Separation of AAH from a PM in a patient who has an adenocarcinoma in the same lobe is difficult for any pathologist. Features of AAH have been described in the literature, but the diagnostic difficulty is that the foci of AAH are just that: they are atypical but lack definitive characteristics of cancer.[1-3]

Suzuki et al. present a rather large study investigating the outcomes of patients with AAH. They show that patients with atypical adenomatous hyperplasia had similar 5-year survival rates, based on cancer stage, as patients with lung cancer without AAH. Thus, even though the separation of atypical adenomatous hyperplasia from PM may be difficult, the pathologists in this study showed that they could make this separation. This is good news, and I infer that even though I may struggle with this difficulty, I will probably be accurate in the separation of metastasis from AAH. Further, interobserver studies need to be done to show that we all can make this separation. In addition, the authors should follow up this study with a second study illustrating the specific features they used (if any!) for the separation. Only then will I feel more comfortable in making this separation.

S. Raab, M.D.

References

1. Kodama T, Biyajima S, Watanabe S, et al: Morphometric study of adenocarcinoma and hyperplastic epithelial lesions in the peripheral lung. *Am J Clin Pathol* 85:146–151, 1986.
2. Mori M, Chiba R, Takahashi T: Atypical adenomatous hyperplasia of the lung and its differentiation from adenocarcinoma: Characterization of atypical cells by morphometry and multivariate cluster analysis. *Cancer* 72:2331–2340, 1993.
3. Nakanishi K: Alveolar epithelial hyperplasia and adenocarcinoma of the lung. *Arch Pathol Lab Med* 114:363–368, 1990.

High c-erbB-3 Protein Expression Is Associated With Shorter Survival in Advanced Non–Small Cell Lung Carcinomas

Yi ES, Harclerode D, Gondo M, et al (Univ of California, San Diego; Baylor College of Medicine, Houston)
Mod Pathol 10:142–148, 1997

1–4

Introduction.—Overexpression of c-erbB-1 and c-erbB-2 proteins has been described in various human carcinomas and often appears to be an adverse prognostic factor. A recently cloned member of this type I receptor family, c-erbB-3, was investigated for the frequency and significance of its overexpression in lung cancer.

Methods.—Paraffin blocks from primary lung carcinoma resection specimens were retrieved from pathology department archives of 1 hospital in Houston. Data obtained on these cases included date of last contact or death, smoking histories, staging information, diagnosis date, pathologic diagnosis, and cause of death. A series of 549 cases were immunostained with a monoclonal anti-human c-erbB-3 antibody. Distinctive membranous staining or punctuate cytoplasmic staining was interpreted as positive and scored on a scale of 0 to 3 according to the proportion of the c-erbB-3–positive tumor cells to the entire tumor cells present on the section.

Results.—Actuarial cumulative survival was performed on the 443 cases that had a single primary site in the lung of pure non–small-cell carcinoma and follow-up data for more than 3 months. Patients in stages III and IV with high c-erbB-3 expression (score of 3, 50% or more of positive cells) survived for a significantly shorter time than did patients with low c-erbB-3 expression. High vs. low c-erbB-3 expression had no significant effect on survival of patients with stage I or stage II non–small-cell carcinomas. In all stages, squamous cell carcinoma showed the highest rate of c-erbB-3 positivity (28.6%), followed by adenocarcinoma (15.9%) and large-cell carcinoma (10.6%).

Conclusions.—This is the first study to report the frequency and clinical significance of c-erbB-3 expression in lung cancers. The finding that high expression of c-erbB-3 might be an adverse prognostic factor in advanced non–small-cell lung carcinomas suggests a potential target for molecular therapy.

▶ It would be important to immunohistochemically stain for c-erbB-3, a growth factor receptor, if it could be shown that upregulation of the receptor correlates with the prognosis of patients with non–small-cell lung carcinomas.[1] The preliminary work by Yi et al. is an attempt to investigate this correlation. It is unfortunate that there was a correlation between high c-erbB-3 expression and survival only in patients with high-stage (stages III and IV) non–small-cell carcinomas, and not in patients with low-stage non–small-cell carcinomas. Patients with these high-stage carcinomas already do poorly, and the significance of predicting survival in these patients is uncertain.

The authors presented only survival curves and not mean length of survival data, so it is uncertain what the real difference in patient survival was. This study depended on observer observation, which is inherently subjective, and future studies should use more quantification (e.g., image analysis or Western blot). The authors also chose to measure protein (receptor) levels instead of message (messengerRNA) levels, which also must be investigated. A last point is that the authors have not validated their scoring system or shown reproducibility. Much more investigation must be done to determine the correlation of c-erbB-3 expression and lung carcinomas before any definitive conclusions may be reached.

S. Raab, M.D.

Reference

1. Plowman GD, Culouscou J-M, Whitney GS, et al: Ligand-specific activation of HER4/p 180 erbB4, a fourth member of the epidermal growth factor receptor family. *Proc Natl Acad Sci USA* 90:1746–1750, 1993.

DNA Cytophotometry and Prognosis in Typical and Atypical Bronchopulmonary Carcinoids: A Clinicomorphologic Study of 100 Neuroendocrine Lung Tumors

Padberg B-C, Woenckhaus J, Hilger G, et al (Univ of Hamburg, Germany; Technical Univ of Dresden, Germany; Bethesda Hosp, Duisburg, Germany; et al)

Am J Surg Pathol 20:815–822, 1996   1–5

Background.—Neuroendocrine lung tumors are subdivided into typical carcinoids (TC), which are usually benign, low-grade malignant atypical carcinoids (AC), and aggressive poorly differentiated carcinomas. Attempts have been made to identify prognostic features of AC, but results are contradictory. Surgical material obtained from 100 patients with TC and AC of the lung was investigated for the relation between static DNA cytophotometry and patient survival.

Methods.—Cases were obtained from the files of different institutes of pathology. The formalin-fixed, paraffin-embedded material represented 100 primary, 4 residual, and 4 metastatic pulmonary carcinoids. Hospital charts and questionnaires were used to obtain information relating to the preoperative history and follow-up data for each patient.

Results.—Patients were 63 women and 37 men with a mean age of 65 years at resection of the primary lung tumor. Sixty primary tumors were histologically classified as TC and 40 as AC. The mean diameter of the tumors was 2.5 cm; 61 were categorized as T1 and 31 as T2. Fourteen patients had initial lymph node involvement. Surgery was done in all but 4 patients, 2 who refused and 2 whose disease was inoperable. There were 8 cases of tumor-related death; all 8 patients had carcinoids measuring 1.4 cm or more. An additional 13 patients died of other causes. Six patients with residual tumor after surgery were alive with persistent disease at a median of 82 months. Seventy-three patients were alive and symptom free at a median of 102 months after surgery. Fifty-eight of the 60 TC, but only 20 of the 40 AC, had euploid DNA histograms. The histologic type of disease (TC vs. AC) and the DNA content of tumors (euploid vs. aneuploid) significantly affected prognosis. Tumor-related deaths occurred only among patients with atypical (8 of 40) or DNA aneuploid carcinoids (8 of 22). As long as the primary tumor or related metastases showed a diploid DNA content, lymph node metastases alone was not associated with a poor prognosis.

Conclusion.—Aneuploid DNA distributions of a primary or secondary bronchopulmonary carcinoid may identify high-risk patients who coud benefit from radical surgery and aggressive adjuvant therapy.

▶ According to Padberg et al. this is the fifteenth study that has examined DNA cytophotometry in carcinoids and ACs to determine whether there is a correlation between ploidy and patient survival. If there is a correlation, then ploidy could be performed for prognostic purposes. The authors abide by the classification using the categories of TC and AC which, according to the article by Dresler et al. (Abstract 1–2), should be trashed. No matter. As the authors indicated, the previous studies using DNA cytophotometry have shown contrasting results regarding ploidy and survival,[1-3] and I do not think that this is the definitive work that settles all questions.

Using univariate analysis, Padberg et al. showed that patients with aneuploid tumors did worse than patients with diploid tumors. However, to show true significance, multivariate analysis, incorporating much more pathologic and clinical data, must be used. Particularly, before we perform flow cytometry for prognostic purposes, it must be shown that ploidy correlates with patient survival beyond the survival correlated with stage of disease.

On a side note, none of the patients with a TC and follow-up died of disease, and only 8 patients with an AC and follow-up died of disease. Although this indicates an extremely good prognosis for patients with TC, I would not consider these tumors as entirely benign. Typical carcinoids are low-grade malignancies, which in some instances, although not shown in this current study, may result in death.

S. Raab, M.D.

References

1. Paladugu RR, Benfield JR, Pak HY, et al: Bronchopulmonary Kultschitsky cell carcinomas: A new classification scheme for typical and atypical carcinoids. *Cancer* 55:1303–1311, 1985.
2. Yousem SA, Taylor SR: Typical and atypical carcinoid tumors of the lung: A clinicopathologic and DNA analysis of 20 tumors. *Mod Pathol* 3:502–505, 1990.
3. Warren WH, Gould VE: Neuroendocrine neoplasms of the lung: A 10 year perspective of their classification. *Zentralbl Pathol* 139:107–113, 1993.

Primary Leiomyosarcomas of the Lung: A Clinicopathologic and Immunohistochemical Study of 18 Cases
Moran CA, Suster S, Abbondanzo SL, et al (Armed Forces Inst of Pathology, Washington, DC; Univ of Miami, Fla)
Mod Pathol 10:121–128, 1997   1–6

Background.—Leiomyosarcomas are rare smooth-muscle tumors usually occurring in the female genital tract, gastrointestinal tract, and soft tissues. However, rarely do they occur as primary lung neoplasms. One series of patients with primary pulmonary leiomyosarcomas was described.

Patients and Findings.—Eighteen patients with primary malignant smooth-muscle tumors of the lung were included in the review. The patients were 11 males and 7 females, aged 5 to 76 years, with a mean age of 50 years. Tumor diameters ranged from 1.7 to 10 cm. Four tumors were classified as low grade; 2, intermediate; and 12, high grade. Low-grade tumors consisted of an orderly proliferation of fascicles of spindle cells intersecting at right angles and showing oval-to-spindle cells with cigar-shaped nuclei, minimal pleomorphism, and low mitotic activity with no bleeding or necrosis. Intermediate-grade lesions also had the fascicular configuration but showed increased cellularity with atypia and a dense chromatin pattern, occasional pleomorphism, and a mild increase in mitotic activity. High-grade lesions were characterized by high cellularity, marked pleomorphism and atypia, many areas of hemorrhage and necrosis, and high mitotic activity. Among 16 patients undergoing immunohistochemical examination, positive staining of tumor cells with smooth-muscle actin was shown in 12, desmin in 5, and co-expression of actin, desmin, or both and keratin in 3. Six patients with lesions of low or intermediate grade were alive and well 2 to 12 years after their diagnosis. Eight patients with high-grade tumors died of disease with widespread metastases 1 to 24 months after diagnosis. The median survival in this group was 5 months. One patient with a high-grade tumor was alive and well 12 years after operation. Another 3 patients with high-grade lesions were lost to follow-up.

Conclusions.—Histologic grade appears to be the best prognostic indicator of clinical behavior in primary leiomyosarcoma of the lung. Smooth-muscle actin is the most sensitive immunohistochemical marker for establishing the diagnosis. Primary leiomyosarcoma should be considered in the differential diagnosis of pulmonary spindle cell neoplasms.

▶ Granted, primary leiomyosarcomas of the lung are rare.[1-5] However, spindle cell neoplasms of the lung are not that uncommon, and leiomyosarcoma always is in the differential diagnosis of a spindle cell neoplasm. Most well to moderately differentiated leiomyosarcomas are fairly easily recognized, and the most obvious separation is from a metastasis. Poorly differentiated leiomyosarcomas are more problematic and may resemble sarcomatous carcinomas, spindle cell mesotheliomas, and other uncommon primary sarcomas.

Moran et al. subclassified 18 primary leiomyosarcomas into 3 groups: low grade, intermediate grade, and high grade. From their data, I am uncertain that the terminology of low grade and intermediate grade is appropriate. Because none of the patients with low-grade or intermediate-grade tumors had metastases or died of disease, why should these tumors even be called sarcomas? For these tumors, why not favor designations of leiomyoma or smooth-muscle tumor of uncertain malignant potential, like the designations used for smooth-muscle tumors of the gynecologic or gastrointestinal tract? Moran et al. showed that patients with high-grade tumors had a poorer prognosis, but good staging data were absent from this study; tumor stage may well be the decisive factor in determining patient outcome, as it is for most other lung malignancies. Immunohistochemically, there were no surprises with these tumors.

What should we do if we encounter a spindle cell neoplasm with smooth-muscle features? We should probably think metastasis first and primary leiomyosarcoma only after excluding everything else.

S. Raab, M.D.

References

1. Yellin A, Rosenman Y, Liberman Y: Review of smooth muscle tumours of the lower respiratory tract. *Br J Dis Chest* 78:337–351, 1984.
2. Ramanathan T: Primary leiomyosarcoma of the lung. *Thorax* 29:482–489, 1974.
3. Schanher PW: Primary pulmonary leiomyosarcoma: Case report with review of literature. *Ann Surg* 181:20, 1971.
4. Guccion JG, Rosen SH: Bronchopulmonary leiomyosarcoma and fibrosarcoma: A study of 32 cases and review of the literature. *Cancer* 30:836–847, 1972.
5. Jimenez JF, Uthman EO, Townsend JW, et al: Primary bronchopulmonary leiomyosarcoma in childhood. *Arch Pathol Lab Med* 110:348–351, 1986.

Lung Carcinoma Surgical Pathology Report Adequacy: A College of American Pathologists Q-Probes Study of Over 8300 Cases From 464 Institutions

Gephardt GN, Baker PB (Kennestone Hosp, Marietta, Ga; Ohio State Univ, Columbus)
Arch Pathol Lab Med 120:922–927, 1996   1–7

Introduction.—There have been no previously published guidelines for evaluating the accuracy of documentation of surgical pathology reports of resected lung carcinomas. To determine the rate of reporting of gross and microscopic pathologic features of resected primary lung carcinomas, a retrospective, multicenter study was conducted.

Methods.—Data for review were provided in more than 8,300 surgical pathology reports from 464 institutions. Variables examined in the study (descriptors) were developed by the authors from their own practices and were discussed before the study was undertaken by the QAS/Quality Assurance Committee of the American College of Pathologists. Twenty-three descriptors provided for the assessment of bronchogenic carcinoma of the lung in surgical pathology reports. These descriptors were grouped into 4 categories: general findings, gross findings, microscopic findings, and other information. Surgical pathology reports were examined for the presence or absence of the 23 descriptors. Data were analyzed for each institution, and institutions were classified according to hospital bed size, teaching status, pathology residency program status, and government association status.

Results.—A standard report form or checklist was used in 20.8% of cases. Most reports included type of procedure (89.6%) and lobe or lung of origin (99.1%). Gross findings commonly reported included tumor size (97.2%), a description of regional nodes attached to the specimen (74.7%), and a description of the parenchyma not involved by neoplasm (80.1%); venous invasion was noted in only 18.3% of cases. A microscopic description appeared in 77.6% of reports. Findings stated included histologic type (99.3%), histologic grade (80.9%), status of lymph nodes (89.0%), the presence or absence of neoplasm at bronchial margin resection (90.8%), the presence or absence of neoplasm in visceral pleura (64.6%), and the status of nonneoplastic parenchyma (72.8%). Frozen sections were used to evaluate the bronchial margin of excision in 38.5% of cases. Certain descriptors were more likely to be used by teaching institutions and those with residency programs (neoplasm at the vascular margin and the sources/sites of the tissue blocks). Nonteaching institutions, smaller institutions, and those without pathology residency programs were more likely to report whether regional nodes were attached to the specimen and to evaluate nonneoplastic parenchyma.

Conclusions.—The rate of reporting gross and microscopic features of resected lung carcinoma varies among institutions. It is important that the surgical pathology report contain all elements of prognostic importance.

▶ The proposed objective of this article was to assess the adequacy of reporting the gross and microscopic findings of resected lung cancers. In my opinion, this article does not really address the issue of adequacy of reports, but actually surveys how lung cancer specimens are reported in different pathology practices. These are different issues. For a report to be adequate or inadequate, it has to be compared to a gold standard report, which does not exist.

Data that should be included on a surgical pathology report should have an effect on patient treatment or prognosis,[1, 2] and as stated in this article, not all of the pathology data that are reported affect patient treatment or prognosis. For example, the presence or absence of tumor at the visceral pleura was reported by 64.6% of laboratories, although these data have not been shown to be clinically significant. Therefore, although it is interesting to see the data that different laboratories report, we should be careful not to consider that the reporting of all this information is mandatory. I think synoptic reports are a good idea, but only if they report the information useful to clinicians.

S. Raab, M.D.

References

1. Myers JL, Askin FB, Yousem SA: Recommendations for the reporting of resected primary lung carcinomas, Association of Directors of Anatomic and Surgical Pathology. *Hum Pathol* 26:937–939, 1995.
2. Nash G, Hutter RVP, Henson DE: Practice protocol for the examination of specimens from patients with lung cancer. *Arch Pathol Lab Med* 119:695–700, 1995.

Bronchioloalveolar Lung Carcinomas: K-*ras* Mutations Are Constant Events in the Mucinous Subtype

Marchetti A, Buttitta F, Pellegrini S, et al (Univ of Pisa, Italy)
J Pathol 179:254–259, 1996

1–8

Background.—Bronchioloalveolar carcinoma (BAC) has been defined as a form of differentiated lung adenocarcinoma that grows as a single layer of malignant cells along the walls of terminal airways. Because of its uncertain histogenesis and its similarity to conventional lung adenocarcinoma (CLA), its existence as a separate clinicopathologic entity is debated. The clinical behavior of BAC seems to depend on its histologic subtype (mucinous, nonmucinous, or sclerosing). The different morphologic patterns and clinical outcomes of the BAC subtypes suggest that their biological behavior may differ from one another as well as from CLA.

Methods and Findings.—Fifty-eight BACs and 50 CLAs were examined for mutations at codon 12 of the K-*ras* oncogene. The BACs included 10 mucinous, 40 nonmucinous, and 8 sclerosing lesions. K-*ras* mutations were found in 36% of the BACs and 26% of the CLAs. These mutations were clearly associated with the mucinous type of BAC. All 10 mucinous tumors had mutations in the K-*ras* gene, whereas only 23% of the nonmucinous and 25% of the sclerosing BACs had the mutation. Nonmucinous BACs, sclerosing BACs, and CLAs had comparable frequencies of K-*ras* mutations.

Conclusion.—K-*ras* mutation appears to be a constant event in mucinous BACs. In the nonmucinous and sclerosing forms, its frequency is comparable to that associated with CLAs. Thus, BAC appears to be a heterogeneous group of lung tumors. Further study is needed to rule out the possibility that, at least in the lung, K-*ras* mutations are generally associated with tumors derived from goblet cells.

▶ The term bronchioalveolar carcinoma is not uniformly used by all pathologists. Clasically, 3 types of BAC have been described: mucinous, nonmucinous, and sclerosing. Most pathologists can easily recognize the mucinous subtype because the large mucin-containing cells lie along unthickened interstitia and stand out even at low power. With the nonmucinous subtype, and particularly with the sclerosing subtype, there is a greater degree of fibrosis and inflammation, and some of these tumors are classified by some pathologists simply as adenocarcinoma or adenocarcinoma with bronchioalveolar features.

Some studies have shown that there are prognostic differences among patients with these different tumor subtypes, indicating that subclassification may have value. Thus, some hypothesize that the term bronchioalveolar carcinoma comprises a heterogeneous group of neoplasms, and this is supported by the study by Marchetti et al. Ten of 10 mucinous BACs had K-*ras* mutations, whereas the percentage was much lower for other bronchioalveolar subtypes and for CLAs.

Currently, this may not have much practical significance, because the mucinous bronchioalveolar subtype is the most easily diagnosed. However, seeing the mucinous subtype indicates worse survival than some other subtypes, and this could be conveyed to clinicians.

S. Raab, M.D.

References

1. Donaldson JC, Kaminsky DB, Elliot CR: Bronchiolar carcinoma: Report of 11 cases and review of the literature. *Cancer* 41:250–258, 1978.
2. Rusch VW, Reuter VE, Kris MG, et al: *Ras* oncogene point mutation: An infrequent event in bronchioalveolar cancer. *J Thorac Cardiovasc Surg* 104:1465–1469, 1992.

Evaluation of Cultures of Percutaneous Core Needle Biopsy Specimens in the Diagnosis of Pulmonary Nodules

Chitkara YK (Carondelet St Mary's Hosp, Tucson, Ariz)
Am J Clin Pathol 107:224–228, 1997

1–9

Introduction.—Many radiologists now use the automated biopsy gun to obtain tissue samples for definitive diagnosis of pulmonary nodules. A portion of the percutaneous core needle biopsy (CNB) is usually submitted for microbiological cultures to isolate and identify the causative infectious agent. To determine the values of cultures of tissue obtained by image-directed CNB of lung nodules, 250 biopsy specimens (248 patients) done during a 5-year period were reviewed.

Methods.—The percutaneous CNBs were done at a hospital in Tucson, Arizona, an area endemic for coccidioidomycosis. Fluoroscopic guidance was used in 237 procedures, and CT, in 13. A portion of the tissue was submitted for culturing and the remaining specimen was fixed in formalin. Frozen section examinations were done in 52 cases at the radiologist's request. Reviews were conducted of hematoxylin-eosin sections of all biopsy samples showing infectious origin. Also reviewed were the medical records of all patients.

Results.—The pulmonary lesion was described as solitary in 221 patients, whereas multiple nodules were seen at radiographic examination in 27 patients. A neoplasm was diagnosed in 145 patients on histologic examination of the specimen. Before biopsy, these lesions were thought to be malignant in 67.6% of cases, indeterminate in 31%, and benign or probably benign in 1.4%. Seventy-one of the 80 granulomas at biopsy had been judged as indeterminate. Spherules of *Coccidioides immitis* were seen in 54 of the biopsy specimens with granulomas; microbiological cultures were positive in 9.6%. Overall, a definite histopathologic diagnosis was made in 90% of patients. Fourteen of the 25 nondiagnostic biopsy specimens yielded no pathogenic organisms. Subsequent open lung biopsies confirmed coccidioidomycosis in 5 cases, large-cell undifferentiated carcinoma in 3, adenocarcinoma in 1, and malignant lymphoma in 1. Cultures were uniformly negative when special stains failed to reveal organisms.

Conclusions.—Microbiological cultures of material obtained by open or needle biopsy of pulmonary nodules are commonly performed, yet the usefulness of this practice is uncertain. In this review of 250 CNBs, positive cultures were seen only in cases in which the stains had previously enabled the causative organism to be identified. Because of their insensitivity, cultures of CNB specimens need not be routinely performed.

▶ This study by Chitkara once again raises the question of how to treat a patient with a solitary pulmonary nodule. Apparently, at Carondelet St. Mary's Hospital in Tucson, Arizona, approximately 50 patients per year undergo a transthoracic CNB. Although it is not reported, it would be interesting to know whether this group of patients represents all patients with solitary nodules, or whether there are other patients who undergo a different procedure. I also wonder why the radiologist chose to do a CNB rather than a fine-needle aspiration.

Chitkara reported that 25 patients had a nondiagnostic CNB; I assume, although it is not directly stated, that all these patients had a follow-up open lung biopsy. If this is the case, malignancy was diagnosed in 145 of 150 specimens, which shows high sensitivity. Some of these patients with high-stage cancer were saved from a more invasive procedure.

Coccidioides immitis was diagnosed in a high percentage of nonneoplastic cases, although the cause of the 19 granulomas in the cases where special stains failed to show *C. immitis* was never truly determined; these cases may have had *C. immitis* that never was cultured or seen by special stains. The authors showed that cultures had low yield in patients with *C. immitis*, but this low culture sensitivity for fungal organisms might not be true in other geographic locations, such as areas endemic for histoplasmosis.

In addition, I question whether fine-needle aspiration with immediate interpretation would have been better than CNB in the nondiagnostic specimens. This study shows that pathologists should be able to interpret radiologic specimens but does not show whether fine-needle aspiration or CNB is better.[1-3]

S. Raab, M.D.

References

1. Renshaw AA: The relative sensitivity of special stains and culture in open lung biopsies. *Am J Clin Pathol* 102:736–740, 1994.
2. Ulbright TM, Katzenstein AL: Solitary necrotizing granulomas of the lung: Differentiating features and etiology. *Am J Surg Pathol* 4:13–28, 1980.
3. Raab SS, Silverman JF, Zimmerman KG: Fine needle aspiration of pulmonary coccidioidomycosis: Spectrum of findings in 73 patients. *Am J Clin Pathol* 99:582–587, 1993.

Calcofluor White Stain for the Detection of *Pneumocystis carinii* in Transbronchial Lung Biopsy Specimens: A Study of 68 Cases

Fraire AE, Kemp B, Greenberg SD, et al (Univ of Massachusetts, Worcester; Baylor College of Medicine, Houston; Baptist Hosp, Orange, Tex; et al)
Mod Pathol 9:861–864, 1996
1–10

Introduction.—Calcofluor white (CFW) is a chemofluorescent agent that causes fungi to fluoresce when viewed with a fluorescent microscope. Although CFW is useful in identifying *Pneumocystis carinii* cysts in respiratory fluids and secretions, its ability to detect *P. carinii* cysts in tissue preparation has not been determined. Formalin-fixed, paraffin-embedded, transbronchial tissue biopsy specimens from HIV-seropositive patients with clinical or radiologic evidence of *P. carinii* pneumonia or both were examined for concordance of the CFW stain and the conventional Gomori methenamine silver (GMS) stain.

Methods.—Sixty-eight transbronchial biopsy specimens were stained with the GMS stain according to standard procedures. The CFW technique included both a deparaffinization and a staining procedure. The CWF stain was interpreted as positive for *P. carinii* cysts if round-to-oval nonbudding structures, 5–7 µm in diameter, were observed to stain an intense double parenthesis–like structure near the center of the cyst. Forty-five minutes were required for the CFW procedure, including deparaffinization, and microscopic evaluation took 5 minutes. The conventional GMS procedure required 3.5 hours to perform and 5 minutes for microscopic evaluation. Total costs for labor, reagents, and expendables were $3.04 for CFW and $4.89 for GMS.

Results.—Thirty-six (52.9%) of the 68 specimens were positive for *P. carinii* cysts by both CFW and GMS; 27 (39.7%) were negative by both techniques. The concordance rate was thus 92.6%. Four of the disparate results were CFW positive and GMS negative; 1 was CFW negative and GMS positive.

Discussion.—A variety of staining methods have been used for the detection of *P. carinii* cysts in respiratory fluids. The CFW stain is rapid, simple, and less expensive than other test methods and can be performed in any laboratory equipped with a fluorescent microscope. Its concordance rate with GMS was high (92.6%) for the recognition of the cysts in tissue preparations. The double parenthesis–like structure provides a reliable and readily identifiable marker for detection of *P. carinii* cysts.

▶ A transbronchial biopsy specimen from a patient suspected of having *P. carinii* pneumonia is sent to pathology. What do you do? I would first wonder why we are receiving a biopsy specimen rather than a wash or a bronchio-alveolar lavage, although bronchoscopy with transbronchial biopsy apparently is the procedure of choice at Ben Taub General Hospital, Houston, Texas. If this is the case, it seems rather aggressive to me, although this may be more of a clinical problem than a pathology problem, because we must deal with what is sent. Do you order a special stain (GMS or CFW) before any stains are out, after slides are out depending on what you see, or not at all? To me, the important question is whether to get a stain, rather than which stain to get. This was not addressed in the study.

Fraire et al. showed that the sensitivity of CFW was similar to that of GMS, although each stain detected 1 or more cases of *P. carinii* that the other stain missed. Thus, it would seem that if you order a stain, it could be either a GMS or a CFW. That the CFW stain was performed faster than the GMS does not really mean much for the particular patient case, because many clinicians generally are not beating down the door for an immediate answer. The real variable that should have been measured is actual technology labor time, rather than overall time to produce the stain. Fraire et al. reported that the CFW procedure cost less than the GMS procedure, but I am curious to know their overall charges for these stains. The take-home message to me is that GMS and CFW are both OK.[1, 2]

S. Raab, M.D.

References

1. Monheit JE, Cowan DF, Moore DG: Rapid detection of fungi in tissues using calcofluor white and fluorescent microscopy. *Arch Pathol Lab Med* 108:616, 1984.
2. Raab SS, Cheville JL, Bottles K, et al: Utility of gomori methenamine silver stains in bronchoalveolar lavage specimens. *Mod Pathol* 7:599–604, 1994.

Bronchiolitis Obliterans-organizing Pneumonia (BOOP)-like Variant of Wegener's Granulomatosis: A Clinicopathologic Study of 16 Cases
Uner AH, Rozum-Slota B, Katzenstein A-LA (State Univ of New York, Syracuse; Crouse Irving Mem Hosp, Syracuse, NY)
Am J Surg Pathol 20:794–801, 1996   1–11

Background.—Wegener's granulomatosis (WG) in the lung is characterized by the classic histologic features of necrotizing granulomatous inflammation and necrotizing vasculitis. Several histologic variants have recently been identified, characterized by bronchocentric inflammation, a marked eosinophil infiltrate, alveolar hemorrhage, and capillaritis or interstitial fibrosis. A new variant, in which bronchiolitis obliterans-organizing pneumonia (BOOP)–like fibrosis represents the main histologic findings, was reported.

Methods and Findings.—Sixteen patients were found to have BOOP. None of these patients had the extensive geographic necrosis that characterizes WG. However, small suppurative granulomas, minute foci of bland necrosis, and microabscesses were common. All patients had the typical necrotizing vasculitis of WG. Also commonly found were darkly staining multinucleated giant cells, prominent acute inflammation, aggregates of epithelioid histiocytes, hemosiderin-filled macrophages, and regions of nonspecific parenchymal fibrosis (Fig 3).

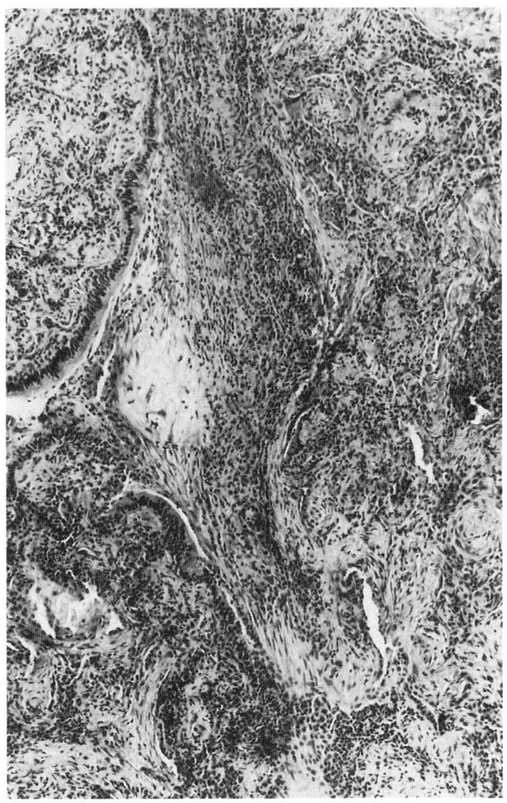

FIGURE 3.—Photomicrograph showing a darkly staining focus of bland necrosis (*top of field*) within an area of otherwise typical bronchiolitis obliterans. (Courtesy of Uner AH, Rozum-Slota B, Katzenstein A-LA: Bronchiolitis obliterans-organizing pneumonia [BOOP]-like variant of Wegener's granulomatosis: A clinicopathologic study of 16 cases. *Am J Surg Pathol* 20:794–801, 1996.)

Conclusions.—This variant of WG has clinical and radiographic features indistinguishable from the classic type. Occasionally, Wegener's granulomatosis can show histologic changes that suggest BOOP. An appreciation of additional features, especially vasculitis, suppurative granulomas, tiny necrotic zones, microabscesses, and multinucleated giant cells, will ensure that the diagnosis is not overlooked.

▶ The article by Uner et al. is one of several published in the past year on BOOP-like histologic changes that may be seen in a variety of conditions. Other articles are listed in the references after this comment. Bronchiolitis obliterans-organizing pneumonia, originally described in 1985 by Epler et al., may be idiopathic or associated with a variety of pulmonary conditions. If associated with other conditions (e.g., infections), the histologic changes may be described as BOOP-like, although they may be identical to the idiopathic BOOP. The histologic findings seen in BOOP include nodules of granulation tissue in the lumen of small airways that extend into alveoli.

Uner et al. did a good job documenting that BOOP-like histologic findings may be seen in WG. In many cases (44%) of WG, the BOOP-like findings are seen at the periphery of the granulomatous foci. In 16 (13%) of the cases, BOOP-like findings were the major histologic finding, and areas of necrosis were absent. Thus, it still may be WG even though it looks like BOOP.

In the article by Siddiqui et al. on BOOP-like findings in lung allograft recipients, BOOP-like findings were associated with both cytomegalovirus pneumonitis and mild or moderate acute rejection. These authors concluded that BOOP-like findings resulted from epithelial injury secondary to rejection or infection and were not a component of, or necessarily predisposed to, chronic rejection. Thus, both these articles stress that BOOP-like findings may be seen associated with other entities.

I conclude that we should only use the diagnosis of idiopathic BOOP if all other conditions that may look like BOOP (and there appear to be a lot of these conditions) have been excluded. Once again, this stresses the need to know the complete history, laboratory, physical, and radiographic findings before signing out a case as BOOP. In addition, it poses the problem that it may be difficult to sign out a transbronchial biopsy specimen as BOOP, because this may represent only the edge of another, more specific process, and the BOOP findings are only secondary.

S. Raab, M.D.

References

1. Epler GR, Colby TV, McLoud TC, et al: Bronchiolitis obliterans organizing pneumonia. *N Engl J Med* 312:152–158, 1985.
2. Travis WD, Hoffman GS, Leavitt RY, et al: Surgical pathology of the lung in Wegener's granulomatosis: Review of 187 open lung biopsies from 67 patients. *Am J Surg Pathol* 15:315–333, 1991.
3. Yousem SA: Bronchocentric injury in Wegener's granulomatosis: A report of five cases. *Hum Pathol* 22:535–540, 1991.
4. Siddiqui MT, Garrity ER, Husain AN: Bronchiolitis obliterans organizing pneumonia-like reactions: A nonspecific response or an atypical form of rejection or infection in lung allograft recipients? *Hum Pathol* 27:714–719, 1996.

Histopathologic Diagnosis Made in Lung Tissue Resected From Patients With Severe Emphysema Undergoing Lung Volume Reduction Surgery
Keller CA, Naunheim KS, Osterloh J, et al (St Louis Univ, Mo)
Chest 111:941–947, 1997   1–12

Background.—Lung volume reduction surgery is now widely performed to relieve severe dyspnea in patients with end-stage emphysema. The histopathologic findings in 1 series of patients undergoing thoracoscopic lung volume reduction surgery or sternotomy were reported.

Methods.—The 80 consecutive patients studied included 75 undergoing lung volume reduction surgery and 5 having sternotomy to improve function and relieve dyspnea. Preoperative pulmonary testing showed severe obstructive lung disease and significant air trapping in all patients. Two groups were identified and compared: 30 patients with histopathologic diagnoses in addition to emphysema, and 50 with emphysema only.

Findings.—Unexpected findings such as interstitial fibrosis, noncaseating granulomatosis, chronic inflammation, and unsuspected neoplasia were noted in 30 patients (37.5%) of the total group. Infiltrative processes were not found on review of these patients' imaging studies. The mean lung weight resected was significantly heavier in this group than in the group with emphysema only, although both groups had the same estimated lung volume. The patients with additional diagnoses also had a significantly greater mean number of days in the hospital and more days requiring chest tubes. The 2 groups did not differ in findings on preoperative pulmonary function tests. The patients with additional histopathologic findings had serious postoperative complications more often than patients with emphysema alone.

Conclusion.—A significant percentage of patients diagnosed as having severe emphysema will have unexpected findings on histopathologic study. When such patients are subjected to lung volume reduction surgery, they will have more serious complications and longer periods of air leaks than patients with emphysema alone, necessitating longer hospital stays.

▶ At more and more hospitals, operations are performed for end-stage emphysema. At my institution, these produce the surgical specimens that, unfortunately, have no clinical history and simply show up in pathology specimen buckets. This study presents the histologic findings in 80 such patients. Keller et al. claim that 30 patients had "unsuspected" findings, although I do not agree that all these patients truly had unsuspected findings or that these findings were clinically significant.

Such findings as interstitial fibrosis (11 patients), chronic inflammations (4 patients), and subpleural fibrosis (3 patients) are completely expected in a patient with chronic obstructive pulmonary disease. Likewise, granulomatous inflammation (12 patients) may or may not have clinical significance and probably is not unexpected in areas endemic for particular organisms, such as *Histoplasma capsulatum* (which is endemic to the Missouri River Valley, part of the cache area for St. Louis University, at which the authors are staff clinicians).

Thus, the most important unsuspected diagnosis is malignancy (3 patients) which, of course, truly affects patient management. I conclude that we should, as usual, carefully look for these tumors and other significant lesions (i.e., emphysema specimens are not "gross only") and also be careful to explain the significance of benign findings. Otherwise, clinicians may think that certain "unsuspected" diseases are important.

S. Raab, M.D.

Reference

1. Cooper JD, Trulock E, Triantafillou A, et al: Bilateral pneumonectomy (volume reduction) for chronic obstructive pulmonary disease. *J Thorac Cardiovasc Surg* 109:106–119, 1995.

p53 Expression and Proliferative Activity Predict Survival in Non-invasive Thymomas

Pich A, Chiarle R, Chiusa L, et al (Univ of Turin, Italy)
Int J Cancer 69:180–183, 1996   1–13

Introduction.—Tumor invasiveness is considered to be the most important factor affecting survival in patients with thymomas. To determine features related to survival in noninvasive tumors, *p53* immunohistochemistry, DNA flow cytometry, and argyrophilic nuclear organizer region (AgNOR) staining was done on formalin-fixed, paraffin-embedded sections from 46 thymomas.

Methods.—Cases of primary noninvasive thymomas, stage I, were collected from pathology files of the study institution. Patients were 27 women and 19 men with a mean age of 50 years; 28 had associated myasthenia gravis (MG). All had undergone gross total tumor resection, and 6 received adjuvant postoperative radiotherapy. The mean follow-up of the patients after surgery was 90 months. Correlations were sought between thymoma clinicopathologic characteristics, *p53* immunoreactivity, DNA content, and AgNOR counts.

Results.—Twenty-one thymoma cases (45.6%) showed *p53* overexpression. This finding was significantly correlated with AgNOR counts but was not associated with any clinicopathologic features or DNA content. The overall 5- and 10-year survival rates were 91% and 87%. No correlations were found between age, sex, histologic type, MG, and DNA content and prognosis. Survival rates were significantly higher, however, for *p53*-negative than for *p53*-positive patients and for patients with low AgNOR counts than for those with high AgNOR counts. At the end of the observation period, all *p53*-negative patients were alive.

Conclusions.—Survival in stage I thymomas showed no correlation with the traditional prognostic factors of age, histologic type, and MG or with DNA content. In contrast, there was a strong correlation between *p53* immunopositivity and survival. In this series, all patients who did not express *p53* protein were alive at the end of the follow-up period. Cell-proliferative activity also was of prognostic value: all patients who died showed very high AgNOR counts at diagnosis.

▶ Tumor invasiveness is the most important histologic feature in predicting the prognosis of patients with thymoma. For patients with a noninvasive thymoma, are there any prognostic indicators? Pich et al. showed that *p53* negativity and low AgNOR counts correlated with longer survival in a study of 46 patients who had a noninvasive thymoma.

The results of this study are dampened because the authors elected to perform univariate rather than multivariate analysis, and because, of the 5 patients who died, none died of thymoma. Thus, I think it is a sleight of hand to suggest that *p53* and AgNOR can be used to determine the prognosis in these patients. In a side note regarding this article, the authors used both the American and European classification schemes to subclassify thymomas.[1, 2]

Although thymomas are relatively rare and most of us probably use the American scheme, it is interesting to see that other descriptive schemes are out there.

S. Raab, M.D.

References

1. Lewis JE, Wick MR, Scheithauer BW, et al: Thymoma: A clinicopathologic review. *Cancer* 60:2727–2743, 1987.
2. Müller-Hermelink HK, Marino M, Palestro G: Pathology of the thymic epithelial tumors, in Müller-Hermelink HK (ed): *The Human Thymus: Histophysiology and Pathology. Current Topics in Pathology,* vol 75. Berlin, Springer-Verlag, 1986, pp 207–268.

Touch Imprints in the Intraoperative Diagnosis of Anterior Mediastinal Neoplasms
Kornstein MJ, Max LD, Wakely PE Jr (Virginia Commonwealth Univ, Richmond)
Arch Pathol Lab Med 120:1116–1122, 1996   1–14

Introduction.—Frozen sections of anterior mediastinal tumors, particularly malignant lymphoma and invasive thymoma, are among the most difficult to interpret. Intraoperative diagnosis often is important, however, for determining the proper extent of excision. To improve the accuracy of intraoperative diagnosis, touch imprints and frozen sections from 21 anterior mediastinal lesions were retrospectively studied and compared for rates of correct diagnosis.

Methods.—Cases for which both touch imprints and frozen sections were available were identified from a search of surgical pathology files for mediastinal tumors. The tumors included 8 thymomas, 2 thymic carcinomas, 6 non-Hodgkin's lymphomas, 3 cases of nodular sclerosing Hodgkin's disease, and 2 seminomas. Imprints and frozen sections were examined separately and in a blinded fashion by 3 independent reviewers. Diagnoses from these reviews were compared with the final surgical pathology diagnosis.

Results.—Review of the touch imprint alone yielded correct diagnoses in 76% to 81% of cases. All 3 observers made the correct diagnosis in 12 (57%) of the cases. Eight of 14 errors consisted of overdiagnosing lymphoma, and there were 6 misdiagnoses: 2 of lymphoma as carcinoma, 2 of lymphoma as a thymoma, 1 of carcinoma as a germ cell tumor, and 1 of thymoma as a carcinoma. On frozen section alone, the correct diagnosis was made in 67% to 86% of cases. The correct diagnosis was made by all 3 reviewers in 10 (48%) of the cases; 9 of 14 errors consisted of overdiagnosing lymphoma. Three identical misdiagnoses were made on both touch imprints and frozen sections. The original intraoperative diagnosis was correct in 67% of cases, incorrect in 14%, and deferred in 19%.

Discussion.—Touch imprints were found to be as useful as frozen sections in the diagnosis of mediastinal tumors, and the 2 techniques are complementary. Depending on the observer, nearly all tumors in this series (86% to 100%) were diagnosed correctly by one or the other technique. Familiarity with the appearance of thymic epithelial cells on touch imprints could improve the accuracy of this simple, inexpensive technique in diagnosing anterior mediastinal lesions.

▶ The take-home message I get from this article is that the intraoperative consultation of mediastinal lesions is full of problems. Of 21 anterior mediastinal lesions, a correct diagnosis was rendered in only 14 (68%) of the cases, and in 4 cases the diagnosis was deferred. The error rate for frozen section of anterior mediastinal lesions is high compared with the error rate for frozen sections of other sites,[1-4] as reported in the article by Novis et al.[4]

I think that the authors are correct in suggesting that touch preparations help in the interpretation of anterior mediastinal lesions, because many of the lesions that occur in the anterior mediastinum are dissociative, and touch preparations may show subtle differences not appreciated on frozen section. I think the main consideration is in separating lesions that are only having a biopsy specimen taken (e.g., lymphoma) from those that the surgeon intends to resect (e.g., thymoma). Thus, if the surgeon has patient consent to do a full resection, try to exclude lymphoma and be certain with the diagnosis of an epithelial neoplasm. I advocate touch preparations for all intraoperative consultations and not just those from the anterior mediastinum.

Note that the authors are fans of the Wright-Giemsa stain, and for those who are not experienced with this stain, this article might be less meaningful. The Wright-Giemsa helps to identify particular features (such as lymphoglandular bodies) that may be commonly seen in some anterior mediastinal lesions and not in others. Hematoxylin-eosin touch preparations also can be done to help identify particular nuclear characteristics of some anterior mediastinal lesions.

S. Raab, M.D.

References

1. Juttner FM, Fellbaum CH, Popper H, et al: Pitfalls in intraoperative frozen section histology of mediastinal neoplasms. *Eur J Cardiothorac Surg* 4:584–586, 1990.
2. Mair S, Lash RH, Siskin D, et al: Intraoperative surgical specimen evaluation: Section analysis, cytologic examination, or both? A comparative study of 206 cases. *Am J Clin Pathol* 96:8–14, 1991.
3. Adler OB, Rosenberger A, Peleg H: Fine-needle aspiration biopsy of mediastinal masses: Evaluation of 136 experiences. *AJR* 140:893–896, 1983.
4. Novis DA, Gephardt GN, Zarbo RJ: Interinstitutional comparison of frozen section consultation in small hospitals: A College of American Pathologists Q-probe study of 18,532 frozen section consultation diagnoses in 233 small hospitals. *Arch Pathol Lab Med* 120:1087–1093, 1996.

2 Breast

Mammary Intraepithelial Neoplasia: A Translational Classification System for the Intraductal Epithelial Proliferations
Tavassoli FA (Armed Forces Inst of Pathology, Washington, DC)
Breast J 3:48–58, 1997   2–1

Background.—Increased use of screening mammography has led to more frequent diagnosis of low-grade ductal carcinoma in situ (DCIS) and atypical intraductal hyperplasia (AIDH). Variable thresholds are applied to separating low-grade DCIS from AIDH, and the methods used to assess the extent of DCIS differ considerably from one laboratory to another. Despite the trend toward conservative management of DCIS, many women diagnosed with DCIS undergo mastectomy and radiation therapy. Some of these cases probably would have been diagnosed as AIDH, had the tissue been examined by another pathologist. The problem of distinguishing AIDH from DCIS is examined in this study.

Definition of AIDH.—In a 1985 report, AIDH was established as a significant risk factor for the subsequent development of invasive breast carcinoma. The lesion is considered to have some, but not all, morphological features of DCIS. Later studies found AIDH to have the cytologic features of low-grade DCIS, thus differing from ordinary intraductal hyperplasia (IDH). From a functional viewpoint, AIDH and low-grade DCIS form a continuum, whereas low-grade DCIS differs significantly from high-grade lesions.

Risk for Invasive Carcinoma.—Among women with AIDH the absolute risk for development of invasive carcinoma is about 10%. In contrast, the risk associated with IDH is less than 3%. Yet some studies of the subsequent risk of invasive carcinoma for low-grade DCIS report an even lower risk. Thus if AIDH is categorized as a precursor for DCIS, then DCIS behaves more indolently than its precursors. Contributing to these contradictions is the magnitude of interobserver variability in separating AIDH from low-grade DCIS. There remain significant differences among experts in breast pathology in the threshold for diagnosis of low-grade DCIS. Consequently, several years ago, the term *mammary intraepithelial neoplasia* (MIN) was suggested as a replacement for various patterns of intraductal epithelial proliferation.

Mammary Intraepithelial Neoplasia.—With MIN as a translational system, all noninvasive proliferations within the mammary ductal system

TABLE 1.—Classification of MIN, Ductal Type (Ductal Intraepithelial Neoplasia)

Proposed DIN classification		Description	Current designation	Pleomorphic nuclear atypia	Necrosis
DIN	1a	IDH	IDH	−	− or +
	1b	-Type 1 AIDH	AIDH	−*	−
		-Type 2 AIDH			
		-Monolayered and minimally hyperplastic moderately atypical cellular proliferations ("Clinging carcinoma")			
	1c	Low-grade DCIS	DCIS, Grade 1	−*	−
DIN 2		Cribriform or micropapillary DCIS with necrosis or atypia	DCIS, Grade 2	− +	+ −
		DCIS with significant cytologic atypia	DCIS, Grade 3	+++	+++
DIN 3		with or without necrosis		+++	−

*No significant pleomorphic nuclear atypia is present, although at least a minor degree of atypia is assumed in all DCIS (as well as AIDH) proliferations.
Abbreviations: AIDH, atypical intraductal hyperplasia; *DCIS*, ductal carcinoma in situ; *DIN*, ductal intraepithelial neoplasia; *IDH*, intraductal hyperplasia; *MIN*, mammary intraepithelial neoplasia.
(Courtesy of Tavassoli FA: Mammary intraepithelial neoplasia: A translational classification system for the intraductal epithelial proliferations. *Breast J* 3:48–58, 1997.)

would qualify as MIN. Their growth pattern would determine further subdivisions, such as ductal, lobular, and papillary. In the case of ductal intraepithelial neoplasia (DIN), various subclasses might be identified that would include lesions now designated as *IDH, AIDH,* or *DCIS* (Table 1). A consensus also is needed on the question of margin involvement.

Conclusion.—There is a need for standardization of terminology for the intraductal proliferations now designated as *IDH, AIDH,* and *DCIS.* One way of achieving this might be to arrive at a consensus for the use of a translational system of classification or a working formulation terminology. The system proposed here could be modified over time according to research findings. With a standardized approach, precise recommendations could be made for the management of intraductal epithelial proliferations.

▶ Much of this article reviews issues in the terminology, incidence, management and diagnostic criteria for AIDH and DCIS. Difficulties in making reproducible distinctions between AIDH and DCIS are then highlighted. When these are compared with the history of similar problems in classification of preneoplastic lesions of the uterine cervix, the leap to what has been called *mammary Intraepithelial neoplasia* (MIN) is not a great one. Ductal lesions are then classified as MIN of various grades. A traslational type of reporting similar to that often used for lesions of the uterine cervix is suggested as a means of improving standardization of diagnoses and interinstitutional comparisons.

M.W. Stanley, M.D.

Suggested Reading

Rosai J: Borderline epithelial lesions of the breast. *Am J Surg Pathol,* 15:209–221, 1991.

Tavassoli FA, Man Y-G: Morphofunctional features of intraductal hyperplasia, atypical intraductal hyperplasia, and various grades of intraductal carcinoma. *Breast J* 1:155–162, 1995.

Cancerization of Small Ectatic Ducts of the Breast by Ductal Carcinoma In Situ Cells With Apocrine Snouts: A Lesion Associated With Tubular Carcinoma
Goldstein NS, O'Malley BA (William Beaumont Hosp, Royal Oak, Mich)
Am J Clin Pathol 107:561–566, 1997   2–2

Background.—Because small ectatic ducts lined by atypical ductal cells with apocrine snouts have been seen occasionally in tubular carcinoma specimens, some pathologists believe that these carcinomas are a form of ductal carcinoma in situ (DCIS). Cases of invasive carcinoma, in situ carcinoma, and fibrocystic change were reviewed to characterize lesions

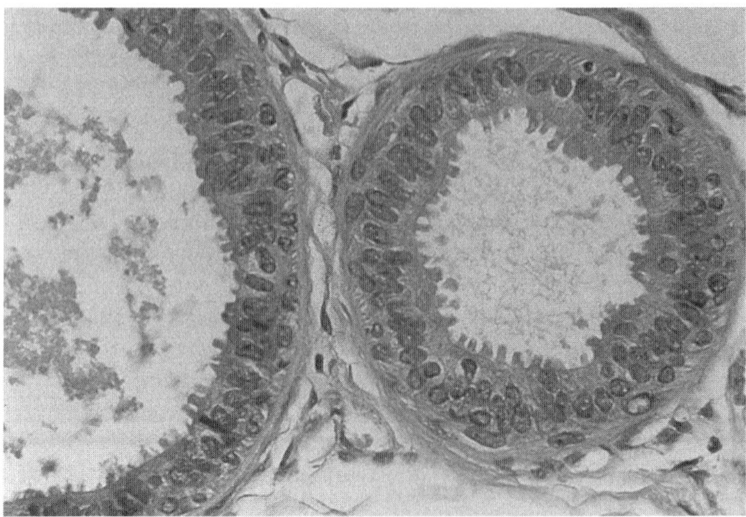

FIGURE 3.—High-power magnification of 2 small ectatic ducts lined by atypical ductal cells with apocrine snouts. Hematoxyline–eosin: original magnification, ×384. (Courtesy of Goldstein NS, O'Malley BA: Cancerization of small ectatic ducts of the breast by ductal carcinoma in situ cells with apocrine snouts: A lesion associated with tubular carcinoma. *Am J Clin Pathol* 107:561–566, 1997.)

formed by atypical ductal cells with apocrine snouts and to determine their relationship with various benign and malignant masses.

Methods and Findings.—The study included 32 cases of tubular carcinoma, 41 cases of invasive grade 1 ductal carcinoma with DCIS, 40 cases of invasive grade 1 ductal carcinoma without DCIS, 40 cases of invasive grade 3 ductal carcinoma, 40 cases of invasive lobular carcinoma, 20 cases of well-differentiated DCIS, and 80 cases of fibrocystic changes. In 17 specimens, lesions were formed by atypical ductal cells with apocrine snouts. Fourteen were associated with tubular carcinoma, and 3 were associated with invasive grade 1 ductal carcinoma. The associated DCIS was formed by cells identical to those in the lesions in 6 invasive carcinomas. These lesions were located at the periphery of the invasive carcinoma, adjacent to the DCIS. These lesions probably consisted of low-grade intraductal malignant epithelial cells that partially involve small ectatic ducts and are frequently adjacent structures as a form of cancerization (Fig 3).

Conclusions.—The cells observed in these 17 breast lesions were identical to those of the associated invasive carcinoma, which was generally of a tubular type. This lesion may be viewed as DCIS or cancerization of small ectatic ducts by well-differentiated intraductal carcinoma cells. Pathologists need to be aware of this microscopic lesion and its association with invasive carcinoma to avoid misinterpreting it as typical columnar changes of small ectatic ducts.

▶ This condition has been incompletely described in the past. The authors begin very appropriately by reminding us that the columnar alterations in small breast ducts are relatively common and usually benign (blunt duct adenosis). In contrast, the lesion they describe features cytologic atypia and apocrine cytoplasmic snouts. The most interesting aspect of this work is that, by searching for this lesion in association with numerous examples of various breast cancers, they are able to highlight its strong association with tubular carcinoma. Their discussion of differential diagnostic possibilities (blunt duct adenosis and apocrine metaplasia in small ducts) is quite good. This intraductal malignancy can be thought of as either a form of DCIS or an example of lobular cancerization. In either scheme, its frequent location at the periphery of an associated carcinoma indicates that it must be carefully sought when lumpectomy margins are examined. Furthermore, if it is found in the absence of an infiltrating carcinoma, the remaining tissue must be thoroughly examined so that a cancer is not overlooked. The authors do not address the next obvious question. Should another surgical procedure be recommended, if this pattern is identified and the pathologist is sure that the biopsy specimen contains no invasive carcinoma?

M.W. Stanley, M.D.

Suggested Reading

Oberman HA, Markey BA: Noninvasive carcinoma of the breast presenting in adenosis. *Mod Pathol* 4:31–35, 1991.

Rasbridge SA, Millis RR: Carcinoma in situ involving sclerosing adenosis: A mimic of invasive carcinoma. *Histopathology* 27:269–273, 1995.

Weidner N: Malignant breast lesions that may mimic benign tumors. *Semin Diagn Pathol* 12:2–13, 1995.

Morphological and Biological Characteristics of Mammogram-detected Invasive Breast Cancer
Moezzi M, Melamed J, Vamvakas E, et al (New York Univ; Massachusetts Gen Hosp, Boston)
Hum Pathol 27:944–948, 1996
2–3

Background.—With mammography, minimal cancers can be detected. The morphological and biological features of tiny invasive breast cancers, measuring 5 mm or less, have not been described in detail.

Methods and Findings.—Thirty-nine invasive breast cancers of 5 mm or less, detected on mammography, were compared with 78 consecutive cancers of 10 mm or larger, detected clinically. Of the small tumors, 13% were tubular carcinomas, compared with 3.8% of the larger tumors, which is a statistically nonsignificant difference. The 2 tumor groups had comparable incidences of other histologic types. The small tumors were of lower overall grade, were of lower architectural and nuclear grades, and had fewer mitotic figures. None of these tumors were lymph-node positive.

The 2 tumor groups had similar estrogen and progesterone receptor expression. The small cancers expressed p53 nuclear protein less often than the large tumors, had lower levels of microvessel density, and were more often diploid. The S-phase of the diploid tumors was similar in the 2 groups, but the S-phase of the aneuploid tumors was lower in the small tumors. Expression of Ki67 in the small tumors was also lower.

Conclusions.—Small invasive breast cancers detected mammographically represent an evolutionary phase of breast cancer, which generally lacks the morphological and biological markers of aggressive behavior. The presence or absence of such markers may account for the influence of tumor size on survival in women with breast cancer.

▶ Many of the mammographically detected breast carcinomas diagnosed today are small (<1 cm), and this low stage (pT1a) is associated with a good prognosis. This interesting paper illustrates that these minimal carcinomas often fail to show a variety of morphological and biological markers of aggressive behavior. The authors conclude that these small malignancies are caught while passing through a less aggressive developmental stage. This leads to the idea that the importance of tumor size on prognosis reflects accumulation of prognostically adverse mutations as the tumor grows. However, the authors also discuss the possibility that mammography may preferentially detect relatively indolent carcinomas. One fact supporting this is that many tumors arising in screened populations that are aggressive ab initio present as clinically apparent interval cancers. One wonders whether at least some subset of these small carcinomas might never grow up to become big lethal cancers. Obviously, the necessary experiment can never be done. However, as our understanding of breast cancer and its prognostically significant markers advances, we may learn to identify such a group of tumors.

M.W. Stanley, M.D.

Suggested Reading

Klemi PJ, Joensuu H, Toikkanen S, et al: Aggressiveness of breast cancers found with and without screening. *Br Med J* 304:467–469, 1992.

Toikkanen S, Dean PB, Joensuu H: Screen-detected breast carcinomas: Do they differ from those diagnosed outside screening programs? *Pathol Ann* 29:261–279, 1994.

Atypical Apocrine Adenosis of the Breast: A Clinicopathologic Study of 37 Patients With 8.7-Year Follow-up

Seidman JD, Ashton M, Lefkowitz M (Armed Forces Inst of Pathology, Washington, DC)
Cancer 77:2529–2537, 1996

2–4

Purpose.—An occasional breast biopsy specimen will show apocrine metaplasia superimposed over sclerosing adenosis. This condition, called apocrine adenosis, is sometimes accompanied by cytologic atypia. The long-term risk of breast cancer associated with this atypical apocrine adenosis is unknown. Thirty-seven patients with atypical apocrine adenosis were followed up to determine their risk of developing breast carcinoma.

Methods.—The patients had a mean age of 50 years. Forty-nine percent had a palpable mass and 35% had an abnormal mammogram. All had atypical apocrine adenosis, defined as apocrine adenosis with enlarged

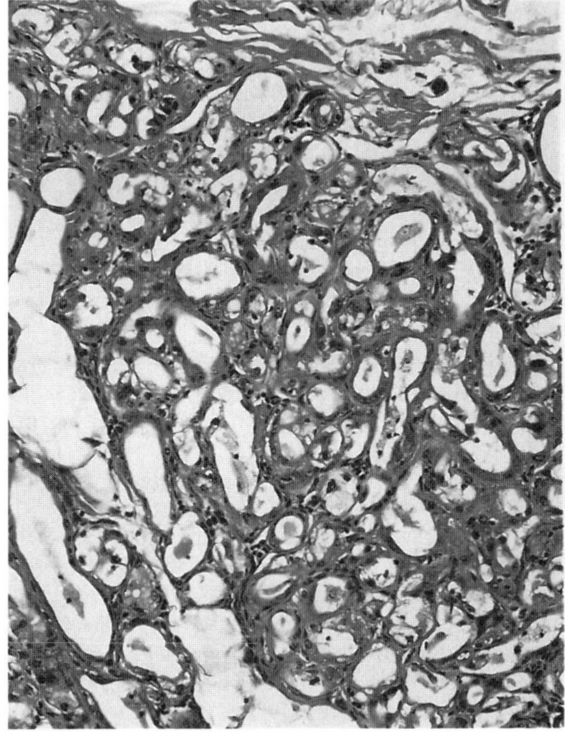

FIGURE 3.—Medium-power view of nonatypical apocrine adenosis. Note the small nuclei with no significant variation in size, and scattered nuclei showing small, prominent nucleoli. Hematoxylin-eosin; original magnification, ×150. (Courtesy of Seidman JD, Ashton M, Lefkowitz M: Atypical apocrine adenosis of the breast: A clinicopathologic study of 37 patients with 8.7-year follow-up. *Cancer* 77:2529–2537. Copyright 1996, American Cancer Society. Reprinted by permission of Wiley-Liss, Inc, a subsidiary of John Wiley & Sons, Inc.)

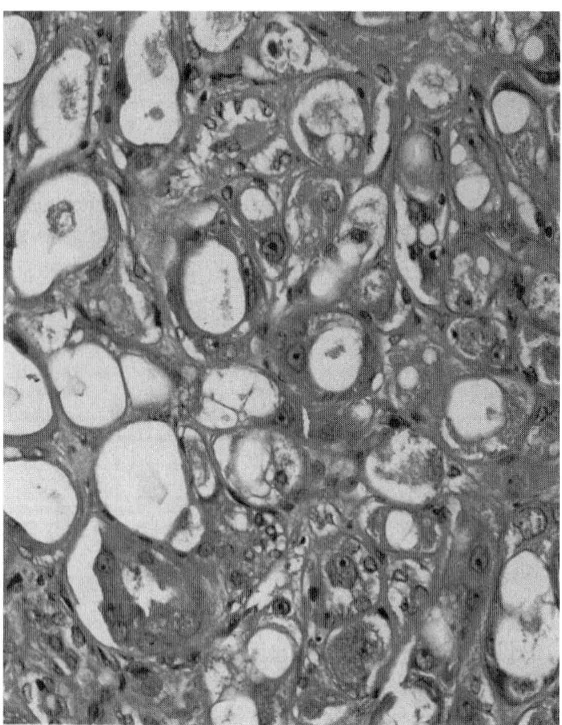

FIGURE 5.—High-power view of atypical apocrine adenosis. Note threefold variation in nuclear size, a few enlarged nucleoli, and clear to foamy cytoplasm and luminal secretions. Hematoxylin-eosin; original magnification, ×300. (Courtesy of Seidman JD, Ashton M, Lefkowitz M: Atypical apocrine adenosis of the breast: A clinicopathologic study of 37 patients with 8.7-year follow-up. *Cancer* 77:2529–2537. Copyright 1996, American Cancer Society. Reprinted by permission of Wiley-Liss, Inc, a subsidiary of John Wiley & Sons, Inc.)

nucleoli and more than a threefold variation in nuclear area (Fig 3). Abundant clear to foamy cytoplasm often appeared in areas of atypia (Figs 5 and 6). The analysis excluded patients with the cytoarchitecture typical of intraductal carcinoma. Relative risk was calculated using data from the Surveillance, Epidemiology, and End Results study.

Results.—The patients were followed up for a mean of nearly 9 years. At a mean of 6 years, 4 patients had invasive ductal carcinoma, 3 in the ipsilateral breast. This translated into a relative risk of 5.5. All patients with carcinoma were older than 60 years at the time atypical apocrine adenosis was diagnosed, with cancer developing at a mean age of 70 years. For the 11 patients who were older than 60 years, the relative risk of developing carcinoma was 14.

Conclusions.—For older women, a diagnosis of atypical apocrine adenosis on breast biopsy carries an increased risk of breast cancer. For younger women, the cancer risk is probably low. Some cases of atypical apocrine adenosis may really be apocrine carcinomas in situ. However, the

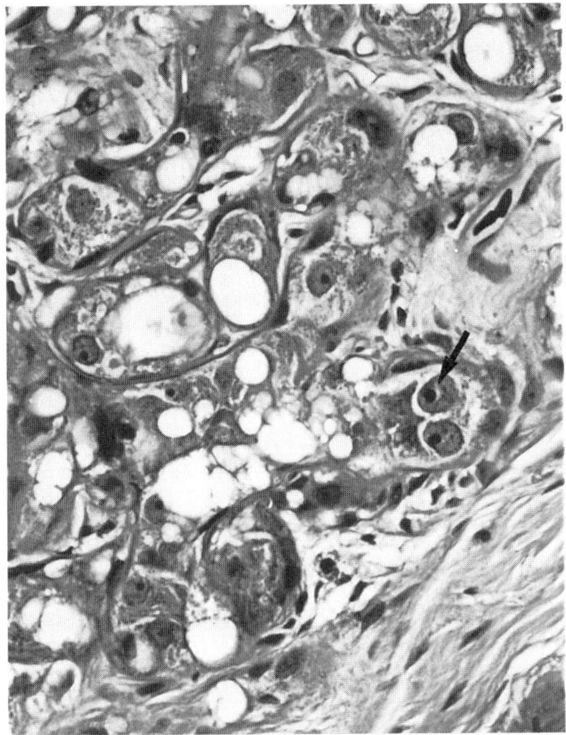

FIGURE 6.—Atypical apocrine adenosis with marked nucleolar enlargement (*arrow*). Hemotoxylin-eosin; original magnification, ×480. (Courtesy of Seidman JD, Ashton M, Lefkowitz M: Atypical apocrine adenosis of the breast: A clinicopathologic study of 37 patients with 8.7-year follow-up. *Cancer* 77:2529–2537. Copyright 1996, American Cancer Society. Reprinted by permission of Wiley-Liss, Inc, a subsidiary of John Wiley & Sons, Inc.)

cancers may go unrecognized because they lack the typical architectural features of intraductal carcinoma.

▶ A number of proliferative and metaplastic lesions usually seen in breast ducts can also involve lobules. These include apocrine change and various types of intraductal carcinoma (DCIS). This paper addresses the potential prognostic significance of "atypical apocrine adenosis" that features nuclear atypia and apocrine cytoplasmic characteristics, lacks the architecture of DCIS, and inhabits a lesion with the low-magnification pattern of sclerosing adenosis.

The definition of atypia is addressed carefully in this study and is based on enlarged nucleoli and a threefold or greater variation in nuclear size. The greatest difficulty probably remains confident recognition of this troublesome entity, that is not uncommonly mistaken for infiltrating carcinoma. The illustrations in this article are very useful in this regard.

The clinical relevance of atypical apocrine adenosis revealed by this investigation is that it was associated with an increased risk of subsequent infiltrating carcinoma, primarily in women older than 60 years (relative risk = 5.5; 95% confidence interval = 1.9–16). Other diagnostic problems involving apocrine cells are reviewed in the discussion.

As our understanding continues to grow, more will no doubt be published about lesions that are now variously termed atypical apocrine hyperplasia, apocrine intraductal carcinoma (with or without involvement of sclerosing adenosis), and atypical apocrine adenosis. These authors leave open questions about whether the lesions they illustrate actually represent apocrine intraductal carcinomas. If so, they are difficult to recognize as such because their confinement within sclerosing adenosis precludes development of architectures usually associated with DCIS.

M.W. Stanley, M.D.

Suggested Reading

Abati AD, Kimmel M, Rosen PP: Apocrine mammary carcinoma: A clinicopathologic study of 72 cases. *Am J Clin Pathol* 94:371–377, 1990.

Carter DJ, Rosen PP: Atypical apocrine metaplasia in sclerosing lesions of the breast: A study of 51 patients. *Mod Pathol* 4:1–5, 1991.

O'Malley FP, Page DL, Nelson EH, et al: Ductal carcinoma in situ of the breast with apocrine cytology: Definition of a borderline category. *Hum Pathol* 25:164–168, 1994.

Rosen PP, Oberman HA: Tumors of the mammary gland, in Rosai J, Sobin LH (eds): *Atlas of Tumor Pathology*. Third series. Fascicle 7. Washington, DC, Armed Forces Institute of Pathology, 1993, pp 54–55.

Tavassoli FA, Norris HJ: Intraductal apocrine carcinoma: A clinicopathologic study of 37 cases. *Mod Pathol* 7:813–818, 1994.

Mammary Mucocele-like Lesions: Benign and Malignant
Hamele-Bena D, Cranor ML, Rosen PP (Mem Sloan-Kettering Cancer Ctr, New York)
Am J Surg Pathol 20:1081–1085, 1996   2–5

Purpose.—Mucocele-like lesions (MLLs) of the breast were originally described as benign tumors. Since then, these lesions have been linked to ductal hyperplasia or carcinoma. The MLLs consist of multiple cysts lined by flat or cuboidal-to-columnar epithelium with focal hyperplasia. Forty-nine patients with MLLs were studied to further characterize this lesion.

Patients.—The review included 53 lesions from 49 patients, (median age 47 years). Four patients had bilateral MLLs. Twenty-five lesions were benign and 28 malignant: 14 in situ and 14 invasive. Age, tumor size, and laterality were similar for patients with benign vs. malignant MLLs. The malignant lesions were more likely to have coarse calcifications and to be detected on mammograms.

Findings.—On pathologic examination, the intraductal carcinomas had a micropapillary or cribriform pattern, whereas most of the invasive carcinomas were mucinous. Benign MLLs were usually not estrogen or progesterone positive, whereas malignant lesions were often positive for HER2/*neu*.

Treatment and Outcomes.—Most patients with benign MLLs were treated by excisional biopsy. Seventeen patients with malignant MLLs underwent excisional biopsy as well; 4 had wider excision, including axillary dissection in 3; and 5 had mastectomy and axillary dissection. At a mean and median follow-up of 4 years, there were 2 recurrences in the breast: 1 benign and 1 malignant. All patients were alive and disease free.

Conclusions.—Malignant MLL of the breast is a low-grade tumor that is clinically very similar to benign MLL. The cancerous lesions have more prominent calcifications, which leads to their detection by mammography. Recommended treatment is excisional biopsy for benign MLL and breast-conserving surgery for malignant MLL. Patients with carcinoma involving the surgical margins or an extensive intraductal component should receive radiotherapy.

▶ Most of us have a clear concept of mucinous breast carcinoma as a neoplasm featuring cellular islands floating in mucinous lakes. Some are sparsely cellular, but the lower limit of this phenomenon can be unclear. Multicystic MLLs with columnar lining cells and variable amounts of stromal mucin complicate this concept considerably. Originally described in the 1980s, MLLs have been considered a benign entity to be distinguished from mucinous carcinoma. However, this paper indicates that about half of all MLLs represent low-grade malignancies, the multicystic component being associated with intraductal carcinoma (micropapillary or cribriform) or infiltrating carcinoma (usually mucinous). Mammography seems to selectively detect more of the malignant lesions because of their more frequent association with coarse calcifications. Conservative therapy is appropriate, but occasional local recurrences may be identified.

This paper illustrates another example of a new entity about which our understanding continues to expand long after its initial description. I very much enjoyed Dr. Rosen's use of the term "mucinous carcinoma with a mucocele-like configuration." This newly clarified spectrum of lesions, ranging from benign to malignant and unified by a continuum of increasing cellular proliferation, is less simple but more satisfying than the old idea of benign mucoceles vs. mucinous carcinomas. The older concept just did not ring true. We've seen this before.

M.W. Stanley, M.D.

Suggested Reading

Benchimol S, Lane DP: p53: Oncogene or anti-oncogene? *Genes Dev* 4:1–8, 1990.

Burger PC, Scheithauer BW: *Tumors of the Central Nervous System*, ed 3. Washington, DC, Armed Forces Institute of Pathology, 1994, pp 25–161.

Cagle PT, Brown RW, Lebovitz RM: p53 immunostaining in the differentiation of reactive processes from malignancy in pleural biopsy specimens. *Hum Pathol* 25:443–448, 1994.

Effects of Chemotherapy on Pathologic and Biologic Characteristics of Locally Advanced Breast Cancer

Honkoop AH, Pinedo HM, De Jong J, et al (Univ Hosp Vrije Universiteit, Amsterdam)
Am J Clin Pathol 107:211–218, 1997

2–6

Introduction.—Neoadjuvant chemotherapy for breast cancer provides a useful in vivo model in which to study the effects of chemotherapy on tumor morphology and biology. However, there are few data on the effects of chemotherapy on tumor architecture and cell biology. The effects of neoadjuvant chemotherapy on the pathologic and biological characteristics of breast cancers were studied.

Methods.—A total of 42 patients with locally advanced breast cancer were studied. All received neoadjuvant chemotherapy, followed by surgery and radiation therapy. The effects of chemotherapy on a wide range of findings was investigated, including tumor architecture, morphometric nuclear and nucleolar characteristics, DNA ploidy, mitotic activity index as an indicator of proliferation, expression of differentiation antigens, and microvessel density. The findings in surgical specimens were compared with those of pretreatment specimens, including subclavicular biopsy specimens obtained before chemotherapy in 9 patients. The other patients only had fine-needle aspiration performed before chemotherapy, so the morphologic and biological features could only be studied after chemotherapy.

Results.—Twenty-three patients were left with no or only microscopic tumor after chemotherapy. In this group, there was a characteristic pattern of relatively cellular fibrous tissue with a lymphocytic infiltrate, iron-laden macrophages, and scattered tumor foci, if any. Lymph nodes showed areas of nodular hyaline fibrosis, sometimes with iron-laden macrophages. The tumors showed reduced mitotic activity and reduced microvessel density. However, the posttreatment specimens showed no consistent alterations of nuclear and nucleolar morphometry, DNA ploidy, or expression of differentiation antigens. There were no pathologic or biological characteristics that predicted response to chemotherapy.

Conclusions.—In patients with no tumor or only microscopic tumor remaining after chemotherapy, the typical morphologic findings include fibrous tissue, lymphocytic infiltrate, and iron-laden macrophages. Cell proliferation and global amount of microvessels are reduced, but there is no consistent pattern of changes in DNA ploidy, nuclear and nucleolar morphometry, or cellular differentiation. The effects of chemotherapy and growth factors on angiogenesis and stromal reactions must be studied further, along with the relationship between these factors and response to chemotherapy.

▶ Preoperative chemical treatment of breast carcinoma (neoadjuvant chemotherapy) is being used with increasing frequency. This article looks at tumor morphology and biology in 42 patients with locally advanced carcinoma after this type of treatment. The preoperative diagnoses had been made by incisional biopsy, supraclavicular lymph node excision, or breast fine-needle aspiration. In half of the cases, there was little or no residual tumor in the definitive resection material. These cases showed regressive alterations with fibrosis, inflammation and hemosiderin-laden macrophages. There were no consistent alterations in nuclear, nucleolar, or DNA ploidy characteristics. Importantly, no pathologic or biological feature was predictive of response to chemotherapy. Those handling specimens of this type need to be aware that little residual tumor may be identified. It is important that careful sampling be directed toward areas of fibrous tissue and to the site known to have been occupied by the tumor before therapy. Although immunohistochemical stains for cytokeratins were performed on initial and on posttreatment samples, the authors do not comment on the potential utility of these methods for identifying small amounts of residual carcinoma.

M.W. Stanley, M.D.

Suggested Reading

Chevillard S, Pouillart P, Beldjord C, et al: Sequential assessment of multidrug resistance phenotype and measurement of S-phase fraction as predictive markers of breast cancer response to neoadjuvant chemotherapy. *Cancer* 77:292–300, 1996.

Frierson HF, Fechner RE: Histologic grade of locally advanced infiltrating ductal carcinoma after treatment with induction chemotherapy. *Am J Clin Pathol* 102:154–157, 1994.

Hortogagyi GN: Multidisciplinary management of advanced primary and metastatic breast cancer. *Cancer* 23:416–423, 1994.

Effects of Preoperative Chemotherapy on the Morphology of Resectable Breast Carcinoma
Sharkey FE, Addington SL, Fowler LJ, et al (Univ of Texas, San Antonio)
Mod Pathol 9:893–900, 1996   2–7

Introduction.—Little has been published regarding the pathologic effects of chemotherapy administered preoperatively in patients with surgically operable tumors. Forty-three patients with surgically operable breast

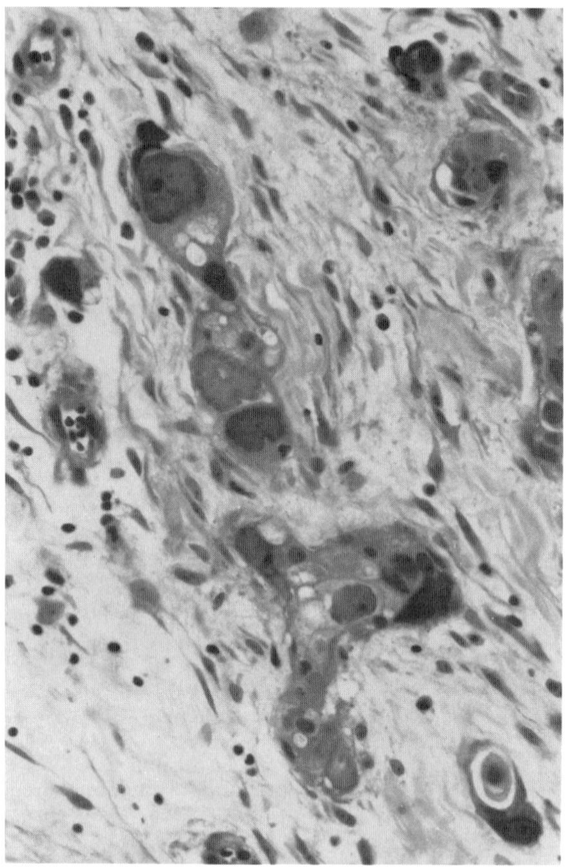

FIGURE 2.—Postchemotherapy cytologic changes. Note pleomorphism, enlarged irregular nuclei and nucleoli, dust-like chromatin, and cytoplasmic vacuolization. Hematoxylin and eosin stain; original magnification, ×250. (Courtesy of Sharkey FE, Addington SL, Fowler LJ, et al: Effects of Preoperative Chemotherapy on the Morphology of Resectable Breast Carcinoma. *Mod Pathol* 9[9]:893–900, 1996.)

carcinoma who received chemotherapy before definitive surgical resection were evaluated.

Methods.—All patients were entered into the National Surgical Adjuvant Breast and Bowel Project B-18 treatment protocol. These women had palpable, operable stage T1, T2, or T3 breast carcinoma, which was treated with 4 intravenous courses of doxorubicin and cyclophosphamide before or after definitive surgery. Either segmentectomy plus axillary node dissection or modified radical mastectomy was performed. Of 89 patients entered into the protocol, 43 were randomized to the preoperative chemotherapy arm. The remaining 46 patients received chemotherapy postoperatively. Complete response was defined as complete disappearance of clinically detected tumor. Partial response was defined as 50% or greater reduction in the product of the 2 greatest perpendicular tumor diameters.

Core needle biopsy and fine-needle biopsy specimens were obtained for initial diagnosis in 28% and 72% of women, respectively.

Results.—Of the 43 patients undergoing the preoperative chemotherapy arm, 36 (84%) had a clinical response. Ten (23%) patients had complete clinical regression. Twenty-three (53%) patients had histologic evidence of regression. The correlation between histologic regression and clinical response was poor. Of 19 tumors that displayed a 90% or greater reduction in clinically measured cross-sectional area, there was even less correlation with histologic evidence of regression. There was an increase in nuclear grade between the initial biopsy, or fine-needle aspiration specimen, and the definitive surgical specimen in 13 (32%) of the 41 women evaluated, compared with only 1 (3%) of women evaluated in the postoperative chemotherapy group (Fig 2). This increase in nuclear grade was noted in 12 of the 13 women in whom a fine-needle biopsy was obtained before treatment. A reduction in nuclear grade was seen in 1 of the women in the preoperative chemotherapy group and in 4 women in the postoperative chemotherapy group. In the preoperative chemotherapy group, intraductal or intralymphatic tumor was unusually prominent in 17 of 43 (40%) women. In 9 women treated in the preoperative chemotherapy wing, there was histologic evidence of tumor regression in the axillary lymph nodes. Regressive changes also were observed in nonneoplastic breast tissue and in lymphoid populations of lymph nodes. The evidence of tumor regression in the lymph nodes correlated with histologic evidence of regression in the primary tumor. There was no significant correlation between histologic regression in the primary tumor and the presence of lymph node metastasis or between clinical regression and lymph node metastases. Residual atypical intraductal proliferations were difficult to evaluate.

Conclusion.—Findings from this cohort provide quantitative evidence for reports that have previously described histologic and cytologic changes related to chemotherapy in primary breast carcinoma. Histologic evidence of downstaging and relative treatment resistance by intraductal and intralymphatic tumor was observed. These findings stress the need for pathologic staging in patients with primary breast carcinoma.

▶ These authors report findings that overlap with some noted by Honkoop, et al. (Abstract 2–6), but they also offer additional observations. These include prominent intraductal or intralymphatic tumor, and frequent increases in nuclear grade. Histologic evidence of regression was not detected in all cases with clinical response. Examples of microscopic residual carcinoma were noted in some instances of apparent complete clinical remission. This paper does a good job of describing patient and study design factors that limit the comparisons that can be drawn among the various published investigations. The information seems heavily weighted toward clinical findings. A few loose ends in the pathologic descriptions are troublesome. Apparent posttherapy diagnosis alterations of infiltrating ductal carcinomas to mucinous carcinoma (2), atypical medullary carcinoma (2), and adenoid cystic carcinoma (1) might have been related in part to sampling error in the initial diagnostic material; but with no explanation, these descriptions are disconcerting.

M.W. Stanley, M.D.

To Freeze or Not to Freeze: A Comparison of Methods for the Handling of the Breast Biopsies With No Palpable Abnormality
Niemann TH, Lucas JG, Marsh WL Jr ((Ohio State Univ, Columbus))
Am J Clin Pathol 106:225–228, 1996   2–8

Background.—Whereas breast biopsy specimens were previously examined by frozen section on a routine basis, it is now generally agreed that frozen section should not be performed on small or nonpalpable lesions. Starting in 1994, the authors' pathology department switched from doing routine frozen sections on breast biopsy specimens to performing frozen sections only on specimens with gross lesions larger than 1 cm. The results of these 2 approaches were compared.

Findings.—In the year before the new policy was instituted, frozen sections were performed on 98% of the 444 breast biopsy specimens submitted, whether or not a gross lesion was present. Fourteen false negative diagnoses were made on frozen section specimens, for a sensitivity of 84% and a false negative rate of 3%.

In the year after the new policy was instituted, 601 specimens were submitted. Frozen section was performed only on the 310 specimens that contained a gross lesion larger than 1 cm. There were only 3 false negative diagnoses in this group, for a sensitivity of 96% and a false negative rate of 1%. No frozen section was performed on the 273 specimens with no gross lesion or on the 18 specimens with gross lesions smaller than 1 cm.

Conclusions.—The accuracy of frozen section diagnosis of breast biopsies is improved by selective freezing of only those specimens with a gross lesion larger than 1 cm. The data support the recommendation in recent editorials that frozen sections should not be performed on small or nonpalpable breast lesions. The selective approach also helps reduce the costs of frozen section.

▶ This study reinforces the thinking that underlies current practice in evaluating excisional breast biopsy samples. The authors compare a "freeze everything" approach to 444 biopsy accessioned in 1 year, with a selective application of frozen sections to 601 biopsies obtained during a subsequent 12-month period. During the latter part of the study, biopsies without a gross lesion or with an abnormality measuring less than 1 cm were not evaluated by frozen section. The paper gives all the appropriate numbers, as well as sensitivity, specificity, and predictive value calculations. For most readers, the most important numbers will be the false negative rates of 3.3% versus 1% for the 2 study periods, indicating improved frozen section accuracy when the methods are selectively applied. In both series, almost all false negative diagnoses were the result of sampling error. (There were no false positive frozen section diagnoses during either part of the study.) These authors point out the well-known benefits of not having to interpret subtle findings in previously frozen tissue. Another advantage of limiting the use of frozen sections is cost-savings under capitated payment plans ($24,000 during the second 1-year series at the authors' institution). Those who are still being pressured by surgeons to freeze too many biopsies of the breast (or of other sites) must resist this pressure and help educate their clinical colleagues. The "freeze everything" approach is wasteful and error prone. Small abnormalities rendered uninterpretable by freezing artifact can be a disaster for the patient as well as for the pathologists' risk management team.

M.W. Stanley, M.D.

Suggested Reading

Fechner RE. Practice parameter: Frozen section examination of breast biopsies. *Am J Clin Pathol* 103:6–7, 1995.

Ferreiro JA, Gisvold JJ, Bostwick DG. Accuracy of frozen-section diagnosis of mammographically directed breast biopsies: Results of 1,490 consecutive cases. *Am J Surg Pathol* 19:1267–1271, 1995.

Oberman HA: Frozen section diagnosis of breast biopsy specimens: A necessary procedure? *Arch Surg* 128:955–956, 1993.

Oberman HA: A modest proposal. *Am J Surg Pathol* 16:69–70, 1992.

Schnitt SJ, Connolly JL: Processing and evaluation of breast excision specimens: A clinically oriented approach. *Am J Clin Pathol* 98:125–137, 1992.

Surgical Biopsy Findings in Patients With Atypical Hyperplasia Diagnosed by Stereotaxic Core Needle Biopsy
Tocino I, Garcia BM, Carter D (Yale Univ, New Haven, Conn)
Ann Surg Oncol 3:483–488, 1996   2–9

Objective.—Mammographically suspicious and indeterminate breast lesions can be diagnosed in specimens obtained by stereotaxic large-core needle biopsy (SCNB). However, the diagnostic and management role of SCNB in such borderline conditions as atypical ductal and lobular hyperplasia is unclear. The SCNB and surgical biopsy results of patients with atypical hyperplasia were compared retrospectively.

Methods.—A total of 323 patients who underwent 358 consecutive SCNBs were studied. On review of the mammograms and pathology reports, 25 lesions in 22 patients were identified as atypical ductal or lobular hyperplasia. The SCNB results in these cases were compared with the histologic findings of surgical biopsy, which were available for 22 lesions in 19 patients.

Results.—In the 22 lesions, the results of surgical biopsy and SCNB were not in agreement in 16 cases, were in partial agreement in 2 cases, and complete agreement in 4 cases. Open biopsy revealed carcinoma in 10 cases: invasive carcinoma in 5 and ductal carcinoma in situ in 5. None of these cancers was apparent on SCNB.

Conclusions.—A diagnosis of atypical ductal or lobular hyperplasia on SCNB does not correlate well with the histologic findings on surgical biopsy. Many patients with atypical hyperplasia diagnosed on SCNB prove to have malignancies. All patients with atypical hyperplasia on SCNB should therefore undergo excisional biopsy.

▶ This article uses a large series of core breast biopsies to find a significant number of such specimens with atypical intraductal hyperplasia (ADH). (Atypical lobular hyperplasia is addressed only as an incidental finding in excised breast biopsies.) A few such cases are described in other large series but are rarely the focus of investigation. Correlation of this biopsy finding with the ultimate pathology in excisional biopsies is of interest because it is not only a marker lesion for subsequent development of invasive carcinoma, but it is also commonly seen adjacent to carcinoma; the latter suggests potentially significant problems related to sampling errors in the core specimens. Problems with the reproducibility of this histopathologic diagnosis have been noted. (In my opinion these are often somewhat overstated.) Importantly, the criteria for ADH used in this article are similar to those of Page and coworkers. The system of Page and colleagues, as well as that of Tavassoli and Norris uses a quantitative criterion (2 spaces vs. 2 mm, respectively) as one of the means to distinguish between ADH and ductal carcinoma in situ (DCIS). One might expect this to frustrate efforts to distinguish between these 2 lesions in core biopsies, but the authors indicate that this was an uncommon problem seen in only 1 of 22 samples. The numbers are useful, but the take-home message is that core biopsies showing ADH can be correct but may either underestimate the excisional biopsy findings (no more ADH identified) or may undercall the final diagnosis (DCIS or invasive carcinoma identified). In the latter instance, patient management will frequently be altered. These noncorrelation events reflect sampling error inherent in the methods and not a quality assurance problem. These authors go on to give a good discussion of factors that influence the rate of ADH in an institution's biopsy material (4% to 20% in the literature cited); these include the patient age distribution, criteria for biopsy based on mammographic findings, interlaboratory agreement, the number of cores obtained, and the completeness of surgical excision. It is also known that many ADH/DCIS lesions extend beyond the area of mammographic abnormality.

M.W. Stanley, M.D.

Suggested Reading

Jackman RJ, Nowels KW, Shepard MJ, et al: Stereotaxic large-core needle biopsy of 450 nonpalpable breast lesions with surgical correlation in lesions with cancer or atypical hyperplasia. *Radiology* 193:91–95, 1994.

Lennington WJ, Jensen RA, Dalton LW, et al: Ductal carcinoma in situ of the breast: Heterogeneity of individual lesions. *Cancer* 73:118–124, 1994.

Liberman L, Evans WP III, Dershaw DD, et al: Atypical ductal hyperplasia diagnosed at stereotaxic core biopsy of breast lesions: An indication for surgical biopsy. *AJR* 164:1111–1113, 1995.

Stomper PC, Cholewinski SP, Penetrante RB, et al: Aytpical hyperplasia: Frequency and mammographic and pathologic relationships in excisional biopsies guided with mammography and clinical examination. *Radiology* 189:667–671, 1993.

Large-gauge Core Needle Biopsy of the Breast

Reynolds HE, Jackson VP, Gin FM, et al (Indiana Univ, Indianapolis)
Breast J 2:370–373, 1996   2–10

Background.—Large-gauge core needle biopsy (LGCNB) of the breast is a very accurate, safe procedure and a less costly alternative to surgical excision. One experience with this procedure was reported.

Methods.—During a 40-month period, LGCNB was performed on 137 lesions in 125 patients. Fifty-nine procedures used stereotactic guidance with a prone table, and 78 used US guidance with a freehand technique. In all procedures, a 14-gauge core needle attached to an automated biopsy device was used.

Findings.—Fifty-three diagnoses were malignant, and 84 were benign. Surgical correlation, available in 46 of the malignant cases, demonstrated no false-positive findings. One lesion was missed at the initial surgical excision but retrieved at re-excision. Surgical or mammographic follow-up was available in 42 of the 84 patients given diagnoses of benign masses on LGCNB. The mean duration of the mammographic follow-up was 13 months. One diagnosis proved to be false negative. The sensitivity of LGCNB was 98%, and the specificity was 100%. Its positive predictive value was 100%, and its negative predictive value was 96%.

Conclusions.—Large-gauge core needle biopsy is a highly accurate procedure that is well accepted by patients. Difficulties include ensuring compliance with follow-up recommendations among patients with benign results and excluding invasive carcinoma.

▶ Technical considerations and limitations, as well as issues of patient comfort, length of procedure, cost, and radiation exposure, vary between stereotactic and US biopsies of nonpalpable breast lesions. These authors applied both methods based on fairly standard selection criteria, which they review. Criteria for following a benign core biopsy diagnosis with surgical excision are also discussed. This is a fairly small study (137 lesions in 125 patients), but 1 example each of a false-negative core and a false-negative excision is described. Those of us who do breast fine-needle aspiration spend a great deal of time worrying about false-negative aspirations, but many physicians, including both pathologists and clinicians, too often forget that every type of biopsy has a false-negative rate.

The following is not meant to reflect on this paper or the authors in any fashion; this just seems like a good time to consider issues that bother some of us in the laboratory. Most of the now copious literature on the safety and efficacy of various breast biopsy methods is in the radiology literature. In real life, many of us apply these methods in a team setting with equal input from surgeons, pathologists, and radiologists. The literature sounds like radiologists interpret the films, select the patients for biopsy (by whatever nonsurgical method), perform the procedure, get a report from the pathologist, interpret the report, elect a follow-up plan, carry out the follow-up, and provide quality control for the entire process. Regardless of whether this is actually what is happening, we can conclude little else from a flood of papers with neither pathologists nor surgeons among the authors.

In reading this literature during the last several years, I find 3 bothersome points in the process. First, the radiologist must interpret the pathology report. My own observations of this process lead me to believe that some conferencing with the pathologist is often needed if optimal understanding of the findings is to be achieved. (For example, I was surprised to find the term *fibrocystic disease* used at all, much less as an unqualified diagnosis for 9 cases in the paper just reviewed.) Next, the radiologist must decide whether the mammogram and the histopathologic findings are sufficiently concordant as to preclude surgical excision. Finally, the follow-up in most of these studies is usually a few months, is based largely on mammography, and falls short of published guidelines describing the length of follow-up for these cases. Is anyone else bothered by this increasingly radiologicocentric system?

M.W. Stanley, M.D.

Suggested Reading

Dershaw DD, Morris EA, Liberman L, et al: Nondiagnostic stereotactic core breast biopsy: Results of rebiopsy. *Radiology* 198:323–325, 1996.

Liberman L, Dershaw DD, Rosen PP, et al: Stereotactic core biopsy of breast carcinoma: Accuracy at predicting invasion. *Radiology* 194:379–381, 1995.

Liberman L, Fahs MC, Dershaw DD, et al: Impact of stereotactic core breast biopsy on cost of diagnosis. *Radiology* 195:633–637, 1995.

Mammographically Directed Breast Biopsies: A College of American Pathologists Q-Probes Study of Clinical Physician Expectations and of Specimen Handling and Reporting Characteristics in 434 Institutions
Nakhleh RE, Jones B, Zarbo RJ (Henry Ford Hosp, Detroit; St John Hosp, Detroit)
Arch Pathol Lab Med 121:11–18, 1997   2–11

Objective.—The breast biopsy is a complex procedure involving sampling of an abnormal area followed by a specimen radiograph report to the surgeon, which may or may not meet expectations. Results of a study examining the specific information surgeons want in a pathology report, how specimens are processed in the laboratory, and the information actually included in pathology reports are presented.

Methods.—Data collected from Clinical Physician Survey forms sent to 1,469 biopsy surgeons by 434 surgical pathology laboratories that are members of the College of American Pathologists' voluntary Q-probes quality improvement program contained information about 7,300 biopsy cases.

Results.—Most physicians were consistent in wanting the following information: whether the diagnosis was benign, ductal carcinoma in situ, or invasive ductal carcinoma. Processing action information showed that the specimen was received fresh in 63% of cases, a radiograph was performed in 60%, the lesion was marked to identify it in 89%, a grossly suspicious lesion was present in 93%, the specimen was inked in 71%, the tissue was taken for special studies in 81%, and the tissue was taken for receptor status in 75%. Radiographs were taken of 5% of the specimens and 4% of the tissue blocks. No biopsy report checklist was used in 65.7% of laboratories, although the percentage of reports containing desired information was signficantly higher for laboratories that did use a checklist. Reports included correlations of mammographic abnormalities and microscopic findings in 62% of cases, margin status in 92%, lesion size in 77%, tumor grade in 83% of invasive malignancies, and extent of intraductal carcinoma in 76%.

Conclusion.—The Q-probes quality improvement programs identified the use of checklists as the factor that significantly influenced the completeness of reports of biopsies of suspicious breast lesions.

▶ This is another large CAP Q-Probes survey based on this organization's now standard methods. The goal was to compare what clinicians who take care of breast-mass patients want from pathologists with what we are actually putting into our reports. This study explores numerous issues, and much of the data are summarized very effectively in tabular form. There is much here that is consistent with the previous ADASP recommendations, many readers' expectations, and the way that many of us are already practicing. Even so, there are some surprises. Examples include clinician desires for flow cytometry in breast cancer and for hormone receptor studies for in situ lesions. On the laboratory side, I was surprised to learn that

TABLE 11.—The Number of Positive Responses Regarding Items in Reports Depending on the Use of Checklists

	CL for all Breast Disease	CL for Invasive Carcinoma	CL for Carcinoma In Situ	CL for In Situ and Invasive Carcinoma	CL Only for Mammographic Biopsies	No CL for Mammographic Biopsies	No CL Used	Any CL Used†
Is clinical information regarding mammographic abnormalities present in the report?	72	66	75	68	74	61	60	69
Is it stated if the tissue was received fresh without any fixative or in a fixative?	65	49	50	58	66	60	62	59
Is it stated if the tissue was physically marked in any way (eg, needle, wire, other) before it was received in Surgical Pathology?	83	79	74	88	81	77	75	80
Does the report mention whether an accompanying radiograph came with the specimen?	55	57	51	48	55	52	51	52
Is the size of the tissue present?	99	99	99	99	99	99	99	99
Is it stated whether a grossly suspicious lesion is present or absent?	87	80	88	85	87	84	83	86
If a grossly suspicious lesion is noted, is its size present?*	90	90	90	94	91	90	90	90
If a grossly suspicious lesion is present, is there a gross assessment of the margin status?*	71	37	46	48	63	49	50	51
Is it noted if the specimen was inked?	58	57	63	64	66	58	58	63
If a grossly suspicious lesion is present, is it stated whether tissue was taken for cytosol estrogen and progesterone receptor assays, flow cytometry, or other studies?*	38	43	40	35	45	43	43	41

Is a microscopic description present?	77	51	53	56	76	65	69	60
Is there correlation of the mammographic abnormality with the microscopic findings?	71	68	61	69	72	60	59	67
If the diagnosis is in situ or invasive carcinoma, is the status of margins stated?*	93	91	93	97	97	88	88	93
If the diagnosis is in situ or invasive carcinoma, is there any estimate of size (eg, no. of slides, actual measurement)?*	83	71	79	87	84	73	73	81
If the diagnosis is an invasive carcinoma, is the grade of the tumor stated?*	90	92	95	86	91	79	79	89
If the diagnosis is an invasive ductal carcinoma, is there a statement regarding the extent of intraductal carcinoma?*	84	62	89	81	87	76	72	83
If the diagnosis is an invasive malignancy and tissue was not taken for biochemical receptor assay, were estrogen and progesterone receptors evaluated by immunohistochemistry?*	83	89	87	84	77	87	81	88

*Responses of "not applicable" were excluded from the analysis.

†For all but 3 items, there is a significant improvement ($P < 0.05$) in reporting with the use of a checklist versus no checklist.

CL, Checklist.

(Courtesy of Nakhleh RE, Jones B, Zarbo, RJ: Mammographically directed breast biopsies: A College of American Pathologists Q-probes study of clinical physician expectations and of specimen handling and reporting characteristics in 434 institutions. *Arch Pathol Lab Med* 121:11–18, 1997.)

approximately 15% of the biopsies were not inked to facilitate assessment of resection margins. Problems with pathology report "content adequacy" are further summarized in Table 11. As in other Q-Probe studies, use of a checklist is suggested as one way to ensure inclusion of all appropriate information. This report clearly offers information about ways in which we might provide education for our clinical colleagues, and it also shows areas in which some laboratory practices can be improved.

I have one quarrel with the authors. They note correctly that many biopsies performed for evaluation of mammographic lesions arrive in the laboratory with a specimen radiograph but no radiologist interpretation. They come to the obvious conclusion that pathologists are looking at these films without help from a radiologist. They go on to state, "It is our opinion that this practice would increase the possibility that a lesion would be missed or misinterpreted, as most pathologists are not trained in radiograph interpretation." I feel that they miss the point. We do not interpret these films in any real diagnostic sense. In most instances, they serve as a simple guide to the location of potential lesions. This does not constitute making a diagnostic interpretation. Furthermore, I would argue that many pathologists are indeed qualified to carry out this function. The authors might have made suggestions for educating our colleagues. They might have given some responsibility to the radiologists to alter their own mode of practice. Instead, they have made a weighty statement about a pattern in pathology practice over which we have little or no control. Would they prefer that we leave the film unexamined and section away at large fatty biopsies without grossly apparent pathology? Statements of this type, by authors of this importance, with organizational sponsorship of this magnitude, in journals of this gravity, cannot be far removed from standard-of-care statements. Describing the current situation would have been helpful; their comment is not. This is especially so, since I find no other editorial statements of such gravity elsewhere in this article.

M.W. Stanley, M.D.

Suggested Reading

Association of Directors of Anatomic and Surgical Pathology: Immediate management of mammographically detected breast lesions. *Am J Surg Pathol* 17:850–851, 1993.

Routine Contralateral Breast Biopsy: Helpful or Irrelevant?: Experience in 871 Patients, 1979–1993
Cody HS III (Mem Sloan-Kettering Cancer Ctr, New York)
Ann Surg 225:370–376, 1997
2–12

Background.—The value of routine contralateral biopsy in patients with breast cancer is still controversial. An experience with a large series was analyzed to further define the role of this procedure.

TABLE 5.—Routine Biopsy of the Normal Contralateral Breast: Summary of Results

Author (year)	No.	Biopsy+, Invasive [no. (%)]	Biopsy+, *In Situ* [no. (%)]	Biopsy+, Total [no. (%)]
Fenig (1975)	314	11 (3.5)	12 (3.8)	23 (7.3)
King (1976)	109	1 (1)	4 (3.7)	5 (4.6)
Urban (1977)	301	5 (1.7)	18 (6.0)	23 (7.7)
Leis (1978)	321	10 (3.1)	14 (4.4)	24 (7.5)
Pressman (1980)	85	0	7 (12)	7 (12)
Andersen (1980)	170	7 (4.1)	3 (1.8)	10 (5.9)
Martin (1982)	100	2 (2)	0	2 (2)
Wanebo (1985)	40	1 (2)	6 (15)	7 (17.5)
Pressman (1986)	226	4 (1.8)	28 (12.4)	32 (14.2)
Smith (1992)	95	2 (2.1)	3 (3.2)	5 (5.3)
Cody (1997)	871	14 (1.6)	40 (4.6)	54 (6.2)
Total	2632	57 (2.2)	135 (5.2)	192 (7.3)

(Courtesy of Cody HS III: Routine contralateral breast biopsy: Helpful or irrelevant? Experience in 871 patients, 1979–1993. *Ann Surg* 225:370–376, 1997.)

Methods and Findings.—Eight hundred seventy-one patients with breast cancer underwent routine contralateral biopsy in the author's practice between 1979 and 1993. Atypical hyperplasia was found in 6.9% of all random biopsy specimens, lobular carcinoma in situ was found in 3.2%, invasive cancers were found in 1.6%, and ductal carcinoma in situ was found in 1.4%. When lobular carcinoma in situ was excluded as a positive result, invasive lobular carcinoma was not significantly more bilateral than invasive duct cancer and in situ tumors were not significantly more bilateral than invasive cancers. Positive results could not be predicted by tumor size, axillary node status, or young age. Four percent of patients older than 50 years had a positive biopsy result compared with 1% of patients younger than 50 years, which was a significant difference. A positive biopsy result was also significantly more frequent in patients with a first-degree relative than those without a family history, the frequency for the former being 6.3% and the frequency for the latter being 2.2% (Table 5).

Conclusions.—Routine contralateral biopsy identified conditions requiring immediate management in 3% of patients and revealed a risk with the potential to affect future decisions in another 10.1%. This practice deserves wider consideration as a screening method for a high-risk population.

▶ This author uses a relatively large experience to argue in favor of routine contralateral breast biopsies in patients being surgically treated for early-stage breast cancer. All biopsies were directed at the upper outer quadrant, and tissue measuring 2–4 cm in greatest dimension was removed. The additional morbidity and expense was minimal. The results indicate that a management-altering lesion will be found in about 3% of these patients who are at high risk for disease in the contralateral breast. The author points out that this is much higher than the 0.2% yield of single-round screening mammography. He goes on to conceptualize contralateral breast biopsy as a screening procedure applied to demonstrably high-risk individuals. The data concerning the bilaterality of lobular carcinoma are interesting. The incidence of bilaterality in infiltrating lobular carcinoma is the same as for infiltrating ductal carcinoma (in situ lobular lesions are excluded from consideration). Regardless of one's opinion regarding routine contralateral breast biopsy, the author reminds us about 2 patient groups who are at extremely high risk and in whom the procedure is to be used frequently. These are women younger than the age of 30 years who have received mantle radiation for treatment of Hodgkin's disease and those with germ line mutations of the *BRCA1* gene.

M.W. Stanley, M.D.

Suggested Reading

Ford D, Easton DF, Bishop DT, et al: Risks of cancer in *BRCA1*-mutation carriers. Breast Cancer Linkage Consortium. *Lancet* 343:692–695, 1994.

Yahalom J, Petrek JA, Biddinger PW, et al: Breast cancer in patients irradiated for Hodgkin's disease: A clinical and pathological analysis of 45 events in 37 patients. *J Clin Oncol* 10:1674–1681, 1992.

Subsequent Breast Carcinoma Risk After Biopsy With Atypia in a Breast Papilloma

Page DL, Salhany KE, Jensen RA, et al (Vanderbilt Univ, Nashville, Tenn; Univ of Pennsylvania, Pa)
Cancer 78:258–266, 1996
2–13

Background.—Although intraductal papillomas are not a common finding in breast biopsy specimens, they are often found in women in whom biopsies are performed for the uncommon indication of bloody nipple discharge. Most authors do not believe that uncomplicated intraductal papillomas are precursor lesions of carcinoma; however, their malignant potential is still open to debate. The risk of subsequent breast cancer was assessed for women with a biopsy finding of papilloma.

Methods.—The case-control study included 122 patients with breast biopsy specimens showing benign papillomas: 31 subsequently had invasive carcinoma and 91 did not. Both groups of biopsy specimens were analyzed for the presence of atypical hyperplasia (AH), not only within the papilloma but also within the surrounding parenchyma. The diagnosis of papilloma with AH was made if the histologic and cytologic features of hyperplastic epithelium came near but fell short of the diagnostic criteria for ductal carcinoma in situ (Figs 2 and 3).

Results.—Invasive breast cancer developed in 19% of cases vs. 2% of controls, for a relative risk of 9.6. Invasive cancer was 4 times more likely for women with papillomas containing AH than in women whose specimens showed no AH within or surrounding the papilloma. Added atypical hyperplasia outside the papilloma appeared to increase risk. Most of the

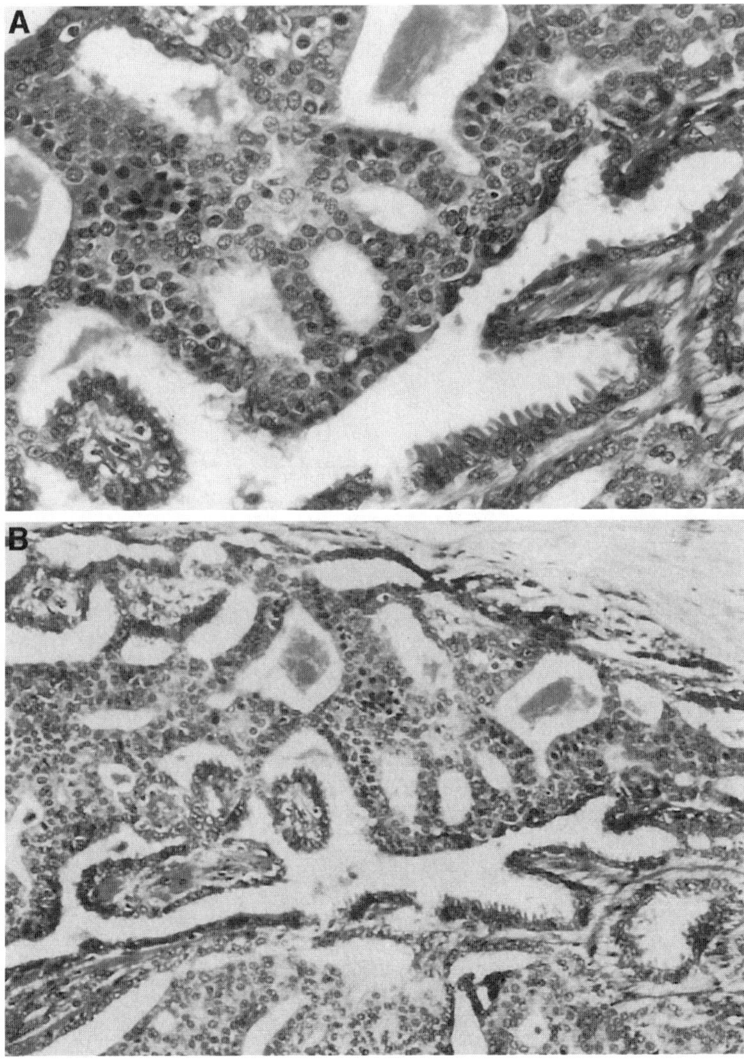

FIGURE 2.—**A,** high-power view of an area within a papilloma showing development of sharply defined spaces between a fairly evenly placed population of similar cells. This was about the full extent of this change and indicated atypical hyperplasia (AH) in this papilloma. **B,** low-power view of an area seen at high power in **A.** This view shows an encysted area with a papillary lesion inside. Note uniform population of proliferated cells with an even pattern of spaces between the cells defining AH, but confined to a small area (<3 mm). (Courtesy of Page DL, Salhany KE, Jensen RA, et al: Subsequent breast carcinoma risk after biopsy with atypia in a breast papilloma. *Cancer* 78:258–266. Copyright 1996, American Cancer Society. Reprinted by permission of Wiley-Liss, Inc, a subsidiary of John Wiley & Sons, Inc.)

invasive cancers occurred in the same breast as the papilloma, and most likely near the site of the papilloma. Risk of cancer was not increased for patients with ordinary patterns of epithelial hyperplasia, without specific evidence of AH within the papillomas.

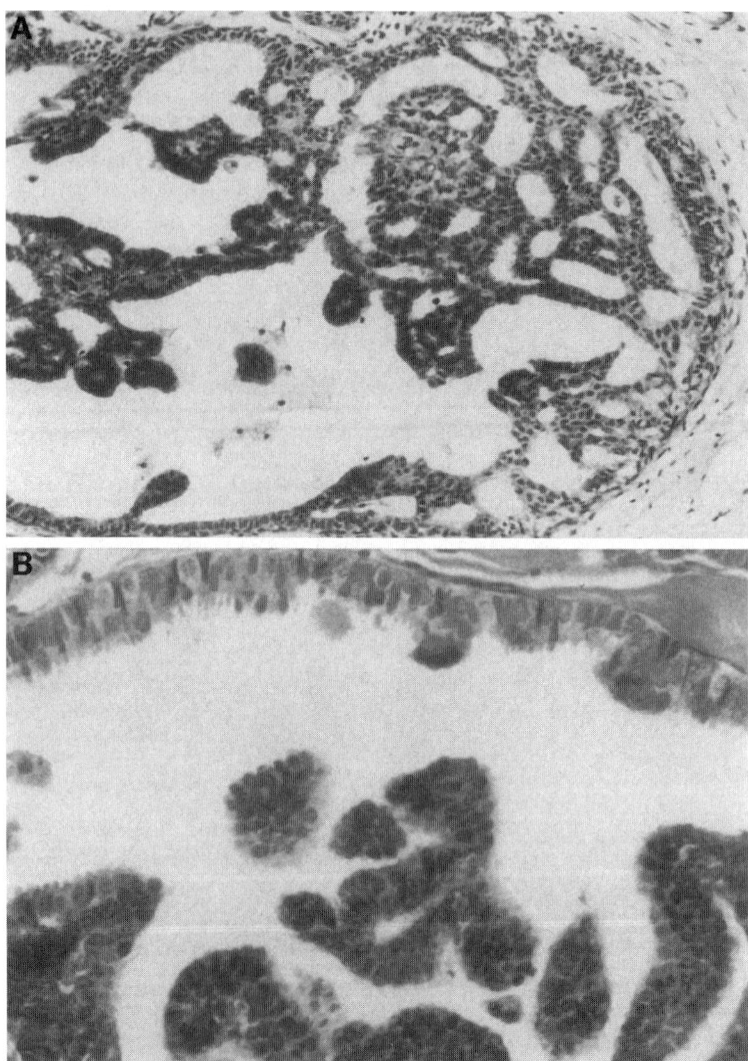

FIGURE 3.—These 2 photographs are from the histologically most atypical of all the cases. **A,** low-power view of most of the atypical area which is continuous with papilloma at left. Note there is a cribriform focus seen at low power and some micropapillae similar to micropapillary ductal carcinoma in situ seen in both the low power (**A**) and high power (**B**) pictures. **B,** high-power photograph of a micropapillary atypia in an adjacent area to that seen as lower power in **A.** (Courtesy of Page DL, Salhany KE, Jensen RA, et al: Subsequent breast carcinoma risk after biopsy with atypia in a breast papilloma. *Cancer* 78:258–266. Copyright 1996, American Cancer Society. Reprinted by permission of Wiley-Liss, Inc, a subsidiary of John Wiley & Sons, Inc.)

Conclusions.—The finding of AH within a breast papilloma is clinically significant, warranting close follow-up. The risk of cancer is 4-5 times higher than in women with other specifically defined patterns of AH within the breast parenchyma (Table 3). Surveillance should pay special attention

TABLE 3.—Relative Risk of Cancer in Women With Papillomas*

Patients	No AH	with AH	No FH	with FH	No AH or FH	No. other PD	With other PDWA
Micropapilloma	3.35†	4.40	3.42†	3.77	3.54†	1.90	4.42
95% CI	(1.94–5.77)	(1.10–17.58)	(1.98–5.88)	(0.94–15.06)	(2.01–6.23)	(0.60–5.74)	(2.38–8.21)
No. Dev. CA/at risk	13/154	2/14	13/46	2/22	12/134	3/59	10/95
Large papilloma	2.30‡	13.1†	3.06†	3.20	2.10	2.27	2.42
95% CI	(1.20–4.42)	(4.93–35)	(1.70–5.53)	(0.80–12.81)	(1–4.40)	(1.08–4.76)	(0.61–9.68)
No. Dev. CA/at risk	9/130	416	11/125	2/21	7/112	7/100	2/30

*Risks are derived relative to women from the Third National Cancer Survey in Atlanta and are adjusted for age at biopsy and length of follow-up.
†P value < 0.001.
‡Two of the 9 women in this group who developed invasive cancer had AH in the original papilloma. If they are removed, risk falls to about 1.8.
Abbreviations: no AH, no atypical hyperplasia in parenchyma surrounding papilloma; *FH*, history of breast carcinoma in at least 1 first-degree relative; *PD*, proliferative disease, *AH*, or any sclerosing adenosis or hyperplasia associated with cancer risk elevation; *PDWA*, PD without any atypical ductal or atypical lobular hyperplasia; *No. Dev. CA*, number of women developing invasive carcinoma in this group; *at risk*, number of women in this group at risk for developing cancer; *CI*, confidence interval.
(Courtesy of Page DL, Salhany KE, Jensen RA, et al: Subsequent breast carcinoma risk after biopsy with atypia in a breast papilloma. *Cancer* 78:258–266. Copyright 1996, American Cancer Society. Reprinted by permission of Wiley-Liss, Inc, a subsidiary of John Wiley & Sons, Inc.)

to the area within the breast in which AH is found. The findings to date do not warrant wider excision after local excision of papillomas with AH.

▶ Papillary proliferations of breast duct epithelium comprise a diverse group of lesions including papillomas, papillomas with atypia, intracystic papillary carcinomas, and papillary proliferations with varying degrees of infiltrating carcinoma. Interpretation of the more complex lesions is often difficult. These authors investigated the risk conveyed by papillary lesions for subsequent development of infiltrating breast carcinoma. Micropapillomas (3 mm or less) and large papillomas were considered separately and each lesion was categorized as being with or without AH, other proliferative lesions, or a family history of breast carcinoma. The data derived are the most useful yet published, because of the careful stratification of various clinical and pathologic conditions, and the use of up-to-date criteria and nomenclature that should be familiar to all readers. The illustrations are of good quality and will serve as a useful starting point for those wishing to think through this difficult problem. Taking criteria that we already use in breast pathology and applying them to this difficult group of lesions is very helpful. The fact that this paper gives the method considerable statistical justification and clinical relevance strengthens this approach considerably.

M.W. Stanley, M.D.

Suggested Reading

Dawson AE, Mulford DK: Benign versus malignant papillary neoplasms of the breast: Diagnostic clues in fine needle aspiration cytology. *Acta Cytol* 38:23–28, 1994.

Lefkowitz M, Lefkowitz W, Wargotz ES: Intraductal (intracystic) papillary carcinoma of the breast and its variants: A clinicopathological study of 77 cases. *Hum Pathol* 25:802–809, 1994.

Vimentin Expression Is Not Associated With Poor Prognosis in Breast Cancer
Seshadri R, Raymond WA, Leong AS-Y, et al (Flinders Univ, Bedford Park, Australia; Inst of Med and Veterinary Sciences, Adelaide, South Australia; South Australian Health Commission, Adelaide)
Int J Cancer 67:353–356, 1996   2–14

Background.—Several pathologic, molecular, and clinical features of primary breast cancer have been studied in the past decade to identify useful prognostic parameters. Vimentin appears to be expressed mainly in hormone receptor-negative, high-grade carcinomas. Thus, vimentin expression may be an indicator of poor prognosis. The clinical significance of this variable in relation to established clinical and pathologic parameters of prognosis in primary breast cancer was investigated.

Methods.—Archival tumor samples from 360 women with primary breast cancer were examined. Samples were embedded in paraffin and analyzed using immunohistochemistry with monoclonal antibodies to vimentin intermediate filament (VIF), p53 protein, and cell proliferation marker MIB-1.

Findings.—The vimentin staining pattern was heterogeneous. However, in vimentin-positive areas, more than 80% of the tumor cells were positive. Vimentin expression was unassociated with tumor size or the number of axillary lymph nodes involved. Significant associations were documented between vimentin expression and high-grade tumors, absence of hormone receptors, increased p53 expression, and high tumor proliferation fraction as estimated by MIB-1 count. However, vimentin expression was not correlated with increases in the risk of relapse or death as a result of breast cancer.

Conclusions.—In this large series, vimentin expression was not associated with an increased risk of relapse or death as a result of breast cancer. Vimentin expression is an epiphenomenon associated with hormone receptor-negative tumors that has no prognostic significance.

▶ This is investigative biology at its most frustrating. Just because A (vimentin expression) is associated with B (high grade, absence of hormone receptors, increased p53 expression, and high tumor cell proliferative fraction) and B is associated with C (tumor aggressiveness), one cannot conclude that A is associated with C. The problem is too complex, and the measurable factors are too interrelated for the methods available. The authors point out that earlier (and smaller) studies found conflicting results. The interpretation of the data is complicated by the fact that the range or mean of the follow-up duration is never clearly stated.

M.W. Stanley, M.D.

Ductal Carcinoma In Situ of the Male Breast: Analysis of 31 Cases
Cutuli B, Dilhuydy JM, De Lafontan B, et al (Centre Paul Strauss, Strasbourg, France; Institut Bergonifé, Bordeaux, France; Centre Claudius Regard, Toulouse, France; et al)
Eur J Cancer 33:35–38, 1997   2–15

Background.—Because of its rarity, ductal carcinoma in situ (DCIS) in men is not well defined. The clinicohistologic features of DCIS in the largest series of men reported to date were described.

Methods and Findings.—Thirty-one men with DCIS of the breast treated at 19 French regional cancer centers between 1970 and 1992 were included in the analysis. These patients comprised 5% of all men with breast cancer treated in that period. The median age was 58 years, and 6 men were younger than 40 years. Twelve lesions were classified as T0, 10 were classified as T1, and 5 were classified as T2. Four were unclassified. Clinical gynecomastia was present in 35.5% of the patients. Ten percent had family histories of breast cancer. Mastectomies were performed in 25 men, and lumpectomies were performed in 6. Nineteen underwent axillary dissection. Radiation therapy was administered postoperatively in 6. Overall, 15 lesions were of the papillary subtype—pure or associated with a cribriform component. The 12 lesions measured ranged in size from 3 to 45 mm. All sampled lymph nodes were negative. At a median follow-up of 83 months, local relapse occurred in 13% (between 12 and 55 months). Three of the 4 patients with local relapses had been treated with lumpectomies. In 1 patient, the recurring lesion was still in situ; in the other 3, it was invasive. Radical salvage surgery was performed in 3 patients who had relapses. However, metastases developed in 1 patient who died 30 months later. In another patient, aged 43 years, a contralateral tumor developed. A metachronous cancer developed in 3 other men.

Conclusions.—Although the etiology and risk factors of male breast cancer remain unknown, gynecomastia may be a predisposing factor. The prognosis of DCIS in men is good, as it is in women. Basic treatment consists of a total mastectomy without axillary dissection. In many patients, the first symptom is bloody discharge from the nipple. The age of DCIS occurence in men is younger than it is for infiltrating carcinoma, which suggests that it is the first step in breast cancer development.

▶ Male intraductal breast cancer is rare, even among carcinomas of this organ in men, often is seen with a bloody nipple discharge, and is associated with a good prognosis. The preferred treatment is a total mastectomy without either axillary dissection or adjuvant treatment. This can be modified for those lesions with a high risk of microinvasion, including masses larger than 2.5 cm and comedo carcinoma. Interestingly, a history of gynecomastia was noted in 36% of 31 cases; this is higher than in previous reports.

M.W. Stanley, M.D.

Suggested Reading

Salvadori B, Saccozzi R, Manzari A, et al: Prognosis of breast cancer in males: An analysis of 170 cases. *Eur J Cancer* 30A:930–935, 1994.

3 Female Genital Tract

Papillary Apocrine Fibroadenoma of the Vulva
Higgins CM, Strutton GM (Princess Alexandra Hosp, Brisbane, Australia)
J Cutan Pathol 23:256–260, 1997   3–1

Background.—Isolated reports of a group of unusual tumors of the vulva and perineum have appeared in the literature. These tumors are morphologically distinct from hidradenoma papilliferum but also show apocrine differentiation. An unusual tumor of the vulva that apparently belongs in this group was described and the current literature reviewed.

Case Report.—Woman, 37, had a 10-year history of a gradually growing, painless, nontender subcutaneous mass in the left labium majus. Before presentation, the mass became painful, and the covering skin had split with protrusion of the underlying lesion. After the tumor was removed, the patient did well with no recurrences.

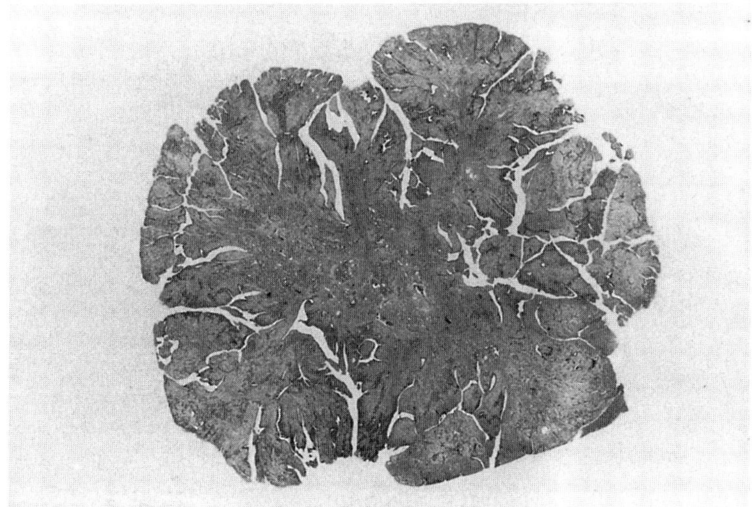

FIGURE 2.—Transverse section through tumor; hematoxylin-eosin; original magnification, ×2. (Courtesy of Higgins CM, Strutton GM: Papillary apocrine fibroadenoma of the vulva. *J Cutan Pathol* 24:256–260, copyright 1997, Munksgaard International Publishers Ltd., Copenhagen, Denmark.)

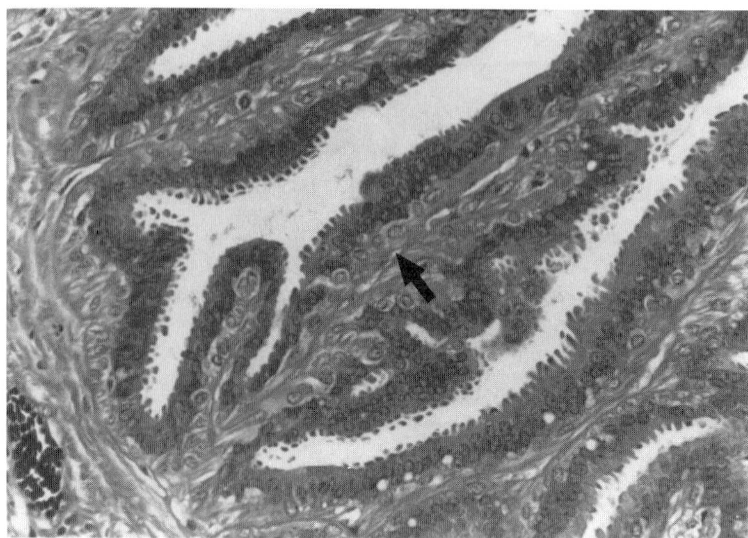

FIGURE 3.—Surface of tumor with external layer showing decapitation secretion and underlying myoepithelial layer (*arrow*); hematoxylin-eosin; original magnification, ×280. (Courtesy of Higgins CM, Strutton GM: Papillary apocrine fibroadenoma of the vulva. *J Cutan Pathol* 24:256–260. Copyright 1997, Munksgaard International Publishers, Ltd., Copenhagen, Denmark.)

Histopathologic Findings.—Histopathologic examination revealed smooth-surfaced, broad papillae with multiple infoldings (Fig 2). The cell shapes varied from spindled to almost cuboidal (Fig 3). Duct structures with a double lining were found to be scattered throughout the stroma. In

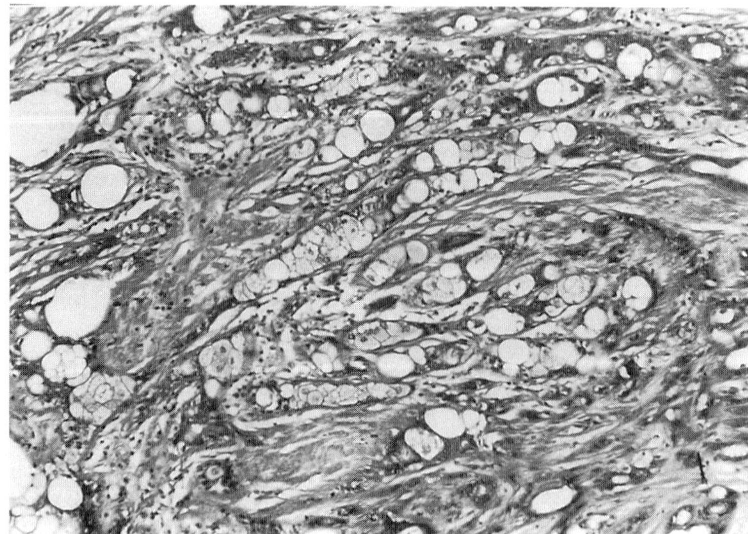

FIGURE 7.—Focus of ducts with sebaceous differentiation; hematoxylin-eosin; original magnification, ×110. (Courtesy of Higgins CM, Strutton GM: Papillary apocrine fibroadenoma of the vulva. *J Cutan Pathol* 24:256–260. Copyright 1997, Munksgaard International Publishers, Ltd., Copenhagen, Denmark.)

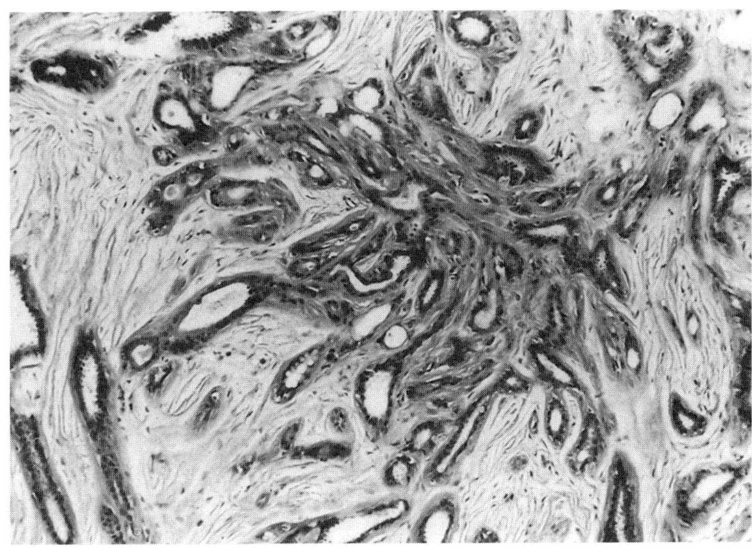

FIGURE 8.—Focus of ducts with sclerosing adenosis-like change with spindled myoepithelial cells; hematoxylin-eosin; original magnification, ×110. (Courtesy of Higgins CM, Strutton GM: Papillary apocrine fibroadenoma of the vulva. *J Cutan Pathol* 24:256–260. Copyright 1997, Munksgaard International Publishers, Ltd., Copenhagen, Denmark.)

1 region, the ducts merged with solid structures consisting of cells with sebaceous differentiation (Fig 7). Foci with closely packed, distorted oval ducts with peripheral spindle cells with eosinophilic cytoplasm were observed beneath the surface layer and within the stroma (Fig 8).

Discussion.—This unusual papillary tumor of the vulva exhibited apocrine features, some areas resembling sclerosing adenosis of the breast, displaying mucinous and sebaceous differentiation. The literature includes reports on a small number of similar lesions of the vulva, many of which have been classified as ectopic breast tissue tumors. In the absence of associated normal breast lobules, these lesions cannot be differentiated from those arising from apocrine sweat glands. This papillary apocrine fibroadenoma may be a distinct cutaneous tumor at this site.

▶ This case illustrates the "Istanbul phenomenon." It is not difficult for us to recognize our neighbor when we see him every day on the other side of our driveway. However, if we see him in a crowd during a trip to a foreign country, we have a hard time accepting the fact that we know that person. A diagnosis of fibroadenoma of the breast is an easy task for a first-year pathology resident. The same diagnosis for a vulvar lesion would probably cause frenetic intradepartmental (if not interdepartmental) consultation activity.

K.E. Sirgi, M.D.

Nodular Fasciitis of the Vulva: A Study of Six Cases and Literature Review

O'Connell JX, Young RH, Nielsen GP, et al (Vancouver Hosp and Health Sciences Ctr, BC; Massachusetts Gen Hosp, Boston; British Columbia Cancer Agency, Vancouver)
Int J Gynecol Pathol 16:117–123, 1997

3–2

Background.—Nodular fasciitis (NF), the most common of a group of reactive mesenchymal proliferations mimicking a variety of benign and malignant soft-tissue tumors, occurs most often in the subcutaneous tissue of the extremities and trunk. Few cases of NF involving the vulva have been reported. Six new patients with this disease and a review of the literature were presented.

Patients and Findings.—The patients, aged 7 to 51 years, were initially seen with a vulvar tissue mass. In the 5 consultation cases, the diagnosis of NF had not been considered. In the 4 patients in whom a specific site was noted, the tumor was confined to the labia. The maximal dimension of the masses ranged from 1.5 to 3.5 cm. All were locally excised. The resection margins were involved in all cases. Typical NF features were observed. In

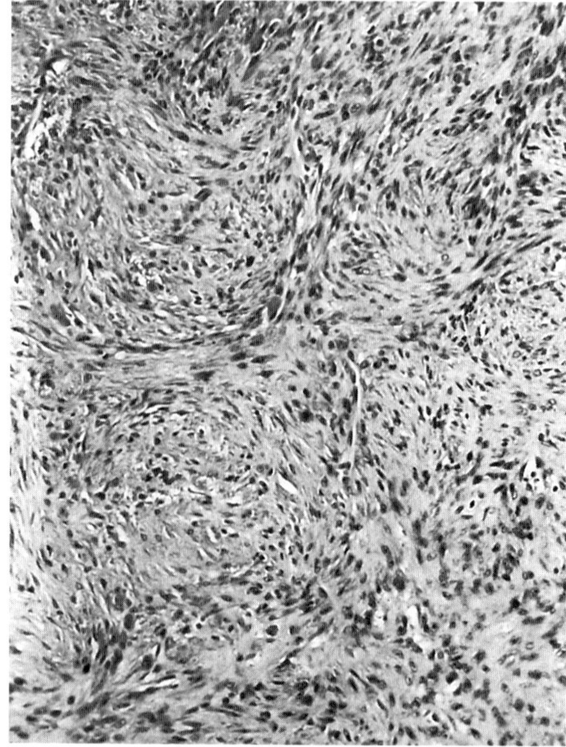

FIGURE 3.—Prominent storiform pattern. (Courtesy of O'Connell JX, Young RH, Nielsen GP, et al: Nodular fasciitis of the vulva: A study of six cases and literature review. *Int J Gynecol Pathol* 16:117–123, 1997.)

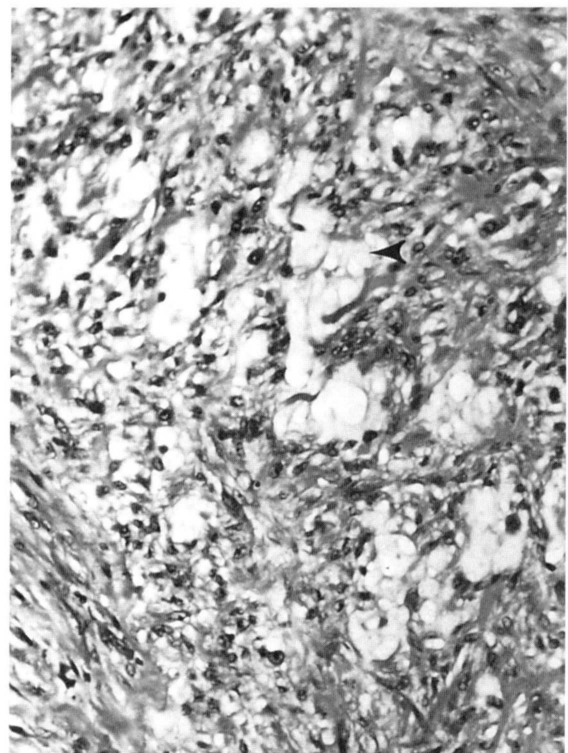

FIGURE 8.—Microscopic stromal mucin-filles "cysts" (*arrowhead*). (Courtesy of O'Connell JX, Young RH, Nielsen GP, et al: Nodular fasciitis of the vulva: A study of six cases and literature review. *Int J Gynecol Pathol* 16:117–123, 1997.)

addition, cleftlike spaces lined by pump synovial-like cells were noted in 2 cases. At a mean 24-month follow-up, 5 patients were free of recurrence. The sixth patient had a recurrence at 4 months and underwent re-excision (Figs 3 and 8; Table 1).

Discussion.—The lesion most closely resembling vulvar NF is the postoperative spindle cell nodule, a rapidly growing mass that develops within weeks to months of a surgical procedure at that site. Also resembling vulvar NF is aggressive angiomyxoma, a neoplasm of myofibroblastic cells that often involves the perineal soft tissue; it occurs most often in women of reproductive age. However, aggressive angiomyxomas are usually larger than 5 cm, unlike NFs. Angiomyofibroblastoma of the vulva also affects the age group affected by vulvar NF, is usually small, and seems to have a predilection for the labial soft tissue. However, angiomyofibroblastoma is usually well circumscribed and is composed of alternating hypocellular and hypercellular regions made up of spindled, plasmacytoid, and epithelioid cells embedded in a variably myxoid or collagenous ground substance. To facilitate the diagnosis of NF, pathologists need to be aware that NF may occur in the vulva and have features that distinguish it from other mesenchymal lesions at this site.

TABLE 1.—Clinical and Pathologic Information From Cases of Vulvar Nodular Fasciitis

Case	Age (yr)	Site	Size (cm)	Signs and symptoms	Favored initial diagnosis	Follow-up
1	31	Left labium majus	3.5	Painful mass ? duration	Atypical leiomyoma	Recurrence 4/12 after incomplete excision. Reexcision, NED at 6/12
2	51	Vulva NOS	2.2	Painless mass 1/12	Nodular fasciitis	NED at 3/12
3	38	Right labium majus	1.5	Painless mass 3/12	? Angiomyofibro-blastoma	NED at 2 yr
4	7	Vulva NOS	2.5	Painless mass ? duration	Rhabdomyosarcoma	NED at 7 yr
5	33	Labium minus	1.5	Painful mass ? duration	Neurofibroma	NED at 10/12
6	43	Left labium majus	2.0	Painful mass 2/12	Fibroma vs aggressive angiomyxoma	NED at 15/12
Previously reported cases (reference)						
1 (2)	NA	Labium majus	NA	NA	NA	NA
2 (4)	19	Right labium minus	2.5	Painless mass	Leiomyosarcoma	Reexcision of area, NED at 2 yr
3 (5)	32	Right labium	3.0	Painless mass 61/2	Nodular fasciitis	Reexcision of area, NED at 6/12
4 (6)	15	Left labium majus	2.5	Painless mass 3/12	Nodular fasciitis	NED at 1 yr
5 (6)	18	Right labium	3.0	Painless mass 6/52	Low-grade sarcoma	NED at 6/12

Abbreviations: NOS, not otherwise specified; *NA*, not available; *NED*, no evidence of disease.
(Courtesy of O'Connell JX, Young RH, Nielsen GP, et al: Nodular fasciitis of the vulva: A study of six cases and literature review. *Int J Gynecol Pathol* 16:117–123, 1997.)

Smooth-Muscle Tumors of the Vulva: A Clinicopathological Study of 25 Cases and Review of the Literature
Nielsen GP, Rosenberg AE, Koerner FC, et al (Harvard Med School, Boston; Massachusetts Gen Hosp, Boston)
Am J Surg Pathol 20:779–793, 1996   3–3

Background.—Smooth-muscle tumors of the vulva are much less common than those of the uterus. A clinicopathologic study of 25 patients with smooth-muscle tumors of the vulva was reported.

Patients and Findings.—The patients ranged in age from 17 to 67 years, and 2 were pregnant. Tumor diameters ranged from 1.5 to 16 cm, with a mean of 5.2 cm. Sixteen tumors were circumscribed, and 6 had focally infiltrative margins. Fourteen tumors consisted primarily of spindle cells; 2 of them had prominent myxoid stroma. Seven tumors were primarily epithelioid, with a prominent hyalinized or myxoid stroma. The cells often had a plexiform pattern. In 4 tumors, there were about equal numbers of epithelioid and spindle cells. Cytologic atypia was mild in 10 tumors, moderate in 9, and severe in 6. All tumors stained for at least 1 muscle marker. Thirteen of 17 tumors were positive for estrogen receptors, and 16 of 18 for progesterone receptors. Four tumors recurred locally during 1 to 19 months of follow-up. One patient with recurrent tumor died of metastases 7 months after initial surgery (Figs 3, 4, 6, and 7).

Discussion.—Expanded criteria are proposed to distinguish between vulvar leiomyomas and leiomyosarcomas. Tumors with 3 or more of the following characteristics should be classified as sarcomas: a greatest dimension of 5 cm or more, infiltrative margins, 5 or more mitotic figures per 10 HPF, and moderate-to-severe cytologic atypia. Tumors with only 1 of these features should be diagnosed as leiomyoma, and those with only 2 as benign but atypical leiomyoma. Sarcomas should be excised with wide negative margins. Conservative treatment is indicated for leiomyomas and atypical leiomyomas, with careful, long-term follow-up.

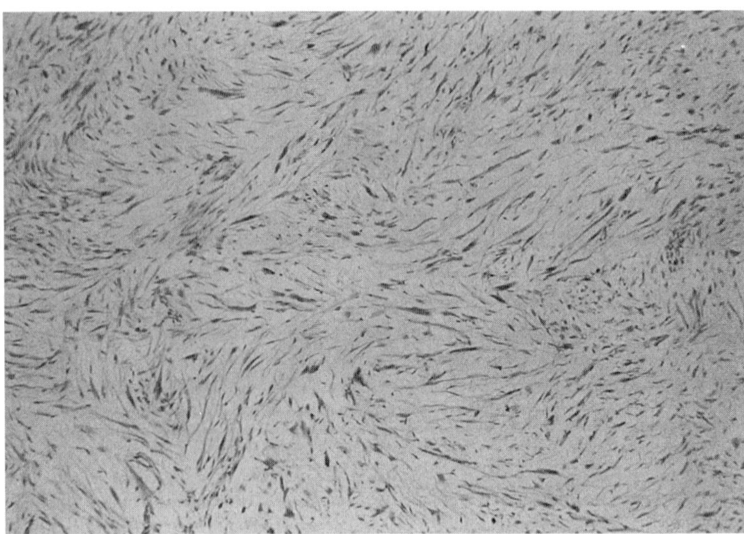

FIGURE 3.—Abundant myxoid stroma separating spindle cells in an atypical leiomyoma. (Courtesy of Nielsen GP, Rosenberg AE, Koerner FC, et al: Smooth-muscle tumors of the vulva: A clinicopathological study of 25 cases and review of the literature. *Am J Surg Pathol* 20:779–793, 1996.)

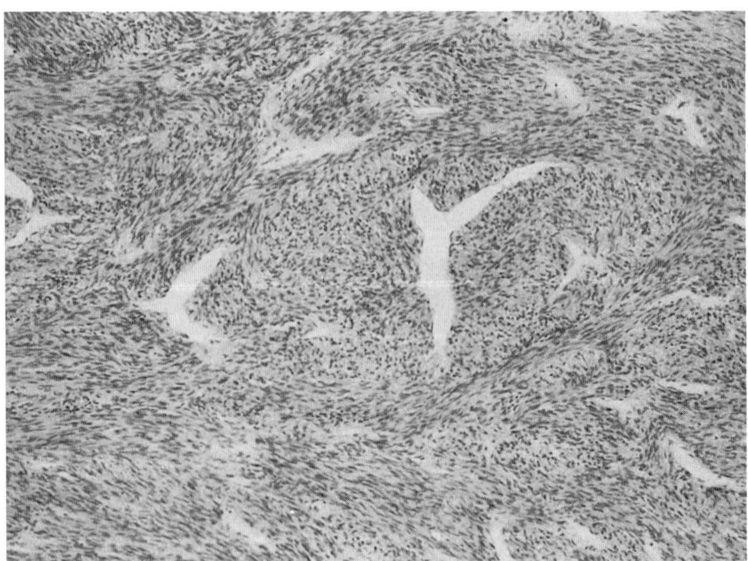

FIGURE 4.—Hemangiopericytoma-like pattern was present in 1 tumor. (Courtesy of Nielsen GP, Rosenberg AE, Koerner FC, et al: Smooth-muscle tumors of the vulva: A clinicopathological study of 25 cases and review of the literature. *Am J Surg Pathol* 20:779–793, 1996.)

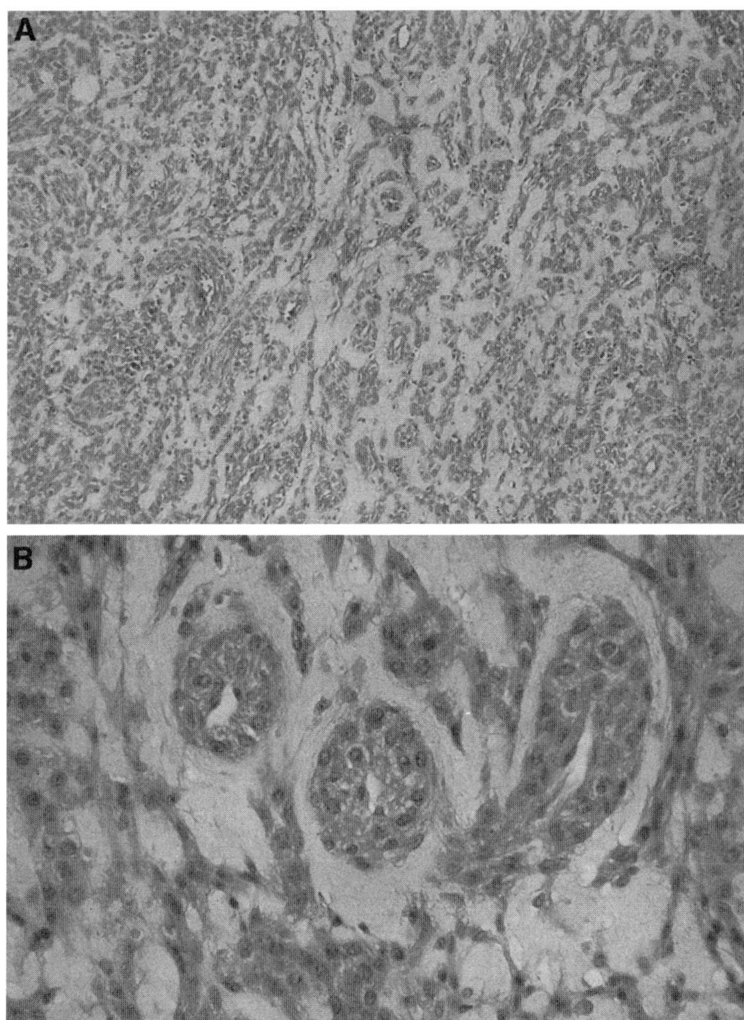

FIGURE 6.—Epithelioid leiomyoma with a plexiform growth pattern, stromal hyalinization, and tumor cells forming perivascular collarettes. (Courtesy of Nielsen GP, Rosenberg AE, Koerner FC, et al: Smooth-muscle tumors of the vulva: A clinicopathological study of 25 cases and review of the literature. *Am J Surg Pathol* 20:779–793, 1996.)

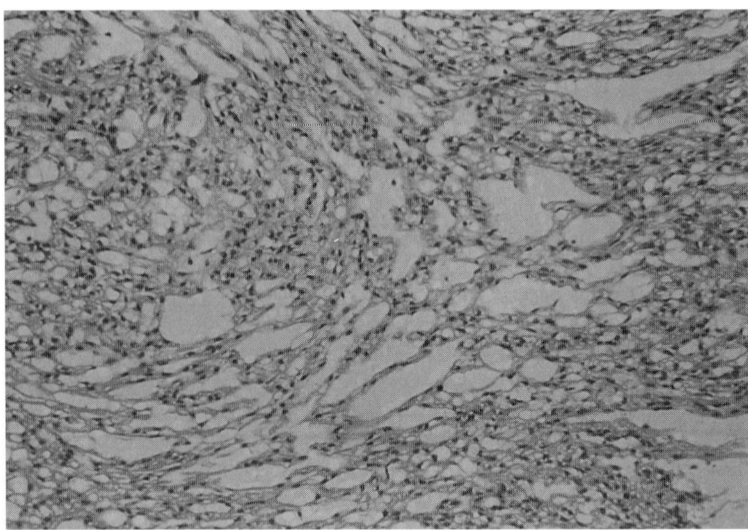

FIGURE 7.—Abundant extracellular mucin in an epithelioid leiomyoma. (Courtesy of Nielsen GP, Rosenberg AE, Koerner FC, et al: Smooth muscle tumors of the vulva: A clinicopathological study of 25 cases and review of the literature. *Am J Surg Pathol* 20:779–793, 1996.)

Aggressive Angiomyxoma: A Clinicopathologic Study of 29 Female Patients

Fetsch JF, Laskin WB, Lefkowitz M, et al (Armed Forces Inst of Pathology, Washington, DC; Natl Naval Med Ctr, Bethesda, Md; Gothenburg Univ, Sweden)
Cancer 78:79–90, 1996   3–4

Background.—Aggressive angiomyxoma, an uncommon mesenchymal tumor preferentially affecting the female pelvic and perineal regions, was initially described in 1983. Since then, about 65 patients have been reported in the English-language literature. A clinicopathologic study of 29 patients was presented.

Patients and Findings.—The patients were identified from the Armed Forces Institute of Pathology between 1960 and 1992 and were aged 16 to 70 years. Tumor affected the soft tissues of the pelvis, perineum, vulva, buttock, retroperitoneum, and inguinal areas. Most lesions were 10 cm or more in greatest dimension. Follow-up data for 22 patients were available, the follow-ups ranging from 8 to 198 months. Ten months to 7 years after the initial resection, 8 patients had recurrences.

Histologic assessment showed neoplasms sparsely to moderately cellular and mostly composed of bland, relatively nondescript, stellate and spindled cells embedded in a loosely collagenized matrix with scattered vessels of varied caliber. A few tumors contained cells with more abundant eosinophilic cytoplasm, suggesting focal smooth muscle differentiation. The tumor matrix was only weakly reactive for mucosubstances. Edema fluid

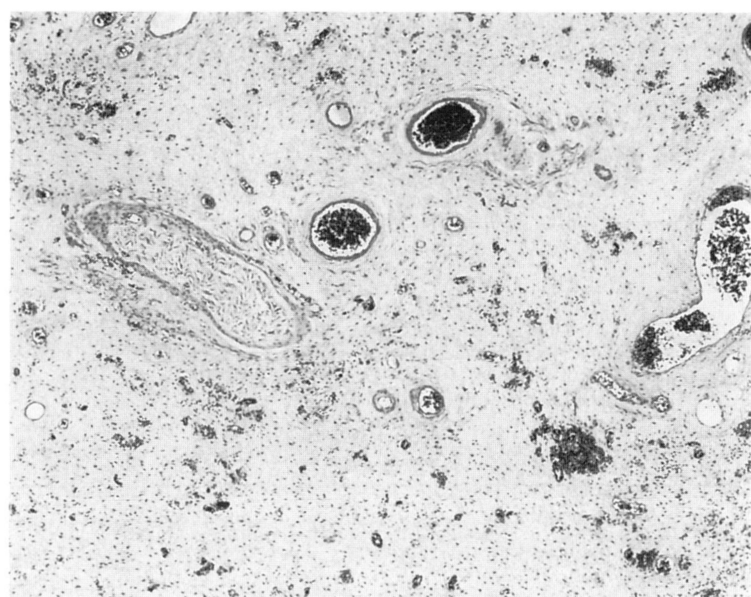

FIGURE 2.—Low power photomicrograph of aggressive angiomyxoma demonstrating a relatively uniform population of small mesenchymal cells, mature vessels of varying caliber, and the entrapment of a medium-sized nerve segment. (Courtesy of Fetsch JF, Laskin WB, Lefkowitz M, et al: Aggressive angiomyxoma: A clinicopathologic study of 29 female patients. *Cancer* 78:79–90. Copyright 1996, American Cancer Society. Reprinted by permission of Wiley-Liss, Inc., a subsidiary of John Wiley & Sons, Inc.)

appeared to be a major component of the noncollagenous stroma. In most tumors, neoplastic cells were at least focally immunoreactive for desmin, smooth muscle actin, muscle-specific actin, vimentin, CD34/QBEND-10, and estrogen and progesterone receptors. All tumors examined were negative for S100 protein. Less than 1% of the 16 tumors tested showed Ki67 immunoreactivity (Figs 2 and 3).

Conclusion.—Aggressive angiomyxoma is a distinctive, locally aggressive mesenchymal tumor that seems to be relatively site specific. In female patients, its incidence peaks in the fourth decade of life. This entity had a strong propensity for local recurrence, although metastatic disease has not been described. Long-term follow-up is necessary, as the first evidence of recurrence may be many years after the initial resection. The neoplastic cells of the tumor display fibroblastic and myofibroblastic features and seem to be affected by hormones. The progenitor cell may have a capacity for smooth-muscle differentiation.

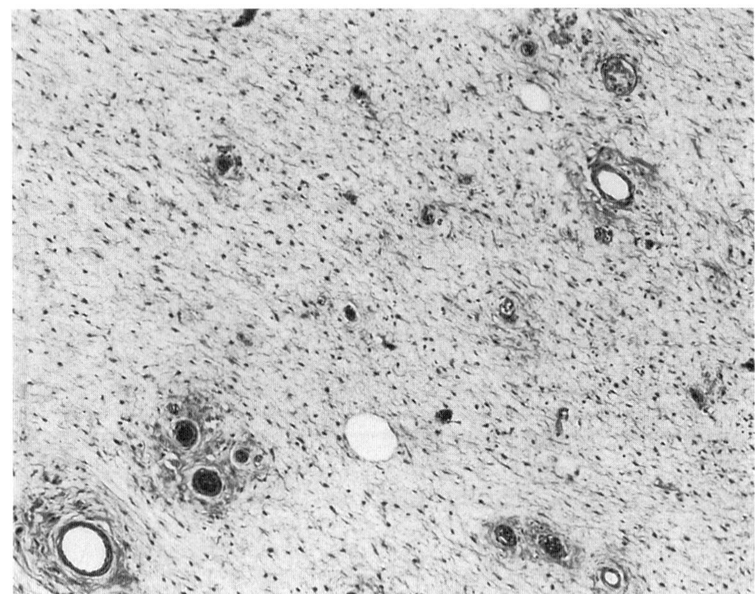

FIGURE 3.—Low power photomicrograph demonstrating cellular uniformity in aggressive angiomyxoma. (Courtesy of Fetsch JF, Laskin WB, Lefkowitz M, et al: Aggressive angiomyxoma: A clinicopathologic study of 29 female patients. *Cancer* 78:79–90. Copyright 1996, American Cancer Society. Reprinted by permission of Wiley-Liss, Inc., a subsidiary of John Wiley & Sons, Inc.)

Vulval Angiomyofibroblastoma: Clinicopathologic Analysis of Six Cases

Fukunaga M, Nomura K, Matsumoto K, et al (Jikei Univ, Toyko; Natl Hirosaki Hosp, Aomori, Japan; Yoshida Gen Hosp, Hiroshima, Japan)

Am J Clin Pathol 107:45–51, 1997

3–5

Background.—Angiomyofibroblastoma (AMFB) of the vulva is a rare neoplasm often clinically diagnosed as a Bartholin's gland cyst and pathologically as aggressive angiomyxoma. The entity is a well-circumscribed tumor that usually arises in the superficial soft tissues of the vulva. The findings of 6 vulvar AMFBs assessed by immunohistochemical, ultrastructural, and flow cytometric analysis were reported.

Patients and Findings.—The patients were 6 women aged 32 to 46 years. The tumors were found to be well circumscribed, ranging from 2 to 9 cm in greatest dimension. Five were diagnosed clinically as Bartholin's gland cysts. Histologically, the lesions were seen to have altering hypercellular and hypocellular edematous regions with abundant blood vessels. The hypercellular regions showed a perivascular proliferation of spindle-shaped and round cells, frequently forming small nests or epithelioid arrangements and a short, fascicular spindle cell pattern. The proliferating vessels were capillary sized with thin walls. No cellular atypia or mitotic figures were observed. An adipose element was noted in 2 tumors, 1 showing a prominent vascular proliferation reminiscent of a capillary

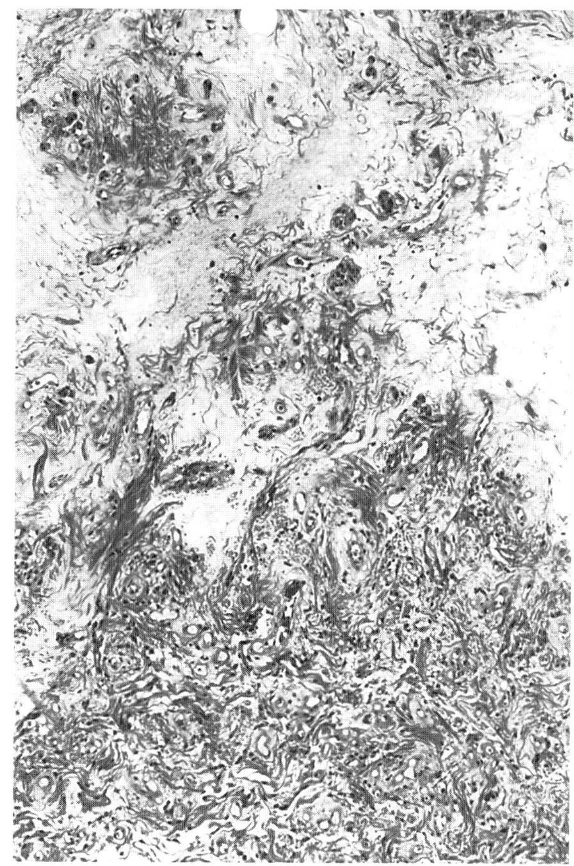

FIGURE 1.—Tumor is characterized by alternating hypercellular and hypocellular edematous areas; hematoxylin-eosin; original magnification, ×100. (Courtesy of Fukunaga M, Nomura K, Matsumoto K, et al: Vulval angiomyofibroblastoma: Clinicopathologic analysis of six cases. *Am J Clin Pathol* 107:45–51, 1997.)

hemangioma. Immunohistochemically, tumor cells were strongly positive for vimentin and desmin, with some weakly positive for HH35 and α–smooth muscle actin. Ultrastructural analysis showed fibroblastic differentiation in 1 neoplasm. Three tumors were DNA diploid and 2 were aneuploid. After excision, none of the tumors recurred (Fig 1).

Conclusion.—These tumors fulfilled the histologic criteria of AMFB as initially described. Epithelioid arrangement of round or spindle-shaped cells was one of the most characteristic histologic findings. The presence of capillary hemangioma-like blood vessel proliferation and an adipose component were also noted.

Genital Angiomyofibroblastoma: Comparison With Aggressive Angiomyxoma and Other Myxoid Neoplasms of the Skin and Soft Tissue

Ockner DM, Sayadi H, Swanson PE, et al (Washington Univ, St Louis)
Am J Clin Pathol 107:36–44, 1997

3–6

Background.—Angiomyofibroblastoma (AMFB), a recently described tumor involving the vulvar soft tissue of young–to–middle-aged women, may mimic aggressive angiomyxoma. Fewer than 40 case reports of AMFB have been published.

Methods and Findings.—Three patients with AMFB were compared with 10 patients with aggressive angiomyxoma and 28 patients with other myxoid tumors with possible morphologic similarities to AMFBs. Examination showed that AMFBs were circumscribed, partially myxoid proliferations with marked variation in cellular density. Cytologically, the neoplastic elements of this entity were bland. Both fusiform and epithelioid profiles were noted, with a tendency to concentrate around intralesional blood vessels. There was no mitotic activity nor necrosis. The vessels had an arborizing configuration and were venule or capillary sized. By contrast, the other tumor types assessed were infiltrative and/or cytologically atypical. Immunoreactivity for vimentin, desmin, actin, and estrogen receptor protein was noted in all AMFBs and most aggressive angiomyxomas and smooth-muscle tumors but not in any other neoplasm studied. Electron microscopic examination showed myofibroblastic differentiation in the AMFB cells (Table 3).

Conclusion.—Conventional morphologic study is essential for recognizing genital AMFB. Immunohistology may also be useful for excluding other differential diagnoses. The data also indicate that AMFB, aggressive angiomyxomas, and superficial smooth-muscle tumors have similar morphotypes and immunohistologic attributes, irrespective of their origin.

TABLE 3.—Differential Diagnostic Findings in Neoplasms of the External Genitalia

Tumor	CC	CA	CK	VIM	DES	ACT*	S100	CD34	CD57	ERP
Angiomyofibroblastoma	+	0	0	+	±	±	0	0	0	±
Myxofibroid polyp	+	±	0	+	0	0	0	±	0	0
Aggressive angiomyxoma	0	0	0	+	±	±	0	0	0	±
Myxoid leiomyoma	+	0	0	+	±	±	0	0	0	±
Myxoid leiomyosarcoma	0	+	0	+	±	±	0	±	±	±
Benign peripheral nerve sheath tumors	+	±†	0	+	0	0	±	±	±	0
Malignant peripheral nerve sheath tumors	0	+	0‡	+	0‡	0‡	±	±	±	0
Myxoid liposarcoma	0	+	0	+	0	0	+§	0	0	0
Posttraumatic spindle cell nodule or nodular fasciitis	±	0	±	+	±	±	0	0	0	0
Paratesticular myxoma	+	0	0	+	0	0	0	0	0	0
Myxoid dermatofibrosarcoma protuberans	0	±	0	+	0	0	0	+	0	0
Myxoid malignant fibrous histiocytoma or myxofibrosarcoma	0	+	0	+	0	0	0	0	0	0
Myxoid melanoma	0	+	0	+	0	0	+	0	±	0
Myxoid sarcomatoid carcinoma	0	+	+	±	0‖	0‖	0	0‖	0	0

*Includes both muscle specific and α-isoform actin.
†So-called ancient neurilemoma may show focal cytologic atypia in the absence of mitotic activity.
‡Malignant nerve sheath tumors may rarely demonstrate aberrant reactivity for keratin, desmin, and actin.
§Univacuolated lipoblasts are positive only for S100 protein in myxoid liposarcoma.
‖Rare examples of sarcomatoid carcinoma may display aberrant reactivity for desmin, actin, and CD34.
Abreviations: CC, circumscribed; CA, cytologic atypia; CK, cytokeratin; VIM, vimentin; DES, desmin; ACT, actin; S100, S100 protein; ERP, estrogen receptor protein.
(Courtesy of Ockner DM, Sayadi H, Swanson PE, et al: Genital angiomyofibroblastoma: Comparison with aggressive angiomyxoma and other myxoid neoplasms of the skin and soft tissue. *Am J Clin Pathol* 107:36–44, 1997.)

Cellular Angiofibroma: A Benign Neoplasm Distinct From Angiomyofibroblastoma and Spindle Cell Lipoma

Nucci MR, Granter SR, Fletcher CDM (Brigham and Women's Hosp, Boston)
Am J Surg Pathol 21:636–644, 1997   3–7

Background.—Some mesenchymal tumors of the vulva cannot be easily classified as aggressive angiomyxoma or angiomyofibroblastoma (AMFB). Four cases of a distinctive benign soft-tissue tumor of the vulva were described. They had histologic features similar to those of spindle cell lipoma and could be mistaken for aggressive angiomyxoma or AMFB.

Methods and Findings.—The 4 patients were 39 to 50 years of age. Preoperatively, the clinical diagnosis was a labial or Bartholin gland cyst in

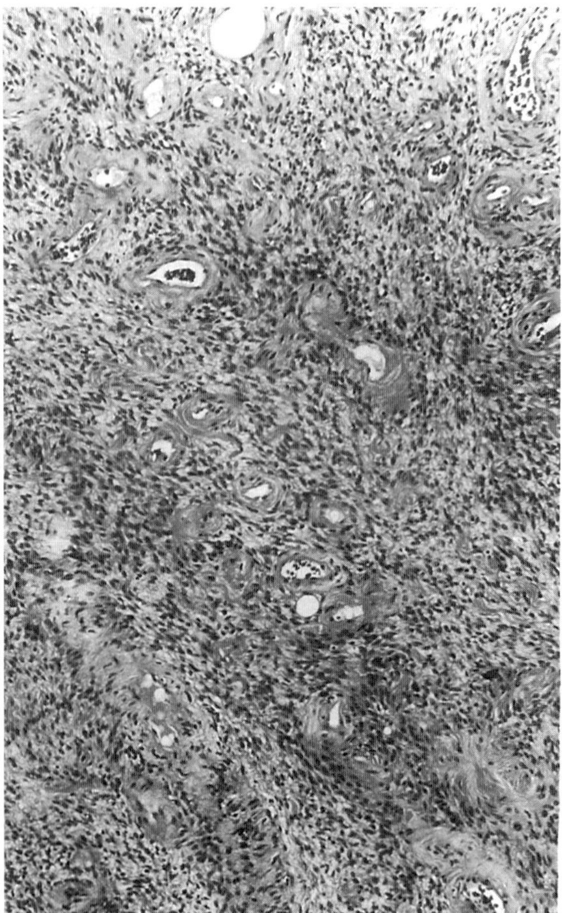

FIGURE 2.—Typical medium power appearance shows a cellular spindle cell component and small vessels with hyaline walls. (Courtesy of Nucci MR, Granter SR, Fletcher CDM: Cellular angiofibroma: A benign neoplasm distinct from angiomyofibroblastoma and spindle cell lipoma. *Am J Surg Pathol* 21:636–644, 1997.)

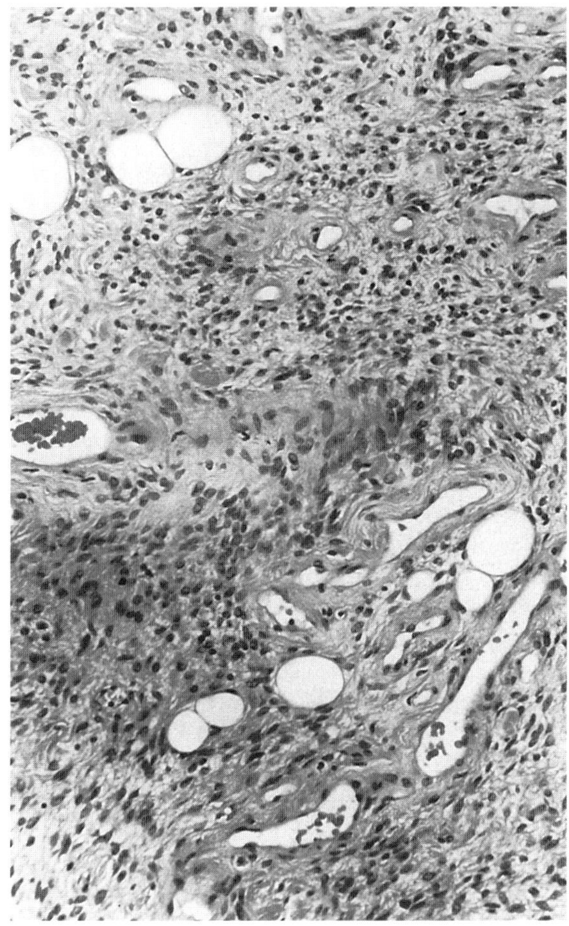

FIGURE 3.—Sparsely distributed adipocytes were present in each tumor. (Courtesy of Nucci MR, Granter SR, Fletcher CDM: Cellular angiofibroma: A benign neoplasm distinct from angiomyofibroblastoma and spindle cell lipoma. *Am J Surg Pathol* 21:636–644, 1997.)

3 patients. The tumors were smaller than 3 cm and usually well circumscribed. Microscopically, the appearance of these tumors was remarkably consistent and was characterized by a cellular neoplasm composed of uniform, bland, spindled stromal cells; many thick-walled and often hyalinized vessels; and a scarce component of mature adipocytes. In 3 tumors, mitotic activity was brisk. The stromal cells were positive for vimentin and negative for CD34, S-100 protein, actin, desmin, and epithelial membrane antigen, which suggested fibroblastic differentiation. In the 2 patients followed up, there was no evidence of recurrence (Figs 2 and 3; Table 3).

Conclusion.—This tumor is a unique, previously undescribed entity. The term "cellular angiofibroma" is proposed to emphasize the cellular spindle

TABLE 3.—Comparison of Cellular Angiofibroma With Angiofibroblastoma and Aggressive Angiomyxoma

	Cellular angiofibroma	Angiomyofibroblastoma	Aggressive angiomyxoma
Clinical features			
Age (yr)	39–50 (median 47.5)	23–71 (mean 42)	16–70 (mean 36)
Sex	F > M	F > M	F > M
Presentation	Vulval/pelvic mass	Vulval/pelvic mass	Vulval/pelvic mass
Duration of symptoms	4–18 mo	2 wk–8 yr	Usually a few months, can be years
Size of lesion	1.2–2.5 cm	0.5–12 cm (usually <5 cm)	3–60 cm (usually >5 cm)
Behavior	NSR after simple exc	NSR after simple exc	Local recurrence in 30%
Pathology			
Borders	Usually well circumscribed; can be focally infiltrative	Well circumscribed	Infiltrative; can be partly circumscribed
Blood vessels	Numerous small to medium sized vessels with hyalinization	Numerous, mostly capillaries	Small to medium sized vessels, many thick walled or hyalinized
Stromal cells	Highly cellular; spindle cells	Spindle, plump and multinucleate cells, perivascular accentuation	Low cellularity; stellate or spindle cells with fine cytoplasmic processes
Stroma	Occasional adipocytes, wispy collagen bundles, can be focally myxoid	Edematous to collagenous	Myxoid to collagenous

Note: Data listed for aggressive angiomyxoma and angiomyofibroblastoma compiled from other sources.
Abbreviations: Exc, excision; *NSR,* no sign of recurrence.
(Courtesy of Nucci MR, Granter SR, Fletcher CDM: Cellular angiofibroma: A benign neoplasm distinct from angiomyofibroblastoma and spindle cell lipoma. *Am J Surg Pathol* 21:636–644, 1997.)

cell component and the prominent blood vessels. The differential diagnosis of this distinctive lesion would include aggressive angiomyxoma, AMFB, spindle cell lipoma, solitary fibrous tumor, perineurioma, and leiomyoma.

▶ I have selected the excellent papers abstracted here (Abstracts 3–2 through 3–7) to address the problematic differential diagnosis of stromal spindle cell lesions of the genital area in general, and of the vulva in particular. The difficulty in correctly diagnosing these lesions for the practicing pathologist is caused by a combination of factors, including their rare occurrence and—for at least 2 of these entities (AMFB and cellular angiofibroma)—their relatively recent discovery. We may all forget to include 1 or more of these entities in our differential diagnostic algorithms, and the potential for overdiagnosis or underdiagnosis is great. Strict adherence to morphologic criteria is crucial because of the relative lack of consensus on the immunophenotypic characteristics of these lesions, as emphasized in these papers. Having stated all of the above, let me add that if you feel confused after reading these papers (or their abstracts), welcome to the club!

K.E. Sirgi, M.D.

Microinvasive Adenocarcinoma of the Cervix: A Clinicopathologic Study of 77 Women

Östör A, Rome R, Quinn M (Royal Women's Hosp, Melbourne, Australia)
Obstet Gynecol 89:88–93, 1997   3–8

Objective.—To present diagnostic criteria and treatment recommendations for microinvasive adenocarcinoma of the cervix.

Methods.—The authors reviewed records for 77 patients who had been treated for microinvasive adenocarcinoma of the cervix between 1971 and 1995. Microinvasion had been defined as penetration of the stroma to a depth of no more than 5 mm. Follow-up ranged from a few months to 12 years, with 29 cases monitored for at least 5 years, but 33 cases were detected in the last 3 years of the period. One author examined slides from 48 punch biopsies, 58 cold-knife conization specimens, and 69 hysterectomy specimens.

Results.—Tumor length ranged from 0.8 to 21 mm, and tumor volume ranged from 3 to 1,000 mm³. Punch biopsies were adequate for definitive diagnosis in only 6 patients. The 58 cold-knife conizations showed that margins were free in 39 cases, involved in 18, and inconclusive in 1. All specimens with free cone margins were found to be free of residual disease after conization. Cold-knife conization was definitive therapy for 16 patients (it was combined with pelvic-node dissection in 4). The other patients required some type of hysterectomy. None of the 26 patients who had radical hysterectomy had parametrial spread, and there were no metastases in the 48 patients who underwent pelvic-node dissection or in the 23 women who had one or both adnexa removed. Adenocarcinoma recurred at the vault in one patient, 5 years after total abdominal hysterectomy. The original tumor had been the largest seen, 21 mm in horizontal spread. A second patient developed squamous cell carcinoma at the vault 9 years after total abdominal hysterectomy.

Conclusions.—Diagnosis of microinvasive adenocarcinoma requires a conization or hysterectomy specimen. Specimens must be extensively sampled so that margins can be assessed carefully and neoplasms can be sized accurately. Conization specimens should be processed by the whole embedding method, or the entire cone should be processed with suspicious blocks sectioned serially. The prognosis of microinvasive adenocarcinoma is the same as it is for squamous cell carcinoma, and the treatment also should be the same. In cases with free margins, conization is adequate treatment. Simple hysterectomy, with or without pelvic-node dissection, is appropriate if the lesion is not removed completely by conization. There seems to be no need for radical hysterectomy (except when an invasive tumor extends to the cone margins) and no need to remove the adnexa, especially in younger women who wish to preserve their fertility.

▶ The definition of microinvasive adeno carcinoma (or squamous carcinoma) of the cervix varies from one study to another. The 2 measurements most often used to define microinvasion are 3 mm and 5 mm. The concept of microinvasion, with its therapeutic implications, has been extensively evaluated for squamous lesions of the cervix but is still under scrutiny for cervical glandular lesions. Based on this well-structured study, the practicing pathologist can now objectively offer to clinical colleagues acutely needed guidance on how to manage the treatment of patients (often young) afflicted with a cervical microinvasive adenocarcinoma. Controlling overtreatment becomes much easier. Also, with the therapeutic implications presented here, it now becomes imperative for the pathologist to clearly indicate in the diagnosis the depth of invasion of malignant cervical glandular lesions, information too often missing from pathology reports of cases received in consultation.

K.E. Sirgi, M.D.

Adenocarcinoma In Situ of the Cervix: Significance of Cone Biopsy Margins
Wolf JK, Levenback C, Malpica A, et al (Univ of Texas, Houston)
Obstet Gynecol 88:82–86, 1996   3–9

Purpose.—Adenocarcinoma in situ of the uterine cervix is a recognized pathologic entity that is believed to be a precursor of invasive adenocarcinoma. There is debate regarding the treatment of these tumors, particularly the role of cone biopsy. The treatment and outcomes of 61 patients with adenocarcinoma in situ of the cervix are reviewed, focusing on the cone biopsy margins.

Methods.—Of 94 patients with adenocarcinoma in situ of the cervix diagnosed between 1984 and 1993, 61 had complete clinical and pathologic material available for review. The mean age of the patients was 36 years. Patients with mixed lesions, consisting of both adenocarcinoma in situ and squamous cervical intraepithelial neoplasia, were included.

Findings.—The diagnosis of adenocarcinoma in situ of the cervix was made by cone biopsy in 55 patients, by cervical biopsy in 5, and incidentally after hysterectomy in 1. Of the patients who had cone biopsy, 80% went on to have a hysterectomy. The in situ cancer was associated with invasive cancer in 13% of patients. The cone biopsy margin status was established in 50 patients—the margins were positive in 46% of patients and negative in 54%. Nineteen of 23 patients with positive margins underwent hysterectomy, and 53% of this group had residual uterine disease. Hysterectomy was performed in 21 of 27 patients with negative margins, and 33% of this group had residual uterine disease. Disease recurred in 2 patients with negative biopsy margins who did not undergo a hysterectomy. At a median follow-up of 57 months, 90% of patients were alive without evidence of disease.

Conclusions.—Adenocarcinoma in situ of the cervix is often associated with residual uterine disease, which can be present even if the cone biopsy margins are negative. Thus, treatment is similar to that recommended for patients with positive cone biopsy margins. Patients who refuse hysterectomy need counseling about the risks of recurrent disease and frequent follow-up Papanicolaou smears.

▶ Glandular abnormalities of the cervix are overshadowed by the high number of their squamous counterparts in a regular gynecology biopsy practice. A glandular "dysplasia" is often associated with other squamous abnormalities, and the temptation, at least with a Pap smear specimen, to interpret atypical glandular cells as reactive to an involvement of the glands by squamous dysplasia is high. The problem is somewhat similar with biopsy and curettage specimens, where squamous intraepithelial abnormalities are usually more "eye-catching" than the glandular ones. This study, with its recommendation for a more aggressive therapeutic management of cervical adenocarcinoma in situ, should remind us to look carefully for glandular abnormalities in routinely sampled cervical material.

K.E. Sirgi, M.D.

Investigation of 100 Consecutive Negative Cone Biopsies
Golbang P, Scurry J, de Jong S, et al (Mercy Hosp for Women, Melbourne, Australia; Victorian Cytology Service, Melbourne, Australia; Cytopath Histology and Cytology, Melbourne, Australia)
Br J Obstet Gynaecol 104:100–104, 1997   3–10

Background.—Although studies have reported a 4.5% to 64% incidence of negative cone biopsies, there has been only 1 investigation of

TABLE 1.—Protocol for Follow-up of Cone Biopsies

Time	Procedure
6 weeks	Routine post-operative visit
3 months	Pap smear
6 months	Colp and Pap smear, biopsy if indicated
12 months	Pap smear

Note: For patients with negative cone biopsy specimens, the 3-month visit includes an extra colposcopy to exclude vaginal abnormality. After 3 negative Papanicolaou smears, patients revert to an annual smear.

(Courtesy of Golbang P, Scurry J, de Jong S, et al: Investigation of 100 consecutive negative cone biopsies. *Br J Obstet Gynaecol* 104:100–104, 1997. Published by Blackwell Science Ltd.)

these biopsies. In that study, the findings of pre-cone assessments in patients with positive and negative cone biopsies were compared. A colposcopic suspicion of invasion, a positive pre-cone smear, 2 severely dyskaryotic smears in 12 months, previous abnormal histology, and previous treatment for cervical intraepithelial neoplasia predicted the presence of intraepithelial neoplasia or invasive malignancy in cone biopsy specimens. The reasons for cone biopsies being reported as not containing intraepithelial or invasive malignancy were determined.

Methods and Findings.—Of 436 consecutive cone biopsies performed, results of 100 were reported as negative. The final diagnoses of these patients were re-evaluated. Reassessment showed that initially negative cone biopsy results were positive in 21 cases, unsatisfactory in 27, and true negative in 51. Positive cases were diagnosed on review in 11 patients and extra levels in 10. All unsatisfactory cases resulted from denudation. Forty-seven of the true negative cases never had histologic confirmation by punch biopsy or endocervical curettage, and 4 had a previously confirmed histologic abnormality (Table 1).

Conclusion.—To decrease the number of negative cone biopsy results, clinicians can take Papanicolaou smears after correction of atrophy and inflammation and carefully perform colposcopy to reduce the number of unsatisfactory or misinterpreted findings. Smear and colposcopic findings can be confirmed by biopsy before cold-knife conization. A large loop excision of the transformation zone can be performed when there is a discrepancy between the smear abnormality and colposcopy/biopsy results. In addition, good quality cone biopsy specimens should be obtained using a method that does not involve handling the mucosa and that is performed after the mucosa has had time to regenerate after colposcopic investigation. All blocks with multiple levels should be exhausted before reporting a cone biopsy finding as negative.

▶ This is an excellent, well-researched paper with important practical applications for the cytopathologist, surgical pathologist, and gynecologist/colposcopist. It is not unusual in pathology departments where the cytology section is physically (and spiritually) separated from the surgical pathology operation to have a suboptimal level of communication between these 2 departmental branches. Cervical cone biopsy results are signed out as negative in total ignorance of the previous Papanicolaou smear results, and vice versa.

To address the frustration that a "negative" cervical cone biopsy report will most probably cause to a gynecologist and to his patient, the pathologist should take great care to address (in writing) the following issues:

* Result of previous Papanicolaou smear(s) review.

* Adequacy of sampling of the transformation zone.

* Extent of tissue blocks examination (number of levels cut per block).

Patient care would also be better served by a monthly cytology/surgical pathology/clinical gynecology correlation conference, a task probably easier for hospital-based pathology practices.

K.E. Sirgi, M.D.

Syphilitic Cervicitis Simulating Stage II Cervical Cancer: Report of Two Cases With Cytologic Findings
Gutmann EJ (Med College of Wisconsin, Milwaukee)
Am J Clin Pathol 104:643–647, 1995　　　　　　　　　　　　　　　　　3–11

Background.—Syphilitic cervicitis can mimic an ulcerated malignancy clinically. It may be characterized by a cervicovaginal smear pattern including lymphocytes, plasma cells, histiocytes, and debris. The 2 patients presented illustrate these points.

Case reports.—The patients were 2 women, 42 and 46 years of age, initially seeking medical care for vaginal discharge. Each was found to have a cervical mass that was clinically grossly compatible with invasive cervical cancer. This clinical impression was supported by colposcopic findings. Cervicovaginal smears and cervical biopsy specimens were obtained. Weeks after the patients were initially examined, the masses were diagnosed as syphilitic cervicitis.

The smears reflecting the correct diagnosis contained evidence of chronic inflammation (Table 1). The lymphocytes formed minute clusters occasionally. Some of the histiocytes contained or were found in amorphous debris. Histopathologic correlation suggests that this finding reflects ulceration. Some minor histiocyte clusters were observed. Epithelioid histiocytes were not found, although classic granulomas were seen in the histopathologic material. In both cases, rare plasma cells and lysed blood were found, suggesting previous bleeding.

Conclusion.—The initial failure of physicians to consider the correct diagnosis in these 2 patients suggests a relative unawareness of the capacity of a common venereal disease to simulate a common gynecologic malig-

TABLE 1.—Cervical Specimens: Comparisons of Initial and "Reviewed" Diagnoses

Specimen	Initial Diagnosis	Diagnosis on Review
Case 1 Smear A (taken approximately 3 weeks before presentation)	"Negative. Moderate acute inflammation."	Rare dense minute clusters of lymphocytes. Rare strands of neutrophils, debris, and histiocytes. One minute cluster of atypical glandular cells of undetermined significance.
Smear B (taken 2 weeks after presentation)	"Rare atypical—favor reactive—squamous and endocervical cells." "Moderate acute and chronic inflammation: the chronic inflammatory component is polymorphic, with a few atypical, possibly reactive, lymphoid cells present. There is no definite evidence of dysplasia/neoplasia."	Fresh and lysed blood. Moderate, obscuring acute inflammation. Rare atypical squamous cells of undetermined significance. Scattered small and large lymphocytes, often admixed with neutrophils. Rare multinucleated histiocytes. Minute clusters of histiocytes. Rare strands of neutrophils, debris, and histiocytes. Rare plasma cells.
Biopsy 1 (taken 2 weeks after presentation, and concurrently with Smear B)	"Chronic active cervicitis with focal dysplasia." "Granulation tissue with intense acute and chronic inflammation." Detached fragment of dysplastic squamous cepithelium. Focal ulceration. [No special stains performed.]	Marked chronic inflammation, including numerous lymphocytes and plasma cells. Endothelial proliferation. Ulcer with fibrin and neutrophils and debris. No definite evidence of dysplasia. Steiner's stain: spirochetes noted.
Biopsy 2 (taken 4 weeks after presentation)	"Chronic granulomatous cervicitis with spirochete infection consistent with syphilis." "A multitude of spirochetes noted" in the Steiner's stain.	Dense acute and chronic inflammation, with a marked predominance of plasma cells. Endothelial proliferation. Focal ulceration. Several granulomas, some of which contain numerous spirochetes (Steiner's stain).
Case 2 Smear (taken upon presentation)	"Negative. Inflammation. Bloody. Reactive changes."	Reactive-appearing atypia of squamous cells. Fresh and lysed blood, moderate obscuring acute inflammation, scattered lymphocytes, rare plasma cells, and numerous scattered histiocytes containing amorphous debris.
Biopsy (taken approximately 1 week after presentation)	"Granulomatous inflammation." "Severe inflammatory infiltrate consisting of neutrophils, plasma cells, and lymphocytes." Steiner's stain: "Negative for organisms."	Granulomas comprised of epithelioid histiocytes, giant cells, and lymphocytes. Admixed with the granulomas, dense clusters of plasma cells. Endothelial proliferation. Detached minute masses of neutrophils, histiocytes containing amorphous debris, and fibrin. Steiner's stain: rare spirochetes noted.

(Courtesy of Gutmann EJ: Syphilitic cervicitis simulating stage II cervical cancer: Report of two cases with cytologic findings. *Am J Clin Pathol* 104:643–647, 1995.)

nancy. Pathologists and clinicians familiar with such cases may be able to provide a timely and accurate diagnosis.

▶ This study emphasizes the paradox of any anatomical pathology examination. On one hand, it is very important to interpret microscopic sections in the context of the patient's clinical and radiographic presentation; on the other hand, it is crucial to keep, at all times, an absolute degree of objectivity and to diagnose "only what is on the slide." Shy pathologists are sometimes tempted to quickly agree in their report with an aggressive clinician "pushing" for an unequivocal diagnosis of cancer.

"Come on, the lesion is fungating and ulcerated, and it is infiltrating the surrounding tissues; it can't be anything else!" they would say, with an unwavering assurance (if not arrogance).

It is the pathologist's role, based on studies similar to the one abstracted above, to remind our clinicians that objectivity and prudence are not synonymous with indecision and ignorance. On the contrary, they are sure signs of an acute awareness of the "great mimickers" of pathology. Syphilis is certainly one of them.

K.E. Sirgi, M.D.

Atypical Oxyphilic Metaplasia of the Endocervical Epithelium: A Report of Six Cases

Jones MA, Young RH (Maine Med Ctr, Portland; Harvard Med School, Boston)
Int J Gynecol Pathol 16:99–102, 1997   3–12

Background.—A number of benign, atypical or metaplastic processes affecting endocervical glandular epithelium may be mistaken for more serious dysplastic or neoplastic conditions. An atypical metaplastic change of endocervical glandular epithelium, designated "atypical oxyphilic metaplasia of the endocervical epithelium," was described in 6 patients.

Methods and Findings.—The 6 women were aged 41 to 62 years. One was postmenopausal. Mean gravidity and parity were 2.8 and 2.7, respectively. One women was taking combined oral contraceptives and 1 was taking tamoxifen for breast cancer at the time of diagnosis. The lesions were discovered incidentally in all women. None had gross abnormality. On microscopic examination, affected endocervical glands were lined by large cuboidal or polygonal epithelial cells with dense, eosinophilic, focally vacuolated cytoplasm, and varying degrees of nuclear atypia. The nuclei were enlarged, hyperchromatic, and often multilobated or multinucleated. Two patients had rare apical snouts. There was no stratification or mitotic activity. All 3 patients tested showed rare, focal periodic acid-Schiff positivity with and without diastase predigestion. In 2 of 3 cases, mucin staining was negative, and in 1 of 3, luminal secretions were focally stained. All 3 patients tested negative for GCDFP-15 and carcinoembryonic antigen (Figs 2 and 4).

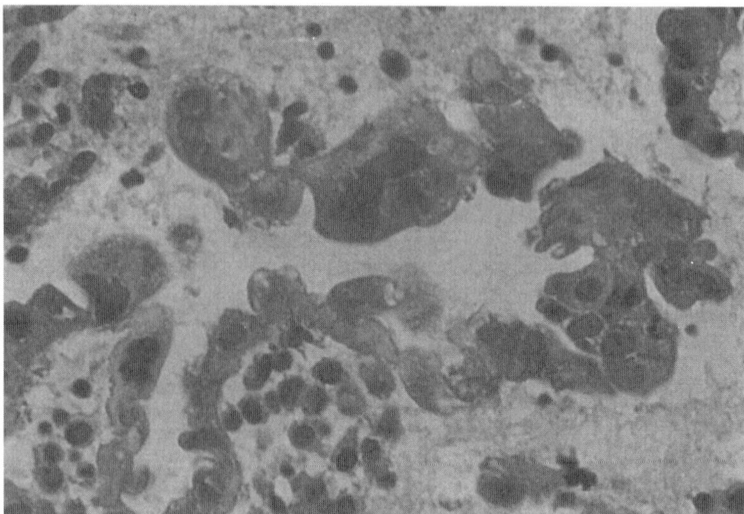

FIGURE 2.—Oxyphilic glandular fragments in a curettage specimen. The cyptolasm is abundant, oxyphilic, and contains rare small vacuoles. The nuclei are variably enlarged, hyperchromatic, and either multilobated or multinucleated. (Courtesy of Jones MA, Young RH: Atypical oxyphilic metaplasia of the endocervical epithelium: A report of six cases. *Int J Gynecol Pathol* 16:99–102, 1997.)

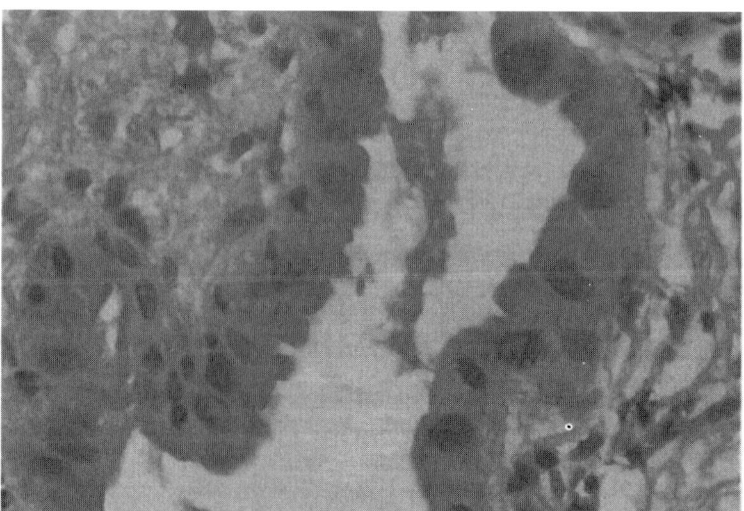

FIGURE 4.—Oxyphilic metaplasia of endocervical epithelum. The cytoplasm is abundant and there is scant eosinophilic secretion in the gland lumen. Nuclei are densely hyperchromatic in this example. (Courtesy of Jones MA, Young RH: Atypical oxyphilic metaplasia of the endocervical epithelium: A report of six cases. *Int J Gynecol Pathol* 16:99–102, 1997.)

Conclusion.—A novel benign atypia of the endocervix is yet another entity that must be distinguished from dysplastic and neoplastic lesions.

Transitional Cell Metaplasia of the Uterine Cervix and Vagina: An Underrecognized Lesion That May Be Confused With High-Grade Dysplasia. A Report of 59 Cases
Weir MM, Bell DA, Young RH (Harvard Med School, Boston)
Am J Surg Pathol 21:510–517, 1997   3–13

Introduction.—In examining surgical specimens of the lower female genital tract, the pathologist's major objective is to recognize intraepithelial neoplasia. Some cases of squamous metaplasia can be misinterpreted as dysplasia; otherwise, there are few pathologic processes that simulate

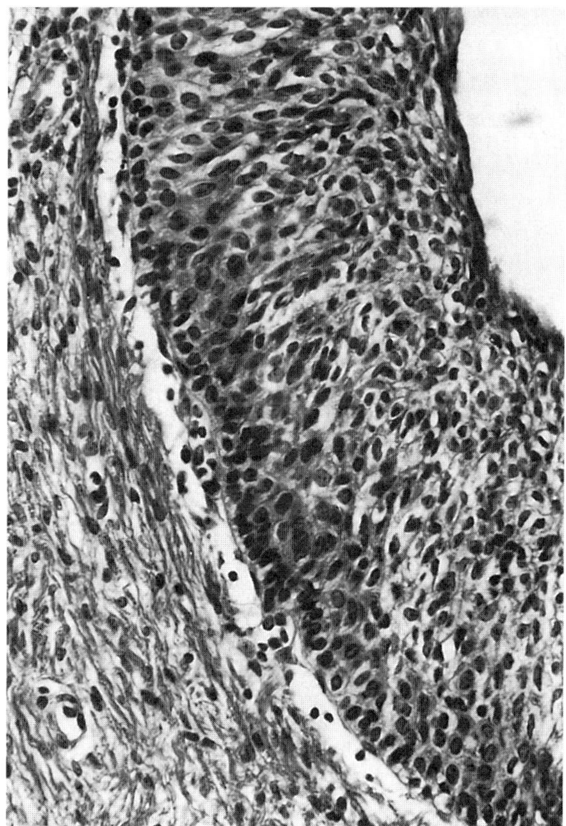

FIGURE 1.—Transitional cell metaplasia involving exocervix. The epithelium is hyperplastic, resembling hyperplastic urothelium. There is only minimal maturation at the surface. Note the lack of cytologic atypia. (Courtesy of Weir MM, Bell DA, Young RH: Transitional cell metaplasia of the uterine cervix and vagina: An underrecognized lesion that may be confused with high-grade dysplasia. A report of 59 cases. *Am J Surg Pathol* 21:510–517, 1997.)

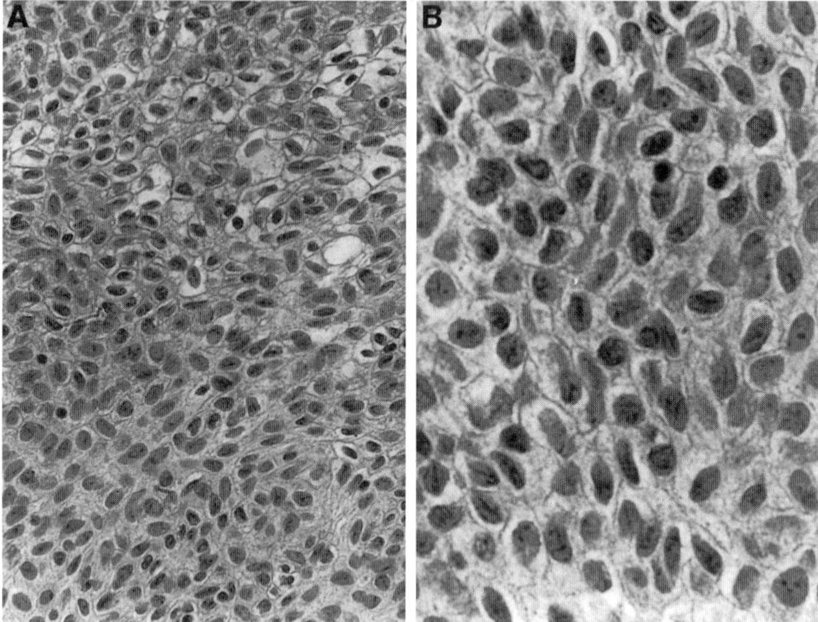

FIGURE 7.—**A**, transitional cell metaplasia showing typical cytologic features. Note the perinuclear halos, spindled nuclei with tapered ends, and low nuclear-to-cytoplasmic ratios. **B**, higher magnification of transitional cell metaplasia, showing characteristic tapered nuclei with longitudinal grooves and wrinkled contours. (Courtesy of Weir MM, Bell DA, Young RH: Transitional cell metaplasia of the uterine cervix and vagina: An underrecognized lesion that may be confused with high-grade dysplasia. A report of 59 cases. *Am J Surg Pathol* 21:510–517, 1997.)

squamous dysplasia. The authors report an abnormality—termed transitional cell metaplasia—that can be misdiagnosed as high-grade dysplasia.

Patients.—A total of 63 cervical or vaginal surgical specimens meeting the criteria of transitional cell metaplasia were analyzed. The patients' average age was 68 years; 57 were postmenopausal and 2 were perimenopausal. Four patients had received hormonal therapy. The surgical specimen was obtained by hysterectomy in 29 patients, endocervical or endometrial curettage in 18, cervical biopsy or cone biopsy in 11, and vaginal biopsy in 5. The transitional cell metaplasia was always an incidental finding.

Findings.—The exocervix was involved in 14 cases, the transformation zone in 33, the vagina in 10, or a combination of these in 4. In the cervical and vaginal specimens, the surface epithelium was most often involved with transitional cell metaplasia. Isolated stromal nests were present in 9 cases and invagination of the surface epithelium into the stroma in 2. Transitional cell metaplasia usually appeared as immature hyperplastic epithelium, made up of spindled nuclei with tapered ends and longitudinal nuclear grooves (Fig 1). Orientation of the nuclei was vertical in the deeper layers, and horizontal with a streaming pattern in the superficial layer. Cell characteristics included low nuclear-to-cytoplasm ratios, perinuclear halos, and few or no mitotic figures (Fig 7). Just 2 cases showed mild-to-moderate atypia.

Conclusions.—Transitional cell metaplasia of the cervix and vagina appears to be a relatively common lesion with the potential for misdiagnosis as high-grade dysplasia. The confusion may arise from the apparent lack of maturation. However, closer inspection of the cytologic detail will reveal the typical findings of transitional cell metaplasia. The lesion usually occurs as an incidental finding in older women. Increased recognition of transitional cell metaplasia will reduce the potential for unnecessary treatment.

▶ The list of metaplastic epithelial cervical lesions that may create diagnostic confusion with more serious dysplastic or neoplastic lesions keeps growing as these articles show (Abstracts 3–12 and 3–13). This really means that the number and variety of diagnostic traps waiting for pathologists to fall into has dramatically increased. In this litigious atmosphere in which pathologists (mainly cytopathologists) are today practicing, it might be a good idea to keep by the microscope a (very) frequently updated list of such look-alikes of malignancy, categorized by the different organs of the body (cervix, prostate, breast…).

K.E. Sirgi, M.D.

Glandular Cells Derived From Direct Sampling of the Lower Uterine Segment in Patients Status Post-Cervical Cone Biopsy: A Diagnostic Dilemma

Heaton RB, Harris TF, Larson DM, et al (Natl Naval Med Ctr, Bethesda, Md)
Am J Clin Pathol 106:511–516, 1996   3–14

Background.—With the use of endocervical brushes for sampling of the endocervical canal, more and more cervical smears are referred to the pathologist as atypical glandular cells. Cells sampled directly from the lower uterine segment endometrium (LUS) may resemble atypical glandular lesions or a high-grade squamous intraepithelial lesion. Such diagnostic problems are especially likely in women who have undergone cervical cone biopsy. The cytologic findings of LUS were analyzed, including their incidence in patients who have undergone cone biopsy.

Methods.—Sixty-four patients were studied who had undergone cervical cone biopsy, either by cold knife conization or loop endocervical evaluation procedure. Cervical smears from these patients were reviewed, and the findings were compared with those of smears obtained before conization. The results of any postcone cervical biopsies or endocervical curettage specimens were analyzed as well.

Results.—Thirty-seven percent of patients were flagged on the initial screen performed for the study, but many of these proved to have only exfoliated endometrial cells, stromal elements, or both. This left 19% of patients showing fragments of LUS on postcone smears. On cytologic analysis, the fragments were often large, with gland openings, branched

TABLE 3.—Features of AIS, ECI, TM, and LUS

	AIS	ECI	TM	LUS
Palisading (peripheral)	+	+	+	++
Palisading (internal)				++
Honeycombing	+	−−	+/+++	++
Nucleoli	++	−−	+	+
Mitoses	+/+++	++	+/−	+
Ciliated cells	−/+	−−	+++	++
Terminal bars	−−	−−	++	+
Rosettes	+/+++	−−	−/+	−/+
Loss of polarity	−−	+++	+/−	−−
Isolated strips	+/+++	−−	−/+	−−
Feathering	+++		+/−	−−

Abbreviations: AIS, adenocarcinoma in situ; *ECI*, endocervical involvement of high-grade squamous intraepithelial lesion; *TM*, tubal metaplasia; *LUS*, endometrial cells from lower uterine segment; −, not present; + to +++, sometimes to often present; +/+++, presence is variable.

(Courtesy of Heaton RB, Harris, TF, Larson DM, et al: Glandular cells derived from direct sampling of the lower uterine segment in patients status post-cervical cone biopsy: A diagnostic dilemma. *Am J Clin Pathol* 106:511–516, 1996.)

glands, and nuclear palisading within. Many of the fragments were accompanied by endometrial stroma. Smaller fragments were common and were densely cellular, with nuclear palisading (Table 3). The postcone smear was more likely to show LUS after cold knife conization than after loop endocervical evaluation procedure. One third of cases with LUS were originally misclassified as squamous dysplasia or glandular atypia.

Conclusions.—In patients who have undergone cervical cone biopsy, particularly cold knife conization, direct sampling of the LUS by endocervical brush is a common occurrence. Unless the presence of these cells is recognized, they can cause diagnostic problems on cytologic examination. The possibility of LUS must be considered before the diagnosis of endocervical glandular dysplasia or atypia is made. When LUS is suspected, a repeat cervical smear and close clinical follow-up are recommended.

▶ The large majority of pap smear specimens consist of squamous and endocervical glandular cells. With time and experience, pathologists have learned to recognize the wide spectrum of variation from typical for these 2 cell types. However, new sampling devices that can better reach the upper endocervical canal, and samplings taken after conization of the cervix are exposing the pathologist to an increasing number of nonendocervical glandular cells with their associated variants. Recognizing these cells as glandular may be a challenge; interpreting these cells as normal is definitely another challenge. Awareness of these normal cells and of their different presentation will help decrease the number of typical glandular cells of undetermined significance in daily practice.

K.E. Sirgi, M.D.

Efficacy of Frozen-Section Evaluation of Uterine Curettings in the Diagnosis of Ectopic Pregnancy

Spandorfer SD, Menzin AW, Barnhart KT, et al (Univ of Pennsylvania, Philadelphia)
Am J Obstet Gynecol 175:603–605, 1996   3–15

Background.—Curettage can be used to distinguish between an abnormal intrauterine pregnancy and an ectopic pregnancy. Frozen-section diagnosis at the time of surgery can markedly reduce the time needed to identify intrauterine chorionic villi and thus exclude the diagnosis of ectopic pregnancy. The accuracy of frozen-section evaluation for identifying products of conception on curettage of patients undergoing surgery for suspected ectopic pregnancy was investigated.

Methods.—Eighty-seven consecutive patients undergoing frozen-section assessment of endometrial curettage specimens were included in the study. The frozen-section diagnosis was considered correct when the final diagnosis concurred with the frozen-section findings.

Findings.—Ninety-three percent of the specimens were identified correctly on frozen-section evaluation. The sensitivity of frozen-section assessment was 78.3%, and the specificity was 98.4% In this population, frozen-section evaluation had a positive predictive value of 94.7% and a negative predictive value of 92.6%. The attending pathologist at frozen-section evaluation, preoperative human chorionic gonadotropin level (Table 2), and time of day at frozen-section assessement (Table 3) were uncorrelated.

Conclusions.—Intraoperative frozen sections can reliably and accurately detect products of conception on endometrial curettage. The accuracy of frozen-section evaluation in identifying products of conception at uterine curettage—93%—compares favorably with the frozen-section accuracy in other surgical procedures.

▶ I cannot remember a single instance in which a frozen-section evaluation was requested on a "products of conception, rule out ectopic pregnancy" order that was not followed by loud rumbling (to put it politely) from the

TABLE 2.—Accuracy of Frozen-Section Diagnosis Depending on Initial hCG Concentration

hCG level (mIU/L)	*No.*	*Correct diagnosis**	*Incorrect diagnosis†*
<2300	60	54 (90%)	6 (10%)
>2300	27	27 (100%)	0 (0%)

Note: Differences are not statistically significant.
*Concordance of frozen section and permanent section.
†Discrepancy of frozen section and permanent section.
Abbreviation; hCG, human chorionic gonadotropin.
(Courtesy of Spandorfer SD, Menzin AW, Barnhart KT, et al: Efficacy of frozen-section evaluation of uterine curettings in the diagnosis of ectopic pregnancy. *Am J Obstet Gynecol* 175:603–605, 1996.)

TABLE 3.—Accuracy of Frozen-Section Diagnosis Depending on Time of Day

Time of day	No.	Correct diagnosis*	Incorrect diagnosis†
Daytime hours (8 AM to 5 PM, Mon.-Fri.)	59	56 (94.9%)	3 (5.1%)
On-call hours (nights or weekends)	28	25 (89.2%)	3 (10.8%)

Note: Differences are not statistically significant.
*Concordance of frozen section and permanent section.
†Discrepancy of frozen section and permanent section.
(Courtesy of Spandorfer SD, Menzin AW, Barnhart KT, et al: Efficacy of frozen-section evaluation of uterine curettings in the diagnosis of ectopic pregnancy. *Am J Obstet Gynecol* 175:603–605, 1996.)

pathologist on duty. The idea of evaluating, by frozen section, bloody, discohesive tissue for sometimes very rare villous structures or, even worse, rare cytotrophoblastic or syncytiotrophoblastic cells is, understandably, not a big favorite among pathologists. Somehow, at least where I work, this has a tendency to happen after regular work hours, that is, when I am alone without appropriate technical help to assist me in cutting and staining (sometimes numerous) tissue blocks. It should be emphasized that *all* of the tissue should be submitted for evaluation. My experience has been that, if the gross specimen is initially carefully examined, products of conception will generally be found in the first 2 blocks submitted. If no villi or syncytiotrophoblastic elements are found, I call the operating room, inform the obstetrician about the preliminary diagnosis, and tell him that the totality of the remaining tissue will be immediately evaluated in additional blocks. This approach has always been well accepted by our clinicians and has helped me save some time by not having to cut and examine all of the tissue at once.

K.E. Sirgi, M.D.

Sertoliform Endometrial Adenocarcinoma: A Study of Four Cases

Eichhorn JH, Young RH, Clement PB (Harvard Med School, Boston; Univ of British Columbia, Vancouver)
Int J Gynecol Pathol 15:119–126, 1996   3–16

Background.—Although endometrioid carcinomas resembling sex-cord stromal tumors in the ovary have been described, only 2 case reports of a comparable tumor of the endometrium have appeared in the literature. Four endometrial carcinomas with a conspicuous component resembling patterns in Sertoli cell tumors were reported.

Methods and Findings.—The 4 patients, aged 44 to 83 years, were multiparous, moderately to markedly obese, and hypertensive. Three women had non–insulin-dependent diabetes mellitus. Three patients initially had abnormal or postmenopausal vaginal bleeding, and 1 had abnormal cervical cytology. On biopsy, 1 tumor was thought to be an endometrial stromal sarcoma with sex-cord–like differentiation. On gross examination of the hysterectomy and bilateral salpingo-oophorectomy specimens, all patients were found to have solid polypoid endometrial tumors. On light microscopic assessment, 3 tumors were

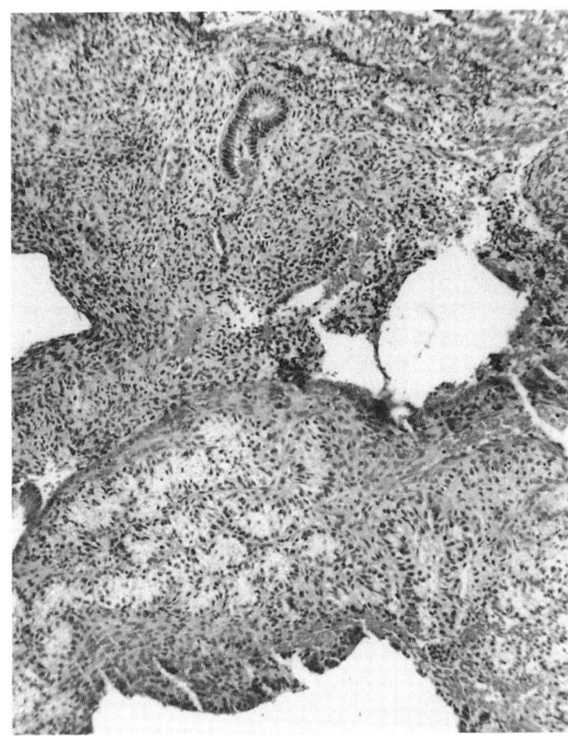

FIGURE 1.—Endometrial biopsy shows cells between glands arranged in tubules and cords, suggesting endometrial stromal sarcoma with sex-cord differentiation; original magnification, ×125. (Courtesy of Eichhorn JH, Young RH, Clement PB: Sertoliform endometrial adenocarcinoma: A study of four cases. *Int J Gynecol Pathol* 15:119–126, 1996.)

superficially invasive of the myometrium and 1 was limited to the endometrium. None of the tumors had the tonguelike pattern of myoinvasive or the angiolymphatic invasion typical of low-grade endometrial stromal sarcomas. The sertoliform component, consisting of uniform small, hollow tubules lined by columnar cells with apical cytoplasm and compact slender cords, predominated in 1 case and was focal in the other 3. Tubules and cords frequently occurred between benign-appearing or carcinomatous glands. In the tumor with predominant sertoliform regions, the lesional cells had clear cytoplasm, which suggested a lipid-rich variant. Special stains of this tumor showed cytoplasmic glycogen but no fat. There was no cytoplasmic mucin, argyrophil granules, or argentaffinity in any tumor. Nonsertoliform tumor regions were composed of typical endometrioid adenocarcinoma. Each tumor also showed concurrent endometrial hyperplasia. Three tumors showed squamous differentiation and minor foci of anaplastic carcinoma with bizarre tumor giant cells. In all tumors, immunoperoxidase stains showed staining for 2 or more markers of epithelial or glandular differentiation in the sertoliform regions, with

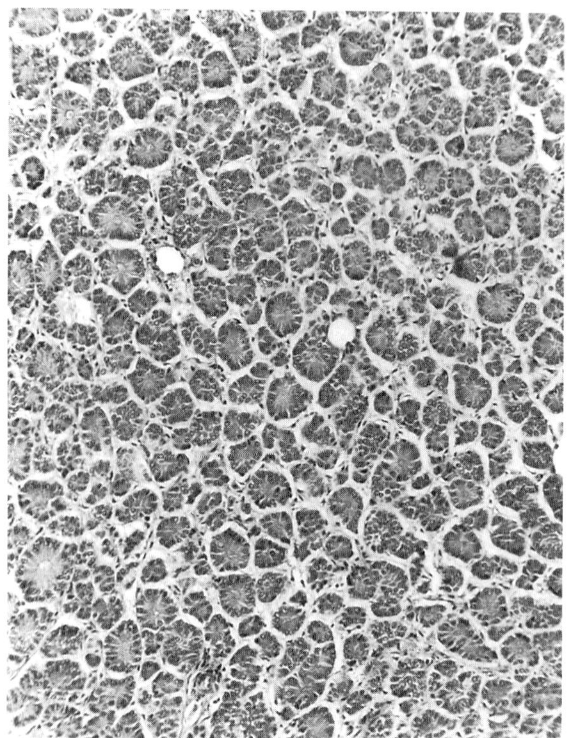

FIGURE 3.—Sertoliform component composed of small hollow tubules lined by columnar cells with apical cytoplasm and small, round nuclei; original magnification, ×125. (Courtesy of Eichhorn JH, Young RH, Clement PB: Sertoliform endometrial adenocarcinoma: A study of four cases. *Int J Gynecol Pathol* 15:119–126, 1996.)

focal expression of vimentin. No desmin or actin staining was noted in any tumors (Figs 1, 3, and 8).

Conclusion.—Sertoliform endometrioid adenocarcinomas occur rarely in the endometrium. These tumors, which appear to be variants of endometrioid adenocarcinoma, are distinct from uterine tumors resembling ovarian sex-cord tumors and stromal sarcomas with sex-cord–like differentiation.

▶ In the World Health Organization classification, gynecologic malignant tumors are neatly categorized in separate paragraphs. However, these paragraphs get longer every few years (or sooner) because of the continuous refinement that Drs. Scully and Young (for the most part) and others keep bringing to the morphologic diagnosis of these tumors... A mixed blessing!

K.E. Sirgi, M.D.

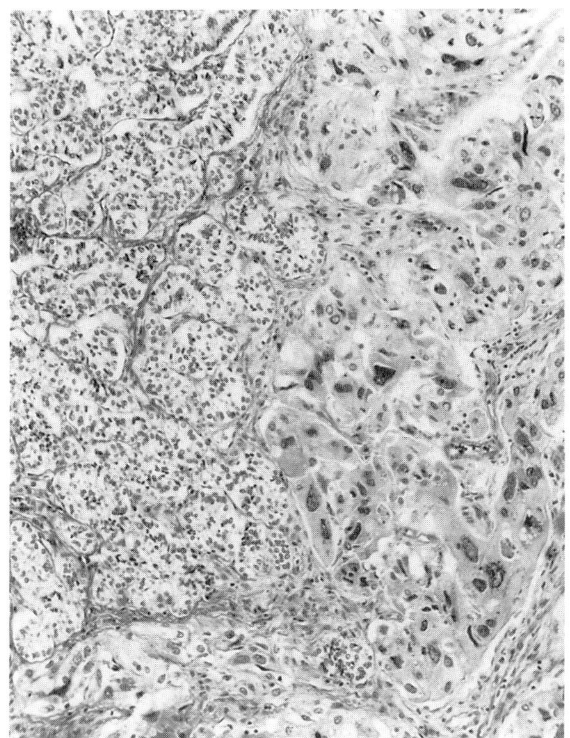

FIGURE 8.—Bizarre tumor giant cells in a predominantly sertoliform tumor; original magnification, ×125. (Courtesy of Eichhorn JH, Young RH, Clement PB: Sertoliform endometrial adenocarcinoma: A study of four cases. *Int J Gynecol Pathol* 15:119–126, 1996).

Epithelioid Smooth-Muscle Tumors of the Uterus: A Clinicopathologic Study of 18 Patients

Prayson RA, Goldblum JR, Hart WR (Cleveland Clinic Found, Ohio)
Am J Surg Pathol 21:383–391, 1997

3–17

Background.—Although epithelioid smooth-muscle tumors of the gastrointestinal tract have been studied thoroughly, few studies have been done on these tumors in the uterus. A clinicopathologic study of 1 group of patients with epithelioid smooth-muscle tumors of the uterus was conducted to determine possible prognostic factors.

Methods and Findings.—Eighteen patients aged 27 to 83 years were studied retrospectively. Three groups were formed based on nuclear grade of the tumor cells. In 2 tumors, both IV leiomyomatosis, the nuclear grade was 1. These tumors had highest mitosis counts of 1 and 3 mitotic figures (MFs)/10 HPF. No tumor cell necrosis was noted. Both patients were alive with no evidence of disease at 5 and 65 months, respectively. Another 10 tumors had grade 2 nuclei. All but 1 had highest mitosis counts of 0 to 3 MF/10 HPF. Nine of the tumors had no cell necrosis, and 1 had an

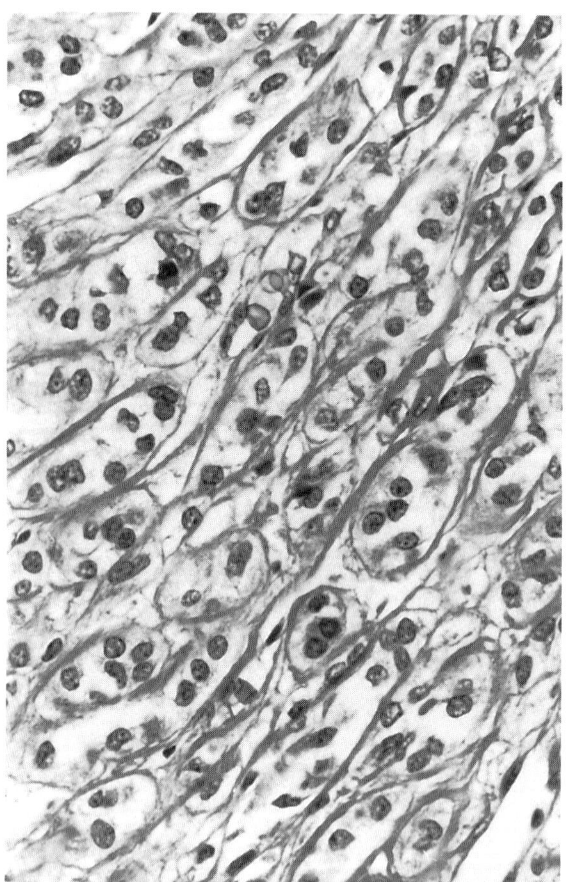

FIGURE 1.—Nuclear grade 1 tumor. Cells have uniform bland nuclei with inconspicuous or absent nucleoli and evenly distributed chromatin. Cytoplasm is of the clear type. (Courtesy of Prayson RA, Goldblum JR, Hart WR: Epithelioid smooth-muscle tumors of the uterus: A clinicopathologic study of 18 patients. *Am J Surg Pathol* 21:383–391, 1997.)

infiltrative border only. Tumor sizes ranged from 1.5 to 14 cm. In 2 tumors, pleomorphic multinucleated giant cells similar to those in bizarre leiomyomas were observed. All 9 patients with follow-up were alive with no disease at 5 to 203 months after surgery. Six tumors had grade 3 nuclei, 5 of which had highest mitosis counts of 4 to 9 MF/10 HPF. Tumors ranged from 4.5 to 13 cm in the maximum dimension. Two showed tumor cell necrosis and 2 had an infiltrative border. Two patients in this group died of disease 11 and 132 months after surgery. Another 2 were alive with no evidence of disease at 48 and 83 months, 1 was alive with an unknown tumor status at 28 months, and 1 was lost to follow-up (Figs 1, 2, and 3).

Conclusion.—Uterine smooth-muscle tumors with a predominance of epithelioid cells are very uncommon. These tumors metastasize infrequently. There is no single histologic finding that predicts metastatic po-

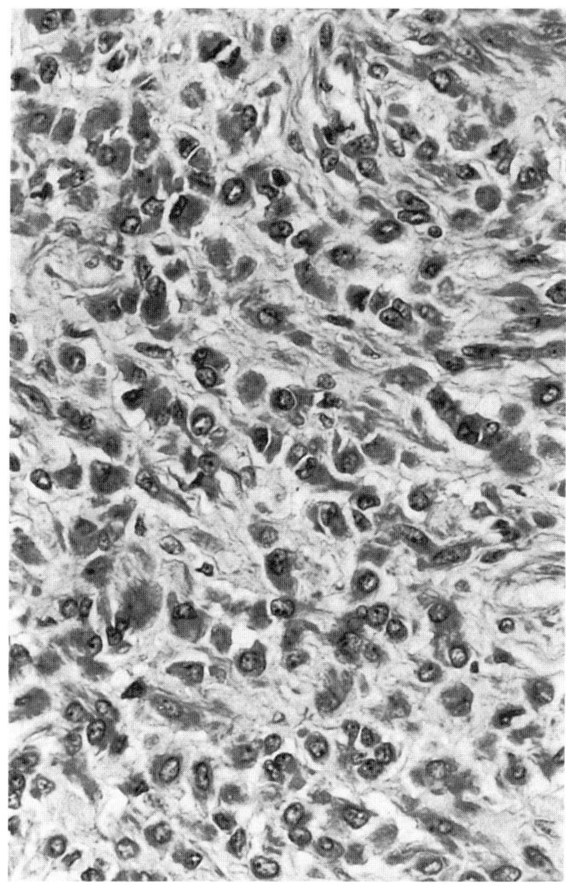

FIGURE 2.—Nuclear grade 2 tumor. Cells have an intermediate degree of nuclear atypia, often with small nucleoli. Cytoplasm is eosinophilic. (Courtesy of Prayson RA, Goldblum JR, Hart WR: Epithelioid smooth-muscle tumors of the uterus: A clinicopathologic study of 18 patients. *Am J Surg Pathol* 21:383–391, 1997.)

tential. Typically, clinically malignant tumors have significant nuclear atypia and some mitotic activity, and most have tumor cell necrosis.

▶ In addition to confirming a more indolent course for the epithelioid variant of uterine leiomyosarcoma, this paper underlines the necessity of evaluating other morphologic parameters than mitotic count in determining the malignant status of a smooth-muscle neoplasm. Nuclear atypia and the presence of necrosis are equally important factors. The synthesis of all 3 findings allows a more accurate prognostication of these neoplasms.

K.E. Sirgi, M.D.

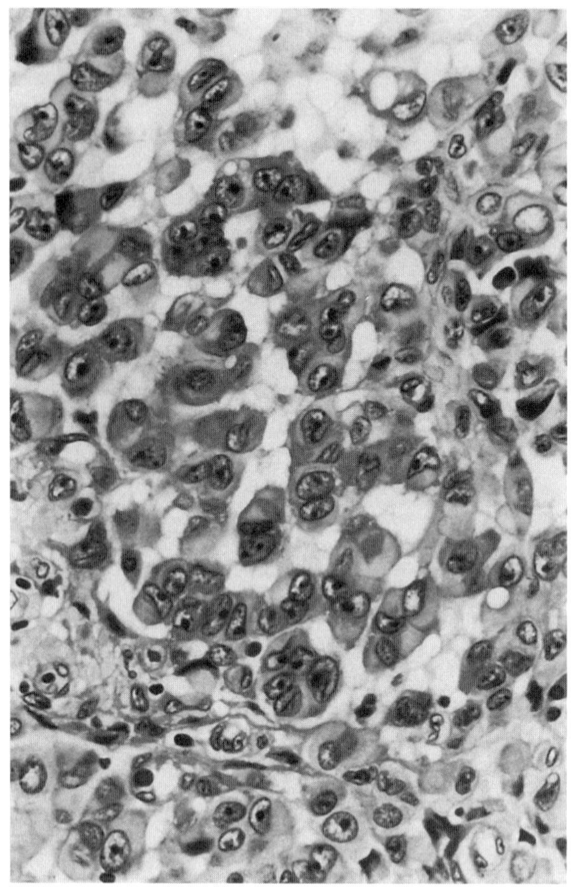

FIGURE 3.—Nuclear grade 3 tumor. Cells have enlarged hyperchromatic nuclei with prominent macronucleoli and unevenly disributed chromatin. Cytoplasm is eosinophilic. These tumor cells have some rhabdoid features. (Courtesy of Prayson RA, Goldblum JR, Hart WR: Epithelioid smooth-muscle tumors of the uterus: A clinicopathologic study of 18 patients. *Am J Surg Pathol* 21:383–391, 1997.)

Retained Trophoblastic Tissue in Fallopian Tubes: A Consequence of Unsuspected Ectopic Pregnancies

Jacques SM, Qureshi F, Ramirez NC, et al (Hutzel Hosp, Detroit; Wayne State Univ, Detroit)
Int J Gynecol Pathol 16:219–224, 1997   3–18

Introduction.—Because tissue specimens are not obtained, histopathologic changes in fallopian tubes are not known in patients with ectopic pregnancies that resolve spontaneously with preservation of fertility. Reported are 5 patients with trophoblastic tissue within the fallopian tubes with characteristics indicative of remote ectopic pregnancies.

Methods.—Retained trophoblastic tissue in the fallopian tubes was detected in tissue samples of 5 women during histopathologic examination. Tissues were routinely processed and stained with hematoxylin-eosin. Selected tissues underwent staining using the immunoperoxidase method. Clinical records were reviewed.

Results.—Four remote ectopic pregnancies were detected in 4 patients undergoing tubal ligation after delivery or during cesarean section (C-section). Of these, 1 patient underwent salpingo-oophorectomy during C-section because a small right ovarian mass and "necrotic area" was detected in the fallopian tube. A 1.0 cm "calcified" nodule was found in the distal fallopian tube in another patient. In a fifth patient undergoing laparotomy, an acute ectopic pregnancy was seen in 1 fallopian tube. A clinically unsuspected 3.0 cm mass detected in the other fallopian tube was an ectopic pregnancy with ghost outlines of chorionic villi and trophoblast. All 5 patients had foci of viable-appearing intermediate trophoblast and surrounding abundant eosinophilic hyalinized material in the fallopian tubes that were detected on histopathologic examination. Four patients additionally had hyalinized ghost outlines of chorionic villi. None of these patients had a previous history of ectopic pregnancy.

Conclusion.—The natural history of clinically unsuspected ectopic tubal pregnancies is not well known. These findings indicate that trophoblasts may persist in fallopian tubes and could cause clinical confusion and possibly tubal pathology.

▶ The number of pregnancies lost in early gestation is not small; figures quoted in textbooks range as high as 60% (many of these pregnancies, of course, are subclinical). While most such pregnancies can be expected to be intrauterine, some will not. What happens to the products of conception in pregnancies at extrauterine sites that end spontaneously in early gestation— to "blighted ova"? Jacques et al. tell us. Once we learn to look for residua of ectopic pregnancies, we probably will see them more often.

A.S. Knisely, M.D.

Malignant Mesotheliomas Presenting as Ovarian Masses: A Report of Nine Cases, Including Two Primary Ovarian Mesotheliomas
Clement PB, Young RH, Scully RE (Univ of British Columbia, Vancouver; Harvard Med School, Boston)
Am J Surg Pathol 20:1067–1080, 1996   3–19

Purpose.—Ovarian involvement is common in women with peritoneal malignant mesothelioma (MM). However, the nature of the ovarian involvement, with tumor confined to the serosa and superficial cortex, in the setting of extensive and often bulky extraovarian disease, does not usually suggest primary ovarian tumor. Nine women with MM presenting as an ovarian mass were described.

Patients.—The 9 patients were identified from a larger series of approximately 60 peritoneal mesotheliomas in women. In each case, the initial clinical, intraoperative, and macroscopic impression was that of a primary ovarian tumor. The referring pathologist either misdiagnosed the lesion or expressed uncertainty about its true nature. Two of the tumors were primary ovarian MMs confined to 1 or both ovaries. The other 7 patients had widespread peritoneal MM, making it impossible to draw any conclusions as to whether the ovarian involvement was primary or secondary. Features suggesting possible primary ovarian MM included ovarian enlargement and/or parenchymal replacement. Clinical features included abdominal or pelvic pain or abdominal swelling. Pelvic examination and/or laparotomy revealed an adnexal mass. One of the tumors was found only at autopsy. None of the patients had a history of asbestos exposure.

Findings.—Pathologic examination showed both serosal and parenchymal involvement of the ovary in 7 cases; the serosa alone and the parenchyma alone were involved in 1 case each. There were 7 exclusively epithelial tumors, with papillary, tubular-glandular, and solid patterns. The other 2 tumors were biphasic. In the epithelial mesotheliomas, the cells were usually moderately atypical, with a low mitotic rate. The stroma was usually hyalinized. Three papillary-type cases had papillae with hyalinized cores. Three cases showed psammoma bodies. Histochemical and immunohistochemical stains confirmed the mesothelial nature of the tumor cells.

Treatment and Outcomes.—Treatment in 8 patients consisted of bilateral oophorectomy, usually with hysterectomy. Four patients received chemotherapy and 1 received radiation. Follow-up was available in 5 patients: 3 had died within 8–44 months after surgery, 1 was alive with tumor at 18 months, and 1 was alive and disease free at 11 years.

Conclusions.—Malignant mesothelioma rarely presents as an ovarian mass, and at least sometimes is a primary ovarian tumor. The pathologist should be aware that ovarian MMs can occur; they can be recognized by their typical microscopic appearance with routinely stained sections and confirmatory histochemical and immunohistochemical studies. The differential diagnosis is an extensive one, including primary and metastatic ovarian tumors with papillary and tubular patterns, as well as other peritoneal mesothelial lesions.

▶ This is an excellent paper written by masters in gynecologic pathology. The line of separation between serous papillary neoplasms of the ovary and peritoneal MMs is often blurred in our mind. A potential source of confusion is that primary serous neoplasms of the peritoneum do occur and may mimic, clinically and morphologically, MMs. The distinction is important because of the differences in behavior and therapy. For the same reasons, the distinction of MM presenting as an ovarian mass from other primary and metastatic ovarian neoplasms is necessary. It is described in this article with great expertise.

K.E. Sirgi, M.D.

Use of Monoclonal Antibody Against Human Inhibin as a Marker for Sex Cord-Stromal Tumors of the Ovary

Rishi M, Howard LN, Bratthauer GL, et al (Armed Forces Inst of Pathology, Washington, DC)
Am J Surg Pathol 21:583–589, 1997   3–20

Objective.—In the ovary, the hormone inhibin is produced by granulosa cells and inhibits secretion of follicle-stimulating hormone. Serum inhibin levels are elevated in patients with granulosa cell tumors (GCT), so inhibin has been measured to detect recurrent tumor. Whether monoclonal inhibin antibody (IAB) could be used to distinguish GCT and primitive gonadal-stromal tumors from small cell carcinoma (SCC) and other poorly differentiated tumors was determined.

Methods.—Monoclonal IAB was used to study 125 paraffin-embedded, microwave-enhanced ovarian tumors and tissues by microwave-enhanced immunohistochemistry. The study material included 32 adult, 7 juvenile, and 4 metastatic GCT; 8 Sertoli-cell or Sertoli-Leydig cell tumors (SCT); 7 SCC of the hypercalcemic type; 6 primitive gonadal stromal tumors (PGST); 5 fibrothecomas, 6 lipid cell tumors (LCT); 5 extrauterine endometrial stromal sarcomas (ESS); 5 hemangiopericytomas (HPC); 1 metastatic malignant melanoma; 1 metastatic malignant lymphoma; and 27 epithelial tumors of various types, including 8 sertoliform endometrioid carcinomas (SEC). Also studied were 7 pregnancy luteomas, 3 corpora lutea, and 2 ovarian follicles. The findings were analyzed to see whether IAB preferentially marked GCT and SCT, thus helping to distinguish GCT from SCC, SCT from SEC, and primitive gonadal-stromal tumors from the various poorly differentiated neoplasms.

Results.—Ninety-seven percent of adult GCT showed a positive reaction to IAB. The average percent of positive cells in this group of tumors was 80%, with a range of 30% to 100%. Positive immunoreactivity with IAB was also noted for all metastatic GCT, all juvenile GCT, 80% of

TABLE 1.—Ovarian Tumors and Tissues Exhibiting Positive Immunostaining With Monoclonal Inhibin Antibody

No. of patients	Tissue sample	Histologic diagnosis	No. of pos. tumors	Staining intensity	% of pos. cells (average)
32	Ovary	Adult GCT	31 (97%)	1–3+	80%
4	Extraovarian	Metastatic GCT	4 (100%)	1–2+	60%
7	Ovary	Juvenile GCT	7 (100%)	2–3+	50%
6	Ovary	Primitive GST	6 (100%)	1–3+	90%
5	Ovary	Fibrothecoma	4 (80%)	1–2+	60%
8	Ovary	Sertoli cell tumor	7 (88%)	2–3+	90%
6	Ovary	Lipid cell tumor	6 (100%)	3+	100%
7	Ovary	Pregnancy luteoma	7 (100%)	1–3+	90%
3	Ovary	Corpora lutea	3 (100%)	3+	100%
2	Ovary	Ovarian follicle	2 (100%)	1–2+	40%

Abbreviations: GCT, granulosa cell tumor; *GST,* gonadal-stromal tumor.
(Courtesy of Rishi M, Howard LN, Bratthauer GL, et al: Use of monoclonal antibody against human inhibin as a marker for sex cord-stromal tumors of the ovary. *Am J Surg Pathol* 21:583–589, 1997.)

TABLE 2.—Tumors Exhibiting Negative Immunostaining With Monoclonal Inhibin Antibody

No. of patients	Tissue sample	Histologic diagnosis	No. with pos. stain	Staining intensity	% of pos. cell (average)
7	Ovary	Small cell carcinoma	0	0	0
8	Ovary	Sertoliform carcinoma	0	0	0
5	Ovary	Endometrial stromal sarcoma	0	0	0
5	Extra-Ovarian	Hemangiopericytoma	0	0	0
1	Ovarian	Malignant melanoma	0	0	0
4	Ovary	Brenner tumor	0	0	0
5	Ovary	Adenocarcinoma	1†	1+	1–2%
2	Ovary	Clear cell carcinoma	1†	1+	1–2%
2	Ovary	Mucinous LMP*	0	0	0
2	Ovary	Mucinous carcinoma	0	0	0
1	Ovary	Mucinous cystadenoma	0	0	0
1	Ovary	Endometrioid LMP*	0	0	0
1	Ovary	Undifferentiated carcinoma	0	0	0

*Low malignant potential LMP (borderline tumor).

†Because of the limited number of positive cells (1% to 2%) and low intensity of immunoreactivity, these cases are best interpreted as basically negative.

(Courtesy of Rishi M, Howard LN, Bratthauer GL, et al: Use of monoclonal antibody against human inhibin as a marker for sex cord-stromal tumors of the ovary. *Am J Surg Pathol* 21:583–589, 1997.)

fibrothecomas, 88% of SCT, 83% of PGST, all LCT, all pregnancy luteomas, all corpora lutea, and all ovarian follicles (Table 1). In all tumor types, the positive reaction was most intense in luteinized stromal cells.

Tumors showing no immunoreactivity to IAB were all SCC, all ESS, all HPC, the metastatic malignant melanoma, and the metastatic malignant lymphoma (Table 2). In the epithelial tumors, including the SEC, the epithelial cells showed no reactivity. In 3 mucinous ovarian tumors with luteinized stromal cells, these cells showed immunoreactivity but the mucinous epithelium did not.

Conclusions.—Monoclonal IAB appears to be a very good indicator of sex cord differentiation in ovarian tumors. It is useful in the diagnosis of GCT, including the distinction of GCT from SCC and other epithelial neoplasms. Monoclonal IAB can also aid in distinguishing between LCT and epithelial malignancies, although not in differentiating between GCT and SCT.

▶ The diagnosis of ovarian sex cord-stromal tumors is often problematic. Morphologic similarities with a variety of other epithelial and stromal neoplasms can mislead even the most experienced pathologist. The commonly used and currently available immunohistochemical stains are not of great help in such a context. If the results described by Rishi et al. are confirmed in future studies, I can predict that the inhibin antibody will quickly become a favorite among pathologists. This study and another have emphasized the higher specificity of the inhibin antibody for sex cord-stromal tumors when using the α subunit of the molecule. Also, in both studies, reactivity of the inhibin antibody was observed with mucinous ovarian neoplasms, a finding which will necessitate further clarification in future studies.[1]

K.E. Sirgi, M.D.

Reference

1. Zheng W, Sung CJ, Hanna I: α and β subunits of inhibin/activin as sex cord-stromal differentiation markers. *Int J Gynecol Pathol* 16:263–271, 1997.

Clinical and Pathological Features of Ovarian Cancer in Women With Germ-Line Mutations of *BRCA1*

Rubin SC, Benjamin I, Behbakht K, et al (Univ of Pennsylvania, Philadelphia; Duke Univ, Durham, NC; Brigham and Women's Hosp, Boston; et al)
N Engl J Med 335:1413–1416, 1996   3–21

Background.—Distinct molecular abnormalities probably contribute to the pathogenesis of hereditary and sporadic ovarian cancers. It was hypothesized that, compared with sporadic ovarian cancers, ovarian cancers associated with germ-line mutations of *BRCA1* have distinct clinical and pathologic characteristics.

Methods and Findings.—The clinical and pathologic features of ovarian cancers in 53 women with documented germ-line mutations of *BRCA1* were studied. The age at onset ranged from 28 to 78 years; the mean was

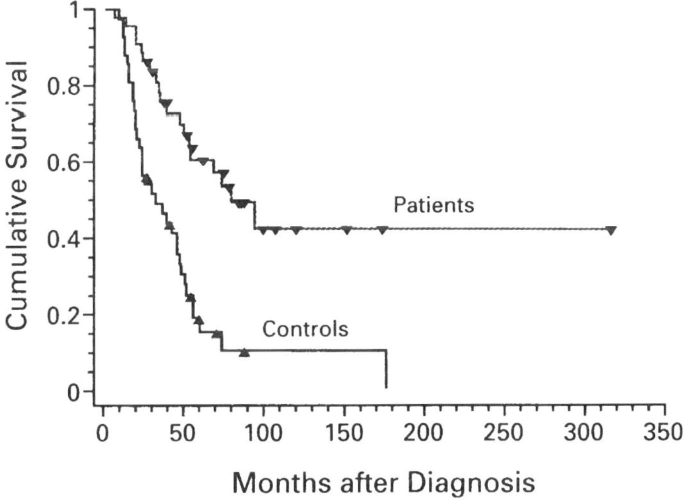

FIGURE 1.—Actuarial survival among 43 patients with advanced-stage ovarian cancer and germ-line *BRCA1* mutations as compared with matched controls without such mutations. *P* < 0.001 by the log-rank test. The *triangles* and *inverted triangles* indicate the durations of follow-up among surviving patients. (Reprinted by permission of *The New England Journal of Medicine* from of Rubin SC, Benjamin I, Behbakht K, et al: Clinical and pathological features of ovarian cancer in women with germ-line mutations of *BRCA1*. *N Engl J Med* 335:1413–1416. Copyright 1996, Massachusetts Medical Society. All rights reserved.)

48 years. Histologic assessment in 43 patients revealed serous adenocarcinoma. Thirty-seven tumors were grade 3, 11 were grade 2, 2 were grade 1, and 3 were of low malignant potential. Tumors were stage III in 38 patients, stage I in 9, stage IV in 5, and stage II in 1. The median follow-up time among survivors was 71 months after diagnosis. By this time, 20 patients had died of their disease, 27 had no evidence of disease, 4 were alive with their disease, and 2 had died of other causes. The 43 patients with advanced-stage disease had an actuarial median survival time of 77 months compared with 29 months among control research subjects matched for age, disease stage, grade, and histologic subtype (Fig 1).

Conclusions.—The clinical course of cancers associated with *BRCA1* mutations appears to be significantly better than that of sporadic ovarian cancers. The reasons for this are not yet clear.

▶ The application of molecular analysis in the medical practice has markedly increased and has greatly contributed to our understanding of numerous neoplastic and nonneoplastic diseases. However, this science is still in its early exploratory phase, and the medical community is still trying to find, in the enormous amount of new information, the minor component that will have relevant clinical, therapeutic, and diagnostic use. Pathologists are regularly bombarded by requests from enthusiastic clinicians who are eager to try for their patients a novel molecular test that they have often read about in an article published in the current issue of their medical journals or in the brochure of a "reference" laboratory that offers this test among a battery of 55 others (with appropriate CPT codes, of course). It is the role of reasonable pathologists to keep informed about new molecular tests and to guide their clinical colleagues toward those tests that have a demonstrated clinical use.

K.E. Sirgi, M.D.

4 Cytopathology

Atypical Squamous Cells of Undetermined Significance Qualified: A Follow-up Study

Kline MJ, Davey DD (Univ of Kentucky, Lexington)
Diagn Cytopathol 14:380–384, 1996   4–1

Introduction.—The Bethesda System recommended the term "atypical squamous cells of undetermined significance" (ASCUS) in 1988. In 1991, it further recommended qualifying the diagnosis when possible to indicate whether a reactive process or a squamous intraepithelial lesion (SIL) is favored. Pathologic diagnoses following a diagnosis of ASCUS quantified as favoring a reactive (FR) or dysplastic (FD) process were reviewed retrospectively to determine the utility and success of the 1991 recommendations.

Methods.—Cervicovaginal smears diagnosed as ASCUS favoring FR or FD were reviewed. Concurrent and follow-up biopsy results were reviewed for 308 cervicovaginal smears diagnosed as ASCUS FR or ASCUS FD and compared with 103 cervicovaginal smears diagnosed as ASCUS without qualification.

Results.—Follow-up diagnosis was SIL in 46.5% of ASCUS FD, 29.5% in ASCUS [FR], and 26.2% of ASCUS unqualified (Table 2). Findings were negative for dysplasia in 30.0%, 48.7%, and 54.4% of ASCUS FD, ASCUS FR, and ASCUS unqualified, respectively. Most SILs diagnosed on follow-up were low-grade squamous intraepithelial lesions (23.1%, 19.4%, and 33.0% for ASCUS FR, ASCUS FD, and ASCUS unqualified, respectively) (Table 3). More numerous cells with enlarged nuclei, slight

---

TABLE 2.—Follow-up Diagnosis According to ASCUS Category

	ASCUS category		
Follow-up result	*Favoring reactive (n = 78)*	*Unqualified (n = 103)*	*Favoring dysplastic (n = 230)*
Negative*	38 (48.7%)	56 (54.4%)	76 (33.0%)
ASCUS	17 (21.8%)	19 (18.4%)	47 (20.4%)
SIL	23 (29.5%)	27 (26.2%)†	107 (46.5%)

Abbreviation: SIL, squamous intraepithelial lesion.
*Includes normal, inflammatory findings on repeated Papanicolaou smear or biopsy.
†Does not include one case with adenocarcinoma in situ.
(Courtesy of Kline MJ, Davey DD: Atypical squamous cells of undetermined significance qualified: A follow-up study. *Diagn Cytopathol* 14:380–384. Copyright 1996, Wiley-Liss, Inc. Reprinted by permission of Wiley-Liss, Inc., a subsidiary of John Wiley & Sons, Inc.)

TABLE 3.—Follow-up Grade of Squamous Intraepithelial Lesion According to
ASCUS Category

| | ASCUS category | | |
| | Favoring reactive | Unqualified* | Favoring dysplastic |
Follow-up result	(n = 78)	(n = 103)	(n = 230)
LSIL	18 (23.1%)	20 (19.4%)	76 (33.0%)
Mild to moderate dysplasia	3 (3.8%)	0	9 (3.9%)
HSIL	2 (2.6%)	7 (6.8%)	22 (9.6%)

Abbreviations: LSIL, low-grade squamous intraepithelial lesions; *HSIL*, high-grade squamous intraepithelial lesions.
*Does not include one case of adenocarcinoma in situ.
(Courtesy of Kline MJ, Davey DD: Atypical squamous cells of undetermined significance qualified: A follow-up study. *Diagn Cytopathol* 14:380–384. Copyright 1996, Wiley-Liss Inc. Reprinted by permission of Wiley-Liss, Inc., a subsidiary of John Wiley & Sons, Inc.)

hyperchromasia, or more irregular nuclear membranes were observed more frequently in ASCUS FD than ASCUS FR. Cells with enlarged pale nuclei and regular nuclear outlines but lacking typical inflammatory changes, such as nucleoli or perinuclear halos, were detected more often in ASCUS FR than ASCUS FD.

Conclusion.—The use of "ASCUS favoring dysplasia" in qualifying the ASCUS diagnosis was supported with these findings. This category may be helpful in identifying patients needing more aggressive follow-up.

▶ This article suggests that what many have been thinking about ASCUS may actually be true: that is, diagnoses at the low end of the ASCUS spectrum don't mean much, but those that really make us think about dysplasia are much more likely to be significant. It is also useful to have this window into the practice of persons who we can regard as experts in the field. We can infer from an ASCUS:SIL ratio of 1.0 that ASCUS is a diagnosis that is used rather sparingly; most of us have higher ratios. Only a minority of the ASCUS interpretations were further qualified (30%). I suspect that this figure would vary widely if we looked at several laboratories. Those expert witnesses ("rogue experts," as I have called them elsewhere in this book) who cite missed ASCUS as negligent practice should reflect on these data.

M.W. Stanley, M.D.

Suggested Reading

Davey DD, Naryshkin S, Nielsen ML, et al: Atypical squamous cells of undetermined significance: Interlaboratory comparison and quality assurance monitors. *Diagn Cytopathol* 11:390–396, 1994.

Robb JA: The "ASCUS" swamp. *Diagn Cytopathol* 11:319–320, 1994.

Young NA, Naryshkin S, Atkinson BF, et al: Interobserver variability of cervical smears with squamous cell abnormalities: A Philadelphia study. *Diagn Cytopathol* 11:352–357, 1994.

Evaluation of the 5-Year Review of Negative Cervical Smears in Patients With High Grade Squamous Intraepithelial Lesions

Tabbara SO, Sidawy MK (George Washington Univ, Washington, DC)
Diagn Cytopathol 15:7–11, 1996

4–2

Objective.—The Clinical Laboratory Improvement Act (CLIA) of 1988 requires reanalysis of all available negative cervical smears in the 5 years preceding a new diagnosis of high-grade squamous intraepithelial lesion (HSIL) or carcinoma. The merit of the regulation was evaluated by a retrospective review of negative cervical smears for 5 years preceding a new diagnosis of HSIL.

Methods.—Smears of 47 patients diagnosed with HSIL were re-examined and classified as unsatisfactory, within normal limits, reactive cellular changes, low grade squamous intraepithelial lesion (LSIL), HSIL, and squamous cell carcinoma. Underdiagnosed SIL was the result of a screening error, where abnormal cells were missed, or an interpretive error, where the abnormal cells were identified but not recognized as possible SIL.

Results.—The re-examination found underdiagnosed SIL in 7 patients at 1 year, 12 at 2 years, 15 at 3 years, and 16 at 5 years. Re-examination of the last smear found 9 of the 16 patients, re-examination of the last 2 smears identified 13, and review of the last 4 smears found 15. In 13 smears interpretive error led to underdiagnosis. Screening error resulted in underdiagnosis in 9 smears. In total, 8 smears were upgraded to a diagnosis of LSIL, and 14 were upgraded to HSIL. No single individual was responsible for the underdiagnosis.

Conclusion.—Whereas the 5-year review does not furnish an evaluation of any individual's diagnostic abilities, it does provide a good quality assurance method that could improve quality. A 3-year review period resulted in detection of 94% of underdiagnosed SIL.

▶ This paper uses a careful approach to confirm 2 things we already know. First, in patients with HSIL, a certain portion of their antecedent negative Pap smears will be false negatives that may show atypical squamous cells of undetermined significance or an SIL. Second, a 2- to 3-year retrospective review is approximately as effective as the CLIA-mandated 5-year review. In the laboratory under study, the problem cases were apparently distributed randomly among the entire cytotechnology and cytopathology staff. This demonstrates the reality of the "irreducible false negative" concept. Furthermore, it indicates that an occasional miss in the setting of otherwise acceptable performance cannot serve as a basis for administrative decision-making in the laboratory.

M.W. Stanley, M.D.

Suggested Reading

Allen KA, Zaleski S, Cohen MB: Review of negative Papanicolaou tests: Is the retrospective 5-year review necessary? *Am J Clin Pathol* 101:19–21, 1994.

Tabbara SO, Sidawy MK: Evaluation of the 10% rescreen of negative gynecologic smears as a quality assurance measure. *Diagn Cytopathol* 14:84–86, 1996.

Frequency of Tumor Diathesis in Smears From Women With Squamous Cell Carcinoma of the Cervix

Rushing L, Cibas ES (Harvard Med School, Boston)
Acta Cytol 41:781–785, 1997   4–3

Background.—The finding of tumor diathesis (TD) alone is not reliable enough to establish a diagnosis of malignancy. The frequency of TD in invasive cancer has not been evaluated in any published studies to date. The prevalence of TD in cervicovaginal smears from patients with squamous cell carcinoma (SCC) was determined.

Methods and Findings.—All 28 smears from 19 patients obtained within 1 year of a biopsy diagnosis of SCC were reviewed. Patients undergoing cervical irradiation before the smear was obtained were excluded from the analysis. Two examiners documented the presence and extent of TD. Fifty-four percent of the smears showed TD. The presence of TD was positively associated with the depth of invasion.

Conclusions.—Although TD is an important criterion of malignancy, it is not found in some cases of SCC, especially in those with less than 5 mm of invasion. Definitively distinguishing between an intraepithelial lesion and a shallow invasive cancer may not be possible on cervicovaginal smears.

▶ We have all been taught to look for a TD when considering a diagnosis of invasive SCC of the uterine cervix. Those who participate in cytology continuing medical education courses will find the presence or absence of a diathesis listed as a diagnostic criterion for or against invasive carcinoma, respectively. Because this pattern represents tissue damage, we are not surprised to find that several things can cause a diathesis, including atrophy, pyometra, cervical stenosis, ulcerative infections, and acute radiation damage (the latter was specifically excluded from this study). These authors have extended our thinking on this subject by noting that almost half of their 28 smears from patients with invasive carcinoma did not show this pattern. Many of these diathesis-negative cases were from tumors that were invasive to depths of less than 5 mm. The concept of microinvasive carcinoma is clinically very important, but it has virtually disappeared from our cytology laboratories' diagnostic lexicon, which is an event celebrated by many of us. Furthermore, we now know that high-grade squamous intraepithelial lesions (HGSIL) that extend into the endocervical glands can show small nucleoli, which further reduces any diagnostically meaningful cytologic differences between HGSIL and many carcinomas with early invasion. When associated with numerous abnormal cells, a TD pattern is still diagnostically useful. However, its absence in a case of HGSIL does nothing to rule out invasion; this can only be accomplished by adequate sampling for histologic study.

M.W. Stanley, M.D.

Suggested Reading

Buckner S-B, England JM, Batheja N: General cytologic principles, in Atkinson B (ed): *Atlas of Diagnostic Cytopathology.* Philadelphia, WB Saunders, 1992, pp 8, 48.

Ehrmann RL: *Benign to Malignant Progression in Cervical Squamous Epithelium.* New York, Igaku-Shoin, 1994, p 150.

Rescreening in Gynecologic Cytology: Rescreening of 8096 Previous Cases for Current Low-grade and Indeterminate-grade Squamous Intraepithelial Lesion Diagnoses—A College of American Pathologists Q-Probes Study of 323 Laboratories
Jones BA (St John Hosp, Detroit)
Arch Pathol Lab Med 120:519–522, 1996   4–4

Background.—The Clinical Laboratory Improvement Amendments of 1988 require rescreening of gynecologic specimens diagnosed as normal or negative in the 5 years preceding a currently identified intraepithelial lesion of high grade or above. This has been an efficient way to identify false-negative cytologic results. Although not required, the rescreening of previous negative smears after a diagnosis of a low-grade squamous intraepithelial lesion has also been reported. The value of such rescreening was investigated.

Methods and Findings.—This College of American Pathologists Q-Probes study included a total of 8,096 smears performed at 323 laboratories. All had been done within 5 years preceding a current examination. Six percent of the rescreened cases were reclassified as atypical squamous cells of uncertain significance, 3.5% were reclassified as squamous intraepithelial lesions or carcinomas, 0.5% were classified as unsatisfactory specimens, and 0.09% were reclassified as atypical glandular cells of uncertain significance or glandular intraepithelial lesions. Ninety-three percent of the false-negative results occurred in cases from the previous 3 years (Table 2; Fig).

Conclusions.—Screening and diagnostic errors can be identified through a policy of rescreening archival cytologic specimens previously diagnosed as within normal limits or diagnosed as benign cellular changes for patients with current diagnoses of low-grade squamous intraepithelial lesions or squamous intraepithelial lesions of indeterminate grade. Many laboratories may find this useful for monitoring quality improvement.

▶ Review of previous negative Pap smears from patients with newly diagnosed high-grade squamous intraepithelial lesions (HGSIL) or carcinomas has been mandated. This time the Q-Probe people are wondering about the yield from reviewing previous negatives from patients with new diagnoses of low-grade lesions (LGSIL) or ungraded dysplasia. Not surprisingly, an array

TABLE 2.—Rescreen Diagnoses for Cases Originally Diagnosed as Within Normal Limits/Negative or Benign Cellular Changes, Distributed by Their Current Diagnoses

| | Cases Originally Diagnosed as WNL/Negative (%) | | Cases Originally Diagnosed as BCC (%) | | |
| | Current Diagnosis SIL-IG | Current Diagnosis LSIL | Current Diagnosis SIL-IG | Current Diagnosis LSIL | Total |
Rescreen Diagnosis	(n = 243)	(n = 6324)	(n = 42)	(n = 1487)	(n = 8096)
WNL	84.8	84.3	2.4	3.3	69.0
BCC	7.8	6.7	81.0	82.9	21.1
ASCUS	3.7	5.5	4.8	7.7	5.9
SIL-IG	1.7	0.2	9.5	0.7	0.4
LSIL	2.1	2.6	2.4	4.7	2.9
HSIL	0.0	0.1	0.0	0.3	0.2
Squamous carcinoma	0.0	0.0	0.0	0.0	0.0
AGUS/GIL	0.0	0.1	0.0	0.1	0.09
Adenocarcinoma	0.0	0.02	0.0	0.0	0.01
Unsatisfactory	0.0	0.5	0.0	0.4	0.5

Abbreviations: WNL, within normal limits; *BCC*, benign cellular changes; *SIL-IG*, squamous intraepithelial lesion of indeterminate grade; *LSIL*, low-grade squamous intraepithelial lesion; *ASCUS*, atypical squamous cells of uncertain significance; *HSIL*, high-grade squamous intraepithelial lesion; *AGUS/GIL*, atypical glandular cells of uncertain significance/glandular intraepithelial lesion.

(Courtesy of Jones BA: Rescreening in gynecologic cytology: Rescreening of 8096 previous cases for current low-grade and indeterminate-grade squamous intraepithelial lesion diagnoses—A College of American Pathologists Q-Probes study of 323 laboratories. *Arch Pathol Lab Med* 120:519–522, 1996.)

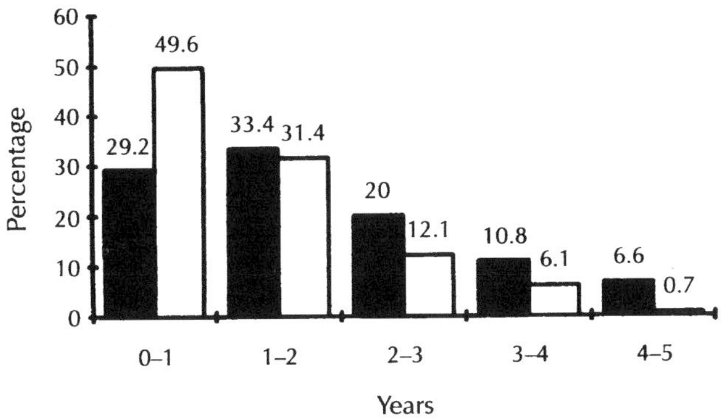

FIGURE.—Distribution of all rescreened cases (*shaded bars*) and false-negative cases (*unshaded bars*) (narrow definition) by the time interval between the original report dates of the rescreened cases and the report dates of the current cases that prompted their rescreening. (Courtesy of Jones BA: Rescreening in gynecologic cytology: Rescreening of 8096 previous cases for current low-grade and indeterminate-grade squamous intraepithelial lesion diagnoses—A College of American Pathologists Q-Probes study of 323 laboratories. *Arch Pathol Lab Med* 120:519–522, 1996.)

of errors was detected. The overall rate of missed abnormalities that would have prompted patient follow-up was 9.9% in contrast to a previously published rate of 20.4% for smears with HGSIL (Jones' article in 1995). Many of these were LGSIL, but, among these 8,096 smears, there were 13 missed HGSILs and 1 missed adenocarcinoma. When cases previously considered normal were evaluated, most errors were a result of screening problems. However, rescreening of cases previously believed to show benign cellular changes frequently revealed interpretive errors. An additional important point is not merely the fact that abnormalities were found among smears previously thought to be negative—that was inevitable. The issue is that the federally mandated standards are minimums and that our profession continues to find ways in which we need to go beyond these guidelines to ensure the best possible quality control and patient care. In this study, 95% of 323 survey-respondent laboratories indicated having a standard procedure for reviewing previous negative smears from patients with new diagnoses of LGSIL or ungraded dysplasia.

M.W. Stanley, M.D.

Suggested Reading

Allen KA, Zaleski S, Cohen MB: Review of negative Papanicolaou test. *Am J Clin Pathol* 101:19–21, 1994.

Hatem F, Wilbur D: High-grade cervical lesions following negative Papanicolaou smears. *Diagn Cytopathol* 12:135–141, 1995.

Jones BA: Rescreening in gynecologic cytology: Rescreening of 3762 previous cases for current high-grade squamous intraepithelial lesions and carcinoma—A College of American Pathologists Q-probes study of 312 institutions. *Arch Pathol Lab Med* 119:1097–1103, 1995.

Glandular Lesions of the Cervix: Validity of Cytologic Criteria Used to Differentiate Reactive Changes, Glandular Intraepithelial Lesions and Adenocarcinoma

DiTomasso JP, Ramzy I, Mody DR (Oregon Health Sciences Univ, Portland; Baylor College of Medicine, Houston)
Acta Cytol 40:1127–1135, 1996   4–5

Background.—Although the incidence of squamous cell carcinoma of the uterine cervix is decreasing because of early detection of a precursor lesion, the incidence of cervical adenocarcinoma is increasing. Factors that may contribute to this increase include a decrease in the incidence of squamous cell carcinoma, resulting in a relative increase in adenocarcinoma; and a possible absolute increase in cervical adenocarcinoma. Improved sampling of the endocervical canal has led to an increase in detection of other lesions that can mimic adenocarcinoma.

Methods.—Twenty-three cytologic criteria were used to evaluate 73 cervicovaginal smears with evidence of glandular lesions. The cases were classified as reactive/benign glandular lesions, low-grade glandular intraepithelial lesions, high-grade glandular intraepithelial lesions, and invasive adenocarcinoma.

Results.—Reactive lesions had well-defined cell borders, normal nuclear/cytoplasmic ratio, little or no nuclear overlapping, round to oval nuclei with fine chromatin, and prominent nucleoli. High-grade glandular intraepithelial lesions had feathered edges, rosettes, cell strips, higher nuclear/cytoplasmic ratio, elongated nuclei, clear nuclear overlapping, and nuclei with hyperchromatic, coarse chromatin. Invasive adenocarcinoma had some features of high-grade glandular intraepithelial lesions, but tended to show a dirty background, single cells, mitotic figures, nuclear pleomorphism, and large nucleoli (Table 1). The odds ratio for predicting invasion was increased by the presence of mitotic figures, a dirty background, and single cells. Low-grade glandular intraepithelial lesions had some features of high-grade lesions, but with more subtle differences. Low-grade lesions were also less cellular and less likely to have cell strips, feathered edges, and rosettes. The low-grade lesions had nuclear overlapping, higher nuclear/cytoplasmic ratio, oval or elongated nuclei, and nuclear hyperchromasia.

Discussion.—The cytologic criteria for various glandular lesions of the cervix overlap. Some of the cytologic criteria can differentiate significant lesions from reactive benign changes in the glandular epithelium. There is a need for defining benign and malignant cervical glandular lesions as new techniques for sampling the endocervical canal are developed.

▶ The first thing to know about this paper is the authors' reclassification of endocervical glandular abnormalities. Invasive adenocarcinoma is unchanged, but adenocarcinoma in-situ (AIS) becomes "high-grade glandular intraepithelial lesion (HGIL)." Between AIS and clearly reactive lesions is a residuum of bothersome abnormalities termed low-grade glandular intraep-

TABLE 1.—Glandular Lesions of the Endocervix: Cytologic Criteria and Results in 73 Cases

Criterion	Reactive (n=29)	LGIL/endocervical glandular dysplasia (n=7)	HGIL/AIS (n=17)	IA (n=20)
General				
Dirty background (%)	7	0	18	55
Cellularity	3+	1–2+	3–4+	3–4+
Supercrowding (%)	10	14	41	45
Cell patterns (%)				
Cell strips	10	29	71	45
Feathered edges	7	29	77	55
Rosettes	3	14	59	80
Papillary groups	0	0	6	5
Single cells	3	0	35	85
Cytoplasmic criteria				
Squamoid cells (%)	21	0	12	15
Cell borders	Well defined	Ill defined	Ill defined	Ill defined
Cell size	Large	Normal to slightly large	Normal to slightly large	Normal to slightly large
Terminal bars/cilia (%)	7	0	0	0
Cytoplasmic vacuoles (%)	7	0	12	20
Apoptosis (%)	7	0	12	10
Nuclear features				
Nuclear overlap (%)	17	86	100	100
Increased N/C ratio	Normal	Mild	Marked	Marked
Increased nuclear size	Mild	Moderate	Marked	Marked
Nuclear shape	Round/oval	Oval to slightly elongated	Oval to elongated	Elongated/pleo-morphic
Chromatin	Fine	Moderate	Moderate/coarse	Coarse, with clearing
Hyperchromasia	Normal to mild	Moderate	Moderate/marked	Moderate/marked
Nucleoli present (%)	60	57	65	80
Nucleolar size	Large	Small	Small	Large
Mitotic figures (%)	3	14	18	60

Note: Percent represents the number of cases showing those criteria. Normal endocervical cells were used as a comparison for changes seen in nucleus and in cell size.
(Courtesy of DiTomasso JP, Ramzy I, Mody DR: Glandular lesions of the cervix: Validity of cytologic criteria used to differentiate reactive changes, glandular intraepithelial lesions and adenocarcinoma. *Acta Cytol* 40:1127–1135, 1996.)

ithelial lesions (LGIL). When all lesions less severe than invasive adenocarcinoma are considered, increasing cellularity, less cytoplasm, increased nuclear size, more elongated nuclear shape, increasing hyperchromasia, greater nuclear overlap, rosettes, cell strips, feathered edges, single cells, chromatin clumping, smaller nucleoli, and more frequent mitoses connote higher grade lesions. None of this is surprising. In this scheme, LGIL is defined as something between reactive and HGIL. The Bethesda System can only place LGIL (and, for that matter, AIS) in the atypical glandular cells of uncertain significance (AGUS) category. These authors recommend appending "favor a low-grade glandular intraepithelial lesion" to cases that fit their LGIL category. Their Figure 5 fits at least one portion of my personal mental image of many AGUS cases. But the literature tells us that many of these cases ultimately show glandular involvement by squamous lesions or tubal metaplasia.

As I understand the current state of our knowledge, preneoplastic lesions of endocervical glandular epithelium that are less advanced than AIS have not been defined in histologic terms. Describing their cytology thus seems problematic indeed. The AGUS classification conveys the uncertainty we have about these lesions. In short, whatever lies between reactive/reparative and AIS is, in my opinion, uncharted territory. Thus, I am bothered by a term like LGIL for a lesion that has no agreed-to histologic correlate and no known biological significance. Those of us who enjoy writing papers must do so with our eyes open. We no longer write only for each other or for other physicians. In another commentary, I mentioned our profession's problem with "rogue experts" testifying in Papanicolaou smear litigation. We are aware of trivial abnormalities having been said to represent problems that might have eventuated in a malignancy. We need to ensure that our literature does not overstate our abilities. Many would agree that such overstatements are in part responsible for the current malpractice crisis.

M.W. Stanley, M.D.

Suggested Reading

Selvaggi SM: Cytologic features of squamous cell carcinoma in-situ involving endocervical glands in endocervical cytobrush specimens. *Acta Cytol* 38:687–692; 1994.

Wilbur DC: Endocervical glandular atypia: A "new" problem for the cytologist. *Diagn Cytopathol* 13:463–469, 1995.

"Arias-Stella Reaction"–like Changes in Endocervical Glandular Epithelium in Cervical Smears During Pregnancy and Postpartum States: A Potential Diagnostic Pitfall

Benoit JL, Kini SR (Henry Ford Hosp, Detroit; Pasqua Hosp, Regina, Sask)
Diagn Cytopathol 14:349–355, 1996   4–6

Introduction.—The Arias-Stella reaction is easily identified histologically (Table 1) in gestational endometrium and extraendometrial sites. Corresponding cytologic appearance has not been well-defined. Endocervical glandular epithelial changes significant enough to cause diagnostic misinterpretations in 11 women during pregnancy and postpartum were described.

Methods.—The cervical-vaginal smears of women with atypical glandular cells during pregnancy were reviewed retrospectively. The cytologic features of each smear were documented.

Results.—Mean patient age at time of smear was 28 years. Duration of pregnancy on initial visit ranged from 3 months gestation to 6 weeks postpartum. Smears from initial visit were interpreted as "suspicious for adenocarcinoma" in 1 patient and "glandular atypia" in the remaining patients. At 4-year follow-up, 1 woman developed endocervical adenocarcinoma in situ. She had 2 negative smears from initial visit to 4-year follow-up. In 9 patients, subsequent cervical smears were negative on multiple follow-up visits. Significant glandular abnormalities were not detected in 4 patients who underwent cervical biopsies or dilatation and curettage. A spectrum of changes involving the endocervical glandular cells were observed (Table 3), ranging from mildly enlarged endocervical cells at the low end of the spectrum (Fig C, 2) to pronounced cellular and nuclear enlargement at the high end of the spectrum (Fig C, 7). All smears had an inflammatory background.

Conclusion.—Clinical history is essential in specimens collected from women of child-bearing age. Since the Arias-Stella phenomenon has been detected as early at 22 days after the last menstrual period, the patient may

---

TABLE 1.—Histologic Features of Arias-Stella Reaction

Presentation	Complex architectural pattern
	Intraluminal budding
	Infolding of hypertrophic cells
	Hypersecretory glands
Cells	Markedly enlarged
	Hyperchromatic with irregular contours
	Hobnail pattern
	(protruding into the lumen)
Nuclei	Ground glass appearance
	intranuclear inclusions
Cytoplasm	Variable, scant to abundant

TABLE 3.—Cytologic Features of the Arias-Stella Reaction–Like Changes and of Poorly Differentiated Endocervical Adenocarcinoma

	Arias-Stella *reaction-like changes*	*Poorly differentiated* *endocervical adenocarcinoma*
Presentation	Cells isolated, in aggregates and in tissue fragments with crowded and overlapped nuclei	Moderate to marked exfoliation of malignant cells; cells isolated; in loosely cohesive groups, or in syncytial-type tissue fragments with or without acinar or papillary pattern
Cell size	Variable; small to large	Cells small to medium sized with high N/C ratio
Nuclei	Enlarged round to oval; N/C ratio variable, generally high; chromatin granular, often smudgy, ground glass appearance, intranuclear inclusions and prominent nuclear grooves	round to oval, with or without irregular borders; chromatin fine to coarsely granular with parachromatin clearing; bizarre in clear cell variant with "giant forms"
Nucleoli	Variable, single/multiple macro/micronucleoli	
Cytoplasm	Variable, scant to abundant; vacuolated, pale to dense leukophagocytosis	Variable, scant to abundant; usually abundant in clear cell variant
Background	Generally inflammatory	Inflammatory, with or without tumor diathesis

Abbreviation: N/C, nuclear to cytoplasmic.
(Courtesy of Benoit JL, Kini SR: "Arias-Stella reaction"–like changes in endocervical glandular epithelium in cervical smears during pregnancy and postpartum states: A potential diagnositc pitfall. *Diagn Cytopathol* 14:349–355. Copyright 1996 by Wiley-Liss, Inc. Reprinted by permission of Wiley-Liss, Inc., a subsidaiary of John Wiley & Sons, Inc.)

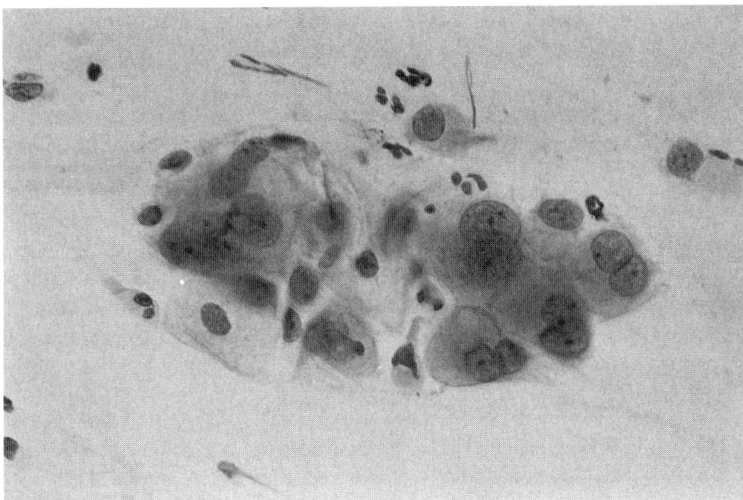

FIGURE C, 2.—Cervical vaginal smear, gestational. Endocervical glandular cells with low nuclear to cytoplasmic ratios, evenly distributed powdery chromatin, and micronucleoli represent Arias-Stella–like changes at the low end of the spectrum (Papanicolaou, ×360). (Courtesy of Benoit JL, Kini SR: "Arias-Stella reaction"–like changes in endocervical glandular epithelium in cervical smears during pregnancy and postpartum states: A potential diagnostic pitfall. *Diagn Cytopathol* 14:349–355. Copyright 1996 by Wiley-Liss, Inc. Reprinted by permission of Wiley-Liss, Inc., a subsidiary of John Wiley & Sons, Inc.)

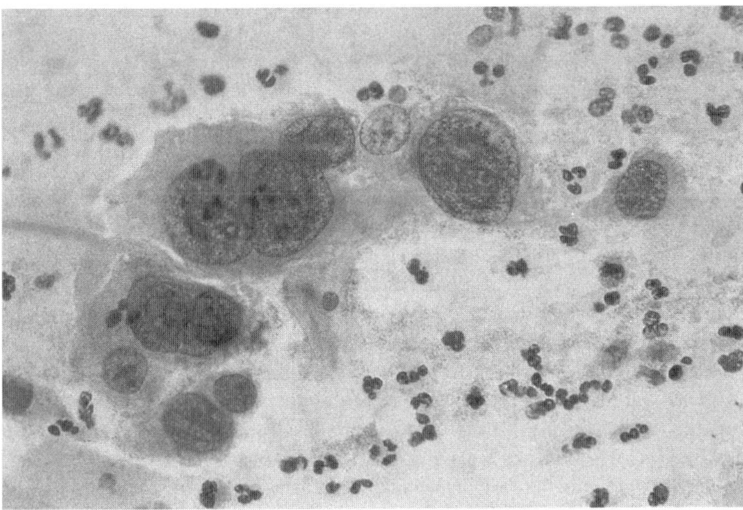

FIGURE C, 7.—Cervical vaginal smear, postpartum. Mrkedly enlarged glandular cells show prominent nuclear grooves and inclusions. Note the binucleation and abundant cytoplasm (Papanicolaou, × 360). (Courtesy of Benoit JL, Kini SR: "Arias-Stella reaction"–like changes in endocervical glandular epithelium in cervical smears during pregnancy and postpartum states: A potential diagnostic pitfall. *Diagn Cytopathol* 14:349–355. Copyright 1996 by Wiley-Liss, Inc. Reprinted by permission of Wiley-Liss, Inc., a subsidiary of John Wiley & Sons, Inc.)

not be aware she is pregnant when giving her history. Diagnostic errors can be averted by taking a pertinent history and being aware of the Arias-Stella reaction.

▶ The authors cite a reference to indicate that this type of reaction can be seen as early in pregnancy as 22 days after the last menstrual period. Although history is very important in interpretation of Papanicolaou smears, the authors point out that, under these circumstances, even the patient herself may not know that she is pregnant. These smears were obtained from women who were pregnant, or who were up to 6 weeks postpartum. One wonders how long cervical Arias-Stella–like changes can persist.

M.W. Stanley, M.D.

Suggested Reading

Holmes EJ, Lyle WH: How early in pregnancy does the Arias-Stella reaction occur? *Arch Pathol* 95:302–303, 1973.

Mulvany NJ, et al: Arias-Stella reaction associated with cervical pregnancy: Report of a case with a cytologic presentation. *Acta Cytol* 38:218–222, 1994.

Cervical Specimens Collected in Liquid Buffer Are Suitable for Both Cytologic Screening and Ancillary Human Papillomavirus Testing
Sherman ME, Schiffman MH, Lorincz AT, et al (George Washington Univ, Washington, DC; Natl Cancer Inst, Bethesda, Md; Digene Corp, Silver Spring, Md; et al)
Cancer 81:89–97, 1997

4–7

Background.—Cervical carcinoma screening using Papanicolaou smears is recognized as an effective screening method, in spite of erroneous and equivocal diagnoses in occasional cases. Equivocal cytologic diagnoses are the most common problem, and are referred to as atypical squamous cells of undetermined significance (ASCUS). Routine referral of women with a diagnosis of ASCUS for colposcopy is impractical because such diagnoses make up 5% to 10% of smears. Detection of human papillomavirus (HPV) DNA is strongly associated with a cervical carcinoma precursor known as squamous intraepithelial lesion. Testing for HPV may help identify women with ASCUS and an underlying squamous intraepithelial lesion.

Methods.—There were 200 cases with cervical abnormalities selected from a screening study of 9,174 women in an area of Costa Rica with a high incidence of cervical carcinoma. All cases had been screened with multiple cytologic and visual methods, ThinPrep slides made from liquid buffer, a computerized slide reading system, and cervicography. Patients with abnormal test results were referred for colposcopy, punch biopsy, or loop excision. Results of ThinPrep cytology and HPV testing were compared to final diagnoses.

Results.—Of the 200 subjects, 7 had a final diagnosis of carcinoma, 44 had high-grade squamous intraepithelial lesions, 34 had low-grade squa-

TABLE 1.—Comparison of ThinPrep Cytologic Diagnoses with Final Case Diagnosis

ThinPrep diagnosis	Final case diagnosis					
	Final-normal	Final-equivocal	Final-LSIL	Final-HSIL	Final-carcinoma	Total
Unsatisfactory	1 (1.6%)	0	0	0	0	1 (0.5%)
Negative	33 (51.6%)	21 (41.2%)	3 (8.8%)	4 (9.1%)	0	61 (30.5%)
ASCUS	30 (46.9%)	19 (37.3%)	6 (17.6%)	6 (13.6%)	2 (28.6%)	63 (31.5%)
LSIL	0	8 (15.7%)	23 (67.6%)	8 (18.2%)	0	39 (19.5%)
HSIL	0	2 (3.9%)	2 (5.9%)	23 (52.3%)	4 (57.1%)	31 (15.5%)
Carcinoma	0	1 (2.0%)	0	3 (6.8%)	1 (14.3%)	5 (2.5%)
Total	64 (100%)	51 (100%)	34 (100%)	44 (100%)	7 (100%)	200 (100%)

Abbreviations: ASCUS, atypical squamous cells of undetermined significance; *HSIL*, high-grade squamous intraepithelial lesion; *LSIL*, low-grade squamous intraepithelial lesion; *SIL*, squamous intraepithelial lesion.

(Courtesy of Sherman ME, Schiffman MH, Lorincz AT, et al: Cervical specimens collected in liquid buffer are suitable for both cytologic screening and ancillary human papillomavirus testing. *Cancer* 81:89–97. Copyright 1997 American Cancer Society. Reprinted by permission of Wiley-Liss, Inc., a subsidiary of John Wiley & Sons, Inc.)

TABLE 3.—Detection of Human Papillomavirus DNA in PreservCyt Using Hybrid Capture, by Final Case Diagnosis

HPV DNA	Final case diagnosis					
	Final-normal (n = 64)	Final-equivocal (n = 51)	Final-LSIL (n = 34)	Final-HSIL (n = 44)	Final-carcinoma (n = 7)	Total (n = 200)
Any type	12 (18.8%)	14 (27.4%)	24 (70.6%)	33 (75.0%)	7 (100%)	90 (45.0%)
Carcinoma-associated	8 (12.5%)	10 (19.6%)	21 (61.8%)	33 (75.0%)	7 (100%)	79 (39.5%)

Abbreviations: HPV, human papillomavirus; *HSIL*, high-grade squamous intraepithelial lesion; *LSIL*, low-grade squamous intraepithelial lesion.

(Courtesy of Sherman ME, Schiffman MH, Lorincz AT, et al: Cervical specimens collected in liquid buffer are suitable for both cytologic screening and ancillary human papillomavirus testing. *Cancer* 81:89–97. Copyright 1997 American Cancer Society. Reprinted by permission of Wiley-Liss, Inc., a subsidiary of John Wiley & Sons, Inc.)

mous intraepithelial lesions, 51 had various equivocal diagnoses, and 64 had normal diagnoses (Table 1). ThinPrep cytology diagnosed squamous intraepithelial lesion or carcinoma in 39 of the 51 subjects with high-grade squamous intraepithelial lesion or carcinoma. In 100% of subjects with carcinoma, 75% with high-grade squamous intraepithelial lesion, 62% with low-grade squamous intraepithelial lesion, 20% with equivocal final diagnoses, and 12% of normal subjects, Hybrid Capture testing detected carcinoma-associated types of HPV DNA (Table 3). If referral for colposcopy had been limited to women with a ThinPrep diagnosis of squamous intraepithelial lesion or ASCUS associated with carcinoma-associated HPV DNA from the same vial, 100% of women with carcinoma and 80% with high-grade squamous intraepithelial lesion would have received examination. Referral of 7% of the population would have been required to achieve this high sensitivity in the entire sample of 9,174 women. The combined screening method would have been marginally better than optimized, conventional screening with referral of any women with abnormal cytologic results.

Discussion.—This new cervical carcinoma screening method uses specimens collected in liquid buffer for cytopathologic diagnosis of thin-layer preparations and HPV testing. This new method would allow clinicians to focus on specimen collection and laboratories to focus on slide preparation, diagnosis, and ancillary testing. The cost-effectiveness of this technique is currently being determined in larger studies.

▶ The problem is ASCUS. In some laboratories, this diagnosis is sufficiently common that referral of all patients for colposcopy is impractical and far from cost-effective. Ironically, some of the newer strategies that are designed to improve identification of abnormal smears do so at the cost of an increased ASCUS burden. Concerted detection of both cytologic abnormalities and the presence of an oncogenic HPV type appears to help identify a subset of ASCUS cases that might harbor a high-grade squamous intraepithelial lesion (HGSIL). These authors take advantage of the fact that, after preparation of a ThinPrep Papanicolaou test slide, the vial still contains cellular material sufficient for HPV testing by an FDA-approved tube test. My impression is that this type of combination cytology/HPV testing will be a part of our practices in the near future. We must note, however, that this type of HPV testing yielded negative results in 5 of 6 women whose ASCUS ThinPrep diagnoses were ultimately shown to represent HGSIL. Furthermore, the authors are candid about an observation that (in my opinion) should inform our public health policy, but that is all too often kept completely out of the conversation by excitement over new machines, with help from marketers and lawyers. On page 95, they write that ". . . the ThinPrep-HPV combination performed only marginally better than the conventional Papanicolaou smear. . . " They go on to describe the extent to which they have optimized the conventional Papanicolaou test during the process of conducting the study. The lesson here seems obvious, but that's just my opinion.

M.W. Stanley, M.D.

Suggested Reading

Bur M, Knowles K, Pekow P, et al: Comparison of ThinPrep preparations with conventional cervicovaginal smears: Practical considerations. *Acta Cytol* 39:631–642, 1995.

Schiffman MH, Kiviat NB, Burk RD, et al: Accuracy and reliability of human papillomavirus DNA testing by Hybrid Capture. *J Clin Microbiol* 33:545–550, 1995.

Wilbur DC, Cibas ES, Merritt S, et al: ThinPrep processor: Clinical trials demonstrate an increased detection rate of abnormal cervical cytologic specimens. *Am J Clin Pathol* 101:209–214, 1994.

Guidelines of the Papanicolaou Society of Cytopathology for the Examination of Fine-needle Aspiration From Thyroid Nodules
Suen K, and the Papanicolaou Society of Cytopathology Task Force on Standards of Practice (Vancouver Hosp & Health Sciences Centre, BC)
Diagn Cytopathol 15:84–89, 1996   4–8

Objective.—Fine-needle aspiration (FNA) of thyroid lesions is a valuable, cost-effective triage procedure. Because a reliable procedure requires low false-negative and false-positive rates, the Papanicolaou Society of Cytopathology has developed guidelines for the examination of FNA thyroid specimens.

Types of Investigations.—The FNA examination is useful in patients with solitary nodules or with autoimmune thyroid disease. It is sometimes used in conjunction with ultrasonographic guidance. Whereas radionuclide scanning is generally not needed, measurement of serum levels of thyroid-stimulating hormone or of antithyroid can provide helpful information.

Proficiency and Technical Aspects.—Adequate sample size, multiple samples obtained by specifically trained, consistently performing individuals, and immediate microscopic evaluation of properly prepared samples are important.

Diagnostic Groups.—The cytopathologist is responsible for determining whether a specimen is suitable for interpretation. Benign, nonneoplastic lesions can be managed conservatively. Cellular follicular lesions, which carry a malignancy rate of 15% to 20%, must be managed individually. Hürthle cell neoplasms may require excision. A diagnosis of malignancy should be based on multiple criteria.

Reporting.—Cytologic reports should be clear and unequivocal. A list of recommended terms is provided. Recommendations for action may be included in the report.

Follow-up.—Patients not requiring thyroidectomy should be followed up by a physician knowledgeable about the course of neoplasms and the limitations of FNA, to decrease the risk of missing a carcinoma.

▶ These suggestions seem useful and practical, and they are based on sound principles of FNA technique and interpretation. Several points stand out as helpful in discussing this method with clinicians. Thyroiditis can be seen as a localized, solitary mass. The most cost-effective approach to evaluation of thyroid nodules begins with FNA; nuclear medicine studies contribute little, but ultrasonography can provide sequential volumetric measurements of masses that are not excised after FNA. One important aspect of this document that is often missing from clinicians' writings on the subject of FNA is the need for training, and for ongoing experience if proficiency in the procedure is to be expected. You cannot dabble in FNA and expect results that approach those in our literature. I enthusiastically applaud the recommendation that 25-gauge needles be used. In my experience, the overwhelming cause of bloody samples and of clinician failures in FNA is the use of unnecessarily large needles. The specimen adequacy suggestions clearly represent a compromise, because the numerous contributors to the final article have a range of opinions that often constitute local standards in their own institutions. The diagnostic criteria, suggestions for report format, and diagnostic terminology are all fairly standard for many of us. All private endocrinologists for whom our laboratory evaluates thyroid FNA smears have been given a copy of this article. We are pleased that it largely confirms methods and thinking already in place in our community. For physicians other than endocrinologists, however, much of this information will be new. In this setting, the force of a consensus document can have a favorable impact on practice standards. We look forward to additional statements from this body.

M.W. Stanley, M.D.

Suggested Reading

Gharib H, Goeliner JR: Fine needle aspiration biopsy of the thyroid: An appraisal. *Ann Intern Med* 118:282, 1993.

Follicular Neoplasms of the Thyroid: Decision Tree Approach Using Morphologic and Morphometric Parameters
Deshpande V, Kapila K, Sai KS, et al (All India Inst, New Delhi)
Acta Cytol 41:369–376, 1997   4–9

Background.—The value of fine needle aspiration of the thyroid is limited in differentiating hyperplastic nodular goiters from true follicular neoplasms and in differentiating follicular adenomas from follicular carcinomas. Whether a panel of morphological and morphometric parameters of the thyroid and ploidy status alone or combined could help distinguish these entities was determined.

Methods and Findings.—Seventy-five smears obtained by fine needle aspiration were reviewed for morphological and morphometric parameters. All had been classified as follicular neoplasms of the thyroid. Of the many parameters investigated, only 2 of the cellular patterns studied—

honeycomb and single dispersed—and the mean maximum nuclear diameter showed trends in differentiating these lesions. On the basis of these patterns and nuclear diameter of less than or greater than μm, a decision tree classification for follicular carcinomas was developed. This decision tree had a sensitivity of 92.8% and a specificity of 57.4% in differentiating benign from malignant lesions.

Conclusions.—The decision tree developed may help distinguish among follicular neoplasms of the thyroid. Other centers now need to assess the efficacy of this classification.

▶ This paper raises a number of questions. In a series of 75 follicular neoplasms, the authors identified 28 (37%) follicular carcinomas. This yield of malignancies is much higher than seen in most experiences, and makes me question the criteria for vascular–capsular invasion. I know that individual thresholds for identifying these key diagnostic features can vary widely. Study of cell cluster patterns (honeycomb, syncytial, etc.) appears to have little utility. Furthermore, those who write about such things seem unable to agree about which lesions most often show which patterns. It is hard to interpret the nuclear diameter information without some idea about the variability within each element of the data set. Most clinicians seem to use thyroid fine-needle aspiration as a screening test. It works well because a large number of masses showing no evidence of thyroiditis or neoplasia can be identified with confidence. With occasional exceptions or embellishments, we could limit our diagnostic lexicon to "operate" vs. "don't operate," and achieve the goals envisioned by most of the physicians who send us slides. Studies that give statistical summaries of morphological information ("cells from disease A have more of something than cells from disease B [P < some number]") are not very useful when we are confronted by a single sample from 1 patient's mass. The situation is little altered by recent investigations: if you see numerous microfollicles and scanty or absent colloid, you should diagnose a follicular neoplasm and inform the clinician that definitive classification requires surgical excision. The good news is that for every one of these unsatisfying reports, you will have sent out approximately 70–90 reports of benign colloid nodules–goiters, and you will have kept most of that majority of patients out of the operating room. After all, fine-needle aspiration is a *very* simple test. As my father used to say, "What do you want for a nickel?"

M.W. Stanley, M.D.

Suggested Reading

Gharib H, Goellner JR: Fine needle aspiration biopsy of the thyroid: An appraisal. *Ann Intern Med* 118:282–290, 1993.

A Method of Teaching Fine Needle Aspiration Biopsy of the Thyroid Gland

Jadusingh IH (Calgary Gen Hosp, Alta; Medical Lab Consultants, Calgary, Alta)
Acta Cytol 41:1156–1158, 1997   4–10

Introduction.—Fine needle aspiration biopsy (FNAB) of the thyroid gland is a standard procedure, but unfortunately, inadequate specimens also seem to be standard procedure. An in vitro method of teaching FNAB is needed that can improve specimen quality and allow microscopic examination.

Biopsy Technique.—A resuscitation manikin, cricothyrotomy simulator, or an airway management trainer can be used for physician education. Needed supplies may be found in most hospitals: needles, syringes, a syringe holder, fixative and glass slides, an unfixed thyroid gland (from an autopsied patient or a less satisfactory formalin-fixed gland), size 8 or bigger latex gloves, a strip of foam about 1.5 cm in thickness, a small pillow, and an examination bed or table. The thyroid gland is positioned in the normal anatomic position on the manikin (Fig 1). The foam is positioned over the gland to imitate subcutaneous fat (Fig 2). The wrist end of the glove is stretched over the head and neck (Fig 3). With the manikin placed on the pillow to simulate a supine patient, the gland is

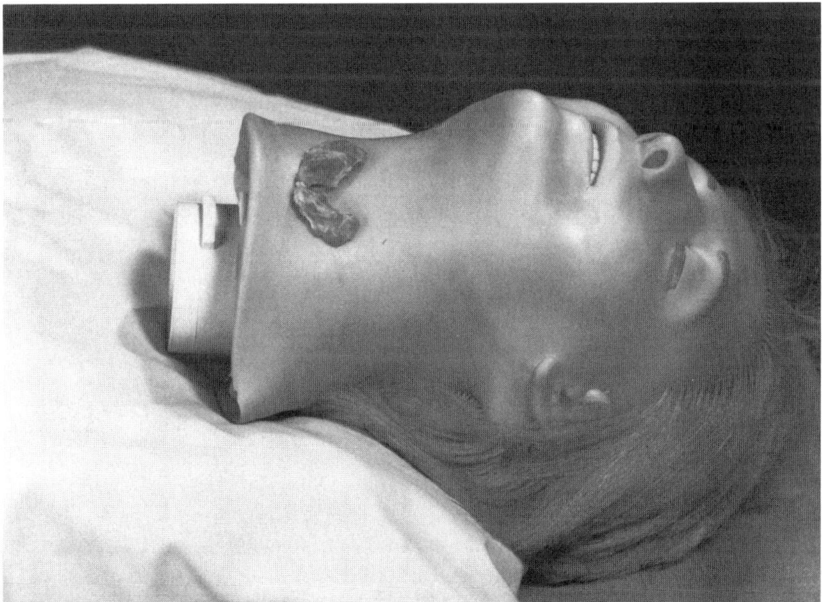

FIGURE 1.—Resuscitation manikin placed on a pillow with a thyroid gland in its anatomic position. (Courtesy of Jadusingh IH: A method of teaching fine needle aspiration biopsy of the thyroid gland. *Acta Cytologica* 41:1156–1158, 1997.)

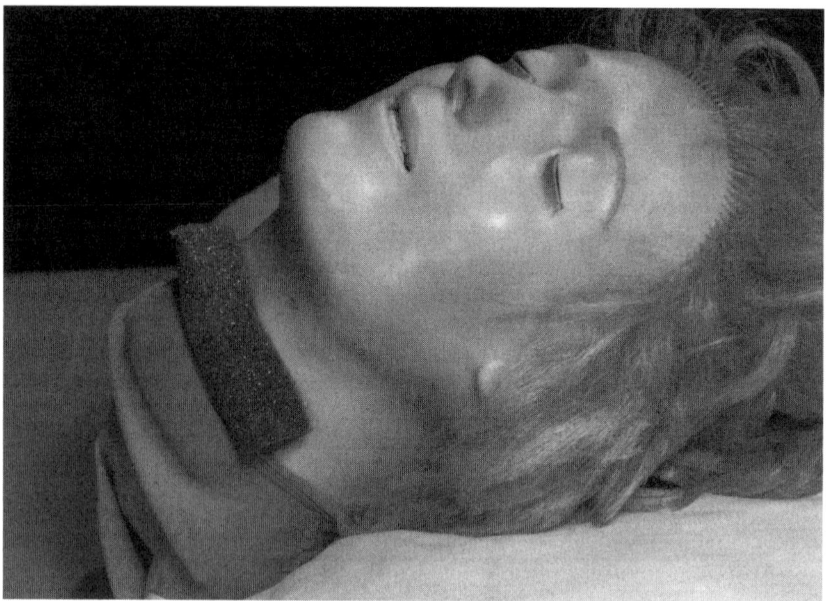

FIGURE 2.—Foam padding, simulating subcutaneous fat. (Courtesy of Jadusingh IH: A method of teaching fine needle aspiration biopsy of the thyroid gland. *Acta Cytologica* 41:1156–1158, 1997.)

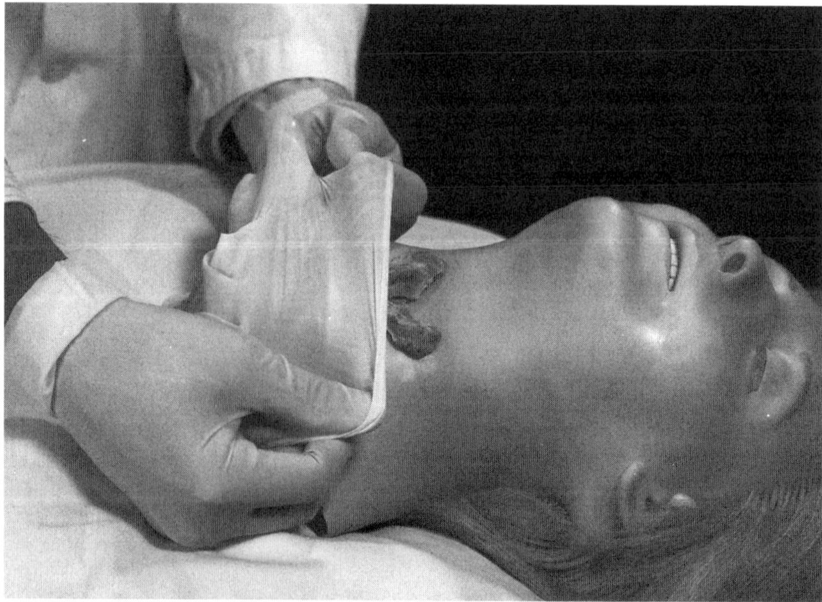

FIGURE 3.—Wrist end of a latex glove stretched over the neck of the manikin. (Courtesy of Jadusingh IH: A method of teaching fine needle aspiration biopsy of the thyroid gland. *Acta Cytologica* 41:1156–1158, 1997.)

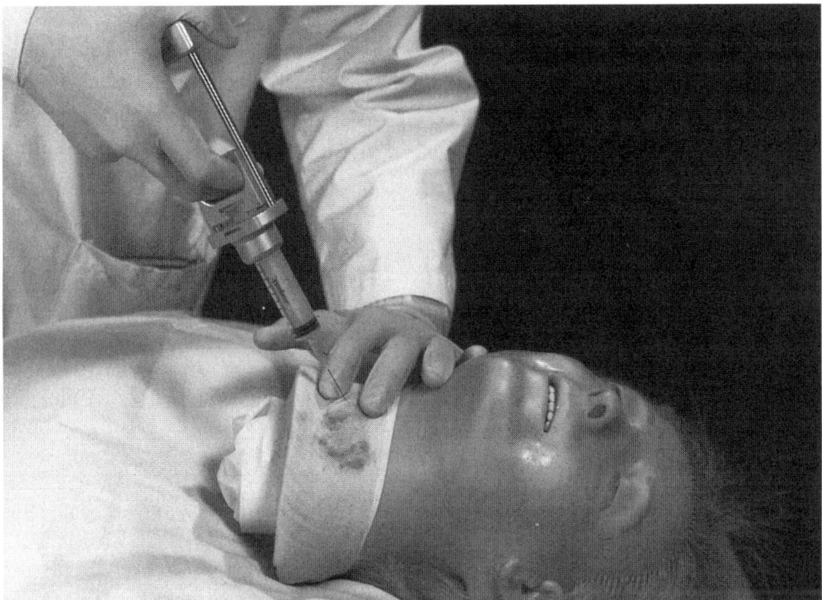

FIGURE 4.—Thyroid gland examined and aspirated (foam material removed for clarity). (Courtesy of Jadusingh IH: A method of teaching fine needle aspiration biopsy of the thyroid gland. *Acta Cytologica* 41:1156–1158, 1997.)

examined and aspirated (Fig 4). When fresh tissue is used, appropriate body and fluid precautions should be followed.

Conclusion.—The proposed method may be used to shorten the learning process for the novice aspirator and hopefully improve the quality of FNAB of the thyroid gland.

▶ The thyroid gland is probably one of the most accessible organs for fine needle aspiration evaluation and certainly one of the most difficult ones to adequately sample for the inexperienced operator. Because of the rich vascularization of the gland, it is not uncommon to receive numerous syringes filled with blood and an accompanying cytology request slip laconically stating: "thyroid tissue." These samples are more appropriate for a complete blood count but rarely yield any relevant glandular diagnostic material. It is a problem very difficult to correct with some clinicians, especially those who will not accept the common sense approach to send their patients to an experienced pathologist for the procedure. Pleading, begging, threatening, and bribing these doctors for better quality samples has consistently failed in my experience. The only system which has worked in our laboratory has been to demonstrate to the clinician, at his or her office, the different steps involved with a successful fine needle aspiration procedure. The method of teaching described above is easy to apply and is transportable to any office, teaching class, or seminar for demonstration purposes. I would certainly recommend using it.

K.E. Sirgi, M.D.

Post–Fine-Needle Biopsy Infarction of Thyroid Neoplasms: A Review of 28 Cases

Kini SR (Henry Ford Hosp, Detroit)
Diagn Cytopathol 15:211–220, 1996   4–11

Objective.—Although fine needle aspiration (FNA) is generally not a traumatic procedure, there have been recent reports of partial or total infarction of thyroid masses after FNA. Reports of 28 cases of thyroid infarctions after FNA and their cytohistologic correlations are presented.

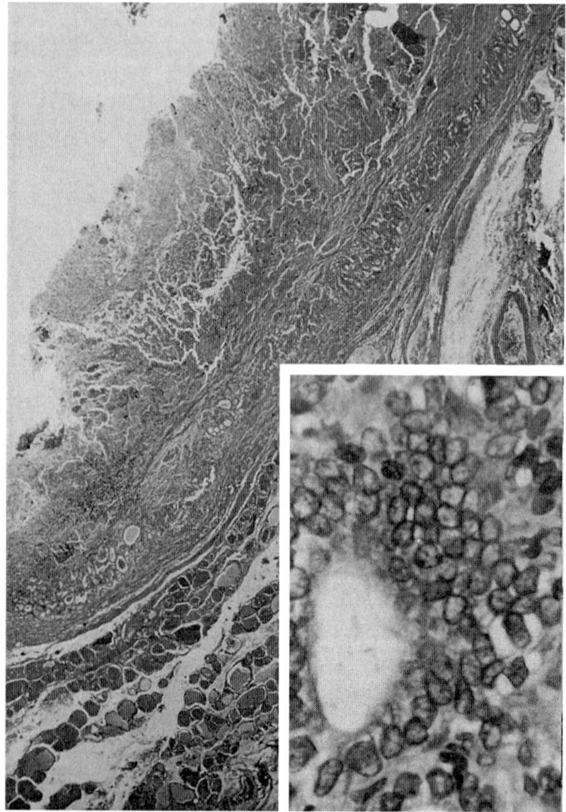

FIGURE 10.—The original histologic diagnosis on excised thyroid was hemorrhagic nodule. The residual tumor at the periphery (*arrow*) was overlooked (hematoxylin and eosin, × 110). **Inset:** Higher magnification of the residual tumor with water clear nuclei confirming the cytologic diagnosis of papillary carcinoma (case #14) (hematoxylin and eosin, × 400). (Courtesy of Kini SR: Post-fine-needle biopsy infarction of thyroid neoplasms: A review of 28 cases. *Diagn Cytopathol* 15:211–220, copyright 1996 by Wiley-Liss, Inc. Reprinted by permission of Wiley-Liss, Inc., a subsidiary of John Wiley & Sons, Inc.)

Methods.—Fine needle aspirations were performed with 20- to 25-gauge needles. Smears were stained by the Papanicolaou method. Large needle biopsies were also performed on 9 patients with lesions larger than 2 cm within 3 weeks of FNA. Surgery followed biopsy within 9 to 90 days in 27 patients.

Results.—Cytologically, there were 15 Hürthle cell tumors, 8 papillary carcinomas, and 5 follicular neoplasms. The 27 surgery patients showed 5 partial and 22 almost complete infarctions. Of the 9 patients who also had a large needle biopsy, 3 showed infarction. Within the infarcted group, the presence of a thin ring of neoplastic tissue at the edge was diagnostic in 8 Hürthle cell tumors and 4 papillary carcinomas. There was no diagnosis in 10 other cases. Three cases were diagnosed as papillary carcinoma. When these 13 cases were retrospectively reviewed, Hürthle cell tumor was diagnosed in 3 cases and papillary carcinomas in 3 (Fig 10). Histologic and cytologic diagnoses were not in agreement in 12 cases because diagnostic elements were obscured or pathologists were not aware of cytologists' findings.

Conclusion.—Cytologic results of thyroid FNA should be available to pathologists so that any neoplasms present are not missed. The presence of either necrosis or infarction should initiate careful examination of the specimen, particularly if neoplasm has been diagnosed.

▶ This is one of those problems that is not very common and that cannot be predicted. As rare as it seems to be, it is apparently more common than spontaneous infarction of thyroid neoplasms. Potential problems in diagnosis are heightened if the surgical pathologist is not aware of the previous procedure and its result, or if one fails to carefully evaluate the thin peripheral rim of viable tissue that frequently remains. We have also seen an example of post-FNA infarction of malignant lymphoma in which an excisional biopsy performed 2 weeks after the FNA showed only a floridly proliferative, fasciitis-like spindle cell lesion. This was initially mistaken for a sarcoma, until correlation with the antecedent FNA was performed. A subsequent biopsy confirmed the initial diagnosis of lymphoma. In this article, there is no mention of post-FNA clinical findings that might have indicated a problem. These authors have focused on neoplasms; most such cytologic diagnoses are followed by surgical excision. On the other hand, a diagnosis of benign colloid nodule/goiter is usually not followed by excision, so that we know less about post-FNA alterations in these conditions. The prominence of Hürthle cell neoplasms in this series is striking. The reason for this is not known, but the authors give some interesting ideas about this observation.

M.W. Stanley, M.D.

Suggested Reading

Batsakis JG: Letters to the editor. *Ann Otol Rhinol Laryngol* 12:484–485, 1993.

LiVolsi VA, Merino MJ: Worrisome histologic alterations following fine-needle aspiration of thyroid. *Pathol Ann* 29:99–120 (part II), 1994.

Us-Krasovec M, Golauth R, Auesperg M, et al.: Tissue damage after fine needle aspiration biopsy. *Acta Cytol* 36:456–457, 1992.

Can Nonproliferative Breast Disease and Proliferative Breast Disease Without Atypia Be Distinguished by Fine-Needle Aspiration Cytology?

Frost AR, Aksu A, Kurstin R, et al (George Washington Univ, Washington, DC)

Cancer 81:22–28, 1997 4–12

Background.—Certain cytologic criteria have been reported to be useful in distinguishing proliferative breast disease without atypia (PBD) from nonproliferative breast disease (NPBD). However, these criteria have not been tested rigorously.

Methods.—Fifty-one air-dried, Diff-Quik[R]-stained fine-needle aspirates of 34 palpable breast lesions with biopsy-proved diagnoses of NPBD and 17 with PBD were reviewed. The criteria evaluated were cellularity, size, and architectural arrangement of the epithelial groups; the presence of single epithelial cells and myoepithelial cells; and nuclear characteristics.

Findings.—A swirling pattern of epithelial cells was the only cytoligic feature that differed significantly between PBD and NPBD. This pattern was noted in 76% of the PBD cases and in 35% of the NPBD cases (Table 1).

Conclusions.—The cytologic features of NPBD and PBD overlap significantly. Thus, fine-needle aspiration is currently not reliable for assessing risk in patients with benign breast disease. Further research on the cytologic identification and subclassification of PBD is needed.

▶ One of the major changes in pathologic practice in the last decade has been a marked improvement in standardized diagnostic criteria and terminology for PBD. We have not achieved perfection, unanimity, or the last word, but things are considerably improved. The concerted consideration of cytologic findings and relatively small-scale architectural derangements suggests that when these lesions are encountered by the aspirating needle, they should yield diagnostic findings that reflect their histopathologic characteristics. In short, many have tried to diagnose and classify PBD in aspirate samples. Some have even suggested that women with no abnormality can be assigned a risk for breast cancer based on blind aspiration of palpably normal breast tissue. The current study finds so much overlap in the cytologic features of proliferative and nonproliferative breast tissue as to render fine-needle aspiration (FNA) virtually useless in addressing these diagnoses. Some previous studies have agreed with this position, whereas other investigators claim striking success in the diagnosis and classification of PBD in aspirate samples. My own opinion has 2 components. First, if you see something "atypical" (whatever that means) on a breast FNA, a surgical

TABLE 1.—Cytologic Features Showing No Statistically Significant Differences

	NPBD	PBD	*p* value
Cellularity			
Low	12/34 (35%)	2/17 (12%)	0.10*
Moderate	12/34 (35%)	5/17 (29%)	
High	10/34 (30%)	10/17 (59%)	0.07†
Size of epithelial groups			
Small	19/34 (56%)	6/17 (35%)	0.24*
Predominantly small	9/34 (25%)	5/17 (30%)	
Large	6/34 (18%)	6/17 (35%)	0.18†
Monolayer	3/34 (9%)	1/17 (6%)	1.00
Cribriform	0/34 (0%)	1/17 (6%)	0.33
Cohesion			
Loose	1/34 (3%)	1/17 (0%)	1.00*
Tight	31/34 (91%)	17/17 (100%)	
Both	2/34 (6%)	0/17 (0%)	0.55†
Single epithelial cells			
None	11/34 (32%)	3/17 (18%)	0.33*
Few	22/34 (65%)	14/17 (82%)	
Many	1/34 (3%)	0/17 (0%)	1.00†
MEC in epithelial groups	32/34 (94%)	17/17 (100%)	0.55
Background MEC			
Few	24/34 (71%)	15/17 (88%)	0.29
Many	10/34 (29%)	2/17 (12%)	
Nuclear size			
$\leq 2\times$ RBC	29/34 (85%)	14/17 (82%)	1.00
$\geq 3\times$ RBC	5/34 (15%)	3/17 (18%)	0.59
Nucleoli			
Absent	2/34 (6%)	0/17 (0%)	0.77*
Micronucleoli	32/34 (94%)	16/17 (94%)	
Macronucleoli	0/34 (0%)	1/17 (6%)	0.59†
Nuclear pleomorphism			
Absent	27/34 (79%)	12/17 (70%)	0.50*
Low	6/34 (18%)	3/17 (18%)	
High	1/34 (3%)	2/17 (12%)	0.26†
Nuclear overlap			
Absent	2/34 (6%)	0/17 (0%)	0.55*
Low	32/34 (94%)	16/17 (94%)	
High	0/34 (0%)	1/17 (6%)	0.33†
Loss of polarity			
Absent	31/34 (91%)	14/17 (82%)	0.39*
Mild	3/34 (9%)	1/17 (6%)	
Marked	0/34 (0%)	2/17 (12%)	0.11†

*Fisher's Exact Test used to compare this cytologic feature with a combination of the 2 immediately below it.
†Fisher's Exact Test used to compare this cytologic feature with a combination of the 2 immediately above it.
Abbreviations: NPBD, Nonproliferative breast disease; *PBD*, proliferative breast disease without atypia; *MEC*, myoepithelial cells; *RBC*, adjacent red blood cell.
(Courtesy of Frost AR, Aksu A, Kurstin R, et al: Can nonproliferative breast disease and proliferative breast disease without atypia be distinguished by fine-needle aspiration cytology? *Cancer* 81:22–28. Copyright 1997 American Cancer Society. Reprinted by permission of Wiley-Liss, Inc., a subsidiary of John Wiley & Sons, Inc.)

biopsy is probably indicated, and detailed statements about PBD have a high probability of turning out to be incorrect. Second, diagnosis and classification of PBD in FNA samples should be considered a purely investigational exercise at this time.

M.W. Stanley, M.D.

Suggested Reading

Masood S, Frykberg ER, McLellan GL, et al: Prospective evaluation of radiologically directed fine-needle aspiration biopsy of nonpalpable breast lesions. *Cancer* 66:1480–1487, 1990.

Stanley MW, Henry-Stanley MJ, Zera R: Atypia in breast fine needle aspiration smears correlates poorly with the presence of a prognostically significant proliferative lesion of ductal epithelium. *Hum Pathol* 24:630–635, 1993.

Thomas PA, Cangiarella J, Raab SS, et al: Fine needle aspiration biopsy of proliferative breast disease. *Mod Pathol* 8:130–136, 1995.

Profileration of Breast Epithelial Cells in Healthy Women During the Menstrual Cycle

Söderqvist G, Isaksson E, von Schoultz B, et al (Karolinska Hosp, Stockholm; Huddinge Univ, Stockholm)
Am J Obstet Gynecol 176:123–128, 1997   4–13

Background.—Hormonal regulation of proliferation in normal breast tissue is not well understood. Proliferation in normal breast epithelial cells obtained from healthy women during the follicular and luteal phases of the menstrual cycle was investigated.

Methods.—Forty-seven women volunteered for the study. Epithelial cells were obtained by fine-needle aspiration biopsy and analyzed for the proliferation marker Ki-67/MIB-1 by immunocytochemical techniques.

Findings.—The proportion of Ki-67/MIB-1–positive cells was 2.04% in the luteal phase, compared with 1.66% in the follicular phase. In women younger than 35years of age, these values were 2.29% and 1.13%, respectively. The proportion of proliferating cells increased from 1.2% in the follicular phase to 2.4% in the luteal phase in ovulating women with 2 aspirates during the same menstrual cycle. Proliferation and serum progesterone levels the day of aspiration were correlated positively.

Conclusions.—These healthy women had a greater proliferation of breast epithelial cells during the luteal phase and a positive association with serum progesterone concentrations. The current findings clearly suggest that progesterone had a proliferative action.

▶ This interesting paper contributes several things to our current thinking about breast fine-needle aspiration cytology. First, it provides clear cell proliferative and endocrinologic evidence of increased cellular activity during the secretory portion of the menstrual cycle. As discussed in the authors' reference 6, this is associated with rather striking morphological alterations. Taken together, this normal physiologic variability could explain many atypical breast aspirates and might suggest that patients should be scheduled for fine-needle aspiration in the first half of the cycle, when possible. Furthermore, these observations are in keeping with the fact that secretory activity has been considered a major source of cytologic atypia in aspirates from fibroadenomas and also has been mistaken for evidence of proliferative breast disease. One is left wishing that the study design could have been expanded to give us a look at these cells in routine fine-needle aspiration smear preparations. We hope that someone will repeat this study of paired follicular and luteal phase aspirations from healthy volunteers and emphasize morphology rather than physiology and endocrinology.

M.W. Stanley, M.D.

Suggested Reading

Longacre TA, Bartow SA: A correlative morphologic study of human breast and endometrium in the menstrual cycle. *Am J Surg Pathol* 10:382–393, 1986.

Stanley MW, Henry-Stanley MJ, Zera R: Atypia in breast fine needle aspiration smears correlates poorly with the presence of a prognostically significant proliferative lesion of ductal epithelium. *Hum Pathol* 24:630–635, 1993.

Stanley MW, Tani EM, Skoog L: Atypical fibroadenoma of the breast: A cause of false positive breast fine needle aspiration. *Diagn Cytopathol* 6:375–382, 1990.

Sialolithiasis: Differential Diagnostic Problems in Fine-Needle Aspiration Cytology
Stanley MW, Bardales RH, Beneke J, et al (Univ of Arkansas, Little Rock; McClellan VA Med Ctr, Little Rock, Ark)
Am J Clin Pathol 106:229–233, 1996   4–14

Introduction.—In the absence of secondary infection, patients with symptomatic sialolithiasis have recurrent pain and swelling related to meals. Chronic obstruction of the salivary gland duct can lead to parenchymal atrophy and periductal chronic inflammation. The fibrotic gland may be very firm, raising clinical suspicion of malignancy. The histologic findings of these pseudoneoplasms include hyperplasia and squamous metaplasia of the epithelium lining the duct, with varying degrees of inflammation. The fine-needle aspiration (FNA) cytology findings of sialolithiasis were reviewed.

Patients.—Five patients with sialolithiasis underwent FNA of a salivary gland mass. There were 3 women and 2 men who had a median age of 65 years. The submaxillary gland was affected in 3 patients and the parotid gland in 2.

Findings.—The cytology specimen showed stone fragments in 3 patients, permitting a diagnosis of sialolithiasis. Two of these patients had surgery. In the other 2 patients, cytology revealed prominent foam cells and metaplastic squamous cells, against a mucoid background that resembled low-grade mucoepidermoid carcinoma. Because these patients did not have stone fragments, the differential diagnosis included low-grade mucoepidermoid carcinoma as well as sialolithiasis. Surgery was performed, revealing sialolithiasis in both cases.

Discussion.—If stone fragments are aspirated, the diagnosis of sialolithiasis is easy to make. When there are no stone fragments, the epithelial changes and mucus accumulation may resemble low-grade mucoepidermoid carcinoma. Sialolithiasis or other lesions obstructing the salivary gland duct should be considered in this situation.

Basal Cell (Monomorphic) and Minimally Pleomorphic Adenomas of the Salivary Glands: Distinction From the Solid (Anaplastic) Type of Adenoid Cystic Carcinoma in Fine-Needle Aspiration
Stanley MW, Horwitz CA, Rollins SD, et al (Univ of Arkansas, Little Rock; McClellan VA Med Ctr, Little Rock, Ark; Abbott-Northwestern Hosp, Minneapolis; et al)
Am J Clin Pathol 106:35–41, 1996   4–15

Background.—In salivary gland fine-needle aspiration (FNA), some uncommon presentations of common tumors, unusual neoplasms, and metastatic deposits may pose diagnostic problems. In the differentiation between basal cell–type monomorphic adenomas and adenoid cystic carcinoma, analysis of the cytologic features of the cell-stroma interface can be helpful. Basal cell adenomas show interdigitation of the collagenous stroma with the adjacent cells, whereas adenoid cystic carcinomas show a sharp, smooth border between the two. Rare spindle cells or capillaries may be found in the stroma of basal cell adenomas, but the cylinders of adenoid cystic carcinoma are acellular. The differentiation between basal cell adenoma and "minimally pleomorphic adenoma" was reviewed in 8 cases.

Methods and Findings.—The analysis included 8 FNA specimens with the cytologic pattern of basal cell adenomas. On histologic analysis, 5 were pure and 3 were minimally pleomorphic adenomas. In the latter group, FNA showed the small blue cell pattern of basal cell adenoma, and histologic examination showed just small foci of typical pleomorphic adenoma. All 8 cases showed the cell-stroma interface pattern of basal cell adenoma, except for 1 cystic case.

The findings of the 2 groups were contrasted with those of 3 cases of solid adenoid cystic carcinoma, with extensive anaplastic areas. The solid carcinomas had both small blue cell pattern and the cell-stroma interface features of basal cell adenoma. The smooth-bordered cylinders associated with adenoid cystic carcinoma were not found in any case. Two of the 3 solid adenoid cystic carcinomas were misinterpreted as benign at FNA.

Conclusions.—Cytologic differentiation between basal cell adenomas and solid adenoid cystic carcinoma can be very difficult. When FNA is performed in solid adenoid cystic carcinoma, the desmoplastic tumor stroma aspirated closely mimics the pattern seen in basal cell adenoma.

When the cytologic diagnosis is adenoid cystic carcinoma, further information must be obtained before definitive surgical therapy is undertaken.

▶ These 2 articles (Abstracts 4–14 and 4–15) remind even the most fanatic supporters (including myself) of the use of FNA biopsies in the diagnostic evaluation of salivary gland lesions that the technique has its limitations, even when the cytopathologist adheres to the strictest morphologic criteria. An unequivocal diagnosis cannot always be established on the basis of FNA alone. Based on the universal medical principle of "first, do no harm," the cytopathologist's role in such a particular setting is to offer an informed differential diagnosis and to avoid the temptation of establishing "kamikaze" diagnosis.

K.E. Sirgi, M.D.

Differential Diagnosis of Adenoid Cystic Carcinoma From Pleomorphic Adenoma of the Salivary Gland on Fine Needle Aspiration Cytology

Lee S-S, Cho K-J, Jang J-J, et al (Seoul Natl Univ, Korea)
Acta Cytol 40: 1246–1252, 1996   4–16

Background.—Although fine needle aspiration (FNA) cytology is 80% to 90% accurate in the diagnosis of pleomorphic adenomas, the most common salivary gland tumor, its sensitivity for diagnosing malignant salivary gland tumors is relatively low. The false-negative findings in this setting may result from difficulty in distinguishing an adenoid cystic carcinoma from a benign mixed tumor on a cytologic smear. Adenoid cystic carcinomas are easy to confuse with high-incidence benign tumors, particularly pleomorphic adenomas. The distinguishing morphological features of these 2 tumors were investigated in a retrospective study.

Methods.—The cytomorphologic features of 9 adenoid cystic carcinomas were compared with that of 12 pleomorphic adenomas of the salivary glands. All cases had been histologically proved.

Findings.—The amount of cytoplasm in individual tumor cells most consistently differentiated adenoid cystic carcinomas from pleomorphic adenomas. A plasmacytoid appearance was a reliable finding that enabled exclusion of an adenoid cystic carcinoma. In all 12 cases of pleomorphic adenomas, tumor cells contained abundant cytoplasm in clusters and isolated cells. A plasma cell-like appearance was noted in 9 cases, especially in isolated cells. Unlike pleomorphic adenomas, little cytoplasm was seen in most adenoid cystic carcinomas. Four adenoid cystic carcinomas and none of the pleomorphic adenomas had hyaline spherical globules, which were specific but not sensitive to adenoid cystic carcinomas. Two thirds of the pleomorphic adenomas showed a fibrillary chondromyxoid ground substance and a mixture of epithelial cells with stroma. The cell cluster pattern helped differentiate pleomorphic adenomas from adenoid cystic carcinomas. The finding of large, loose clusters with spindle cell cores suggested pleomorphic adenomas, whereas small, dense trabeculae with smooth margins and dense clusters containing clear, round spaces were more suggestive of adenoid cystic carcinomas. Overall cellularity, the proportion of isolated cells, the orientation of cellular clusters, and the degree of cellular overlapping were almost no value in helping to differentiate between these lesions.

Conclusions.—A plasmacytoid appearance of individual tumor cells with abundant cytoplasm in pleomorphic adenomas reliably distinguishes them from adenoid cystic carcinomas. Nuclear features did not adequately distinguish between these lesions in isolated cases.

▶ In my opinion, much of the cytologic literature is very good about describing classic findings in many lesions but is often almost silent about diagnostic limitations. The FNA literature seems to foster considerable overconfidence in our ability to diagnose or subclassify all sorts of uncommon entities. One of the areas of most serious overconfidence seems to be that addressed by this paper; some examples of benign mixed tumors (BMTs) (I would add basal cell adenomas) and occasional instances of adenoid cystic carcinomas (ACC) are virtually indistinguishable in FNA samples. (This need not detract from the fact that the majority of BMTs are successfully diagnosed by FNA.) These authors note that cells with minimal cytoplasm typify ACC, whereas, in BMTs, at least some cells have more generous cytoplasmic rims. Plasmacytoid myoepithelial cells are also useful in recognizing BMTs. They found extracellular matrix spheres only in ACCs. The study includes only 12 BMTs; a larger series might have uncovered such material in examples of the well-known pitfall of cylindromatous mixed tumors. Furthermore, nuclear features were not helpful; this confirms our own experience. We do not practice FNA in a vacuum, and additional information can add considerable confidence to the cytologic diagnosis. Pain, seventh nerve damage, or radiographic (CT) evidence of invasive or destructive growth all point strongly toward a malignant diagnosis. Also, if sites other than the major salivary glands are considered, an ACC becomes a much more likely diagnosis than a BMT.

M.W. Stanley, M.D.

Suggested Reading

Hood IC, Qizilbash AH, Salama SSS, et al: Basal cell adenoma of parotid: Difficulty of differentiation from adenoid cystic carcinoma on aspiration biopsy. *Acta Cytol* 27:515–520, 1983.

Stanley MW, Horwitz CA, Rollins SD, et al: Monomorphic and minimally pleomorphic adenomas of the salivary glands (SG): Distinction from the solid (anaplastic) type of adenoid cystic carcinoma in fine needle aspiration (FNA): *Am J Clin Pathol* 106:35–41, 1996.

Squamous Cells in Fine-Needle Aspiration Biopsies of Salivary Gland Lesions: Potential Pitfalls in Cytologic Diagnosis
Mooney EE, Dodd LG, Layfield LJ (Duke Univ, Durham, NC)
Diagn Cytopathol 15:447–452, 1996   4–17

Objective.—The finding of squamous cells in fine needle aspirations (FNAs) of salivary gland lesions is common. Differentiating benign from malignant neoplasms is sometimes difficult. Thirteen of 600 cases of FNAs of salivary gland lesions with squamous elements that represented difficulties in cytologic diagnosis are discussed.

Methods.—Fine needle aspirations performed between January 1984 and July 1995 used the Zajicek method. Air-dried smears were stained with a modified Romanowsky procedure, and alcohol-fixed smears were stained using the Papanicolaou method.

Results.—Thirteen smears had epidermoid features and included chronic sialadenitis, lymphoepithelial cyst, pleomorphic adenoma, Wartin's tumor, mucoepidermoid carcinoma, and squamous cell carcinoma. Careful study of nuclear attributes and other cellular aspects is important for accurate diagnosis after a finding of squamous cells. Proper investigation of a mucoepidermoid carcinoma requires reaspiration of the solid tumor. A finding of intermediate-sized cells containing a bland nucleus and an occasional nucleolus confirms the diagnosis. Keratin pearls and keratinization are absent in mucoepidermoid carcinoma, whereas in squamous cell carcinoma these features are common. Nuclear atypia, anucleate squames, and inflammatory debris are also present in squamous cell carcinoma. Sheets of atypical cells and single atypical epidermoid cells are frequently present. Warthin's tumor requires reaspiration of the solid tumor to find the characteristic oncocytic and lymphoid cells in a background of debris. Hyperchromatic cells may be present. Pleomorphic adenoma aspirates show epithelial and myoepithelial cells and stroma, sometimes confused with mucin. A high threshold for diagnosis is recommended. Lymphoepithelial cysts usually occur in the parotid gland or intraparotid lymph nodes and are associated with HIV infection. These cysts are identified by their cuboid or squamous epithelium and contiguous or infiltrating lymphocytes, histiocytes, and plasma cells. Chronic sialadenitis may be found in a gland bordering a neoplasm. The smear shows hypocellular elements, chronic inflammatory cells, and epidermoid cells with sharp edges. The cell yield is usually low, has tight clusters, and few free epithelial cells. Branchial cleft cysts have squamous or columnar epithelial linings with some degree of inflammatory cell infiltration. There is keratinous debris with a low nuclear-cytoplasmic ratio.

Conclusion.—Evaluation of cellularity, cellular cohesion, the presence of squamous cells, and other cell types is necessary for an accurate differential diagnosis of FNAs of salivary lesions.

▶ In my experience, the salivary glands are second only to the ovary in the number and diversity of neoplasms that they host. This is due in part to the presence of epithelial, myoepithelial, and stromal cells, each of which contributes to this organ's neoplasms in a variety of ways. Diagnosis of these lesions is further complicated by 2 additional factors. First, many of these conditions are quite rare, so that none of us has an opportunity to accumulate significant experience. Second, many are susceptible to a wide range of secondary alterations, including cystic change, chronic inflammation, infarction, squamous metaplasia, and oncocytic alterations. Furthermore, a mass that clinically appears to represent a salivary gland swelling may actually be seated in the gland itself, in the surrounding soft tissues, within a lymph node, or in a branchial cleft-related structure. These authors have concentrated on squamous metaplasia that is 1 complicating factor that can be superimposed on many underlying lesions. When one is dealing with a salivary gland mass in a patient with no other problems, diagnostic difficulty in separating several benign or low grade malignant entities may be of little clinical consequence, as the majority of such lesions share a common surgical approach. On the other hand, if one investigates a mass in this area in a patient with a history of head and neck squamous cell carcinoma (a fairly common event in our practice), squamous cells may occasion considerable diagnostic anxiety. Antecedent radiation therapy only makes matters worse. These authors emphasize sparse cellularity, degenerative features, and background material suggestive of a specific benign diagnosis as helpful diagnostic clues. Some cases will remain very difficult, requiring excision for definitive diagnosis.

M.W. Stanley, M.D.

Suggested Reading

Gottschalk-Sabag S, Glick T: Necrosis of parotid pleomorphic adenoma following fine needle aspiration. *Acta Cytol* 39:252–254, 1995.

Kern SB: Necrosis of a Warthin's tumor following fine needle aspiration. *Acta Cytol* 32:207–208, 1988.

Layfield LJ, Rezniecek M, Lowe M, et al: Spontaneous infarction of a parotid gland pleomorphic adenoma. *Acta Cytol* 36:381–386, 1992.

Fine-needle Aspiration of the Adult Kidney

Renshaw AA, Granter SR, Cibas ES (Harvard Med School, Boston)
Cancer 81:71–88, 1997   4–18

Background.—Fine-needle aspiration of the adult kidney can be an excellent diagnostic tool. In more than 90% of patients with a discrete renal lesion, management is based entirely on radiographic features. The results of renal fine-needle aspiration can affect treatment in 3 specific situations: patients with malignant lesions who may not be suitable for resection, patients with radiographically indeterminate lesions, and patients for whom partial nephrectomy may be preferred over radical nephrectomy. A review of the literature in English on indications and criteria for, and usefulness of, renal fine-needle aspiration was performed.

Findings.—The indications for renal fine-needle aspiration are changing as radiologic imaging of cystic lesions improves and is able to identify more renal lesions incidentally. Cytologic criteria and problems in diagnosing various benign and malignant lesions have been defined. Partial nephrectomy is being performed more and more for some small renal lesions, suggesting that accurate distinction of renal masses may be important to patient management.

Discussion.—Cytopathologists must be able to identify benign lesions and to grade and subtype renal cell carcinomas. The literature offers the criteria for doing this and specifies when those criteria are unreliable. Other topics that are discussed in this extensive article include diagnostic and prognostic criteria of renal fine-needle aspiration in the 3 situations listed above, the value of fine-needle aspiration of cystic lesions, cytologic features and prognostic implications of various subtypes of renal cell carcinoma, and cytologic features of benign and other malignant lesions.

▶ This is a rather lengthy review article, but it is very useful as an update in this complex field. In recent years, several new entities have been described, and the cytology laboratory must keep up with our colleagues' expectations for accurate diagnosis. (Not discussed here is the new cytogenetics-based nosology or renal neoplasia.) Warnings about diagnostic pitfalls abound and include tips about normal tissue (glomeruli and tubular cells of various types), adult congenital polycystic disease, acquired cysts in the setting of renal failure, and cysts with atypia. The problem of renal cortical "adenoma" is handled very well. These authors do an uncommonly wonderful job of pointing out the limitations of fine-needle aspiration. Much of the cytologic literature fails to accomplish this most important goal.

M.W. Stanley, M.D.

5 Urinary Bladder and Male Genitourinary Tract

Papillary Urothelial Hyperplasia: A Precursor to Papillary Neoplasms
Taylor DC, Bhagavan BS, Larsen MP, et al (Johns Hopkins Hosp Med Insts, Baltimore, Md; Sinai Hosp, Baltimore, Md; Good Samaritan Hosp, Baltimore, Md; et al)
Am J Surg Pathol 20:1481–1488, 1996   5–1

Background.—Precursor lesions of papillary urothelial neoplasms have not been well described in the literature. The histologic features of this entity and its relationship to papillary neoplasms were reported.

Methods.—Eleven men and 5 women, aged 40 to 89 years, with papillary hyperplasia (defined as undulating urothelium arranged into thin mucosal papillary folds) were studied. Nine patients had a history of papillary urothelial neoplasms, 1 of whom had subsequent papillary urothelial neoplasms and 2 of whom had concurrent papillary urothelial neoplasms with papillary hyperplasia. Papillary hyperplasia arose in the scar of a previous papillary urothelial neoplasm in 1 of these 9 patients. Another 2 patients had concurrent papillary urothelial neoplasms, yet had no previous history of them. Multiple resections showed papillary hyperplasia over time in 3 of these 11 patients. A twelfth patient had a history of moderate urothelial atypia. In the remaining 4 patients, there was no history of papillary urothelial neoplasms or urothelial atypia.

Conclusion.—Papillary hyperplasia is a well-defined, typically asymptomatic entity. Generally discovered on routine follow-up cytoscopy for papillary urothelial neoplasms, it appears to be a precursor lesion of low-grade papillary urothelial neoplasms.

▶ This article, based on a small number of cases, concludes that papillary hyperplasia "appears to be" a precursor lesion of low-grade urothelial (transitional cell) neoplasms. This is an intriguing proposal, but it is preliminary. It seems reasonable that papillary lesions exist which are not malignancies and which may also represent a precursor lesion. In reality, however, the morphologic distinction between papillary hyperplasia, papilloma, and low grade papillary carcinoma is poorly defined and, I would suspect, very subjective.

The real answer to this question must await molecular-level studies. It should also be pointed out that in an animal model (rat) used by Murphy more than a decade ago,[1] papillary lesions could be induced by instilling distilled water into the bladder. These would regress after the insult was removed.

M.B. Cohen, M.D.

Reference

1. Akaza H, Murphy WM, Soloway MS: Bladder cancer induced by noncarcinogenic substances. *J Urol* 131:152–155, 1984.

Small Cell Neuroendocrine Carcinoma of the Urinary Bladder: A Clinicopathologic Study With Emphasis on Cytologic Features

Ali SZ, Reuter VE, Zakowski MF (Mem Sloan-Kettering Cancer Ctr, New York)
Cancer 79:356–361, 1997   5–2

Purpose.—Pure primary small-cell neuroendocrine carcinoma (SCNEC) of the urinary bladder is a rare, clinically distinct tumor. Its prognosis and treatment are different from that of the more common transitional cell carcinoma, so prompt recognition is important. The cytopathologic features of SCNEC of the bladder were reported.

Patients.—Sixty-one urine specimens from 23 patients with SCNEC of the urinary bladder were investigated. Histologic correlation was available in 16 cases. The patients were 20 men and 3 women, with a mean age of 69 years. The tumor diagnosis was pure SCNEC in 21 patients and high-grade undifferentiated carcinoma with neuroendocrine features in 2 patients. None of the patients had a false-positive or false-negative result on urine cytologic studies. However, several had been initially misdiagnosed as having high-grade transitional cell carcinoma.

Findings.—All patients had hematuria, some with and some without dysuria. On cytologic examination, all cases showed isolated single cells and mostly naked nuclei with scant or absent cytoplasm. Most cases also showed minimal pleomorphism or anisonucleosis, hypercellularity, nuclear molding, and nuclear hyperchromasia with inconspicuous nuclei (Table 2). Less frequent findings included a high mitotic karyorrhectic index, and a bloody inflamed background.

Conclusions.—Cytologic findings in patients with SNEC are distinct and enable an accurate urinary cytologic diagnosis to be made. Other diagnoses to consider are metastatic small-cell carcinoma, high-grade transitional cell carcinoma, and malignant lymphoma. In difficult-to-diagnose cases, immunocytochemistry may be helpful.

TABLE 2.—Cytologic Features (With Approximate Incidence in 61 Urine Specimens)

1) Isolated single cells/lack of nesting or grouping (100%)
2) Mostly naked nuclei seen: rare cells with scant cytoplasm (100%))
3) Minimal pleomorphism or anisonucleosis (90%)
4) Hypercellularity (90%)
5) Nuclear molding (75%)
6) Nuclear hyperchromasia and inconspicuous nucleoli (75%)
7) High mitotic karyorrhectic index (45%)
8) Blood, necrotic, or inflamed background (40%)

(Courtesy of Ali SZ, Reuter VE, Zakowski MF: Small cell neuroendocrine carcinoma of the urinary bladder: A clinicopathologic study with emphasis on cytologic features. *Cancer* 79:356–361. Copyright 1997, American Cancer Society. Reprinted by permission of Wiley-Liss, Inc., a subsidiary of John Wiley & Sons, Inc.)

► This article summarizes the Memorial Sloan-Kettering experience of the urinary cytology of small-cell carcinoma (SCC) of the bladder. It is based on a relatively large experience of 61 urine specimens collected from 23 patients. It should be noted that only a subset of patients (16 of 23) had histologic confirmation of the diagnosis. Important information, however, is missing from this report; for example, (1) were all the cases truly primary bladder carcinomas? (2) were there other histologic types present or were they all pure SCC? (3) what type of urine specimens were examined (voided, bladder wash, etc.)? and (4) were there differences between the cytospin and Thin-prep preparations. Although it is stated that the diagnosis of SCC is accurate, there is another pitfall not fully discussed—namely degenerative changes in both benign and malignant cells.

M.B. Cohen, M.D.

Expression of the CD44 Cell Adhesion Molecule in Urinary Bladder Transitional Cell Carcinoma

Ross JS, del Rosario AD, Bui HX, et al (Albany Med College, NY; Samuel S. Stratton VA Hosp, Albany, NY)
Mod Pathol 9:854–860, 1996   5–3

Background.—The polymorphic integral membrane glycoprotein CD44 cell adhesion molecule is involved in cell matrix adhesion and in lymphocyte activation, recirculation, and homing. Expression of this protein—alternatively known as PgP-1, ECM III, and Hermes antigen—has been reported in malignant lymphoma and various epithelial human cancers. However, its potential role as a prognostic indicator in transitional cell carcinoma of the urinary bladder (UBTCC) has not been studied. Expression of the CD44 cell adhesion molecule in UBTCC was studied and correlated with tumor grade and stage and DNA content.

Methods.—Studies were performed in Feulgen-stained tissue sections from 44 cases of UBTCC. Qualitative and image analysis–quantitated immunohistochemical techniques using the A3D8 monoclonal antibody were used to measure expression of the standard 85- to 95-kDa macromolecule CD44s. Qualitative immunohistochemical techniques using the 2F10 monoclonal antibody were used to measure expression of CD44v6, a splice variant exon of CD44s.

Results.—Grade I tumors showed a 61% positive staining intensity for CD44s, compared with 43% in grade II and 30% in grade III tumors. Area of positive staining intensity was 59% for noninvasive tumors vs. 30% for deeply invasive tumors. Aneuploid DNA content was significantly correlated with loss of CD44s staining. The results of CD44v6 staining were similar, with lesser degrees of staining for high-grade and high-stage aggressive tumors compared with low-grade nonaggressive tumors.

Conclusions.—Expression of the CD44 cell adhesion molecule in UBTCC is related to tumor grade, pathologic stage, and DNA content. Expression of the CD44s and CD44v6 molecules is parallel to that of other cell adhesion molecules that show loss of immunoreactivity with tumor dedifferentiation, advancing pathologic stage, and abnormal DNA content. With further study, the CD44 cell adhesion markers may prove clinically relevant to the treatment of patients with bladder cancer.

▶ The cellular adhesion molecule (CAM) CD44 has received a lot of attention recently in the pathology literature, particularly as a prognostic marker in solid tumors such as bladder cancer (transitional cell carcinoma). In this well-performed and straightforward study, the expression of the standard form of the molecule (CD44s) and one of its variants (v6) were immunohistochemically studied in formalin-fixed, paraffin-embedded sections. As with other tumors, the authors noted decreased expression of CD44s with respect to increasing grade, increasing stage, and aneuploidy. Interestingly, v6 expression also decreased. At other sites, v6 has been noted to increase with more advanced/aggressive tumors.

M.B. Cohen, M.D.

---

p53 Mutations in Multiple Urothelial Carcinomas: A Molecular Analysis of the Development of Multiple Carcinomas

Goto K, Konomoto T, Hayashi K, et al (Kyushu Univ, Fukuoka, Japan)
Mod Pathol 10:428–437, 1997   5–4

Background.—Urothelial carcinoma is a multifocal tumor that can be synchronous, metachronous, or both. It is unclear whether the multifocal tumors originate from a single focus or independently. It has been proposed that the tumors arise from a field defect, from intraluminal seeding and implantation, or from both. These hypotheses were tested in a study of 84 multiple urothelial carcinomas.

Methods.—The tumors were 78 urinary bladder carcinomas and 6 ureteric or renal pelvic carcinomas from 42 patients. The specimens were studied by polymerase chain reaction single-strand conformation polymorphism, DNA sequencing, and immunohistochemical studies for p53 mutations. If p53 mutations were the same in cancer cells from different sites within the same patient, this was evidence for a common origin of multiple tumors. If the p53 mutations differed, this was evidence that the cancers arose independently.

Results.—Forty-two cancers from 22 patients had p53 mutations. The presence of these mutations was strongly linked to tumor grade but not tumor stage. Nine of the 22 patients had the same mutation—sometimes with additional mutations—in multiple cancers, suggesting a common origin for the cancers. However, 11 patients had different mutations in different cancers, and 2 had a mutation in 1 cancer but not the other. In these groups, the evidence pointed to an independent origin of the multiple tumors.

Nine patients had double mutations. Transitions were more common than transversions in this group, in contrast to reported data on urothelial carcinomas. There was a 74% concordance between p53 nuclear reactivity and p53 mutations demonstrated by single-strand conformation polymorphism analysis.

Conclusions.—Multifocal urothelial cancers may have either a common or independent origin. The spectra of p53 mutations observed in this series could reflect the incidence of other possible mutations than those involved in single urothelial carcinomas. Tumors with abnormalities of p53 and other genes might exhibit differences in biological behavior, possibly leading to new treatment approaches.

▶ One of the fundamental questions in bladder cancer biology is whether the high incidence of recurrences is caused by a field effect or is a result of implantation of tumor cells after being released from the index tumor site. One powerful technique to address this question is to analyze the p53 mutational pattern in tumors from the same patient. This can be performed by extracting DNA from fixed, embedded blocks, polymerase chain reaction amplification of the p53 exons (in this case 5–9, which contain most of the described mutations), and sequence analysis. Although there are a number of questions, including technical ones, that arise from this work, I believe this is an interesting study. The conclusions suggest that both mechanisms of tumor recurrence may occur.

M.B. Cohen, M.D.

Endocervical Type Glands in Urinary Bladder: A Clinicopathologic Study of Six Cases

Nazeer T, Ro JY, Tornos C, et al (Univ of Texas, Houston)
Hum Pathol 27:816–820, 1996   5–5

Background.—The urinary bladder can be affected by a variety of hyperplastic, metaplastic, and neoplastic glandular lesions. Recently, the cases of 6 women of reproductive age with endocervical-type glands in the urinary bladder, termed "endocervicosis," were described. Another 6 cases of endocervical-type glands in the urinary bladder were presented to better define the significance of this lesion and to make pathologists aware of its existence.

Methods and Findings.—The 6 women with glandular lesions consisting of endocervical-type glands in the urinary bladder were aged 34 to 65 years. Two patients initially had dysuria and of the next 3, 1 each had painless hematuria, complaints of pelvic discomfort and hematuria, and vaginal discharge. In the sixth patient, who was asymptomatic, a pelvic mass was found during routine gynecologic examination. Three women had masses between the bladder and the uterus. Four masses were in the posterior wall of the urinary bladder, 1 was in the dome, and 1 was in the trigone. Biopsy of the bladder tumor was performed in 4 patients, 1 of whom had had a hysterectomy 10 years earlier. One woman with a pelvic mass between the bladder and uterus had a hysterectomy, bilateral salpingo-oophorectomy, and partial cystectomy. The sixth patient underwent a transurethral resection of the bladder tumor and left oophorectomy.

On histologic examination, all patients had intermediate-to-large irregularly shaped endocervical-type glands in the muscularis propria of the urinary bladder. Cystic dilatation and mucinous secretions were observed in some glands. No desmoplastic tissue reaction occured in the glands. Polymorphonuclear leukocytes were often found in the intraluminal mucin. The glands were lined by tall, mucinous columnar cells in all cases, and less commonly by flattened-to-cuboidal cells. Rare admixed ciliated cells were noted. In 5 tumors, the lining epithelium was bland, although moderate nuclear atypia was present in 1. There were no mitoses. Associated lesions were endometrial-type glands surrounded by elastotic stroma, exuberatnt cystitis glanduralis, and a pseudodiverticulum of the bladder in 1 patient each. All patients are alive and well 6 to 60 months after diagnosis, suggesting that the lesion is benign.

Conclusion.—Endocervical-type glands occur occasionally in the urinary bladder, representing a benign lesion. Although the histogenesis of this tumor is not completely clear, at least some cases appear to be of mullerian origin. Recognizing this lesion is important for avoiding misdiagnosis and inappropriate treatment.

Müllerianosis of the Urinary Bladder
Young RH, Clement PB (Harvard Med School, Boston; Univ of British Columbia, Vancouver)
Mod Pathol 9:731–737, 1996   5–6

Background.—Until recently, endometriosis was the only benign proliferation of müllerian glandular epithelium that seemed to involve the urinary bladder. However, 6 patients with vesical endocervicosis were reported in 1992. This benign müllerian lesion is characterized by bland endocervical-type glands that could be confused with adenocarcinoma. Three patients with striking endosalpingiosis of the urinary bladder that also contained less conspicuous components of endometriosis and/or endocervicosis were reported.

Patients and Findings.—The 3 women, aged 37 to 46 years, had masses up to a maximum of 4 cm involving the posterior wall of the urinary bladder. All underwent transurethral resection. Microscopic examination revealed prominent involvement of the lamina propria and muscularis propria by tubules and cysts lined by müllerian-type epithelium. In 2 patients, the latter focally replaced the urothelium, forming polypoid projections into the bladder lumen. Typically, the tubules and cysts were round to oval, although prominent branching was noted occasionally. The glands were lined primarily by tubal-type epithelium, including ciliated, intercalated, and peg cells, which represented endosalpingiosis. In addition, a minor component of glands lined by columnar mucinous cells was noted in all cases, including a minor component of typical endometriosis in 1 case and endometrioid epithelium associated with prominent pseudoxanthoma cells in adjacent stroma in another case.

Conclusion.—Striking endosalpingiosis of the urinary bladder is usually associated with endocervicosis and/or endometriosis. Thus, the term "müllerianosis is appropriate. This condition can be differentiated from adenocarcinoma and various nonneoplastic glandular lesions of the urinary bladder by a variety of architectural and cytologic findings.

Florid Cystitis Glandularis of Intestinal Type With Mucin Extravasation: A Mimic of Adenocarcinoma

Young RH, Bostwick DG (Harvard Med School, Boston; Mayo Clinic, Rochester, Minn)
Am J Surg Pathol 20:1462–1468, 1996   5–7

Background.—The intestinal variant of cystitis glandularis may be confused with cancer when florid and associated with extravasation of mucin into the stroma, a phenomenon that has not been well described in the literature. Six cases of this sometimes striking phenomenon were described and its benign nature emphasized.

Methods and Findings.—Florid cystitis glandularis of the intestinal type, associated with focal mucin extravasation into the stroma, occurred in 6 men aged 27 to 65 years. Distinguishing it from adenocarcinoma was a major problem in several patients. In 5 patients, the masses simulated bladder neoplasm. All patients complained of hematuria or irritative symptoms. In 4 patients, treatment consisted only of transurethral resection. One patient had a partial cystectomy because of the erroneous diagnosis of adenocarcinoma, and another had total cystectomy because of a neurogenic bladder. Microscopic assessment showed many glands lined with intestinal-type epithelium, consistent with the appearance of the intestinal variant cystitis glandularis. A minor component of typical cystitis glandularis was noted in all patients, being prominent in 4. Foci of basophilic mucin in the stroma, prominent in 4, was noted in all cases. Rounded aggregates of mucin occasionally surrounded by compressed connective tissue cells, simulating mucinous cysts, were noted. Supporting a benign interpretation were the absence of epithelial cells in the extravasated mucin, the lack of atypicality of the cells lining the intestinal-type glands in 5 cases, the generally disorderly distribution of the glands, and their lack of infiltration of the muscularis propria (though they abutted the latter in several cases). Three patients have been followed for 2 to 14 years. Their course has been uneventful.

Conclusion.—Cystitis glandularis may greatly mimic a neoplasm on gross examination. Mucin extravasation, a finding rarely reported to date, tends to make diagnosis difficult.

▶ With the increasing attention being paid to urologic pathology, there have been increased numbers of articles identifying "new" lesions. The article by Nazeer et al. (Abstract 5–5) discusses 6 cases of a glandular lesion in the bladder of women that has morphologic similarities to endocervical mucosa. The most important reason for awareness of this and related lesions is to not confuse them with adenocarcinoma. This particular lesion is thought to be of Müllerian origin, although this is speculative. There has been recent reporting of other glandular lesions in this anatomical location, including "Müllerianosis [i.e., endosalpingiosis] of the urinary bladder" (Abstract 5–6) and "Florid cystitis glandularis of intestinal type with mucin extravasation." (Abstract 5–7). Hopefully, a synthesis will soon bring these entities together as variant forms of glandular metaplasia.

M.B. Cohen, M.D.

Clear Cell Adenocarcinoma of the Urethra: A Clinicopathologic Analysis of 19 Cases

Oliva E, Young RH (Harvard Med School, Boston; Massachusetts Gen Hosp, Boston)
Mod Pathol 9:513–520, 1996   5–8

Background.—Clear cell adenocarcinoma of the urethra is uncommon but distinctive. The histologic spectrum of this tumor, the extent to which it mimics nephrogenic adenoma, its possible relationship with adenocarcinoma and nephrogenic adenoma, and the extent of its association with a urethral diverticulum were documented in the current study.

Methods and Results.—Nineteen patients, aged 35 to 80 years, were studied; 18 were women. The clinical presentation and gross findings were similar to those of urethral carcinomas. However, 12 tumors (all in women) arose in a urethral diverticulum. Microscopically, the tumors showed the classic triad of tubulocystic, papillary, and diffuse patterns characterizing this tumor. The cytologic features were typical of clear cell adenocarcinoma: hobnail cells, flattened cells, and cells with abundant clear cytoplasm. Typically, nuclear pleomorphism was at least moderate and was marked in nearly half the specimens. Mitotic figures were found easily in almost all specimens. In all 13 tumors immunostained for prostate-specific antigen and prostatic acid phosphatase, results were negative. Follow-up data were available for 13 patients. Six had no evidence of recurrence up to 10 years after surgery, and 4 died of disease 5 to 42 months after surgery. Another 3 patients had recurrences but were alive up to 6.5 years after initial assessment.

Conclusions.—Urethral clear cell adenocarcinoma typically occurs in adults, mostly women. This tumor has a particular association with urethral diverticulum, found in 56% of the patients. The tumor is indistinguishable from clear cell adenocarcinoma of the female genital tract but is not related to endometriosis. It probably does not arise by malignant transformation of nephrogenic adenoma. Usually it can be distinguished from the latter by its greater cytologic atypicality and mitotic activity. It does not stain for prostate-specific antigen or prostatic acid phosphatase.

▶ This article describes a retrospective review of a series of 19 cases, 18 of which were from two consultation files (Drs. Scully and Young). Eighteen of the 19 patients were women, and all the tumors occurred in adults (>35 years). Insufficient detail is available to provide meaningful information about the gross findings except to say that slightly more than half of the tumors were found in association with a urethral diverticulum. Microscopically, there was heterogeneity in both the architecture and the cytologic findings. Nuclear "atypia" and mitoses were usually prominent enough to recognize this as malignant and distinguish it from its key differential diagnostic consideration—nephrogenic adenoma—which is also not thought to be a precursor lesion. It should be recognized, however, that this series is essentially based on referred material, and the submitting pathologists presumably did not find the histopathologic findings so straightforward.

M.B. Cohen, M.D.

Transitional Cell Carcinoma Involving the Prostate With a Proposed Staging Classification For Stromal Invasion
Esrig D, Freeman JA, Elmajian DA, et al (Univ of Southern California, Los Angeles; Yale Univ, New Haven, Conn)
J Urol 156:1071–1076, 1996   5–9

Purpose.—The origin and incidence of transitional cell carcinoma involving the prostate are unclear. Disease-free survival appears to be influenced by prostatic stromal invasion and the stage of the primary bladder tumor. However, previous studies have not differentiated between stromal involvement secondary to urethral or ductal basement membrane invasion and extravesical extension. The survival effects of these differences were investigated, including a proposed staging classification for stromal invasion in transitional cell carcinoma involving the prostate.

Methods.—The patients were drawn from a series of 489 men undergoing radical cystoprostatectomy for transitional cell carcinoma during an 18-year period. Of this group, 143 had prostate involvement by transitional cell carcinoma, as demonstrated by the cystectomy specimen. Nineteen patients were classified as having P4a disease, with primary bladder tumor extending full thickness through the bladder wall to invade the prostate (group 1). The other 124 patients had prostate involvement arising from within the prostatic urethra (group 2) (Fig 1). Differences between these 2 groups were analyzed.

Results.—At 5 years, recurrence-free survival was 25% in group 1 vs. 64% in group 2. Overall survival was 21% vs. 55%, respectively. Within group 2, survival was no different for patients with prostatic urethral tumors or carcinoma in situ and ductal tumors, without stromal invasion. Five-year overall survival was 71% for patients with stromal invasion and 36% for those without. Involvement of the prostatic urethra or ducts did not affect survival as predicted by primary bladder stage alone.

Survival was significantly reduced in patients with prostatic stromal invasion arising via the urethra—survival decreased from 65% for patients in stage P1 to 31% for those in stage P2/P3a, to 14% for those in stage P3b. Survival was 65% for P1 bladder tumors with prostatic invasion arising intraurethrally vs. 21% for P4a tumors. Survival for patients with P3b bladder tumors with stromal invasion was similar to that for patients with P4a tumors.

Conclusions.—For patients with transitional cell carcinoma involving the prostatic urethra or duct, survival is no different than that predicted by primary bladder stage alone. These tumors should not be classified as P4a. Survival is significantly reduced for patients with prostatic stromal in-

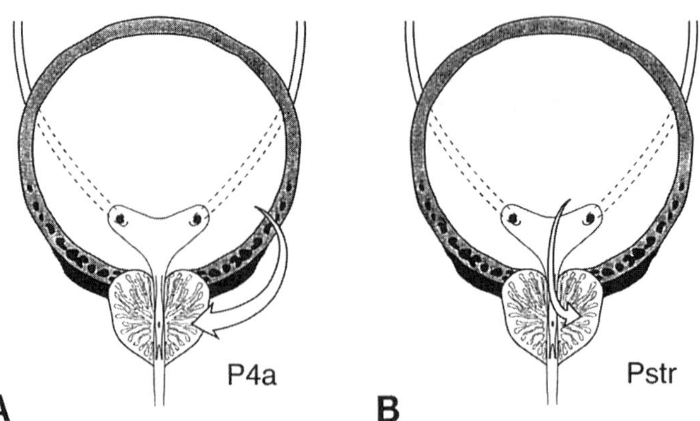

FIGURE 1.—A, prostatic stromal invasion via extension through bladder wall (*P4a*) B, prostatic stromal invasion arising intraurethrally with invasion of basement membrane of prostatic urethra or ducts (*Pstr*). (Courtesy of Esrig D, Freeman JA, Elmajian DA, et al: Transitional cell carcinoma involving the prostate with a proposed staging classification for stromal invasion. *J Urol* 156(3):1071–1076, 1996.)

volvement arising via the urethra. Survival is better for patients with P1 bladder tumors with prostatic stromal invasion arising intraurethrally than for patients with P4a tumors; the former group should be classified P1str. Similarly, survival is better for muscle invasive bladder tumors with stromal invasion (P2str) than for P4a tumors. No significant difference was found between P3b bladder tumors with prostatic stromal invasion arising intraurethrally and P4a tumors.

▶ The current staging of transitional cell carcinoma (TCC) of the urinary bladder is based on the depth of invasion through the bladder wall, including into adjacent structures such as the prostate (pT4). In addition, the possibility that invasive TCC into the prostate can arise from intraprostatic ducts (also pT4) prompted the authors to investigate whether there was a difference in the biology of these 2 types of high-stage TCC. The results of their study indicate that there is a difference, and that those TCCs invading the prostate from intraprostatic ducts have a better prognosis and should therefore be separated out from the mixture of pT4 tumors. It will be important for these results to be confirmed by others.

M.B. Cohen, M.D.

Adenocarcinoma of the Prostate With Atrophic Features
Cina SJ, Epstein JI (Johns Hopkins Univ, Baltimore, Md)
Am J Surg Pathol 21:289–295, 1997   5–10

Objective.—In the diagnosis of prostate cancer, errors can occur if the tumor lacks the classic histologic pattern. The authors have noted an increasing number of prostate adenocarcinomas with attenuated cytoplasm. They designate this picture, which looks like benign atrophy, "adenocarcinoma of the prostate with atrophic features." There have been no formal studies of this variant. The histologic findings in adenocarcinoma of the prostate with atrophic features were described.

Methods.—Forty-four cases of adenocarcinoma of the prostate with atrophic features—42 needle biopsy specimens and 2 transurethral resection specimens—were studied. All cases showed a paucity of cytoplasm of the component cells with at least 50% of the glands showing atrophy, compared with normal benign glands or nonatrophic carcinoma. The clinical and histologic features of these cases were analyzed.

Findings.—The outside diagnosis, known in 30 cases, was atypical/suspicious for carcinoma in 19 cases, correctly interpreted as carcinoma in 8, and considered benign in 3. Just 2 of the 44 patients were receiving hormone therapy when the biopsy was performed. The average amount of carcinoma in each specimen was 1.9 mm. Atrophic features made up an average of 83.5% of each lesion. Findings that contributed to the diagnosis of malignancy included the pattern of growth, the presence of enlarged nucleoli, adjacent nonatrophic cancer, and increased nuclear size (Fig 7). In some cases, the diagnosis was established by the finding of negative im-

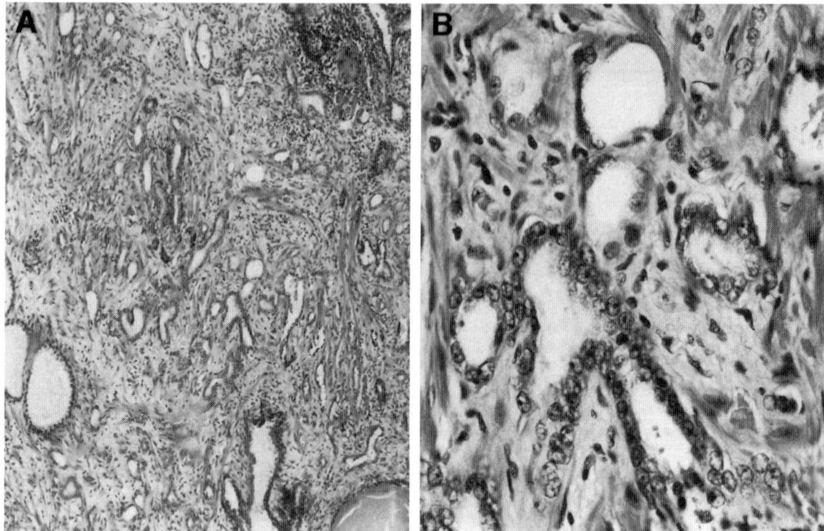

FIGURE 7.—**A**, atrophic adenocarcinoma at radical prostatectomy. Note the extensive infiltrative nature of small atrophic glands. **B**, higher magnification demonstrating atrophic glands lined by large nuclei with huge nucleoli diagnostic of adenocarcinoma. (Courtesy of Cina SJ, Epstein JI: Adenocarcinoma of the prostate with atrophic features. *Am J Surg Pathol* 21:289–295, 1997.)

munohistochemical staining for high–molecular weight cytokeratin. The pattern of tumor growth was infiltrative in 41 cases. The Gleason grade was 3 + 3 = 6 in 89% of cases. Eighty-nine percent of tumors showed increased nuclear size, and 48% showed macronucleoli.

Conclusions.—It may be difficult to distinguish atrophy from adenocarcinoma of the prostate with atrophic features. The prognostic implications of this histologic picture remain to be determined; however, until longitudinal data are available, atrophic carcinoma should be treated as a fully malignant neoplasm.

▶ More and more pitfalls for the diagnosis of prostatic adenocarcinoma are being identified. Here's another one for the list. Traditionally, atrophy was included in the differential diagnosis of prostatic adenocarcinoma, but this article describes a series, of primarily consults, that showed prostatic adenocarcinoma with atrophy. Based on the illustrations (see Fig 7), this diagnosis can be difficult. The 2 key criteria appear to be nuclear enlargement and nucleoli, seen in 80% and 89% of the cases of adenocarcinoma of the prostate with atrophic features, respectively.

M.B. Cohen, M.D.

Single Focus of Adenocarcinoma in the Prostate Biopsy Specimen Is Not Predictive of the Pathologic Stage of Disease

Bruce RG, Rankin WR, Cibull ML, et al (Univ of Kentucky, Lexington; VA Med Ctr, Lexington, Ky)
Urology 48:75–79, 1996

5–11

Introduction.—Patients with a high volume of tumor in their prostate needle biopsy specimen are likely to have a high volume of tumor in the surgical specimen, and have a high incidence of disease outside the prostate. This suggests that patients with a small focus of cancer in the biopsy specimen might be likely to have disease confined to the prostate. The ability of a small focus of tumor in prostate biopsy specimen to predict organ-confined disease—or other favorable prognostic factors—was evaluated.

Methods.—A total of 598 prostate needle biopsies performed during a 4.5-year period were studied. Of these, 49 had a microscopic focus of adenocarcinoma, i.e., one measuring less than 2 mm in length of the entire biopsy core specimen. The clinical and pathologic features of these patients were analyzed, including the pathologic tumor stage after radical prostatectomy, the cancer recurrence rate after external beam radiotherapy, and the presence of bony metastases at diagnosis.

Results.—Treatment consisted of radical prostatectomy in 27 patients, 26 of whom had pelvic lymph node dissection. Twenty-six percent of surgically treated patients had extraprostatic disease, 19% had positive surgical margins, and 1 each had lymph node involvement and invasion of the seminal vesicles. Treatment was by radiotherapy in 10 patients and hormonal therapy in 12. In the radiotherapy group, 20% of patients had relapse at a mean interval of 11.5 months. One fourth of patients receiving hormonal therapy had bony metastases at diagnosis. Overall, about one fourth of patients had some form of unfavorable disease.

Conclusions.—Patients with only a microscopic focus of prostatic adenocarcinoma in their needle biopsy specimen do not necessarily have favorable prognostic factors. This finding is not a reliable predictor of insignificant tumor; its true significance, in combination with other factors, needs further study. Patients with a single focus of adenocarcinoma at biopsy, clinically localized prostate cancer, and a life expectancy of longer than 10 years should receive radical prostatectomy or radiation therapy.

▶ This study, as well as its conclusion, is straightforward: a single microscopic focus on biopsy does not predict stage or outcome. It is possible that other parameters might add to better predictions regarding optimal patient management, but such data are not currently available. From a pathologist's perspective, one should be careful in not overinterpreting nor underinterpreting single foci of small acinar proliferations.

M.B. Cohen, M.D.

Adequate Tissue Sampling of Prostate Core Needle Biopsies

Renshaw AA (Harvard Med School, Boston; Brigham and Women's Hosp, Boston)

Am J Clin Pathol 107:26–29, 1997

5–12

Introduction.—With recent trends in the diagnostic evaluation of prostate cancer, the diagnosis is increasingly made on the basis of small foci in core needle biopsy specimens. Although this situation increases the importance of adequate sampling, there are few data on what constitutes adequate sampling of prostate core needle biopsy specimens. Factors important for adequate sampling of such specimens were assessed retrospectively.

Methods.—A total of 229 patients undergoing prostate core needle biopsy were studied. Of the cores reviewed, 47 had atypical foci, 22 had high-grade prostatic intraepithelial neoplasia (PIN), and 533 had cancer. For each case, 6 cores were obtained for preparation of 2 blocks containing 3 cores each. Each block was used to prepare at least 3 slides containing multiple serial sections. The review sought to determine how much of a sample was needed to detect all atypical, high-grade PIN, and carcinomatous foci.

Results.—The percentage of the core made up of abnormal foci was less than 5% in 97% of atypical foci, 25% of carcinomatous foci, and 0% of high-grade PIN foci. These foci measured less than 1 mm in their greatest dimension. The first slide did not show 13% of atypical foci, 3% of carcinomatous foci, and 0% of high-grade PIN foci (Table).

Conclusions.—This review of prostate core needle biopsy specimens suggests that 13% of atypical foci and 3% of carcinomatous foci are not present on the first slide because the tissue containing these foci has simply not been cut yet. The findings suggest that at least 3 slides should be examined to avoid missing atypical or diagnostic foci. Measures to improve tissue sampling may be helpful.

▶ The issue of appropriate sampling of prostate tissue specimens seems to be an ongoing saga. It began with transurethral prostatectomy specimens more than a decade ago. In this article, the issue of how to handle biopsy samples is addressed. The conclusion is that 3 slides, with about 4 sections per slide, will identify all cases of carcinoma (see Table). It is not clear whether the entire block was consumed during sectioning of the embedded tissue.

TABLE.—Percentage of Lesions Detected on Each Slide

Lesion	*Slide 1*	*Slide 2*	*Slide 3*
Atypical foci	87	9	4
High-grade PIN	100	0	0
Carcinoma	97	2	1

Abbreviation: PIN, prostatic intraepithelial neoplasia.
(Courtesy of Renshaw AA: Adequate tissue sampling of prostate core needle biopsies. *Am J Clin Pathol* 107:26–29, 1997.)

Also, it would have been interesting to know how many sections were actually needed, and at what levels. Lastly, I doubt we have heard the last of this issue.

M.B. Cohen, M.D.

Recommendations for the Reporting of Resected Prostate Carcinomas
Amin MB, Grignon D, Bostwick D, et al (Univ Virginia, Charlottesville, VA)
Am J Clin Pathol 105:667–670, 1996   5–13

Background.—Several committees named by the Association of Directors of Anatomic and Surgical Pathology (ADASP) have developed recommendations on the content of the surgical pathology report for common malignant tumors. Four major areas are covered: items providing an informative gross description; additional diagnostic features that should be in every report if possible; optional features; and checklist.

Recommendations for the Reporting of Resected Prostate Carcinomas.— Among the recommendations is that the Gleason system be used for tumor grade. Of note is that, when more than 2 patterns are seen in a needle biopsy specimen and the worst grade is neither the predominant nor secondary pattern, the predominant pattern and the highest grade should be used in scoring. In reporting the amount of tumor, percentage of the prostate involved by carcinoma should be given in relation to the weight of the specimen in radical prostatectomy specimens. For needle biopsy specimens of prostatic intraepithelial neoplasia (PIN), the presence of grades 2 and 3 should be reported. Low-grade PIN (grade 1) is not reported. Reporting PIN for radical prostatectomies is optional. In specifying the type of extracapsular tissue involved in radical prostatectomies, pathologists should be aware that skeletal muscle may not indicate extracapsular involvement. In reporting on seminal vesicles, the presence or absence of carcinoma should be noted, specifying whether it is in the wall or adventitia. Tumor in the adventitia of the seminal vesicle does not qualify as true seminal vesicle invasion. The amount of tumor in needle biopsy specimens may be reported if desired. If reported, the amount of tumor should be given in millimeters, along with a measure of the length of each core involved, and tumor location should be specified as being at the tip or within the center of the core. Extracapsular extension of carcinoma in a lymph node metastasis and its measurement may also be described if desired.

Conclusions.—These recommendations were developed to provide an informative report for clinicians. They are intended as suggestions and are in no way mandatory. These recommendations may not be applicable in special circumstances.

▶ The importance of this article is self-evident and is probably already in the files of most surgical pathologists. The Appendix is a checklist of features that ADASP believes should be included in the pathology report.

M.B. Cohen, M.D.

Do Close But Negative Margins in Radical Prostatectomy Specimens Increase the Risk of Postoperative Progression?

Epstein JI, Sauvageot J (Johns Hopkins Hosp, Baltimore, Md)
J Urol 157:241–243, 1997
5–14

Objective.—Because of the anatomical location of the prostate, a true radical resection is rarely achieved. The tumor often extends very close to the margin of resection—within 1 or 2 mm—but not to the inked edge of the gland. In this situation, the pathologist may note that the "margins are free of tumor yet microscopically close," implying that there may be an increased risk of progression. The effects of close but negative margins on risk of progression after radical prostatectomy were analyzed.

Methods.—A total of 104 radical prostatectomy specimens with tumor-free margins were examined. Fifty-two of the patients had disease progression and 49 did not. The disease was clinically confined in all patients, i.e., stage T1 or T2; all seminal vesicles and lymph nodes were tumor free on pathologic examination. The patients without progression had been followed up for at least 5 years with no evidence of disease. No radiotherapy or hormonal therapy was given until progression occurred. Follow-up included serum prostate specific antigen testing. The distance between the most peripheral tumor and the surgical margin of resection was measured in each case to see whether it was related to the risk of postoperative progression.

Results.—In the patients without progression, the distance between the tumor and margin was 0.5 mm or less in 82% of cases, and less than 1.0 mm in all cases. The tumor was no closer to the margin in patients with progression than in patients without progression. A regression analysis was performed to assess how progression was affected by Gleason score, distance between tumor and margin, location of closest margin, and pathologic stage. The only factor related to progression was tumor grade. In 97% of cases, the narrowest margin was at the posterior aspect.

Conclusions.—In patients undergoing radical prostatectomy, having close but negative margins does not influence the risk of postoperative progression. The prognosis is just as good as in patients with wider margins. Pathologists need not report these margins as close, and physicians should not alter therapy according to the closeness of the margins.

▶ I believe the conclusion from this article is important: "It is not necessary for pathologists to designate the margin as close, since biologically this term has no significance." It is very similar to a previous article by one of the authors.[1]

M.B. Cohen, M.D.

Reference

1. Epstein JI: Evaluation of radical prostatectomy capsular margins of resection: The significance of margins designated as negative, closely approaching, and positive. *Am J Surg Pathol* 14:626, 1990.

Histologic Grade Heterogeneity in Multifocal Prostate Cancer: Biological and Clinical Implications

Ruijter ETh, van de Kaa CA, Schalken JA, et al (Univ Hosp Nijmegen, The Netherlands; Univ of Utrecht, The Netherlands)
J Pathol 180:295–299, 1996　　　　　　　　　　　　　　　　　5–15

Background.—As the incidence and prevalence of prostatic carcinoma continue to increase, the debate over staging and management intensifies. The tumor biological and clinical implications of prostate cancer heterogeneity and multifocality were further investigated.

Methods and Findings.—Histologic grade heterogeneity and tumor multifocality were mapped in a series of 61 completely sectioned whole-mount radical prostatectomy specimens with clinical stage T2 prostate cancer. Fifty-five prostate biopsy specimens were also examined to determine the accuracy of preoperative grading. Only 28% of all prostates had a single tumor. In 16%, 1 histologic grade of cancer was observed. Extracapsular invasion did not only occur in the largest tumor in each case. Rather, it occurred in tumors of relatively small volume and low histologic grade. Histologic grade variability was directly proportional to tumor volume. Neither grade heterogeneity nor tumor multifocality of the prostatectomy specimen was significantly associated with the grade accuracy of biopsy specimens. Biopsy grading error was highest among small, well-differentiated tumors.

Conclusion.—Whole-mount sectioning of prostatectomy specimens of patients with clinically localized adenocarcinoma shows that grade heterogeneity is most closely associated with tumor volume. In addition, the largest (index) tumor may not be representative of the pathologic stage. Grading error of prostate needle biopsy specimens is only partially explained by grade heterogeneity or tumor multifocality.

▶ This article highlights several important aspects of prostate cancer. First, prostate cancer is a heterogeneous disease, both with respect to location (i.e., multifocality) and grade. Second, tumor volume does not necessarily predict pathologic stage. Third, the correlation between grading of biopsy and prostatectomy specimens was far from perfect and is only in part attributable to tumor heterogeneity.

M.B. Cohen, M.D.

Increasing Incidence of Minimal Residual Cancer In Radical Prostatectomy Specimens

DiGiuseppe JA, Sauvageot J, Epstein JI (Johns Hopkins Med Inst, Baltimore, Md)
Am J Surg Pathol 21:174–178, 1997　　　　　　　　　　　　　5–16

Introduction.—Many cases of early prostate cancer are now detected at screening by means of prostate-specific antigen and transrectal US. Surgical resection in such cases has sometimes yielded residual cancer that is histologically difficult to identify. In a review of radical prostatectomies performed at the study institution between 1988 and 1995, the incidence of minimal residual cancer, described in some reports as the "vanishing cancer phenomenon," was examined.

Methods.—During the period under review, 3,038 consecutive radical prostatectomies were performed; excluded were cases with a history of transurethral resection or previous hormonal therapy and those with a focal Gleason grade of 4 or 5, capsular penetration, or positive surgical margins. Excluded from further analysis were cases with a focus of carcinoma greater than 0.1 cc. Specimens with 1 or 2 foci of carcinoma having no focus greater than 0.05 cc were termed "difficult to find;" those with 1 or 2 foci measuring between 0.05 and 0.1 cc or with 3 or 4 foci less than 0.1 cc were classified as "minute."

Results.—Eighty-four resection specimens (2.8%) were found to have minimal residual cancer. Sixty met criteria for "difficult to find" (mean total volume 0.03) cancers and 20 were considered "minute" (mean total volume 0.07 cc); no residual cancer was identified in 4. Seventeen cases of minimal residual cancer consisted of a single microscopic focus of carcinoma measuring 0.01 cc or less; most of those were detected only at review. The incidence of minimal residual cancer increased significantly over the study period, from 0.5% of radical prostatectomies in 1988 to between 3% and 4% since 1993. Patients with minimal residual cancer were similar in age distribution to other parties who undergo radical prostatectomy at the study institution.

Discussion.—The increase in minimal residual cancer over the course of the study period can be attributed to more aggressive screening for early prostate cancer and to better criteria for diagnosing minute cancer on needle biopsy. Most of the cases identified in this review were "difficult to find," having a mean aggregate tumor volume more than 10-fold smaller than that viewed as clinically significant. Complete submission of the specimen for review should identify carcinoma in most cases initially described as without residual cancer.

▶ Minimal residual cancer, the vanishing cancer phenomenon, etc., are all euphemisms for a real problem for pathologists. In the first true systematic study of this phenomenon, it is clear that this is a true phenomenon, and includes both no cancer (0.07%) at prostatectomy and very small volume cancer (~4%). Interestingly, its incidence has increased from 0.5% in 1988 to 4% in 1993. The authors do recommend complete submission of the prostate in the event no carcinoma is identified in the initial sections; this is a costly exercise but fortunately a rare occurrence, at least at Hopkins.

M.B. Cohen, M.D.

Spread of Adenocarcinoma Within Prostatic Ducts and Acini: Morphologic and Clinical Correlations

McNeal JE, Yemoto CEM (Stanford Univ, Calif)
Am J Surg Pathol 20:802–814, 1996

5–17

Background.—Malignant epithelial masses in prostatic duct lumens have been interpreted as being several different entities, including Gleason cribriform grade 3 carcinoma and cribriforming dysplasia. However, there is no convincing evidence that these various diagnostic alternatives represent anything other than a single morphologic entity in different situations and at different stages of development.

Methods and Results.—Fifty-one of 130 radical prostatectomy cancers containing intraductal lesions were investigated. Total cancer volumes ranged from 4 to 10 cc. Such lesions with duct lumen-sparing septa or masses were rarely found in areas away from invasive cancer. However, dysplasia was common. Thus, these lesions were viewed as part of the evolution of invasive carcinoma rather than precursors and were designated *intraductal carcinoma* distinct from dysplasia. Areas of intraductal cancer within invasive carcinoma usually represented extension of cancer in the branches of a single segment of the duct-acinar system from near the urethra to the gland capsule. The invasive component produced large tumor masses in perineural spaces in 51% of the cancers. This was correlated strongly with extensive capsule penetration and frequent positive surgical margins selectively at the superior nerve pedicle. Postprostatectomy cancer progression was apparently associated with the amount of grade 4/5 cancer, the amount of intraductal carcinoma, and large perineural tumor mass.

Conclusions.—Intraductal prostatic adenocarcinoma is a common morphologic entity with clear histologic criteria and a unique biologic significance. It has an increased capacity for extensive spread within ducts and perineural spaces. The current data support a unitary concept that may be applied to all glandular dysplastic lesions with intraluminal cribriform growth.

▶ This is another careful study by a long-standing prostate cancer pathologist. It focuses on distinguishing Gleason grade 3 adenocarcinoma (cribriform pattern) from PIN and intraductal adenocarcinoma, representing spread from a tumor embedded within the prostatic stroma. The latter, which is the focus of this article, is probably something akin to cancerization of ducts (and lobules) in ductal adenocarcinoma of the breast. It is implied that intraductal adenocarcinoma may have a more aggressive biologic course, but this is difficult to isolate as an independent prognostic factor. Nonetheless, this lesion can, and should, be separated from both PIN and a cribiform pattern of adenocarcinoma. It will be interesting to see if this can reliably be done on biopsy material.

M.B. Cohen, M.D.

Molecular Biology of Prostatic Intraepithelial Neoplasia

Bostwick DG, Pacelli A, Lopez-Beltran A (Mayo Clinic/Mayo Med School, Rochester, Minn; Univ of Cordoba, Spain)
Prostate 29:117–134, 1996

5–18

Introduction.—In the ongoing search for precursors of prostatic adenocarcinoma, much attention has been focused on prostatic intraepithelial neoplasia (PIN). This term represents a spectrum of microscopic changes—including progressive basal cell layer disruption, changes in markers of secretory differentiation, nuclear and nucleolar abnormalities, and increasing cell proliferation, DNA content, and allelic loss—that is strongly associated with prostatic carcinoma. The biopsy finding of PIN is highly predictive of adenocarcinoma and should spur a search for concurrent invasive carcinoma. The available molecular biological data on PIN were reviewed.

Findings.—Studies have shown that PIN is related to progressive phenotypic and genotypic abnormalities, falling somewhere in between normal prostatic epithelium and cancer. Taken together, these findings suggest impaired cell differentiation and regulatory control as the process of prostatic carcinogenesis advances. Biomarkers are lost or gained, including morphometric, differentiation, and stromal markers; growth factors and their receptors; oncogenes; tumor suppressor genes; and chromosomes. Most of these biomarkers are amplified as the abnormality progresses from high-grade PIN to cancer—localized, metastatic, and hormone refractory (Fig 1). The available evidence suggests that the genesis of prostate cancer involves selection of various genetic changes, which modify the expression or function of the genes that control cell growth and differentiation.

Discussion.—There is considerable evidence that high-grade PIN is a precursor lesion of prostatic adenocarcinoma. In clinical practice, the finding of high-grade PIN in a prostatic biopsy specimen suggests the need for close surveillance and follow-up biopsy. Future research will provide additional information on the function and prognostic value of oncogene expression in the prostate: normal and before and after the development of cancer. In studies of chemoprevention for prostatic carcinoma, PIN may be a useful intermediate end point.

▶ This review article summarizes the literature up until about the end of 1995. Prostatic intraepithelial neoplasia remains the putative precursor lesion for prostatic adenocarcinoma, and evidence is in large part based on circumstantial evidence—i.e., similarities in the (molecular biological) profile between the two. In addition, much of this focuses on high-grade PIN, which has reasonable interobserver and intraobserver agreement; the same cannot be said about low-grade PIN and consequently raises doubts about its importance in prostatic carcinogenesis.

M.B. Cohen, M.D.

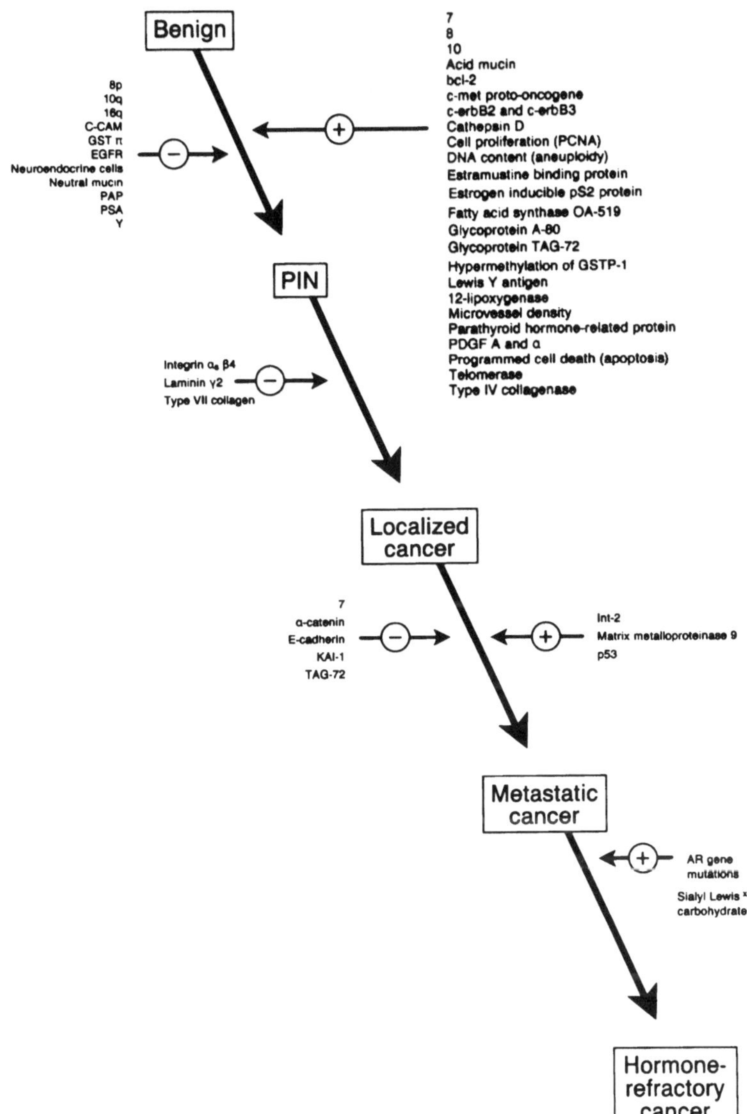

FIGURE 1.—Genetic changes and other changes associated with progression of prostate cancer. Some biomarkers show upregulation or gain (indicated by *plus sign*), whereas others are downregulated or lost (*minus sign*). There is a prominent clustering of changes in expression for many biomarkers between benign epithelium and high-grade prostatic intraepithelial neoplasia (PIN), indicating that this is an important threshold for carcinogenesis in the prostate. A small number of other changes are introduced in the progression from high-grade PIN to localized cancer, metastatic cancer, and hormone-refractory cancer. The model indicates the initial change in expression of a biomarker; most of these changes become magnified in subsequent steps. This model is based chiefly on studies of human prostatic tissue and excludes many biomarkers that have not been evaluated in PIN or different stages of cancer. (Courtesy of Bostwick DG, Pacelli A, Lopez-Beltran A: Molecular biology of prostatic intraepithelial neoplasia. *Prostate* 29:117–134. Copyright 1996 by Wiley-Liss, Inc. Reprinted by permission of Wiley-Liss, Inc., a subsidiary of John Wiley & Sons, Inc.)

Malignant Cytological Washings From Radical Prostatectomy Specimens: A Possible Mechanism for Local Recurrence of Prostate Cancer Following Surgical Treatment of Organ Confined Disease

Ward JF, Nowacki M, Sands JP, et al (Naval Med Ctr, San Diego, Calif)
J Urol 156:1381–1385, 1996   5–19

Background.—Reports have appeared of local prostate cancer recurrence after complete and successful resection of organ-confined disease. Whether secretions from the cut distal urethra during radical prostatectomy contain malignant prostatic epithelial cells, possibly contributing to this problem, was determined.

Methods.—Prostate cytologic specimens from 50 consecutive men were studied prospectively. All patients had clinically organ-confined adenocarcinoma of the prostate treated by radical retropubic or radical perineal prostatectomy. Direct cytologic assessment was performed by 1 examiner to identify malignant or benign cells in these washings.

Findings.—Organ confinement was confirmed in 58% of the 33 radical perineal and 17 radical retropubic prostatectomy specimens. Twenty-four percent of all cytologic specimens had malignant prostatic epithelial cells. Seventeen percent of the cytologic washings from prostates with pathologically confirmed organ-limited cancers had malignant cells. Perineural invasion was observed in most tumors with positive washings, but only Gleason grade significantly predicted recurrence. The operative approach did not change the rate of positive cytology.

Conclusion.—The prostatic washings from men with pathologically organ-confined prostate cancer can contain malignant prostatic epithelial cells. The cytologic findings were unaffected by operative approach. Gleason grade significantly predicts cytologic malignancy. Such cells may be a mechanism of failure after successful radical prostatectomy.

▶ This study is similar to one published by Kassabian et al.[1] One major conclusion from both of these studies is that manipulation of the prostate during surgery may be a mechanism for local recurrence. This is a premature conclusion, although the tenet to not (overly) manipulate the prostate is embedded within the surgical field. There are several other concerns regarding this study, but pathologists should be aware of the study because they may be called on to examine prostatic "secretions" for cytologic evidence of malignancy.

M.B. Cohen, M.D.

Reference

1. Kassabian VS, Bottles K, Weaver R, et al: Possible mechanism for seeding of tumor during radical prostatectomy. *J Urol* 150:1169, 1993.

The Microscopic Pathology of Peyronie's Disease

Davis CJ Jr (Armed Forces Inst of Pathology, Washington, DC)
J Urol 157:282–284, 1997

5–20

Background.—There are few data on the microscopic pathologic findings in Peyronie's disease, or "penile fibromatosis." Physicians may be

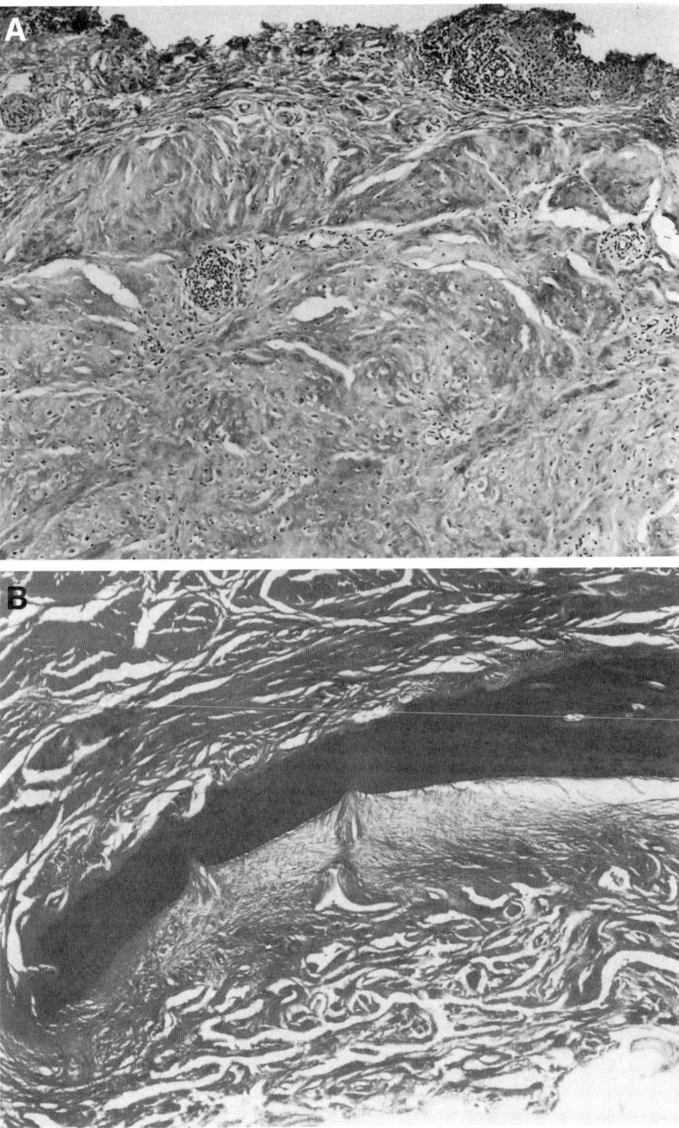

FIGURE 1.—A, external to tunica albuginea (*top*) and within tunica albuginea (*left center*) are perivascular lymphocytes. Hematoxylin-eosin, reduced from ×75. **B,** ossification of tunica albuginea in Peyronie's disease (corpus cavernosum *below*). Hematoxylin-eosin, reduced from ×40. (Courtesy of Davis CJ Jr: The microscopic pathology of Peyronie's disease. *J Urol* 157[1]:282–284, 1997.)

uncertain about the microscopic alterations present and the anatomical structures involved. The specific microscopic findings in Peyronie's disease were reported.

Methods.—Nineteen cases of Peyronie's disease were reviewed. The researchers analyzed hematoxylin and eosin sections, with Masson trichrome used to highlight alterations of collagen structure. Other stains used in selected cases were Movat elastic stain and fibrinogen immunostain for fibrin.

Results.—Thirty-two percent of cases showed a perivascular lymphocytic infiltrate, located within or on either side of the tunica albuginea. Twenty-six percent of cases showed a linear band of ossification in the tunica (Fig 1). The major feature, present in all 19 cases, was disorganization of the collagen of the tunica, most often with some increase in cellularity. These changes were sometimes extremely subtle, and sometimes had to be compared with unaffected tunica to be appreciated. Of 10 cases studied with fibrinogen immunostain, 3 showed fibrin in the affected area of the tunica.

Conclusions.—The major microscopic finding in Peyronie's disease is an alteration in the appearance and cellularity of the collagen of the tunica albuginea. Other findings may include ossification of the middle or inner aspect of the tunica, sometimes with a perivascular lymphocytic infiltrate. Questions remain as to whether these features are specific for Peyronie's disease.

▶ This article describes the experience of the Armed Forces Institute of Pathology with 19 cases of this form of fibromatosis. Besides the relatively acellular collagenous deposition in the tunica albuginea, perivascular lymphocytic infiltrate (32%), linear ossification (26%), and fibrin deposition (16%) may be seen.

M.B. Cohen, M.D.

Anaplastic Variant of Spermatocytic Seminoma

Albores-Saavedra J, Huffman H, Alvarado-Cabrero I, et al (Univ of Texas, Dallas; Hosp de Oncologia, Mexico City; Univ of Texas, Houston)
Hum Pathol 27:650–655, 1996   5–21

Objective.—An anaplastic variant of spermatocytic seminoma has been identified in malignant testicular tumors. The clinical, pathological, immunohistochemical, and ultrastructural findings of 4 cases of anaplastic variant of spermatocytic seminoma are compared with those of conventional spermatocytic seminomas, classic seminoma, and pure embryonic carcinoma.

Methods.—Four of 1303 germ cell tumors from men, aged 33 to 43, were identified as an anaplastic variant of spermatocytic seminoma. Fea-

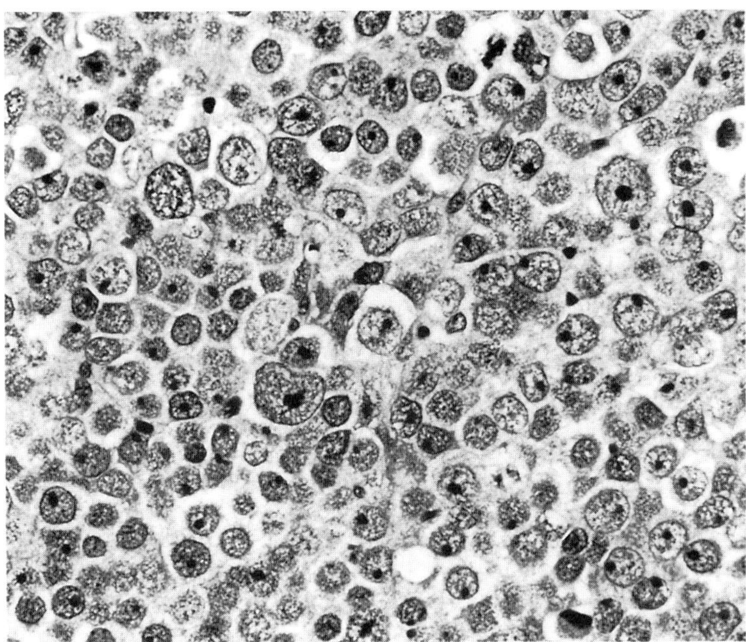

FIGURE 4.—Anaplastic component. Although most cells have prominent nucleoli, they remain the characteristic coarsely granular and filamentous chromatin pattern of spermatocytic seminoma. (Hematoxylin-cosin strain; original magnification ×400.) (Courtesy of Albores-Saavedra J, Huffman H, Alvarado-Cabrero I, et al: Anaplastic variant of spermatocytic seminoma. *Hum Pathol* 27:650–655, 1996.)

tures of this variant were compared with those of 7 conventional spermatocytic seminomas.

Results.—The clinical features included no history of cryptorchidism. Masses appeared 3 to 18 months before surgery, and serum alpha-fetoprotein and human chorionic gonadotropin measurements were negative. Histological examination showed areas of spermatocytic seminoma (10% to 30%) with small, medium, and large cells. The main anaplastic component had cells with prominent nucleoli (Fig 4). All tumors had sheets of cells with large nuclei and prominent nucleoli resembling embryonal carcinoma. Abundant giant cells with strange nuclei were common. There were many normal and abnormal mitotic figures. All tumors showed tunical and vascular invasion and widespread intratubular growth. Necrosis and edema were present in all tumors. Many cells contained large, ropelike nucleoli and plentiful granular and dispersed chromatin. p53 was overexpressed in 2 tumors. Placenta-like alkaline phosphatase, vimentin, leukocytc common antigen, alpha-fetoprotein, neuron-specific enolase, human chorionic gonadotropin, and cytokeratins AE1/AE3 and cytokeratin 18 were not detected. Metastases did not develop in any of the patients.

Conclusion.—This discrete variant of spermatocytic seminoma should be studied thoroughly to learn more about its natural history.

▶ Spermatocytic seminoma is a relatively unusual testicular germ cell tumor that has only very rarely been reported to metastasize. In this report, the authors describe four cases of an anaplastic variant (defined by nuclear atypia and *not* increased mitotic activity). However, none of these tumors metastasized. Consequently, not unlike the case of classic seminoma, the distinction of an anaplastic subset may not be clinically important. In all fairness, though, since this is the first report of this subtype, the experience of others will need to be critically assessed before a definitive conclusion can be drawn.

M.B. Cohen, M.D.

International Germ Cell Consensus Classification: A Prognostic Factor-based Staging System for Metastatic Germ Cell Cancers
Mead GM, for the International Germ Cell Cancer Collaborative Group (Royal South Hants Hosp, Southampton, England)
J Clin Oncol 15:594–603, 1997
5–22

Background.—The incidence of seminomatous and nonseminomatous germ cell tumors (GCT), the most frequent cancers of young men, is increasing rapidly. Mortality from metastatic GCTs was high until the introduction of cisplatin-containing chemotherapy; now, overall cure rates of GCT are better than 80%. A simple prognostic factor-based staging classification system for metastatic GCTs was developed for use in clinical practice and collaborative trials.

Methods.—The study included clinical data on 5,202 patients with nonseminomatous GCT (NSGCT) and 660 patients with seminoma, all treated with cisplatin-containing chemotherapy. The patients were treated by collaborative groups from 10 countries; the median follow-up was 5 years. Multivariate analyses were performed to identify prognostic factors for progression and survival. The multivariate models were then validated in an independent data set of more recently treated patients.

Results.—Independent adverse factors for patients with NSGCT were mediastinal primary site, alfa-fetoprotein level, human chorionic gonado-tropin level, lactic dehydrogenase level, and the presence of nonpulmonary visceral metastases. The latter was the main adverse prognostic factor for patients with seminoma. A model constructed from these factors identified 3 risk groups (Fig 4). Sixty percent of patients were in the good prognosis group, which had a 5-year survival of 91%. Twenty-six percent were in the intermediate prognosis group, which had a 5-year survival of 79%. The remaining 14% of patients, all of whom had NSGCT, were in the poor prognosis group, which had a 5-year survival of 48%.

Conclusions.—A clinically based prognostic classification system for GCT is reported. This system has been agreed to by all major clinical trial

GOOD PROGNOSIS	
NON-SEMINOMA	**SEMINOMA**
Testis/retroperitoneal primary *and* No non-pulmonary visceral metastases *and* Good markers - all of *AFP < 1000 ng/ml and* *hCG < 5000 iu/l (1000 ng/ml) and* *LDH < 1.5 x upper limit of normal* **56% of non-seminomas** **5 year PFS 89%** **5 year Survival 92%**	Any primary site *and* No non-pulmonary visceral metastases *and* Normal AFP, any hCG, any LDH **90% of seminomas** **5 year PFS 82%** **5 year Survival 86%**
INTERMEDIATE PROGNOSIS	
NON-SEMINOMA	**SEMINOMA**
Testis/retroperitoneal primary *and* No non-pulmonary visceral metastases *and* **Intermediate markers - any of:** *AFP ≥ 1000 and ≤ 10,000 ng/mL or* *hCG ≥ 5000 iu/l and ≤ 50,000 iu/l or* *LDH ≥ 1.5 x N and ≤ 10 x N* **28% of non-seminomas** **5 year PFS 75%** **5 year Survival 80%**	Any primary site *and* **Non-pulmonary visceral metastases** *and* Normal AFP, any hCG, any LDH **10% of seminomas** **5 year PFS 67%** **5 year Survival 72%**
POOR PROGNOSIS	
NON-SEMINOMA	**SEMINOMA**
Mediastinal primary *or* **Non-pulmonary visceral metastases** *or* **Poor markers - any of:** *AFP > 10,000 ng/ml or* *hCG > 50,000 iu/l (10000 ng/ml) or* *LDH > 10 x upper limit of normal* **16% of non-seminomas** **5 year PFS 41%** **5 year Survival 48%**	**No patients classified as poor prognosis**

FIGURE 4.—Definitinon of the germ cell consensus classification. (Courtesy of Mead GM, for the International Germ Cell Cancer Collaborative Group: International germ cell consensus classification: A prognostic factor-based staging system for metastatic germ cell cancers. *J Clin Oncol* 15:594–603, 1997.)

groups currently active worldwide. Use of the classification in clinical practice and research will facilitate international communication regarding the assessment and treatment of GCTs.

▶ This, I believe, is an important article which is directly relevant to pathologists. It has unfortunately been published in a journal not widely read by pathologists, hence its inclusion here. The outcome of this consensus paper is a prognostic classification scheme for germ cell tumors, as indicated in the included figure from the article. It highlights a few aspects, including the need to distinguish seminomas from non-seminomatous germ cell tumors and the importance of serum tumor markers (alpha-fetoprotein and human chorionic gonadotrophin).

M.B. Cohen, M.D.

6 Kidney

The Nonspecificity of Focal Segmental Glomerulosclerosis: The Defining Characteristics of Primary Focal Glomerulosclerosis, Mesangial Proliferation, and Minimal Change
McAdams AJ, Valentini RP, Welch TR (Univ of Cincinnati, Ohio)
Medicine 76:42–52, 1997   6–1

Introduction.—Approximately 1 in 5,000 children is found with primary nephrotic syndrome each year. Many children who are unresponsive to corticosteroids have a glomerular lesion characterized by segmental sclerotic alteration of the glomerular tuft. This lesion is referred to as focal segmental glomerulosclerosis. Previous classifications did not consider the absence of mesangial proliferation, generalized foot process changes, basement membrane thickness, or the presence of tubuloreticular inclusions. A detailed clinical review and re-evaluation of biopsy material from 134 children and adolescents was conducted to derive a classification system.

Methods.—Biopsy specimens from children and adolescents who had nephrotic syndrome or asymptomatic proteinuria were studied. Pathologic analysis included histology, immunohistology, and ultrastructure. Classification of biopsy materials included segmental hyalinosis/sclerosis, primary focal sclerosis, mesangial proliferation, and minimal change.

Results.—Among the biopsies studied, 29 had primary focal segmental glomerulosclerosis, 49 had minimal change, and 56 had mesangial proliferation. Among those with minimal change, 41% had 1 or more segmental sclerotic lesions. Children with primary focal segmental glomerulosclerosis were primarily black (76%), with a mean age at clinical onset of 13 years. Tubular atrophy was a feature in 90% of these children, 62% had isolated proteinuria, and 38% had microscopic hematuria. After transplantation, focal segmental glomerulosclerosis does not tend to recur. In the mesangial proliferation group, 79% were white. In these children, 98% had nephrotic syndrome, 52% had microscopic hematuria, and 55% had at least 1 segmental sclerotic lesion. In the minimal change group, 67% were white. Of these, 98% had nephrotic syndrome and 51% had microscopic hematuria. Those with minimal change had generalized fusion of podocyte foot processes. Those with minimal change and mesangial proliferation tended to have recurrences after transplantation.

Conclusion.—The segmental glomerular lesion reflects the progressive nature of a number of disease processes rather than serving as a specific marker for a subtype of primary nephrotic syndrome. Focal segmental sclerotic lesions do not define a unique disorder in children. The histologic appearance of the rest of the glomeruli, rather than the presence or absence of focal sclerosis, should be the focus of concentration in classifying disorders associated with nephrotic syndrome or asymptomatic proteinuria.

▶ This article is an up-to-date review of the experience of focal segmental glomerulosclerosis at Children's Hospital of Cincinnati; it includes 29 cases. The salient conclusion from this study is that the presence of focal sclerotic lesions does not define a distinct entity in children. The differential diagnosis includes focal segmental glomerulosclerosis, minimal change disease, and mesangial proliferation (debatable as a distinct entity). Like most glomerulopathies, a careful clinical-pathologic correlation is necessary to accurately diagnose these disease entities.

M.B. Cohen, M.D.

Mast Cells in Acute Cellular Rejection of Human Renal Allografts
Lajoie G, Nadasdy T, Laszik Z, et al (Univ of Oklahoma, Oklahoma City)
Mod Pathol 9:1118–1125, 1996   6–2

Introduction.—T lymphocytes play a major role in mediating acute cellular rejection of renal allografts; both cytotoxic T-cell and delayed-type hypersensitivity reactions participate in this rejection. In delayed type hypersensitivity reactions in rodents, mast cells were shown to degranulate, and evidence suggests that mast cell proliferation is partly dependent on T lymphocytes. Mast cells are bone marrow–derived hematopoietic cells that share immunophenotypic homology with monocytes/macrophages. Mast cells may have important roles in a variety of inflammatory processes. The detection of mast cells in tissue is greatly facilitated by the recent development of a commercially available monoclonal antibody against mast cell tryptase that recognizes mast cells.

Methods.—To evaluate the presence of mast cells and their participation in the acute rejection of renal allografts, an anti–mast cell tryptase antibody was used to study 28 biopsy specimens from renal allografts transplanted for various lengths of time. The renal biopsy specimens were quantitatively evaluated for the number of mast cells, eosinophils, and plasma cells present. Each specimen was assigned a semiquantitative grade for the degree of cellular rejection, interstitial fibrosis, edema, and hemorrhage. The possible association between the number of mast cells and the degree of acute interstitial rejection, edema, interstitial fibrosis, and hemorrhage, and the number of eosinophils and plasma cells was also examined.

Results.—A positive correlation was found between the number of mast cells and the time since transplantation. The number of mast cells was also positively correlated with the severity of interstitial fibrosis and interstitial edema. In patients with moderate and severe rejection, mast cells were increased in number when compared with patients with mild acute rejection and normal kidneys. In patients with severe rejection, there were 12.20 mast cells per 10 HPFs, whereas patients with mild rejection had 2.44 mast cells per 10 HPFs.

Conclusion.—Mast cells might play a role in the process of acute rejection of renal allografts and in the development of interstitial fibrosis.

▶ Mast cells are enigmatic. Much of their basic (patho) biology continues to be worked out; see, for example, the work of Steve Galli. The article by Lajoie, et al.[1] makes 2 useful observations. First, the identification of mast cells in routinely stained sections may be difficult. In this study, the authors obtained excellent results with an anti–mast cell tryptase monoclonal antibody (Chemicon; Temecula, CA). Second, the authors found a statistically significant correlation between the number of mast cells and the time since transplantation, as well as the severity of interstitial fibrosis and interstitial edema. One obvious conclusion is that mast cells play a role in the pathogenesis of interstitial fibrosis. Clearly, additional studies are necessary.

M.B. Cohen, M.D.

Reference

1. Galli SJ: The Paul Kallos Memorial Lecture. The mast cell: A versatile effector cell for a challenging world. *Int Arch Allergy Immunol* 113:14–22, 1997.

Renal Medullary Carcinoma: Clinical and Therapeutic Aspects of a Newly Described Tumor

Avery RA, Harris JE, Davis CJ Jr, et al (Dwight D Eisenhower Army Med Ctr, Ft Gordon, Ga; Rush Presbyterian St Luke's Med Ctr, Chicago; Armed Forces Inst of Pathology, Washington, DC; et al)
Cancer 78:128–132, 1996   6–3

Objective.—To describe the clinical signs and symptoms and treatment outcome of patients with renal medullary carcinoma.

Background.—Most renal carcinomas occur in individuals between 50 and 70 years, but they also occur in younger patients. Hartman et al. reported that 50% of renal tumors in patients between 10 and 20 years were Wilms' tumor and 50% were renal cell carcinoma. Davis et al recently described a rare kidney tumor in young black patients with sickle cell trait or hemoglobin sickle cell disease. This carcinoma is aggressive, unresponsive to treatment, and causes death within 1 year. It has been named renal medullary carcinoma.

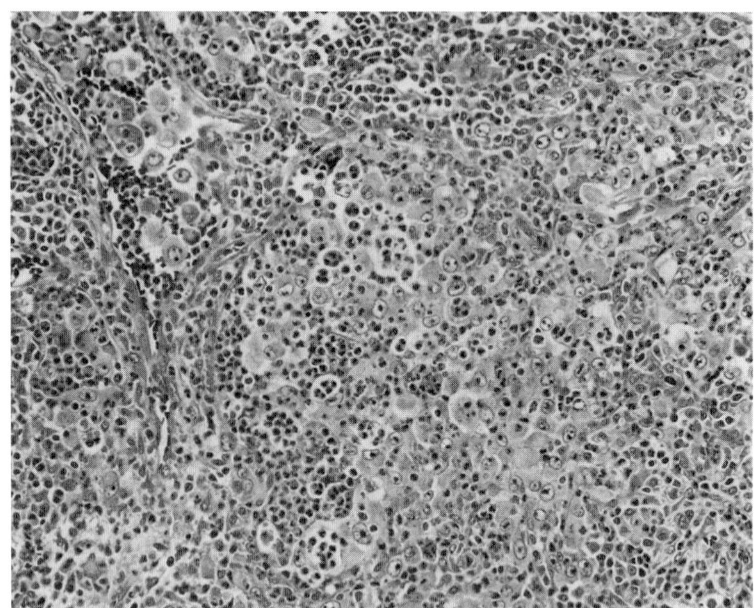

FIGURE 3.—Undifferentiated area of tumor is shown. Note dark cells with pale nuclei and prominent nucleoli. The tumor is richly admixed with inflammatory cells, chiefly polymorphonuclear leukocytes (H & E, original magnification ×200). (Courtesy of Avery RA, Harris JE, Davis CJ Jr, et al: Renal medullary carcinoma: Clinical and therapeuric aspects of a newly described tumor. *Cancer* 78:128–132. Copyright 1996 American Cancer Society. Reprinted by permission of Wiley-Liss, Inc., a subsidiary of John Wiley & Sons, Inc.)

Methods.—Information was collected from patient records and various other sources on 6 patients with renal medullary carcinoma. Cytogenetic studies were performed in fresh frozen tissue from 1 patient.

Results.—All 6 patients had sickle cell trait. Patient age ranged from 24 to 36 years. Five patients were male. The average survival from diagnosis to death was 3 months. The following chemotherapies and immunotherapies were attempted: cyclophosphamide, doxorubicin, cisplatin; methotrexate, vinblastine, doxorubicin, and cisplatin; single-agent interferon; single-agent paclitaxel; and single-agent vinblastine. No objective response to treatment was seen. Investigational therapies included topotecan, doxorubicin, and filgrastim; α-interferon, interleukin-2, and 5-fluorouracil; and single-agent paclitaxel. Cytogenetic studies showed various structural and numerical anomalies. Of karyotyped cells, 2 had abnormalities of chromosome 3 and all had monosomy 11 (Fig 3).

Conclusions.—Renal medullary carcinoma is an aggressive tumor. It is resistant to many chemotherapies and immunotherapies and causes death in a very short time. The disease may have an unidentified genetic component because all patients have sickle cell trait and are young.

▶ Renal medullary is a newly recognized carcinoma arising in the kidney. The first significant report was by Charles Davis, from the Armed Forces

Institute of Pathology (AFIP), who reported a series of 34 such tumors.[1] By far the most striking aspect of this neoplasm is its intimate association with sickle cell disease, more specifically SC trait or SC disease. The histopathology, although variegated, has some specific characteristics, which have been well described by the group at AFIP. It is believed that these tumors arise from calyceal epithelium, and may have a very aggressive course; in Davis' report the mean duration was 15 weeks after surgery. In this report, another 6 cases are reported. Despite aggressive chemotherapy the survival was comparable. Although rare, this tumor should be separated from other "renal cell carcinomas".

M.B. Cohen, M.D.

Reference

1. Davis CJ Jr, Mostofi FK, Sesterhenn IA: Renal medullary carcinoma: The seventh sickle cell nephropathy. *Am J Surg Pathol* 19:1–11, 1995.

Renal Oncocytoma: A Reappraisal of Morphologic Features With Clinicopathologic Findings in 80 Cases
Amin MB, Crotty TB, Tickoo SK, et al (Henry Ford Hosp, Detroit; Mayo Clinic, Rochester, Minn)
Am J Surg Pathol 21:1–12, 1997   6–4

Background.—Several features of renal oncocytoma overlap with those of other renal neoplasms that have a preponderance of granular cytoplasm, such as chromophobe, granular, and papillary renal cell carcinomas. The current literature contains some misconceptions about renal oncocytoma, including the need to grade oncocytomas, the metastatic potential of oncocytomas, and the notion that renal oncocytoma is usually low grade and lacks prominent nucleoli.

Methods and Findings.—Ninety-three tumors from 80 patients were examined to further characterize the histologic features of renal oncocytoma. On gross assessment the tumors were seen to be mahogany brown, to lack necrosis, and to average 4.4 cm. Histologically, the tumors consisted of an exclusive or predominant component of acidophilic cells. Three architectural patterns of disposition were noted: the classic pattern, composed of a characteristic nested or organoid arrangement of cells, each surrounded by a distinct reticulin framework (evident in 57.5% of the cases); a tubulocystic pattern with many closely packed, cystically dilated tubular structures (in 6.3%); and a mixed pattern, showing both the organoid and tubulocystic patterns (in 36.2%). In 53.8% of the tumors, a gross or microscopic scar was observed. Histologically, a distinctive myxoid and/or hyalinized stroma separated cell nests. The nuclei of renal oncocytoma were typically round, with uniform nuclear contours. Nucleoli were prominent in nearly half the tumors. Pleomorphism was absent in half the cases but conspicuous in 12.5%, including foci of bizarre cells. Other atypical features were perinephric fat involvement, present in

---

TABLE 3.—Approach to Histopathologic Diagnosis of Renal Oncocytoma

I. Adequate sampling of tumor (at least 1 per cm of tumor)
II. Gross appearance
    Well circumscribed, homogeneous cortical tumor
    Mahogany brown appearance
    Central scar
    Absence of gross necrosis
    Absence of gross renal vein invasion
III. Architectural features
    Classic
      Nested or organoid arrangement including "solid"
        sheets, tubules, and trabeculae
      Investment of nests by distinct reticulin framework
      Myxoid, edematous, and hyalinized stroma
    Tubulocystic
      Variably sized tubules and cysts with minimal
        intervening stroma; very focal papillary arrangement
        is acceptable
    Mixed
IV. Cytoplasmic features
    Exclusive or predominantly eosinophilic and finely
      granular cytoplasm
    Focal clearing of cytoplasm may be present
      Should not be promiment, confluent or conspicuous
        (like clear-cell renal cell carcinoma)
      Should not be perinuclear with peripheral
        accentuation of cytoplasmic granularity (like
        chromophobe cell carcinoma)
V. Nuclear features
    Round nuclei with regular nuclear contours
    Even chromatin distribution
    Absent to prominent nucleoli
    Absent to vanishingly rare mitotic activity
    Intranuclear holes
    Pleomorphism, hyperchromasia
      Degenerated, smudged nuclear chromatin with
        marked variation of size
      Evidenced in foci, but may be extensive
VI. Permissible "atypical features"
    Perirenal fat involvement
    Hemorrhage
    Minimal microscopic necrosis
    Rare typical mitosis
    Microvascular invasion
VII. Impermissible features
    Extensive papillary architecture
    Areas of clear-cell carcinoma
    Sarcomatoid or spindle-cell areas
    Gross or prominent microscopic necrosis
    Frequent mitoses, including atypical mitoses
    Gross involvement of renal vein

(Courtesy of Amin MB, Crotty TB, Tickoo SK, et al: Renal oncocytoma: A reappraisal of morphologic features with clinicopathologic findings in 80 cases. *Am J Surg Pathol* 21:1–12, 1997.)

11.3%; renal parenchymal invasion unrelated to desmoplasia, in 10%; and hemorrhage, in 31.3% (Tables 3 and 4).

Conclusion.—Renal oncocytoma is a benign neoplasm that does not warrant a nuclear grading scheme. Its unique histologic features are an organoid and tubulocystic architecture; myxoid or hyalinized stroma; and

TABLE 4.—Comparison Between Renal Oncocytoma and Chromophobe Renal Cell Carcinoma

	Renal oncocytoma	Chromophobe renal cell carcinoma
Incidence	5% (27)	5% (27)
Sex distribution	M:F = 3.1:1	M:F = 1.1:1
Presentation		
Asymptomatic	87%	52% (6)
Gross		
General	Homogenous, solid	Homogenous, solid
Color	Mahogany brown	Beige to light brown
Central scar	Common: 54%	Rare: 7% (26)
Necrosis	Very rare	Present: 33%
Multicentricity	Yes	Rare (25)
Bilaterality	Yes	Rare (25)
Microscopic		
Pattern	Compact, nested, alveolar, and tubulocystic	Sheets, broad alveolar growth pattern
Cell types	One cell type	Two cell types
Cytoplasm	Copious, granular ecsinophilic	Voluminous, clear and reticular or eosinophilic and finely granular
Nuclear outlines	Smooth	Irregular
Nuclear chromatin	Regular	Irregular, often clumped
Binucleation	Rare	Frequent
Pleomorphism	Foci of atypical cells	Dependent on nuclear grade
Nuclear grade	Not applicable	Usually Fuhman grade 2, occasionally grade 3
Sarcomatoid transformation	No	Yes (rare) (2,16)
Ultrastructure	Abundant microchondra	Cytoplasmic vesicles and mitochondra (1,3,33)
Histochemistry		
Hales colloidal iron	Weak, focal (9)	Positive (3,33)
Carbonic anhydrase C	Positive	Positive (3)
Immunohistochemistry	Cytokeratin positive	Cytokeratin positive
	Vimentin negative	Vimentin negative
Band 3P analysis	Positive (4)	Negative
Cell of origin	Intercalated cells of collecting duct	Intercalated cells of collecting duct (2)
Chromosomal abnormalities	No recurrent aberration; translocations involving chromosome 11 and loss of chromosome Y and 1 reported (7,13,22,34,35)	Multiple chromosomal losses Most common: loss of chr 1, 2, 10, 13 (31)
Mitochondral DNA	Abnormal restriction fragment pattern	Abnormal restriction fragment pattern (22)
DNA ploidy	Usually diploid or near-diploid aneuploid (11,17,24,29)	Aneuploidy 60–77% (1,3,6)
Disease progression	None	7.5% (4.5%, DOD, 3% AWD) (1,3,6,33)
Outcome	Benign	Low malignant potential

Abbreviations: DOD, dead of disease; *AWD,* alive with disease.
(Courtesy of Amin MB, Crotty TB, Tickoo SK, et al: Renal oncocytoma: A reappraisal of morphologic features with clinicopathologic findings in 80 cases. *Am J Surg Pathol* 21:1–12, 1997.)

the occasional atypical findings of nuclear pleomorphism, prominent nucleoli, and adjacent renal parenchymal and perinephric fat involvement.

▶ The interest in renal oncocytomas continues. In this collaborative study between Henry Ford Hospital and the Mayo Clinic, a series of 80 cases are documented in significant detail. The 2 tables, in particular, included with the abstract, should be useful to the surgical pathologist in making this diagnosis without the routine use of ancillary studies, such as electron microscopy and immunohistochemistry.

M.B. Cohen, M.D.

Cytodifferentiation of a Wilms' Tumor Pulmonary Metastasis: Theoretic and Clinical Implications

Seemayer TA, Harper JL, Shickell D, et al (Univ of Nebraska, Omaha)
Cancer 79:1629–1634, 1997   6–5

Introduction.—An earlier study lead to the theory that neoplasms in very young infants had a benign clinical evolution, an example being neuroblastoma which tended to regress, independent of therapy. Despite a substantial body of experimental work on the biology of cancer, it is unknown whether drugs and/or irradiation induce cytodifferentiation of a malignant tumor. On occasion, a malignant neoplasm may be induced to mature with therapy. A child of 3½ years of age had clinical National Wilms' Tumor Study stage IV Wilms' tumor. Her extensively necrotic blastemic Wilms' tumor was removed after systemic chemotherapy and irradiation. In 1996, at age 16 years, the patient had new, small pulmonary nodules which were discovered by MRI. Several of these nodules were biopsied.

Methods.—To identify similar cases from 1966 to the present, a literature review was conducted using key words such as Wilms' tumor, therapy, relapse, metastasis, maturation, and cytodifferentiation. Completely mature, cytodifferentiated pulmonary metastases of Wilms' tumor after chemotherapy was found in 4 patients. One of these patients also had received irradiation to the pulmonary metastasis.

Results.—The case patient had a primary extremely necrotic blastemic Wilms' tumor that was devoid of maturation. A scar and nodule composed of bland epithelium and tubules admixed with mature smooth muscle was the evidence of lung metastases examined 13 years later. A nearly negligible proliferation index was found after immunohistochemical stains were used to assess the proliferative rate of these cells.

Conclusion.—On occasion, complete cytodifferentiation of Wilms' tumor pulmonary metastasis may be caused by chemotherapy and/or irradiation. Because few patients with metastatic pulmonary Wilms' tumor are subjected to biopsy, the true incidence of such an event is unknown. The notion of surgical biopsy should be entertained for children receiving chemotherapy who have radiologically stable Wilms' lung metastases, as determined by imaging studies. In some instances, therapy could perhaps be halted because it would be deemed unnecessary.

▶ The pathology of primary Wilms' tumor has been well described. One relatively recent source is the new Armed Forces Institute of Pathology fascicle which was co-authored by Bruce Beckwith. The study reported in the abstract above describes the pathology of a case of metastatic Wilms' tumor. What is unusual about this particular case is that mature elements were identified in the resected pulmonary nodules. These nodules were resected more than a decade after the primary tumor was removed and after the patient received protocol chemotherapy. This has been reported previously, albeit rarely. The finding is similar to what has been described with other primitive tumors such as germ cell tumors of the testis. As pointed out by the authors, this finding could have both theoretical and clinical implications regarding the biology of the tumor and the need for additional therapy.

M.B. Cohen, M.D.

7   Head and Neck

Markers for Assessment of Nodal Metastasis in Laryngeal Carcinoma
Takes RP, Baatenburg de Jong RJ, Schuuring E, et al (Univ Hosp Leiden, The Netherlands)
Arch Otolaryngol Head Neck Surg 123:412–419, 1997   7–1

Introduction.—Regional metastasis determines treatment and prognosis in patients with head and neck squamous cell carcinoma. Current imaging techniques are not adequate and ultrasound-guided fine-needle aspiration biopsy has a sensitivity of only 76%. Results of histologic, immunohistochemical, and molecular biological analysis were correlated with clinical and histopathologic data to determine whether biological markers could be identified that could predict the presence of metastases, based on features of the primary tumor, in 31 patients with laryngeal carcinoma.

Methods.—Several histologic features and biological markers were analyzed. These markers were used because of their putative role in the process of metastasis and were analyzed by immunohistochemical and/or Southern blot techniques: proliferating cell nuclear antigen, *p53*, retinoblastoma tumor-suppressor gene (*Rb*), *myc*, *bcl-2* (inhibitor of apoptosis), epidermal growth factor (*EGF*), *EGF*-receptor, *neu*, *nm23* (also known as *NME1*, putative metastasis suppressor) *desmoplakin*, neuron cell-adhesion molecule (*N-CAM*), epithelial cell-adhesion molecule (*Ep-CAM*), E-cadherin, cyclin D1 (*CCND1*), and *EMS1*.

Results.—Nodal metastasis was correlated with the presence of an inflammatory reaction surrounding the tumor, eosinophilic infiltration, positive immunostaining for *Rb*, negative immunostaining for *Ep-CAM*, and amplification of *CCND1* and EMS1. There were no correlations between differentiation and growth pattern and lymph node metastasis. No correlation was determined between *p53*, *E-cadherin*, *EGF*, *nm23*, desmoplakin, or *N-CAM* staining and the presence of lymph node metastasis.

Conclusion.—It is feasible to predict and exclude lymph node metastasis by evaluating the features of the primary tumor only. Use of immunohistochemical staining was easy, quick, and cost effective in evaluating the markers analyzed in this trial.

▶ This study first caught my attention because of the following statement made by the authors: " ... examination with ultrasound-guided fine-needle aspiration biopsy (the most accurate technique to detect lymph node metastases to date) identifies clinically occult metastases ..." This is a European study and I wonder how many of my American-trained surgical pathologists or surgery colleagues agree with that statement. Too many pathologists around me still feel uncomfortable with the concept of rendering a definitive diagnosis on the basis of a cytology specimen alone.

These authors and others[1] are investigating the role of biological markers in predicting tumor behavior. This might some day eliminate the need for radical surgery for staging purposes (and give the pathologists even less tissue to examine).

K.E. Sirgi, M.D.

Reference

1. Tartour E, Deneux L, Mosseri V, et al: Soluble interleukin-2 receptor serum level as a predictor of locoregional control and survival for patients with head and neck carcinoma. *Cancer* 79:1401–1408, 1997.

A Monoclonal Antibody KIS-1 Recognizing a New Membrane Antigen on Human Squamous-Cell Carcinoma
Toh U, Yamana H, Fujita H, et al (Kurume Univ, Japan)
Int J Cancer 66:600–606, 1996   7–2

Introduction.—One of the most common cancers is squamous cell carcinoma. The most effective therapeutic approach is surgical excision because squamous cell carcinoma is relatively resistant to the available chemotherapy or radiation therapy regimens. To expand this treatment modality, it is important to better understand the antigens on squamous cell carcinoma cells. For staining of the surface antigens expressed on squamous cell carcinoma, a relatively large number of monoclonal antibodies are available. It is necessary to establish new monoclonal antibodies for immunodiagnosis or for immunotargeting because the available monoclonal antibodies also recognize normal squamous tissues. A monoclonal antibody, KIS-1, that recognizes squamous cell carcinoma was developed to understand their antigenicity.

Methods.—An esophageal squamous cell carcinoma was used as an immunogen to help understand how a KIS-1 monoclonal antibody recognizes a membrane antigen on human squamous cell carcinomas. Immunofluorescence staining, immunohistochemical study, immunoprecipitation, and immunoblot analysis were conducted on tumor cells and cell lines to test the reactivity of the KIS-1 monoclonal antibody.

Results.—Most esophageal, lung, and oral-cavity squamous cell carcinoma was recognized by the KIS-1 monoclonal antibody, as evidenced by immunofluorescent and immunohistochemical analyses. There was little reactivity with adenocarcinomas from various organs, and there was no reactivity to keratinocyte cell lines. This monoclonal antibody showed reactivity in the basal layer of the normal esophageal epithelium adjacent to the esophageal squamous cell carcinoma, but no reactivity was evinced

TABLE 1.—Summary of the Reactivity of KIS-1 Monoclonal Antibody to Tumor and Normal Tissues

Tissues (histology)	Positive cases per total cases (%)
Cancer tissues	
Esophageal cancer (squamous-cell carcinoma)	101/116 (87%)
Esophageal neoplasm (sarcoma)	0/3 (0%)
Stomach cancer (adenocarcinoma)	3/42 (7%)
Colorectal cancer (adenocarcinoma)	1/18 (6%)
Lung cancer (squamous-cell carcinoma)	9/10 (90%)
well differentiated	3/3 (100%)
poorly differentiated	6/7 (86%)
Lung cancer (adenocarcinoma)	2/6 (33%)
Lung cancer (large-cell carcinoma)	0/1 (0%)
Oral cancer (squamous-cell carcinoma)	5/8 (63%)
Ovarian cancer (adenocarcinoma)	0/1 (0%)
Cervix cancer (squamous-cell carcinoma)	2/3 (67%)
Esophageal dysplasia	5/5 (100%)
Normal tissues	
Esophagus	
adjacent to SCC (<2 cm)	16/16 (100%)
far from SCC (7 cm–10 cm)	0/6 (0%)
Others*	0 (0%)
oral mucosa (2), skin (2), lung (3), breast (2), stomach (5), liver (2), spleen (1), pancreas† (1), gall bladder (2), colon (4), ureter (2), Kidney (2), ovary (1), adrenal gland† (1), neural tissues of normal esophagus and stomach (24), endothelium (16), lymph node (7), PBMC (4), red blood cells (3), bone-marrow cells (3)	

*Number of cases examined appears in parentheses.
†Includes endocrine glands.
Abbreviations: SCC, squamous cell carcinoma; *PBMC*, peripheral blood mononuclear cell.
(Courtesy of Toh U, Yamana H, Fujita H, et al: A monoclonal antibody KIS-1 recognizing a new membrane antigen on human squamous-cell carcinoma. *Int J Cancer* 66:600–606. Copyright 1996, Wiley-Liss, Inc. Reprinted by permission of Wiley-Liss, Inc., a subsidiary of John Wiley & Sons, Inc.)

on any of the other normal tissues, including esophageal epithelium far from squamous cell carcinoma or tissue from patients with nonmalignant disease (Table 1). In nonreducing and in reducing conditions, the KIS-1 monoclonal antibody immunoprecipitated a 46-kDa membrane protein of esophageal squamous cell carcinoma. Immunoblot analysis showed that the antibody recognized the 46 and the 40-kDa proteins of the esophageal squamous cell carcinoma.

Conclusion.—A 46-kDa surface antigen expressed on squamous cell carcinoma was recognized by this monoclonal antibody, which also recognized only the cells in the basal layer of esophageal epithelium adjacent to squamous cell carcinoma. The KIS-1 monoclonal antibody may be a new tool for understanding the antigenicity of squamous cell carcinoma.

▶ I certainly could use such an antibody when cornered by demanding clinicians insisting on knowing the precise squamous or glandular nature of a non–small-cell carcinoma of the lung, although such knowledge would not necessarily help their patient in any useful manner. In practice, I cannot think of many useful *diagnostic* applications for such an antibody. The potential for future specific immunotherapy against malignant and dysplastic squamous epithelium, as indicated in the article, is definitely worth investigating further.

K.E. Sirgi, M.D.

Expression of Epstein-Barr Virus–encoded RNAs as a Marker for Metastatic Undifferentiated Nasopharyngeal Carcinoma

Chao T-Y, Chow K-C, Chang J-Y, et al (Natl Defence Med Ctr, Taipei, Republic of China; Veterans Gen Hosp, Tapei, Republic of China)
Cancer 78:24–29, 1996   7–3

Introduction.—Much research has been conducted to show the close association between Epstein-Barr virus and human diseases such as infectious mononucleosis, Burkitt's lymphoma, and nasopharyngeal carcinoma. The presence of Epstein Barr virus in a metastatic tumor of unknown origin could serve as a potential marker for tumor cells in metastatic lesions of nasopharyngeal carcinoma, as Epstein Barr virus is present in primary and metastatic lesions of undifferentiated nasopharyngeal carcinoma. To detect Epstein Barr virus–infected nasopharyngeal carcinoma cells, Epstein Barr virus–encoded nonpolyadenylated RNAs are often used as a marker. The expression of Epstein Barr virus–encoded nonpolyadenylated RNAs in nasopharyngeal carcinoma cells at various metastatic sites was documented and their significance determined.

Methods.—Twenty-one patients with nasopharyngeal carcinoma participated in this study in which an in situ hybridization technique was used to identify the presence of Epstein Barr virus–encoded nonpolyadenylated RNAs in paraffin embedded tissues from primary and metastatic sites. Two patients had squamous cell carcinoma and 19 had undifferentiated lesions. A comparison was made with controls which were composed of 150 specimens of normal tissues and tissues from patients with a variety of benign and malignant diseases other than nasopharyngeal carcinoma. Immunohistochemistry was used to examine the expression of latent membrane protein and a lytic protein, BZLF-1, in the nasopharyngeal carcinoma specimens.

Results.—Epstein Barr virus–encoded nonpolyadenylated RNAs were contained in the malignant cells of tissues from all patients with undifferentiated nasopharyngeal carcinoma and 1 patient with squamous cell carcinoma. The other patient with squamous cell carcinoma had a negative result. In 18% of tissues (4 of 22), latent membrane protein was expressed in metastatic nasopharyngeal carcinomas, whereas BZLF-1 was not expressed in any of the tissues. In the 43 patients with normal tissues and benign lesions, Epstein Barr virus–encoded nonpolyadenylated RNAs were not detected. Epstein Barr virus–encoded nonpolyadenylated RNAs were detected in only 2 of the 12 patients with non-Hodgkin's lymphoma, in 1 of 2 patients with Hodgkin's lymphoma, and in 1 of 6 patients with gastric cancer, the group composed of malignant diseases other than nasopharyngeal carcinoma.

Conclusion.—Epstein Barr virus–encoded nonpolyadenylated RNAs can be used as a sensitive marker to identify nasopharyngeal carcinoma cells at various metastatic sites by in situ hybridization. The demonstration of Epstein Barr virus–encoded nonpolyadenylated RNAs in lesions of undifferentiated histology may be useful as a diagnostic adjunct for nasopharyngeal carcinoma presenting as metastatic cancer of unknown origin.

▶ Undifferentiated nasopharyngeal carcinoma is frequently seen clinically as a lymph node metastasis in the absence of an obvious primary neoplasm. The availability of a safe (nonradioactive) and reliable marker for identifying Epstein-Barr virus–encoded RNA is a nice addition to the diagnostic armementarium of the surgical pathologist.

K.E. Sirgi, M.D.

Desmoid Fibromatosis of the Sinonasal Tract and Nasopharynx: A Clinicopathologic Study of 25 Cases
Gnepp DR, Henley J, Weiss S, et al (Brown Univ, Providence, RI; Rhode Island Hosp, Providence; Univ of Michigan, Ann Arbor; et al)
Cancer 78: 2572–2579, 1996   7–4

Introduction.—Desmoid fibromatoses are a group of nonmetastatisizing, well differentiated, nonencapsulated fibrous tissue proliferations having a tendency toward local invasion and recurrence. The head and neck are the site of up to 23% of all extra-abdominal desmoid fibromatoses, and this figure increases to one third for children. The soft tissues of the neck are involved in 61% of patients who have desmoid fibromatoses of the head and neck. This study was conducted to provide more information on desmoid fibromatoses in this region as these lesions are rarely found in the upper respiratory tract and there is little written of their biological potential.

Methods.—There were 25 patients, ranging in age from 8 months to 62 years, who were found to have fibromatosis involving the sinonasal and nasopharyngeal areas in the files of the Armed Forces Institute of Pathology between 1885 and 1985. Histologic materials were reviewed, clinical data was tabulated, and follow-up information was obtained for each patient. The range of follow-up was 1 year to 20 years and 7 months, with a median of 6 years and 9 months.

Results.—In 18 patients, a single site was involved, and in 7 patients, multiple contiguous adjacent sites were involved. The most frequently involved site was the maxillary sinus (22 patients), followed by the nasal cavity (5 patients), the ethmoid sinus (4 patients), orbit (4 patients), sphenoid and frontal sinuses (2 patients each), and nasopharynx (1 patient). The last follow-up showed that 18 patients were alive with no evidence of disease, 2 were alive with unknown disease histories, and 3 were alive with recurrent or residual disease. One patient died with no evidence of disease. Recurrences developed in 5 patients (21%). One recurrence occurred at 6 months, another at 16 months, and a third at 34 months. One patient had recurrences at 3.5 months and 5.5 months. At 6.5 years, 1 patient was alive with recurrent disease.

Conclusion.—Desmoid fibromatoses involving the sinonasal tract and nasopharynx appears to have lower recurrence rates and morbidity than desmoid fibromatoses found in other areas of the body. Because of the low recurrence rates for desmoid tumors involving the sinonasal tract, it appears prudent to surgically excise the primary and/or recurrent tumors and reserve radiation or chemotherapy for the exceptional tumor that may not be amenable to complete surgical excision.

▶ Until recently, most articles researching desmoid fibromatosis used a variable (and often colorful) terminology to describe these lesions: "fibrous tissue proliferation," "unchecked fibroblastic reparative process," "tumor-like condition," "exuberant pseudoneoplastic proliferation"... to name a few. Recently, the clonal (hence tumoral) nature of desmoid fibromatosis was demonstrated.[1, 2] The term tumor can now be safely applied to these lesions.

K.E. Sirgi, M.D.

References

1. Maomi LI, Cordon-Cardo C, Gerald WL, et al: Desmoid fibromatosis is a clonal process. *Hum Pathol* 27:939–943, 1996.
2. Lucas DR, Shroyer KR, McCarthy PJ, et al.: Desmoid tumor is a clonal cellular proliferation: PCR amplification of HUMARA for analysis of patterns of X-chromosome inactivation. *Am J Surg Pathol* 21:306–311, 1997.

Salivary Gland Cystadenocarcinomas: A Clinicopathologic Study of 57 Cases

Foss RD, Ellis GL, Auclair PL (Armed Forces Inst of Pathology, Washington, DC)

Am J Surg Pathol 20:1440–1447, 1996   7–5

Introduction.—Cystadenocarcinoma is a term that was applied to salivary gland neoplasia and encompassed a variety of salivary tumors showing cystic and papillary-cystic patterns of growth. A subset of papillary and cystic lesions remained unclassified and then became known as cystadenocarcinomas on the basis of recognizable, recurring histomorphologic patterns of cystic and papillary growth without the features of other well-defined salivary gland tumors. A review of 57 cases of cystadenocarcinomas was conducted to ascertain more fully the clinicomorphologic spectrum and biologic behavior of this tumor class.

Methods.—The files of the Armed Forces Institutes of Pathology were searched for cases of major and oral minor salivary gland adenocarcinomas that demonstrated cystic or papillary-cystic features. Fifty-seven patients, ranging in age from 20 to 85 years met the criteria for inclusion. The criteria were occurrence within a major salivary gland or associated with an intraoral minor salivary gland tumor, invasive growth; predominantly cystic pattern of growth; and absence of acinar or mucoepidermoid differentiation and showing evidence of having originated in a benign mixed tumor. Assessments were made for extent of invasive growth, mitoses, cellular composition, anaplasia, tumor-associated lymphoid proliferation, perineural and vascular invasion, and reactive changes, such as hemorrhage and stromal desmoplasia.

Results.—Patients older than 50 years comprised 71% of the group. Major salivary glands were the source of 37 tumors (65%); 35 were found

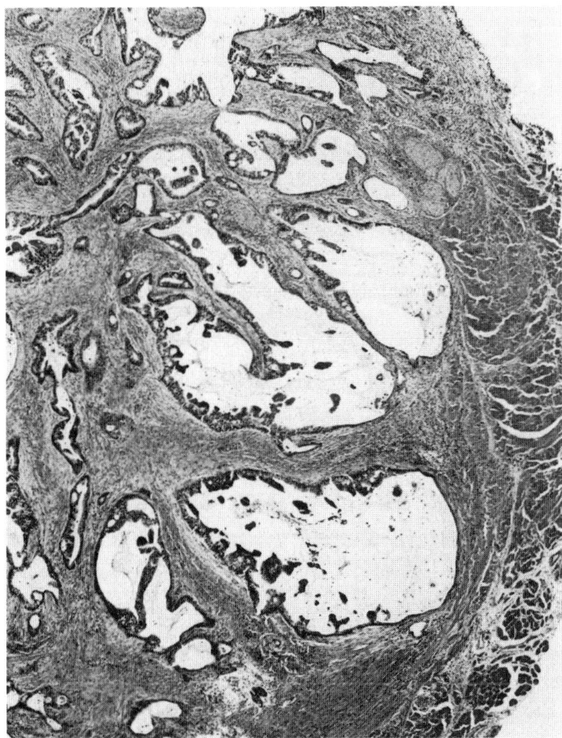

FIGURE 2.—A salivary gland cystadenocarcinoma from the lower lip invades skeletal muscle and induces a desmoplastic stromal response. The tumor metastasized to a submental lymph node. (Courtesy of Foss RD, Ellis GL, Auclair PL: Salivary gland cystadenocarcinomas: A clinicopathologic study of 57 cases. *Am J Surg Pathol* 20:1440–1447, 1996.)

in the parotid and 2 in the sublingual glands. There were 20 minor salivary gland tumors (35%) and they involved the lips (Fig 2), buccal mucosa, palate, tongue, retromolar area, and floor of mouth. Ranging in size from 0.4 to 6.0 cm, the lesions were grossly cystic or multicystic. Seventy-five percent of tumors had a conspicuous papillary component; microscopically, all tumors demonstrated an invasive cystic growth pattern. There was a variance in the predominant cell type, with 35 having small cuboidal cells, 9 having large cuboidal cells, and 7 having tall columnar cells. An admixture of cell types was found in 6 patients. It was common to find ruptured cysts with hemorrhage and granulation tissue. At a mean of 59 months after initial surgery, the 40 patients with follow-up data were either alive or had died of other causes and were free of tumor. There was a local recurrence of 3 tumors at a mean of 76 months. At the time of diagnosis, 3 tumors were metastatic to regional lymph nodes. A regional lymph node metastasis developed in 1 patient after 55 months.

Conclusion.—Salivary gland cystadenocarcinomas represent a distinct group of malignancies with an indolent biological behavior.

▶ This is an interesting neoplasm. Its specificity is defined primarily by its lack of it. Architecturally, it has an invasive cystic and sometimes papillary arrangement (a pattern shared by other salivary gland neoplasms), and cytologically it is recognized by, as the authors state, its "requisitely absent...identifying features that characterizes these other [salivary gland] carcinomas." The good news is that this type of neoplasm is associated with an indolent clinical course. The bad news is that it is associated with second (non–salivary gland) malignant tumors in approximately 20% of cases.

K.E. Sirgi, M.D.

Well-differentiated Acinic Cell Carcinoma of Salivary Glands Associated With Lymphoid Stroma

Michal M, Skálová A, Simpson RHW, et al (Charles Univ in Pilsen, Czech Republic; Univ of Exeter, England; Univ of Helinski; et al)
Hum Pathol 28:595–600, 1997   7–6

Background.—Acinic cell carcinomas may be associated with abundant lymphoid tissue in tumor stroma. A recent study showed that a proportion of cases had such a stroma with well-developed germinal centers, each enveloped by a fibrous pseudocapsule. The sestamibe (MIB1) indices were consistently low in all these tumors. This subgroup was further investigated in a larger series of acinic cell carcinomas in which the stroma contained germinal centers, and the histopathologic findings were correlated with the MIB1 indices and clinical outcomes.

Methods and Findings.—Sixty-nine acinic cell carcinomas of the salivary glands were examined. Twelve appeared to constitute a distinct subgroup. The most notable feature of these 12 tumors was a dense lymphoid stroma with well-developed germinal centers surrounding a

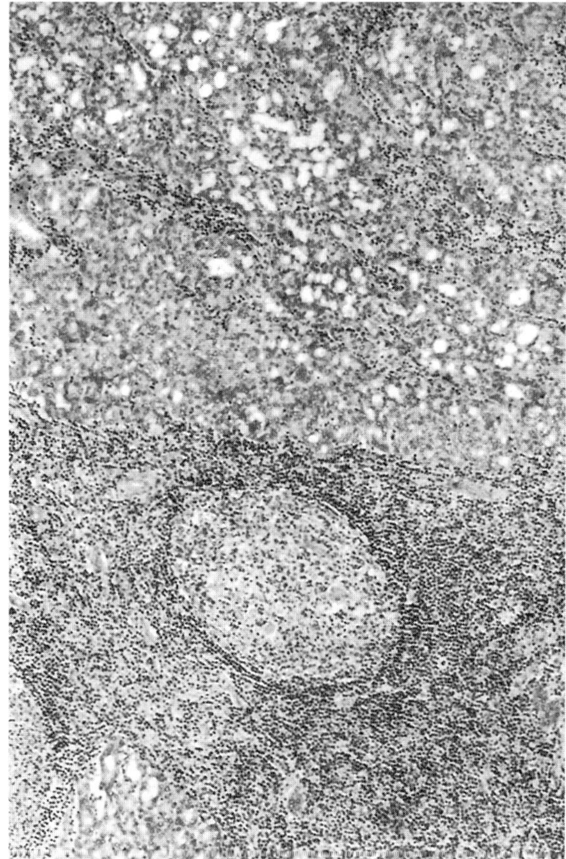

FIGURE 1.—Well-differentiated acinic cell carcinoma of the parotid gland shows microcystic growth pattern and lymphoid stroma with well-developed germinal centers; hematoxylin-esoin; original magnification, ×90.) (Courtesy of Michal M, Skálová A, Simpson RHW, et al: Well-differentiated acinic cell carcinoma of salivary glands associated with lymphoid stroma. *Hum Pathol* 28:595–600, 1997.)

sometimes scanty epithelial component. In each case, a microcystic growth pattern was observed. All 12 tumors were enveloped by a thin fibrous pseudocapsule, mimicking an intraparotid lymph node containing a metastasis; they showed low MIB1 proliferative activity (with a mean index of 1.7%). During the 19-month to 14-year follow-up, all patients remained well with no recurrences or metastases. Another subgroup of 9 acinic cell carcinomas also had a heavy lymphoid stroma with germinal centers, although its distribution was more patchy than in the initial subgroup. Also, the fibrous pseudocapsule was incomplete or absent. In addition, the epithelial growth patterns in these tumors was not microcystic, and the tumors had significantly greater MIB1 indices. Only 3 of 9 patients in this second subgroup remained well. Recurrences or metastases developed in the remaining 6, 2 of whom died from disseminated disease (Figs 1 and 2).

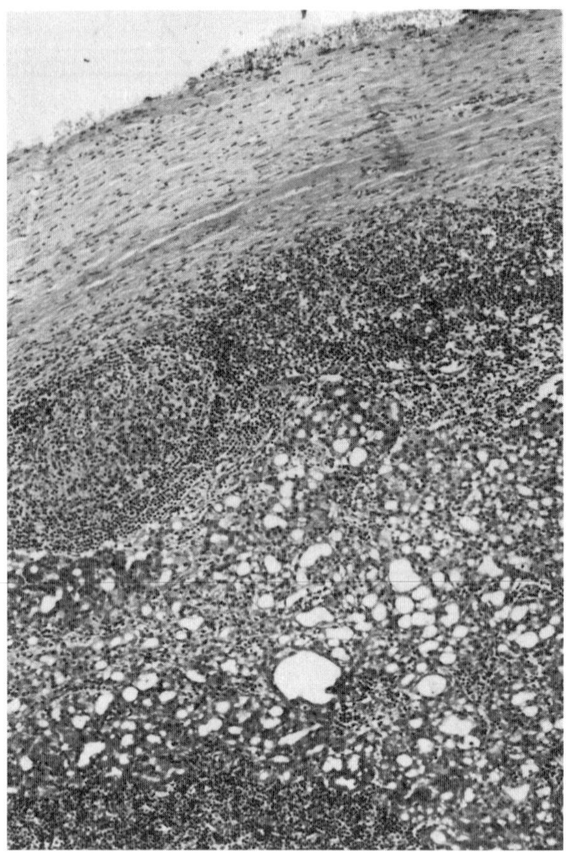

FIGURE 2.—Tumor is entirely surrounded by lymphoid stroma and enveloped by a thin fibrous capsule. No marginal sinuses can be observed; hematoxylin-eosin; original magnification, ×90.) (Courtesy of Michal M, Skálová A, Simpson RHW, et al: Well-differentiated acinic cell carcinoma of salivary glands associated with lymphoid stroma. *Hum Pathol* 28:595–600, 1997.)

Conclusion.—Well-differentiated acinic cell carcinoma with lymphoid stroma is characterized by a microcystic epithelial growth pattern. It is of low histologic grade with little, if any, metastatic potential. Its microscopic picture—that of an epithelial tumor in a dense lymphoid infiltrate with germinal centers surrounded by a fibrous pseudocapsule—must not be mistaken for primary or metastatic acinic cell carcinoma in an intraparotid lymph node.

▶ It is important to remind ourselves from time to time that different types of salivary gland neoplasms have a mixed lymphoid and epithelial component. More specifically, it is important to remember that all salivary gland neoplasms composed of a mixed lymphoid and epithelial proliferation are not Warthin's tumors. This is a potential pitfall for the inexperienced pathologist interpreting fine-needle aspiration biopsy specimens of salivary gland neo-plasms.

In addition, this paper clearly identifies a subtype of acinic cell carcinoma associated with an excellent clinical outcome. The features described in the paper should be specifically looked for and, if present, should be noted in the final pathology report of an acinic cell carcinoma.

K.E. Sirgi, M.D.

8 Gastrointestinal System

Basaloid Squamous Cell Carcinoma of the Esophagus: Diagnosis and Prognosis
Sarbia M, Verreet P, Bittinger F, et al (Heinrich Heine Univ, Düsseldorf, Germany; Johannes Gutenberg Univ, Mainz, Germany)
Cancer 79:1871–1878, 1997   8–1

Background.—Basaloid squamous cell carcinoma is a rare variant of squamous cell carcinoma that can occur in the anus, thymus, and uterine cervix, though most occur in the upper aerodigestive tract in the region of the hypopharynx, oral cavity, and larynx. Basaloid squamous cell carcinoma of the upper aerodigestive tract is considered a high-grade neoplasm because it is associated with low survival. Basaloid squamous cell carcinoma is associated with dysplastic squamous cell epithelium, in situ squamous cell carcinoma, invasive squamous cell carcinoma, and islands of squamous cell carcinoma among the basaloid cells. The chief differential diagnoses of basaloid squamous cell carcinoma are adenoid cystic carcinoma and small cell carcinoma. There is little information on the incidence and outcome of basaloid squamous cell carcinoma of the esophagus.

Methods.—The clinical and pathologic features of 17 biopsy specimens of basaloid squamous cell carcinomas and 133 specimens of typical squamous cell carcinomas were compared. Light microscopy, electron microscopy, and immunohistochemistry were performed.

Results.—In basaloid squamous cell carcinoma, light microscopy revealed relatively small tumor cells arranged in solid lobules with abundant comedo-type necrosis. Basaloid squamous cell carcinoma was almost always accompanied by areas of typical squamous cell carcinoma, foci of squamous cell differentiation, and/or severe squamous cell dysplasia or carcinoma in situ of adjacent mucosa. The ultrastructure of basaloid squamous cell carcinoma had inconsistent features of squamous cell differentiation. Immunohistochemical examination showed poor reactivity to antibodies against wide-range cytokeratins and cytokeratin subtypes typical of squamous cell epithelia. There was infrequent expression of Leu7, smooth muscle actin, and S-100 protein. Characteristic features of basaloid squamous cell carcinoma were older patient age, higher proliferative

TABLE 3.—Comparison of the Clinical and Pathologic Features of 17 Basaloid Squamous Cell Carcinomas and 133 Typical Squamous Cell Carcinomas With Fisher's Exact Test

Parameter	No. (%) of BSCCs	No. (%) of typical SCCs	P value
Gender			NS
Male	13 (76.5%)	108 (81.2%)	
Female	4 (23.5%)	25 (18.8%)	
Tumor size			NS
≤5 cm	10 (58.8%)	89 (66.9%)	
>5 cm	7 (41.2%)	44 (33.1%)	
pT calssification			NS
pT1/pT2	4 (23.5%)	47 (35.3%)	
pT3/pT4	13 (76.5%)	66 (64.7%)	
pN classification			NS
pN0	7 (41.2%)	65 (48.9%)	
pN1	10 (58.8%)	68 (51.1%)	
Lymphatic vessel invasion			NS
Absent	13 (76.5%)	83 (62.4%)	
Present	4 (23.5%)	50 (37.6%)	
Blood vessel invasion			NS
Absent	12 (70.6%)	101 (75.9%)	
Present	5 (29.4%)	32 (24.1%)	
Neural invasion			NS
Absent	14 (82.4%)	99 (74.4%)	
Present	3 (17.6%)	34 (25.6%)	

Abbreviations: BSCC, basaloid squamous cell carcinoma; *NS*, not significant; *SCC*, squamous cell carcinoma.
(Courtesy of Sarbia M, Verreet P, Bittinger F, et al: Basaloid squamous cell carcinoma of the esophagus: Diagnosis and prognosis. *Cancer* 79:1871–1878. Copyright 1997 American Cancer Society. Reprinted by permission of Wiley-Liss, Inc., a subsidiary of John Wiley & Sons, Inc.)

activity, and higher apoptotic indices compared to typical squamous cell carcinoma. There were no differences in pT classification, pN classification, tumor size, blood vessel invasion, lymphatic vessel invasion, neural invasion, or patient gender (Table 3). Survival rates were also similar (Table 5).

Discussion.—These findings indicate that basaloid squamous cell carcinoma is a histopathologic variant of squamous cell carcinoma. Light microscopic, electron microscopic, and immunohistochemical findings can distinguish basaloid squamous cell carcinoma from small cell carcinoma

TABLE 5.—Survival Rates (%) of 13 Patients with Basaloid Squamous Cell Carcinoma and 117 Patients with Typical Squamous Cell Carcinoma of the Esophagus

	2-year (SE)	5-year (SE)
BSCC	38.5 (±13.5)	19.2 (±11.8)
SCC	39.3 (±6.1)	19.0 (±4.5)

Abbreviations: BSCC, basaloid squamous cell carcinoma; *SCC*, squamous cell carcinoma; *SE*, standard error.
(Courtesy of Sarbia M, Verreet P, Bittinger F, et al: Basaloid squamous cell carcinoma of the esophagus: Diagnosis and prognosis. *Cancer* 79:1871–1878. Copyright 1997 American Cancer Society. Reprinted by permission of Wiley-Liss, Inc., a subsidiary of John Wiley & Sons, Inc.)

and adenoid cystic carcinoma. The prognosis of patients with basaloid squamous cell carcinoma and typical squamous cell carcinoma of the esophagus is similar.

▶ Basaloid squamous cell carcinoma occurs in several sites, but is most common in the upper aerodigestive tract. This paper more than doubles the previously reported examples from esophageal sites. These authors found that, after complete resection, the outcome does not differ from that of typical squamous cell carcinomas. For us in the laboratory, the major differential diagnostic problems are adenoid cystic carcinoma and small-cell undifferentiated carcinoma. Evidence of squamous differentiation is usually detected and may involve either the adjacent epithelium (dysplastic squamous epithelium or squamous cell carcinoma in-situ) or the tumor itself (areas of invasive squamous cell carcinoma or islands of squamous cell carcinoma among the basaloid cells). However, these foci may be rare or absent altogether. Other light microscopic, immunohistochemical, and ultrastructural findings help to exclude small-cell neuroendocrine carcinoma. Different therapeutic approaches for these 2 neoplasms makes accurate diagnosis important. The solid ("anaplastic") type of adenoid cystic carcinoma may represent a difficult diagnostic distinction. Mitoses, nuclear pleomorphism, and squamous differentiation are useful clues to the correct diagnosis. The authors add necrosis to this list, but our own experience indicates that it can be prominent in either entity.

M.W. Stanley, M.D.

Suggested Reading

Banks ER, Frierson HF, Mills SE, et al: Basaloid squamous cell carcinoma of the head and neck: A clinicopathologic and immunohistochemical study of 40 cases. *Am J Surg Pathol* 16:939–946, 1992.

Barnes L, Ferlito A, Altavilla G, et al: Basaloid squamous cell carcinoma of the head and neck: Clinicopathological features and differential diagnosis. *Ann Otol Rhinol Laryngol* 105:75–82, 1996.

Klijanienko J, El-Naggar A, Ponzio-Prion A, et al: Basaloid squamous carcinoma of the head and neck: Immunohistochemical comparison with adenoid cystic carcinoma and squamous cell carcinoma. *Arch Otolaryngol Head Neck Surg* 119:887–890, 1993.

Luna MA, El-Naggar A, Parichatikanond P, et al: Basaloid squamous carcinoma of the upper aerodigestive tract. *Cancer* 66:537–542, 1990.

Gastrointestinal Stromal Tumors With Prominent Signet-ring Cell Features

Suster S, Fletcher CDM (Univ of Miami, Fla; Brigham and Women's Hospital, Boston; Harvard Med School, Boston)
Mod Pathol 9:609–613, 1996
8–2

Background.—Gastrointestinal stromal tumors are uncommon lesions with unknown pathogenesis. They are characterized by spindle or epithelioid cell proliferation within the muscle wall, submucosa, or neural plexus of the gastrointestinal tract. Immunohistochemical and electron microscopic examination has shown myogenic, neural, and mixed neural and smooth muscle features. Myxoid types and distinctive round eosinophilic collagen globules have also recently been described.

Findings.—Three gastrointestinal stromal tumors were found incidentally within the muscle wall of resected specimens of stomach, small bowel, and rectosigmoid colon. The patients were 3 women between 45 and 74 years old. The lesions were smaller than 2.5 cm and were well-circumscribed, serosal nodules. Histologic examination showed proliferation of large, round-to-oval cells with abundant clear cytoplasm. The nuclei were displaced toward the periphery, which gave the appearance of a signet-ring cell. The signet-ring cells merged with short fascicles of spindle cells in some areas and were associated with prominent deposition of myxoid matrix in other areas. In 2 cases, histochemical examination showed glycogen granules within the tumor cell cytoplasm. Immunohistochemical analysis showed heterogeneous staining with strong positivity for actin, vimentin, and CD34 in 1 case; strong positivity for vimentin and S-100 protein, and weak, focal positivity for actin and CD34 in another case; and positivity for vimentin alone in the third case.

Discussion.—There is controversy surrounding gastrointestinal stromal tumors because of their histogenetic heterogeneity and range of morphological appearances. These 3 specimens of gastrointestinal stromal tumors had unusual morphological features. These lesions should be differentiated from primary and metastatic mucin-secreting carcinoma and other neoplasms with clear cell or signet-ring cell features.

▶ First there were leiomyomas. Then came gastrointestinal stromal tumors, which were myogenic, neural, or mixed, and might show spindle cell or epithelioid patterns. As noted in the introduction to this paper, tumors with skeinoid fibers and now, signet-ring cells have been added. (Other cytologic and architectural embellishments are nicely reviewed in this paper.) These 3 cases were distributed from the stomach to the rectum, and all were small (less than 2.5 cm). Other histopathologic findings included extracellular myxoid material and a variable component of spindle cell growth. Any prognostic significance of this rare alteration is very difficult to appreciate. In this study, 1 patient is alive at 10 years, another is lost, and the last died of an unrelated malignancy. The literature reviewed by these authors provides no additional insights, in large measure because of the great rarity of this finding. As long as one thinks of this possibility, the major differential diagnostic considerations (gastrointestinal tract carcinoma and metastatic carcinoma) can be excluded with fairly standard immunohistochemical evaluations.

M.W. Stanley, M.D.

Suggested Reading

Franquemont DW, Frierson HF: Muscle differentiation and clinicopathologic features of gastrointestinal stromal tumors. *Am J Surg Pathol* 16:947, 1992.

Lauwers GY, Erlandson RA, Casper ES, et al: Gastrointestinal autonomic nerve tumors: A clinicopathologic, immunohistochemical and ultrastructural study of 12 cases. *Am J Surg Pathol* 17:887, 1993.

Min K-W: Small intestinal stromal tumors with skeinoid fibers: Clinicopathological, immunohistochemical and ultrastructural investigations. *Am J Surg Pathol* 16:145, 1992.

Suster S, Sorace D, Moran CA: Gastrointestinal stromal tumors with prominent myxoid matrix: Clinicopathologic, immunohistochemical and ultrastructural study of nine cases of a distinctive morphologic variant of myogenic stromal tumor. *Am J Surg Pathol* 19:59, 1995.

***Helicobacter pylori* and Primary Gastric Lymphoma: A Histopathologic and Immunohistochemical Analysis of 237 Patients**
Nakamura S, Yao T, Aoyagi K, et al (Kyushu Univ, Fukuoka, Japan; Kawasaki Med School, Kurashiki, Japan)
Cancer 79:3–11, 1997   8–3

Background.—It is believed that *Helicobacter pylori* is involved in gastroduodenal diseases. An association between infection with *H. pylori* and primary gastric lymphoma, especially the lymphoma of mucosa-associated lymphoid tissue type, has recently been described. It has also been reported that low-grade gastric mucosa-associated lymphoid tissue lymphoma may regress after *H. pylori* is eliminated. There have been few studies of the relation between *H. pylori* and primary gastric lymphoma in large samples.

Methods.—The presence of *H. pylori* was examined in 237 formalin-fixed, paraffin-embedded specimens of primary gastric lymphoma. Hematoxylin and eosin stain, modified Giemsa stain, and immunohistochemical staining were used. Specimens were compared with specimens of chronic active gastritis, peptic ulcer, and gastric carcinoma.

Results.—Of the 237 specimens, 145 were positive for *H. pylori*. Positivity for *H. pylori* was more common in patients with lymphoma restricted to the mucosa and submucosa than in patients with lymphoma beyond the submucosa (Table 1). Positivity was also higher in patients

TABLE 1.—Frequency and Grading Scores of *Helicobacter pylori* in Primary Gastric Lymphoma

	HP-positive cases (%)	P value*	HP grading score	P value[†]
All patients (n = 237)	145 (61)	—	0.9 ± 1.0	—
Phenotype				
B cell (n = 216)	132 (61)	0.45	0.9 ± 0.9	0.89
T cell (n = 15)	11 (73)		0.9 ± 1.2	
Histologic type				
MALT (n = 198)	125 (63)	0.23	0.9 ± 1.0	0.08
Others (n = 39)	20 (51)		0.7 ± 1.0	
Grade of MALT				
Low (n = 99)	71 (72)	<0.05	0.9 ± 0.9	0.55
High (n = 99)	54 (55)		0.9 ± 1.0	
Macroscopic type				
SS type (n = 97)	70 (72)	<0.01	1.0 ± 1.0	<0.05
Other types (n = 140)	75 (54)		0.8 ± 0.9	
Size of tumor				
<8.2 cm (n = 129)	83 (64)	0.34	1.0 ± 1.0	<0.01
≥8.2 cm (n = 108)	62 (57)		0.7 ± 0.8	
Depth of invasion				
Not beyond sm (n = 111)	84 (76)	<0.001	1.1 ± 1.0	<0.001
Beyond sm (n = 126)	61 (48)		0.7 ± 0.9	

*Determined by the chi-square test.
[†]Determined by the Mann-Whitney test.
Abbreviations: HP, Helicobacter pylori; MALT, mucosa-associated lymphoid tissue; sm, submucosa; SS, superficial-spreading.
(Courtesy of Nakamura S, Yao T, Aoyagi K, et al: *Helicobacter pylori* and primary gastric lymphoma. *Cancer* 79:3–11. Copyright 1997 American Cancer Society. Reprinted by permission of Wiley-Liss, Inc., a subsidiary of John Wiley & Sons, Inc.)

with low-grade mucosa-associated lymphoid tissue lymphoma than in patients with high-grade tumors. Positivity for *H. pylori* in patients with lymphoma was lower than in patients with chronic active gastritis and peptic ulcer. Positivity for *H. pylori* in patients with lymphoma restricted to the mucosa and superficial submucosa was as high as in patients with chronic active gastritis and peptic ulcer. In patients with lymphoma, the *H. pylori* grading score was lower than in patients with chronic active gastritis, peptic ulcer, or gastric carcinoma.

Discussion.—*Helicobacter pylori* is more common in the early stages of primary gastric lymphoma than in advanced stages and may disappear during disease progression. More studies with long-term follow-up may help define the role of *H. pylori* in the pathogenesis of primary gastric lymphoma.

▶ *Helicobacter pylori* is strongly associated with development of chronic active gastritis, peptic ulcer, and gastric carcinoma. Previous studies have noted its association with malignant lymphoma, and there have been suggestions that low-grade malignant lymphomas of mucosa-associated lymphoid tissue (MALT) may resolve after eradication of the organism. The higher frequency of *H. pylori* involvement in gastric MALT lymphoma may relate in part to the somewhat variable criteria for this diagnosis and on the extent to which various investigators are forced to rely on small biopsy samples. Furthermore, these authors note that there is decreasing association between lymphoma and *H pylori* as the neoplasm extends more deeply into the gastric wall. When lymphomas restricted to the mucosa are examined, the incidence of identifiable organisms equals the very high rate associated with chronic active gastritis. The authors interpret these findings to indicate that the strongest association between infection and malignant lymphoma is demonstrable early in the lymphoma's development.

M.W. Stanley, M.D.

Suggested Reading

Bayerdörffer E, Neubauer A, Rudolph B, et al: Regression of primary gastric lymphoma of mucosa-associated lymphoid tissue type after cure of *Helicobacter pylori* infection. *Lancet* 345:1591–1594, 1995.

NIH Consensus Development Panel on *Helicobacter pylori* in Peptic Ulcer Disease: *Helicobacter pylori* in peptic ulcer disease. *JAMA* 272:65–69, 1994.

Parsonnet J, Hansen S, Rodriguez L, et al: *Helicobacter pylori* infection and gastric lymphoma. *N Engl J Med* 330:1267–1271, 1994.

Roggero E, Zucca E, Pinotti G, et al: Eradication of *Helicobacter pylori* infection in primary gastric lymphoma of mucosa-associated lymphoid tissue. *Ann Intern Med* 122:767–769, 1995.

Synchronous Mucosa-associated Lymphoid Tissue Lymphoma and Adenocarcinoma of the Stomach
Goteri G, Ranaldi R, Rezai B, et al (Ancona Univ, Italy)
Am J Surg Pathol 21:505–509, 1997   8–4

Background.—Although adenocarcinoma and primary lymphoma of the stomach are rarely associated, a causal relationship between these 2 neoplasms and common etiologic factors has recently been proposed. A possible etiopathogenetic role of *Helicobacter pylori* has been suggested. The clinicopathologic findings of synchronous primary gastric lymphoma and adenocarcinoma were reviewed.

Methods.—Of 2,203 gastrectomies for adenocarcinoma and 137 gastrectomies for primary lymphoma, 8 cases with both neoplasms were identified. Of those 8 cases, 6 were total gastrectomies and 2 were stump resections. In the 2 cases of stump resection, tumors were seen 24 and 34 years after gastric resection of a duodenal ulcer.

Results.—The lymphoma and carcinoma formed a single lesion (collision tumor) in 4 cases and were separated in 4 cases. Histologic examination showed that all the lymphomas could be classified as B-cell mucosa-associated lymphoid tissue lymphoma; 6 were low-grade and 2 were low-grade with a high-grade component. The adenocarcinomas were intestinal type in 4 cases, diffuse in 3 cases, and mixed in 1. Four carcinomas were early gastric cancers and 4 were advanced cancers. All 4 of the collision tumors showed early gastric cancer. The association of *H. pylori* with gastric lymphoma and carcinoma was confirmed in 4 cases. One case had spiral bacteria with features of *H. heilmannii.*

Discussion.—The previously unreported presence of 2 different tumors in a gastric stump indicates that postgastrectomy gastritis may have a role in both gastric lymphoma and carcinoma.

▶ Synchronous occurrence of gastric carcinoma and lymphoma of mucosa-associated lymphoid tissue is rare; this report describes 8 cases. *Helicobacter pylori* was identified in one half of these. However, many of them were deeply invasive, and information presented elsewhere in these commentaries indicates that this might be the expected rate of demonstrable infection for such cases.

M.W. Stanley, M.D.

Suggested Reading

von Herbay A, Schreiter H, Rudi J: Simultaneous gastric adenocarcinoma and MALT-type lymphoma *Helicobacter pylori* infection. *Virchows Arch* 427:445–450, 1995.

Wotherspoon AC, Doglioni C, Diss TC, et al: Regression of primary low-grade B-cell gastric lymphoma of mucosa-associated lymphoid tissue type after eradication of *Helicobacter pylori. Lancet* 342:575–577, 1993.

Wotherspoon AC, Isaacson PG: Synchronous adenocarcinoma and low grade B-cell lymphoma of mucosa associated lymphoid tissue (MALT) of the stomach. *Histopathology* 27:325–331, 1995.

Can Ischemic Colitis Be Differentiated From *C Difficile* Colitis in Biopsy Specimens?

Dignan CR, Greenson JK (Univ of Michigan, Ann Arbor)
Am J Surg Pathol 21:706–710, 1997   8–5

Background.—Pseudomembranous colitis is often used to describe the colitis caused by *Clostridium difficile,* although pseudomembranes are also often found in ischemic colitis. Colitis caused by *C. difficile* can occur after broad-spectrum antimicrobial therapy; it is believed that pseudomembranes form from bacterial toxin-mediated mucosal necrosis. Nearly identical clinical and histopathologic features can occur from ischemia resulting from atherosclerosis, thromboemboli, vasculitis, and other occlusive factors, as well as from cardiac failure, septic shock, and other low-flow states. There are no reliable histologic criteria to distinguish colitis caused by *C. difficile* or ischemia in endoscopic biopsy specimens with pseudomembranes.

Methods.—There were 49 biopsy specimens of pseudomembranous colitis; 25 were from patients with *C. difficile* colitis and 24 were from

TABLE 1.—Histologic Findings in *Clostridium difficile* and Ischemic Biopsies

	Hyalinized LP H&E stain	Hyalinized LP trichrome stain	Atrophic crypts	Diffuse pseudomembranes*	Lamina propria hemorrhage	Full-thickness mucosal necrosis
C difficile	0/25	0/25	6/25	1/25	9/25	7/25
Ischemia	16/24	19/24	18/24	6/24	18/24	14/24
Statistical data	$p < 0.0001$	$p < 0.0001$	$p < 0.0006$	$p < 0.05$	$p < 0.01$	$p < 0.05$

*Refers to the surface area of the biopsy specimens rather than distribution within the colon.
Abbreviations: LP, lamina propria; *H&E*, hematoxylin-eosin.
(Courtesy of Digran CR, Greenson JK: Can ischemic colitis be differentiated from *C difficile* colitis in biopsy specimens? *Am J Surg Pathol* 21:706–710, 1997.)

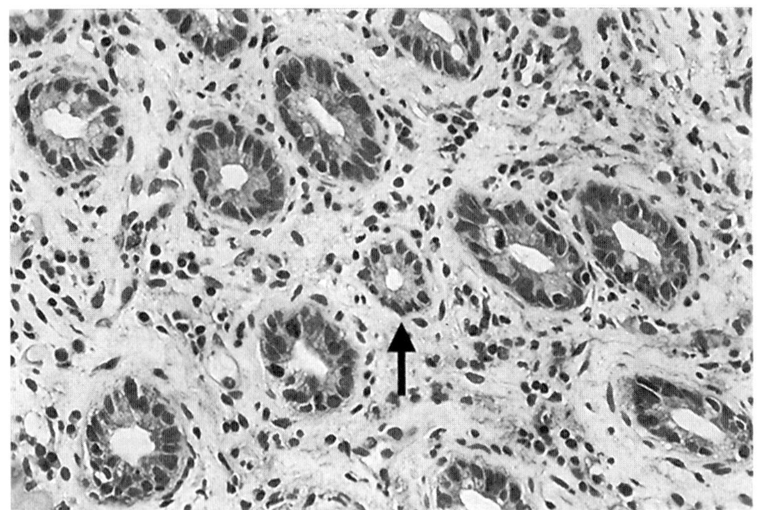

FIGURE 3.—High-power view of hyalinized lamina propria with atrophic microcrypts (*arrow*) in ischemic colitis. (Courtesy of Dignan CR, Greenson JK: Can ischemic colitis be differentiated from C *difficile* colitis in biopsy specimens? *Am J Surg Pathol* 21:706–710, 1997.)

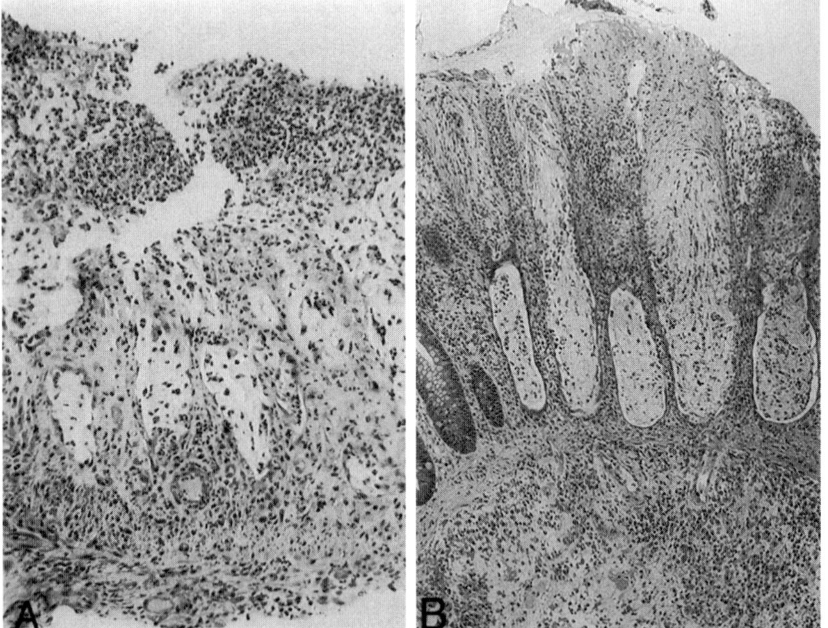

FIGURE 2.—Low-power view of pseudomembranous colitis with full-thickness mucosal necrosis in (**A**) C. *difficile colitis* and (**B**) ischemic colitis. Full-thickness mucosal necrosis was seen more frequently in ischemia than in C. *difficile*. (Courtesy of Dignan CR, Greenson JK: Can ischemic colitis be differentiated from C *difficile* colitis in biopsy specimens? *Am J Surg Pathol* 21:706–710, 1997.)

TABLE 2.—Clinical Features of Patients With *Clostridium difficile* and Ischemic Colitis

	Patient age range (mean)	Time interval range in days* (mean)	Pseudomembranes on endoscopy	Localized process on endoscopy	Polyp or mass on endoscopy
C difficile	26–80 (58.4)	1–105 (15.5)	21/22	1/22	0/22
Ischemia	28–89 (66.7)	1–913 (51.7)	3/24	24/24	7/24
Statistical data	p < 0.051	p < 0.39	p < 0.0001	p < 0.0001	p < 0.01

*Interval between symptom onset and endoscopic biopsy.
(Courtesy of Dignan CR, Greenson JK: Can ischemic colitis be differentiated from *C difficile* colitis in biopsy specimens? *Am J Surg Pathol* 21:706–710, 1997.)

patients with ischemic colitis. The specimens were coded, randomized, and examined for differentiating histologic features.

Results.—Hyalinization of the lamina propria was noted in 19 of the 24 specimens of ischemic colitis, but was not seen in specimens of *C. difficile* colitis (Table 1). Atrophic microcrypts were seen in 18 cases of ischemic colitis (Fig 3) and 6 cases of *C. difficile* colitis. There was significantly more lamina propria hemorrhage, full-thickness mucosal necrosis (Fig 2), and diffuse distribution of pseudomembranes in ischemic colitis than in *C. difficile* colitis. Pseudomembranes were seen significantly more often in *C. difficile* colitis than in ischemic colitis. Masses or polyps were seen only in cases of ischemia. In colon biopsies with pseudomembranes, a hyalinized lamina propria was a specific and sensitive marker of ischemia. Other markers of ischemia were atrophic microcrypts, lamina propria hemorrhage, full-thickness mucosal necrosis, diffuse involvement of all surfaces of all biopsy specimens by pseudomembranes, and endoscopic impression of a localized process, polyp, or mass (Table 2). Endoscopic identification of diffuse pseudomembranes was a marker of *C. difficile* colitis.

Discussion.—In biopsies showing pseudomembranous colitis, features such as a hyalinized lamina propria, atrophic microcrypts, and a localized process, mass, or polyp strongly indicate ischemic colitis. Diffuse, but discrete 0.2- to 0.3-cm pseudomembranes indicate *C. difficile* colitis. Patients with pseudomembranous colitis may have abdominal pain, fever, guaiac-positive stools, history of antibiotic use, and evidence of previous ischemic disease.

▶ The tables highlight the different clinical and histologic findings in these 2 conditions. Lamina propria hyalinization emerges as a specific marker for ischemia. The authors recommend using a trichrome stain to accentuate this finding. The presence of atrophic microcrypts also typifies ischemia, but is a less specific criterion. Endoscopic findings of a polyp or mass, as well as localization of the disease process, also suggest ischemia; the pseudomembranous appearance tends to be more diffuse in cases associated with *C. difficile*. The authors caution that in 2 of their 49 cases, none of these features was noted. Thus, an etiologic factor can be assigned in a majority of pseudomembranous colitis cases, but not in all.

M.W. Stanley, M.D.

Suggested Reading

Bower TC: Ischemic colitis. *Surg Clin North Am* 73:1037–1053, 1993.

Haggitt RC: Differential diagnosis of colitis, in Goldman H, Appelman HD, Kaufman N (eds): *Gastrointestinal Pathology.* Baltimore, Md, Williams & Wilkins, 1990, pp 325–355.

Collagenous Colitis: Histopathology and Clinical Course

Goff JS, Barnett JL, Pelke T, et al (Univ of Michigan, Ann Arbor)
Am J Gastroenterol 92:57–60, 1997   8–6

Background.—Collagenous colitis was first described in 1976. It is a chronic diarrheal disease characterized histopathologically by chronic inflammatory cell infiltration of the lamina propria, damage to the surface epithelium, and excessive intraepithelial lymphocytes. A distinct, thickened layer of subepithelial collagen identifies and defines the disease and differentiates it from similar diarrheal diseases, such as lymphocytic colitis. The relationship between the histopathologic changes and the course of the disease was studied.

Methods.—The records of 31 patients with collagenous colitis were reviewed; 27 patients were also interviewed by telephone at least 2 years after initial diagnosis. The mean patient age was 66 years. Biopsy specimens were also reviewed. The mean duration of symptoms was 5.4 years at time of diagnosis.

Results.—Of the 31 patients, 18 had arthritis, and 22 were using nonsteroidal anti-inflammatory drugs at the time of diagnosis. Patients were classified into 2 groups that were similar regarding sex, age, associated diseases, and use of medication: those with symptom resolution and those with ongoing or intermittent symptoms. Patients with symptom resolution had received treatment with antidiarrheal agents, sulfasalazine, discontinuation of nonsteroidal anti-inflammatory drugs, reversal of jejunoilial bypass, or no treatment. Patients with ongoing symptoms had a range of symptom severity; 2 patients needed only antidiarrheal agents, but 5 needed or had failed treatment with steroids, azathioprine, or sandostatin. Collagen thickness, epithelial damage, and inflammation were similar in both groups. Paneth cell metaplasia was more common in patients with ongoing symptoms. Diagnostic changes were present in left-sided biopsy specimens in 24 of 27 patients.

Discussion.—Most of these patients with collagenous colitis had spontaneous or treatment-induced symptom resolution. Although a longer history of symptoms, Paneth cell metaplasia, and severe inflammation in the lamina propria were more common in patients with ongoing symptoms, clinical variables and histologic findings were not predictive of severity or course of disease.

▶ Collagenous colitis has gone from a case report of a new entity to a commonly discussed condition reported hundreds of times in a period of about 20 years. Clinically, it features chronic diarrhea and endoscopically normal mucosa. Its histopathology shows lymphocytic infiltration of the lamina propria, surface epithelial cell damage, increased intraepithelial lymphocytes, and a thickened subepithelial collagen plate. This latter finding differentiates collagenous colitis from clinically similar entities including lymphocytic colitis. This paper addresses the long-term outlook for these patients. Most cases resolve, but some do not. The point is made clearly that our study of initial biopsy findings does not provide any information that can help predict who will get well spontaneously, who will respond to therapy, and who will go on to longer term disease.

M.W. Stanley, M.D.

Suggested Reading

Lee E, Schiller LR, Vendrell D, et al: Subepithelial collagen table thickness in colon specimens from patients with microscopic colitis and collagenous colitis. *Gastroenterology* 103:1790–1796, 1992.

Zins BJ, Sandborn WJ, Tremaine WJ: Collagenous and lymphocytic colitis: Subject review and therapeutic alternatives. *Am J Gastroenterol* 90:1394–1400, 1995.

Zins BJ, Tremaine WJ, Carpenter HA: Collagenous colitis: Mucosal biopsies and association with fecal leukocytes. *Mayo Clin Proc* 70:430–433, 1995.

Recommendations for the Reporting of Resected Large Intestinal Carcinomas

Ridell RH, for the Association of Directors of Anatomic and Surgical Pathology
Am J Clin Pathol 106:12–15, 1996   8–7

Introduction.—The Association of Directors of Anatomic and Surgical Pathology (ADASP) has developed recommendations for the reporting of resected large intestinal carcinomas. Four major areas that ADASP recommends should be considered for the final report are described.

Gross Description.—For the gross description, these points should be included: how the specimen was received, how the specimen was identified, parts of the intestine included, length of each segment, and other structures included.

Tumor Description.—It is recommended that the diagnostic information include site of tumor and part of bowel resected, histologic type (World Health Organization classification recommended), lymph node metastases, presence of mesenteric deposits, other sites biopsied for metastatic disease, histologic grade, and depth of infiltration. Recommendations are based on the TNM (tumor, node, metastasis) system, with the exception of preferring the term *high-grade dysplasia* over *carcinoma in situ/severe dysplasia*. The adequacy of local excision, other significant disease, and availability of information needed for prognosis or therapy may also be considered for inclusion in the final report.

Optional Features.—Some features are optional because they represent specific institutional preferences. If stage is included in the final report, the staging system should be specified. Results of ancillary investigations may also be included.

Checklist.—It is recommended that a checklist be used to prevent accidental exclusion of information.

Conclusion.—The ADASP recommendations are meant as suggestions for the clinician. Adherence to them is voluntary. The recommendations may not be applicable in special clinical circumstances. These recommendations are meant to be used as an educational resource, not a mandate.

▶ The ADASP continues to look carefully at preparation, description, and reporting of gross and microscopic findings in specimens with a common type of malignancy. This succint article follows the outline established in this group's previous publications. Earlier pronouncements by the World Health Organizations and the TNM system are followed for the most part. The major exception is that *high-grade dysplasia* is preferred over *carcinoma in situ* or its TNM equivalent of *Tis*. It is also clear that while in the colon, the antimesenteric serosal surface is not considered a resection margin, the rectal surface overlying the deepest area of tumor penetration is a margin and should be inked for proper assessment. This type of rectal margin is variously designated as lateral, deep, or radial. These guidelines will be useful for ensuring the best possible prognostic assessment of colorectal carcinomas.

M.W. Stanley, M.D.

Lymph Node Recovery From Colorectal Resection Specimens Removed for Adenocarcinoma: Trends Over Time and a Recommendation for a Minimum Number of Lymph Nodes to Be Recovered
Goldstein NS, Sanford W, Coffey M, et al (William Beaumont Hosp, Royal Oak, Mich; Duke Univ, Durham, NC)
Am J Clin Pathol 106:209–216, 1996   8–8

Introduction.—The prognostic significance of lymph node metastases from colorectal carcinoma has been realized since Charles Mayo noted its importance in a 1904 address to the Oregon State Medical Association. The incidence of regional metastases has recently decreased. This decrease may have resulted from improvements in early cancer detection procedures or may have occurred because pathologists are not performing lymph node dissections with the same care as in earlier years. Pericolorectal lymph nodes were evaluated to ascertain whether the number of lymph nodes recovered and the proportion of specimens with pericolonic lymph node metastases from colorectal carcinoma specimens have changed over time.

Methods.—Slides and reports of the first 20 consecutive pT3 colorectal carcinoma resections in each year from 1955 to 1995 that were not known to be associated with liver or distant metastases at the time of surgery were evaluated. The number of lymph nodes sampled and number of metastases in pericolonic lymph nodes were counted from slides. Data on specimen length, tumor location, and size were collected from pathology reports.

Results.—Slides and pathology reports from 750 stage pT3 colon carcinomas were reviewed. No apparent change was seen in the distribution of tumor location in the time period evaluated. The mean number of lymph nodes detected per specimen over the 41-year period was 9.8. The mean number of lymph nodes recovered per specimen and the incidence of detected lymph node metastases increased over time, particularly during 1992–1995. Detection of lymph node metastases was highest in patients for whom 17 to 20 lymph nodes were recovered per specimen (Fig 2). Detection of lymph node metastases was not increased in specimens with more than 20 lymph nodes.

Conclusion.—A strong positive correlation was seen between the proportion of specimens with metastases detected and the number of lymph nodes recovered. Pathologists should attempt to recover as many lymph

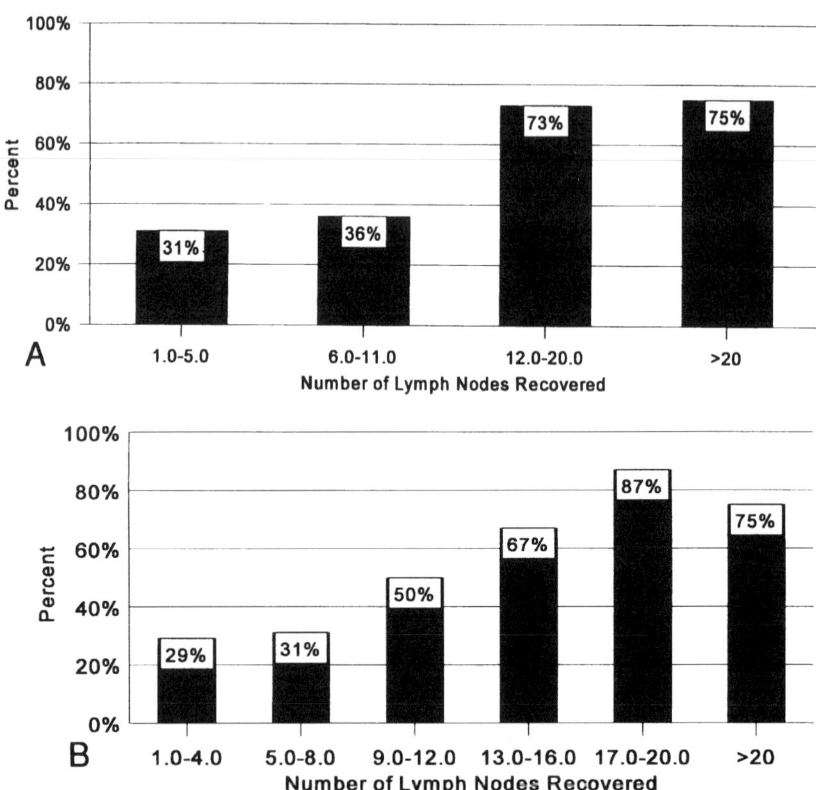

FIGURE 2.—**A,** percentage of specimens with lymph node metastases increased when at least 12 lymph nodes were recovered per case compared with the recovery of 11 or fewer lymph nodes per case. No appreciable change occurred between the 12 to 20 and >20 lymph node groups. **B,** the same cases shown in part A, separated into narrower intervals of lymph node recovery. The percentage of specimens with lymph node metastases was greater in the 17 to 20 group than in the 9 to 12 group and in 13 to 16 lymph node groups. (Courtesy of Goldstein NS, Sanford W, Coffey M, et al: Lymph node recovery from colorectal resection specimens for adenocarcinoma: Trends over time and a recommendation for a minimum number of lymph nodes to be recovered. *Am J Clin Pathol* 106:209–216, 1996.)

nodes as possible in patients with colorectal resection. At least 17 lymph nodes should be recovered to assure accurate documentation of nodal metastases.

▶ The availability of adjuvant therapy for some patients with regional lymph node metastases of colonic carcinoma places renewed emphasis on the importance of accurate assessment in the surgical pathology laboratory. It is clear that if we find more lymph nodes, the number of cases with metastases increases. Previous recommendations that certain numbers of nodes should be sought can be evaluated quickly by referring to Figure 2. This paper also provides a useful review of the relevant literature. The authors argue that because *any* positive node will result in consideration of adjuvant therapy, careful dissections are essential. Literature reviewed in this article also indicates that even small lymph nodes may harbor metastases, so that there are truly no short cuts in the gross room. In the breast, we have moved from dissections to sampling, whereas in the large intestine, we seem to be moving in the opposite direction.

M.W. Stanley, M.D.

Suggested Reading

Fielding LP, Arsenault PA, Chapuis PH, et al: Working party report to the World Congress of Gastroenterology, Sydney 1990. *J Gastroenterol Hepatol* 6:325–344, 1991.

Jass JR: Prognostic factors in rectal cancer. *Eur J Cancer* 31A:862–863, 1995.

Carcinoid Tumors of the Rectum: Effect of Size, Histopathology, and Surgical Treatment on Metastasis Free Survival

Koura AN, Giacco GG, Curley SA, et al (Univ of Texas, Houston)
Cancer 79:1294–1298, 1997   8–9

Background.—Rectal carcinoid tumors make up 11% to 50% of all carcinoid tumors of the alimentary tract. Rectal carcinoid tumors are less aggressive and slower growing than carcinoids at other sites, but they usually metastasize when they are larger than 2 cm. The biological behavior of rectal carcinoids that are 1–2 cm is unpredictable; those smaller than 1 cm and greater than 2 cm behave predictably. Tumors that are 1–2 cm are associated with a 10% to 20% incidence of metastasis.

Methods.—The medical records of 44 patients with rectal carcinoid tumors were reviewed. The mean patient age was 50 years, and median follow-up was 84 months in patients without metastasis. Primary carcinoid tumors were classified by size and by typical or atypical histopathologic features.

Results.—Of the 44 patients, 13 had metastatic disease. Metastasis-free survival at 5 years for patients without metastatic disease was 100% in patients with tumors smaller than 1 cm, 73% in patients with tumors 1–2 cm, and 25% in patients with tumors larger than 2 cm; data on tumor size were unavailable for 3 patients. Metastasis-free survival at 5 years for patients without metastatic disease was 100% in cases of tumors with typical histologic characteristics and 50% in cases of tumors with atypical histologic characteristics, regardless of tumor size. Extensive surgery was performed in 9 patients, but this did not change survival.

Conclusion.—Rectal carcinoid tumors with atypical histopathologic characteristics and that are larger than 1 cm are associated with metastatic disease. Patients with such tumors without evidence of metastasis do not have longer survival after extensive surgery and should be encouraged to participate in studies of adjuvant chemotherapy.

▶ All carcinoid tumors are regarded as at least potentially malignant, but predicting the behavior in an individual case can be very difficult. This is especially true when we consider carcinoids that arise in the rectum, because of their rarity. Small tumors (less than 1.0 cm) often do well, whereas larger ones (greater than 2.0 cm) metastasize frequently. This study looked at a group of 44 rectal carcinoid tumors that included 11 between 1.0 and 2.0 cm and found that this intermediate group also has a marked proclivity for aggressive behavior. This seems to have been accentuated when the term "atypical" was used in the pathology reports that are the substance of this article. The major message of this paper is that extensive surgery offers no advantages over local resection for treatment of most rectal carcinoid tumors. The definition and criteria for "atypical carcinoid" (a term that is rejected by some) are somewhat variable, so the information on that topic in this paper is difficult to interpret. One wonders why, in an institution so rich in diagnostic pathology expertise, a group of nonpathologists would attempt to review a group of uncommon tumors and extract meaningful clinicopathologic conclusions without the involvement of a colleague in the laboratory. Perhaps there will be a companion paper in the pathology literature.

M.W. Stanley, M.D.

Suggested Reading

Felderspiel BM, Burke AP, Sobin LH, et al: Rectal and colonic carcinoids. *Cancer* 65:135–140, 1990.

Enteropathies Associated With Protracted Diarrhea of Infancy: Clinico-pathological Features, Cellular and Molecular Mechanisms
Cutz E, Sherman PM, Davidson GP (Univ of Toronto; Women's and Children's Hosp, Adelaide, Australia)
Pediatr Pathol Lab Med 17:335–367, 1997   8–10

Introduction.—Chronic diarrhea in the neonatal period is challenging diagnostically to both clinicians and pathologists. The various entities associated with protracted diarrhea in infancy were examined, with a focus on conditions with distinct clinicopathologic features.

Classification.—Protracted diarrhea in infancy is typified by 2 mucosal morphologic types: those with preserved villus architecture and those with various degrees of villous atrophy. The villus architecture is preserved in ion transport defects; primary defects of brush border enzymes; and diarrhea secondary to bile acid malabsorption, short bowel syndrome, and acrodermatis enteropathica. Diagnostic considerations for protracted diarrhea in infancy and villous atrophy include: bacterial or viral infections, postinfectious enteropathy, small-bowel bacterial overgrowth, enteropathy secondary to mild protein allergy, underlying immunoregulatory abnormalities, enteropathy with mitochondrial diarrhea rearrangement, and enteropathy associated with trichorrhexis nodosa.

Microvillous Inclusion Disease.—The major clinical feature of microvillous inclusion disease is onset at birth or within the neonatal period of severe, watery diarrhea associated with chronic intravascular volume depletion and impaired growth. This invariably fatal disease is probably inherited in an autosomal recessive manner. The somatostatin analog octreotide may help control diarrhea, but no effective treatment is available. The morphologic type is villous atrophy with findings of crypt hypoplasia and microvillous inclusions in enterocytes and colonocytes.

Tufting Enteropathy.—Tufting enteropathy develops within the first month of life. This autosomal recessive disease is characterized by watery diarrhea. Prolonged survival is possible and growth can be near normal when total parenteral nutrition is used. Histopathologic findings include moderate to severe villous atrophy and normal or hyperplastic crypts. Epithelial cell tufting of enterocytes is the most striking finding. No effective treatment is known.

Autoimmune Enteropathy.—Age at onset of autoimmune enteropathy varies but is usually within the first year of life. It is not known whether the condition is hereditary. Patients often have a family history of autoimmune disease, type I diabetes, glomerulonephritis, hepatitis, hemolytic anemia, asthma, or eczema. Villous atrophy varies from mild to severe. Crypt hyperplasia and inflammatory cell infiltrate in lamina propria may be observed. Most patients respond to immunosuppressive therapy.

Conclusion.—Small-bowel biopsy is important in the diagnosis and management of the enteropathies associated with protracted diarrhea of infancy. The clinicopathologic features of microvillous inclusion disease, tufting enteropathy, and autoimmune enteropathy are distinctly different and are useful in the differential diagnoses of protracted diarrhea of infancy.

▶ This is one of those subjects that has expanded considerably over the past few years. Using a review article format, these authors provide a useful update on conditions previously classified together as "intractable diarrhea of infancy." Microvillous inclusion disease, tufting enteropathy, and autoimmune enteropathy are all rare conditions with variable response to treatment. Microvillous inclusion disease is the most common of these three;

distinctive pathologic findings that are most apparent at the ultrastructural level allow specific identification of this uniformly fatal condition.

M.W. Stanley, M.D.

Suggested Reading

Cutz E, Rhoads JM, Drumm B, et al: Microvillous inclusion disease: An inherited defect of brush-border assembly and differentiation. *N Engl J Med* 320:646–651, 1989.

9 Hepatobiliary System and Pancreas

Banff Schema for Grading Liver Allograft Rejection: An International Consensus Document
Demetris AJ, Batts KP, Dhillon AP, et al (Univ of Pittsburgh, Pa)
Hepatology 25:658–663, 1997   9–1

Introduction.—As the use of hepatic transplantation grows, more physicians without special training in transplantation biology will be taking part in the care of liver transplant recipients. There is a need for some common approach to recognizing, naming, and grading the severity of acute liver allograft rejection. An international panel of specialists met for the purpose of establishing such criteria.

Methods.—The panel consisted of noted experts from the fields of liver transplantation pathology, hepatology, and surgery. Their goal was to create a simple, reproducible, and clinically relevant consensus document for the grading of acute liver allograft rejection. The recommendations were based on published data and the panel's combined experience. The document was completed in a meeting in Banff, Canada in 1995.

Consensus Document.—Organ allograft rejection was defined as an immunologic reaction to foreign tissue or a foreign organ with the potential to cause graft dysfunction and failure. The recommendations for grading considered grading as a measure of the severity of the necroinflammatory process, along with some estimation of vascular or ischemic damage. The panel agreed on a verbal grading system, based on the overall appearance of the liver biopsy specimen. Specimens showing a portal inflammatory infiltrate but not meeting the criteria for acute rejection were classified as indeterminate. The criterion for mild rejection was generally mild rejection infiltrate in a minority of triads, confined to the portal spaces. When rejection infiltrate had expanded to most or all of the triads, rejection was considered moderate. Severe rejection was said to be present when the rejection infiltrate spilled over into the periportal areas. The severe category also included moderate-to-severe perivenular inflammation extending into the hepatic parenchyma and associated with perivenular hepatocytic necrosis.

The panel described its preferred method of reporting liver allograft rejection as well. The report should start with the type of specimen and time after transplantation, followed by the histopathologic diagnoses. For each biopsy specimen, the presence or absence of acute rejection should be stipulated. A rejection activity index—including the categories of portal inflammation, bile duct inflammatory damage, and venous endothelial inflammation—should be used as well. The presence of bile duct loss, obliterative arteriopathy, or other chronic injury should be noted. The findings should be compared with those of the most recent previous biopsy, if appropriate.

Discussion.—Standardized criteria for the grading of acute liver allograft rejection should be useful for all physicians involved in the care of allograft recipients. Use of this system in scientific reports will avoid problems associated with multiple grading systems, and facilitate comparisons between centers.

▶ Liver transplantation shows continuing success as the only treatment for a variety of conditions. These authors noted that, at the time of their writing, it was offered in more than 100 centers, and that 5-year survival rates are generally greater than 50%. If you are involved in this activity as a pathologist, you will be very interested in this consensus statement. I found it to be concise and effectively illustrated.

M.W. Stanley, M.D.

Suggested Reading

Belle SH, Beringer KC, Detre K: Trends in liver transplantation in the United States 1993, in Terasaki PI, Cecka JM, (eds): *Clinical Transplants*. Los Angeles, UCLA Tissue Typing Laboratory, 1994, pp 19–36.

International Working Party: Terminology for hepatic allograft rejection. *Hepatology* 22:648–654, 1995.

Histological Features Predictive of Liver Fibrosis in Chronic Hepatitis C Infection
Paradis V, Mathurin P, Laurent A, et al (Hôpital de Bicêtre, Paris; Groupe Hospitalier Pitié-Salpétrière, Paris; Faculté de Pharmacie, Paris)
J Clin Pathol 49:998–1004, 1996   9–2

Objective.—Liver fibrosis occurs in about 1 in 5 cases of hepatitis C. There are currently no reliable biological or clinical indicators to predict in which patients fibrosis will develop. Such indicators would be useful in selecting patients for antiviral therapy. Transforming growth factor (TGF) β1 is a cytokine that plays a major role in liver fibrogenesis. With the use of TGF β1 RNA as a marker of liver fibrogenesis, the pathologic findings associated with fibrotic potential in hepatitis C were determined.

Methods.—Liver biopsy specimens were obtained from 28 patients with chronic hepatitis C and 5 controls. A quantitative reverse transcription–polymerase chain reaction (RT-PCR) assay was used to measure type I collagen mRNA and TGFβ1 mRNA in each specimen. The RT-PCR results were then correlated with the results of semiquantitative histologic scoring.

Results.—Liver samples from patients with hepatitis C showed stronger expression of type I collagen mRNA than did the control samples. Although type I collagen mRNA level was correlated with degree of fibrosis, it was unrelated to the presence of necroinflammatory lesions (i.e., portal inflammation, piecemeal necrosis, or lobular necrosis). Concentrations of TGFβ1 mRNA was also greater in patients than in controls. This concentration was significantly correlated with the histologic grade of activity and lobular necrosis. Expression of type I collagen mRNA was correlated with expression of TGFβ1 mRNA. On in situ hybridization, TGFβ1 mRNA was expressed mainly in areas of focal lobular necrosis.

Conclusions.—Transforming growth factor β1 mRNA, a sensitive marker of fibrogenesis in chronic hepatitis C, is correlated with the histologic features of fibrosis but not with those of necroinflammation. These 2 features must be examined separately when reporting on liver biopsy specimens from patients with chronic hepatitis C. The finding of lobular necrosis is strongly correlated with TGFβ1 mRNA expression and is an important predictor of prognosis.

▶ Current biopsy-based classifications of chronic hepatitis give a grade (degree of necroinflammatory activity) and a stage (degree of fibrosis). At first, it seems natural to suggest that advanced fibrosis must be the outcome of increased activity. This is contradicted by the fact that in hepatitis C, biopsy specimens often show very low activity, but the liver still goes on to significant fibrosis. These authors used very elegant molecular laboratory methods combined with retrospective review of liver biopsy specimens to reach the circular conclusion that "fibrosis . . . is associated with fibrogenesis." In other words we still do not know what leads to fibrosis, because necroinflammatory activity did not predict increased early molecular evidence of collagen production. It seems that livers in which a biopsy specimen shows fibrosis will probably get more fibrosis. They go on to tell us that lobular necrosis appears to be correlated with increased production of TGF-β1 mRNA, which is itself related to type I collagen mRNA. No doubt there will be more to this story as time goes on. For now, these findings indicate the importance of giving separate assessments for stage and grade in liver biopsy reports.

M.W. Stanley, M.D.

Suggested Reading

Desmet VJ, Gerber M, Hoofnagle JH, et al: Classification of chronic hepatitis: Diagnosis, grading and staging. *Hepatology* 19:1513–1519, 1994.

Scheuer PJ, Ashrafzadeh P, Sherlock S, et al: The pathology of hepatitis C. *Hepatology* 15:567–571, 1992.

A Reappraisal of Hepatic Siderosis in Patients With End-Stage Cirrhosis: Practical Implications for the Diagnosis of Hemochromatosis

Deugnier Y, Turlin B, le Quilleuc D, et al (Hôpital Pontchaillou, Rennes, France)
Am J Surg Pathol 21:669–675, 1997   9–3

Objective.—It can be difficult to differentiate between the various iron overload syndromes. The hepatic iron index (HII) is an accepted test for distinguishing between homozygous hemochromatosis and heterozygous hemochromatosis or alcoholic siderosis. Its use in evaluating iron concentration in patients with end-stage cirrhosis has been questioned, however. The histologic patterns of iron distribution were studied in patients with end-stage cirrhosis, and the reliability of the HII in excluding or confirming the presence of associated hemochromatosis was tested.

Methods.—Specimens of resected liver from 30 patients undergoing transplantation for alcoholic and/or viral end-stage cirrhosis were studied. Histologic assessment of iron distribution was performed. Also, biochemical assessments were done for hepatic iron concentration in the least and most iron-overloaded nodules in each specimen. The marker for the hemochromatosis gene was HLA-A3.

Results.—Twenty-three cases showed intranodular parenchymal siderosis: spotty in 12 cases and diffuse in 11. Only 2 patients had diffuse intrabiliary iron deposits. Fourteen patients had an HII of greater than 1.9, suggesting hemochromatosis. However, these results were not consistent with homozygous hemochromatosis as shown on HLA-A3 antigen testing.

Conclusions.—A high rate of parenchymal siderosis was found in liver specimens from patients with end-stage cirrhosis of various causes. This finding may lead to an HII greater than 1.9, thus mimicking hemochromatosis. In patients with end-stage cirrhosis, the diagnosis of hemochromatosis is a clinical and histologic one, even when the HII is higher than 1.9. Quantitative iron analysis is an adjunct to histologic examination, not a substitute for it.

▶ The differential diagnosis of hepatic iron overload syndromes is difficult. This is especially important, because there is no genetic test for primary hemochromatosis. Thus, the authors suggest that this important condition be addressed by a combination of clinical and histologic findings. The hepatic iron index (HII) was assessed in a group of patients who lack the primary hemochromatosis gene associated marker HLA-A3 and who had iron overload associated with viral or alcohol-induced liver disease. (The HII is the hepatic tissue iron content to age ratio expressed as micromoles iron/gram dry liver tissue weight/year of age.) Values over 1.9 have been taken as evidence of primary hemochromatosis, but in this study were associated frequently with other causes of siderotic cirrhosis. The authors conclude that tissue iron studies are not a substitute for clinical and histopathologic assessment of possible primary hemochromatosis.

M.W. Stanley, M.D.

Suggested Reading

Deugnier Y, Loreal O, Turlin B, et al: Liver pathology in genetic hemochromatosis: A review of 135 homozygous cases and their bioclinical correlations. *Gastroenterology* 102:2050–2059, 1992.

George P, Conaghan C, Angus H, et al: Comparison of histological and biochemical hepatic iron indexes in the diagnosis of genetic hemochromatosis. *J Clin Pathol* 49:159–163, 1996.

Hepatic Epithelioid Hemangioendothelioma: Biological Questions Based on Pattern of Recurrence in an Allograft and Tumor Immunophenotype
Demetris AJ, Minervini M, Raikow RB, et al (Univ of Pittsburgh, Pa; Università degli Studi Bari, Italy)
Am J Surg Pathol 21:263–270, 1997   9–4

Background.—Epithelioid hemangioendothelioma is a vascular neoplasm of intermediate malignancy that is usually progressive, but has an unpredictable clinical course. Most reports have been of lesions of the soft tissues, lung, bone marrow, and liver. Orthotopic liver transplantation has been successful in patients with hepatic involvement. Five cases of epithelioid hemangioendothelioma were analyzed.

Methods.—An immunophenotypic analysis of 5 cases of epithelioid hemangioendothelioma was performed. One case was in a 46-year-old woman who had orthotopic liver transplantation because of extensive, hepatic epithelioid hemangioendothelioma limited to the liver, initially occurring as an insidious seeding of individual tumor cells in areas of perivenular inflammation. Four additional cases of hepatic epithelioid hemangioendothelioma were analyzed.

Results.—In these 5 cases, CD34 was more sensitive than factor VIII for recognizing the disease. Staining for CD34 was diffuse and distinct in epithelioid and dendritic tumor cells. Staining for factor VIII was focal, indistinct, and showed a high background. The tumor cells were negative for CD1a, S-100 protein, Mac 387, CD68, and LN3. There was substantial infiltration of hepatic epithelioid hemangioendothelioma by factor XIIIa+, Mac 387+, CD68+, and LN3+ macrophages and dendrocytes, most considered reactive. The reactive macrophage and dendrocyte populations were seen throughout the fibrotic stroma and mingled with epithelioid clusters of tumor cells. A small number of factor XIIIa+ dendritic-shaped cells had intracytoplasmic lumens (Fig 2). Coexpression for CD34 or factor VIII and XIIIa was seen in a small subgroup of tumor cells.

Discussion.—The known association of factor XIIIa+ dendrocytes with granulation tissue, repair and fibrogenesis, and the modulation of expression of Factor XIIIa and VIII by inflammatory cytokines led to a hypothesis that epithelioid hemangioendothelioma lesions may result from prim-

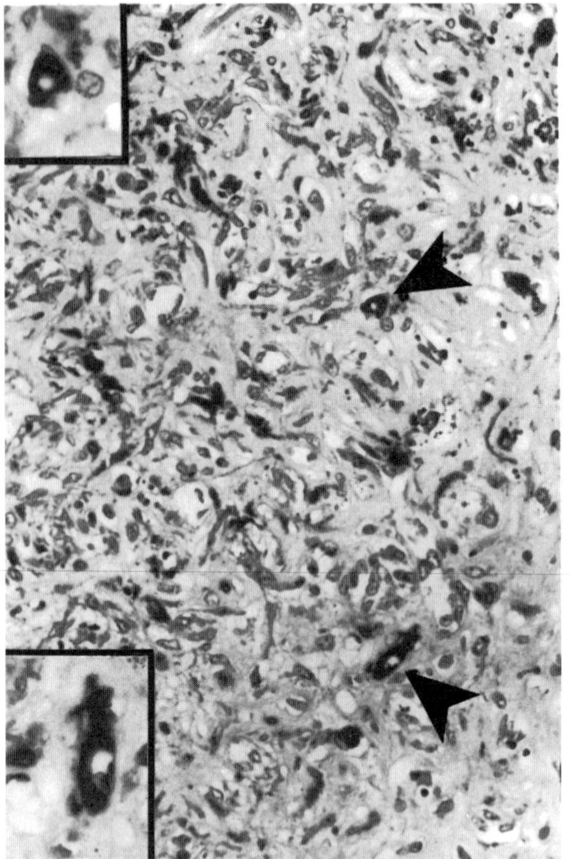

FIGURE 2.—Factor XIIIa staining of an epithelioid hemangioendothelioma lesion. Note the numerous positively stained cells (*arrows*) that contain intracytoplasmic lumens. These cells are shown at a higher magnification in the insets. (Courtesy of Demetris AJ, Minervini M, Raikow RB, et al: Hepatic epithelioid hemangioendothelioma: Biological questions based on pattern of recurrence in an allograft and tumor immunophenotype. *Am J Surg Pathol* 21:263–270, 1997.)

itive reticuloendothelial cells that differentiate along endothelial and dendritic pathways. These lesions may be a neoplastic analogue of wound healing. There may an important biological basis to the variation in factor VIII staining, strong expression of CD34, infiltration with factor XIIIa+ dendrocytes, and coexpression of CD34 and factor XIIIa on the subgroup of tumor cells.

▶ Epithelioid hemangioendothelioma is a vascular neoplasm of intermediate grade that can originate in many sites. The greatest difficulty is accurate diagnosis, as many examples are initially mistaken for carcinoma or missed altogether. Hepatic primaries can be associated with slow growth and long survival, so that liver transplantation has been used as therapy. These authors describe recurrence of the tumor in a hepatic allograft, and use this observation as an impetus for further study of this neoplasm. One interesting observation that may have diagnostic relevance for all of us is their finding that immunostaining with CD 34 is more sensitive than factor VIII related antigen. They provide a very useful review of this tumor's immunohistochemistry, including discussion of the minority that are cytokeratin-positive or CD 34-negative.

M.W. Stanley, M.D.

Suggested Reading

Eckstein RP, Ravich RBM: Epithelioid hemangioendothelioma of the liver: Report of two cases histologically mimicking venoocclusive disease. *Pathology* 18:459–462, 1986.

Ishak KG, Sesterhenn IA, Goodman MZD, et al: Epithelioid hemangioendothelioma of the liver: A clinicopathologic and follow-up study of 32 cases. *Hum Pathol* 15:839–852, 1984.

Kelleher MB, Iwatsuki S, Sheahan DG: Epithelioid hemangioendothelioma of liver: Clinicopathological correlation of 10 cases treated by orthotopic liver transplantation. *Am J Surg Pathol* 13:999–1008, 1989.

Marino IR, Todo S, Tzakis AG, et al: Treatment of hepatic epithelioid hemangioendothelioma with liver transplantation. *Cancer* 62:2079–2084, 1988.

Milchgrub S, Compazano M, Casillas J, et al: Intraductal carcinoma of the pancreas. *Cancer* 69:651–656, 1992.

Morohoshi T, Kanda M, Asanuma K, et al: Intraductal papillary neoplasms of the pancreas: A clinicopathologic study of six patients. *Cancer.* 64:1329–1335, 1989.

Ratcliffe N, Terhune PG, Longnecker DS: Small Intraductal Papillary–Mucinous Adenomas of the Pancreas. *Arch Pathol Lab Med* 120:1111–1115, 1996.
▶ As reviewed by the authors, small intraductal papillary-mucinous tumors of the pancreas were first described in 1989, and so far, this entity has acquired almost as many names as case reports. Larger examples may be associated with recurring pancreatitis, but the small examples in this report of incidental autopsy findings were asymptomatic. Atypia and carcinoma in-situ have been noted in some examples, but few have shown invasion and metastases. Extensive sampling is essential for proper classification. The relationship of these tumors to pancreatic adenocarcinoma is not entirely clear, and has been the subject of discussions that are nicely reviewed in this paper. Some investigators consider all these tumors to represent stages in the development of adenocarcinoma, whereas others retain the designation "adenoma" for well-differentiated examples that are completely intraductal and that have been adequately sampled for histologic study. Furthermore, the authors of this paper suggest that a division of these tumors into benign, borderline, and malignant categories might facilitate under-

standing of the prognosis associated with various histologic findings. The criteria for doing so are not yet entirely clear. It is important to distinguish this entity from the more common mucinous cystic neoplasms, virtually all of which should be considered malignant.

M.W. Stanley, M.D.

10 Soft Tissue and Bone

Malignant Vascular Tumors of the Serous Membranes Mimicking Mesothelioma: A Report of 14 Cases
Lin BT-Y, Colby T, Gown AM, et al (City of Hope Natl Med Ctr, Duarte, Calif; Mayo Clinic, Scottsdale, Ariz; Univ of Washington, Seattle; et al)
Am J Surg Pathol 20:1431–1439, 1996   10–1

Introduction.—It is rare to find endothelial sarcomas arising from or secondarily involving the serous membranes. There have been few cases documented of angiosarcoma occurring in pericardium, omentum, or other serous membranes. Described were patients with malignant endothelial-derived tumors which had a clinical presentation and gross and microscopic appearance that closely resembled malignant mesothelioma or diffuse carcinomatosis of the peritoneal, pleural, or pericardial cavities.

Methods.—The 14 patients in the retrospective review covering an 8-year period had mesothelioma or carcinoma. They ranged in age from 34 to 85 years, with a mean age of 52 years. Immunohistochemical evaluation and electron microscopy were conducted. Peritoneal tumors were found in 2 women and 1 man; pleural tumors were found in 8 men; and pericardial tumors were found in 3 men. Four endothelial markers were used in the study: CD31, CD34, von Willebrand factor, and *Ulex europaeus* agglutinin-I. As a control group, the same antibody panel was used for 39 mesotheliomas and more than 60 adenocarcinomas of various origins.

Results.—A diffuse sheet-like and clustered pattern of tumor growth with variable degrees of vascular differentiation was a shared histologic appearance. Four tumors had a tubulopapillary sarcoma growth pattern similar to mesothelioma. Spindle cells were seen in 9 tumors. Mesothelioma, adenocarcinoma, and leiomyosarcoma were the initial interpretations. All 14 patients had strong vimentin staining and negative or weak-to-moderate cytokeratin staining on immunohistochemical analysis (Table 3). At least 2 of the 4 endothelial markers were coexpressed by the tumor cells. The control group showed strong keratin staining and moderate or negative vimentin staining. None of the markers were expressed in this group. These endothelial tumors were highly aggressive, with 12 patients having disseminated disease. Most died within months of presentation.

Conclusion.—The differential diagnosis of serous membrane neoplasms with features of malignant mesothelioma should include epithelioid he-

TABLE 3.—Results of Immunohistochemical Studies

	1	2	3	4	5	6	7	8	9	10	11	12	13	14	No. of reactive cases
Vimentin	+	+	+	+	+	+	+	+	+	+	+	+	+	+	14/14
Keratin	−	−	−	−	−	+/−	−	+	+	+/−	+/−	+/−	−	−	6/14
CD31	+	+	+	+	+	+	−	−	+/−	+	+/−	+/−	+	−	11/14
CD34	−	+	−	−	−	+/−	−	+	+	−	−	+	+	+	7/14
UEA-1	+	+	+	−	+	+	+	−	+	+	+	+	+	−	11/14
VWF	+/−	+	+/−	+	+	+	+/−	+	+/−	+	−	−	+	+	12/14
Collagen IV*	+	+	+	+	+	+	−	−	+	+	+	+	+	+	12/14

Note: Other markers (number reactive/total number): HMFG-2 (0/4), HBME-1(0/3), carcinoembryonic antigen (0/7), BerEp4 (0.4), B72.3 (0/3), epithelial membrane antigen (0/4), CD15 (0/7), HMB45 (0/3), S100 (0/4), and muscle-specific actin (0/2A).

*Stains basal lamina and outlines the tumor cell clusters.

Abbreviations: UEA-1, Ulex europaeus agglutinin I; *VWF,* von Willebrand factor; +, positive; −, negative; +/−, focal positive.

(Courtesy of Lin BT-Y, Colby T, Gown AM, et al: Malignant vascular tumors of the serous membranes mimicking mesothelioma: A report of 14 Cases. *Am J Surg Pathol* 20:1431–1439, 1996.)

mangioendothelioma and epithelioid angiosarcoma. The presence of abortive vessel formation and strong expression of vimentin should prompt suspicion of endothelial neoplasm. The diagnosis can be confirmed by 2 or more endothelial-associated markers.

▶ Because of its association with occupational health hazard exposure, the diagnosis of malignant mesothelioma carries with it serious medicolegal compensatory implications. In the last decade, a number of antibodies with selective reactivity to various epitopes of glandular carcinoma have assisted the pathologist in the difficult task of differentiating malignant mesothelioma from adenocarcinoma. Sometimes, the good old electron microscope gathering dust in an obscure area of the department is the life saver in such a situation. It seems that from now on, our life is going to get a bit more complicated by adding epithelioid malignant vascular neoplasms to the already crowded differential diagnosis of malignant mesothelioma. In this article, the authors describe the best panel of antibodies for simplifying our diagnostic task.

K.E. Sirgi, M.D.

Lesions of the Bones of the Hands and Feet
Ostrowski ML, Spjut HJ (Baylor College of Medicine, Houston; Methodist Hosp, Houston; Texas Orthopedic Hosp, Houston)
Am J Surg Pathol 21:676–690, 1997   10–2

Background.—Many primary skeletal lesions and neoplasms are site specific. Some are rarely found in the hand and foot bones, whereas others typically occur there. Knowledge of which lesion types commonly affect the hand and foot bones aids in the assessment of tumors at these sites.

Methods and Findings.—The clinical, radiologic, and pathologic findings of 240 lesions in the bones of the hands and feet were reviewed. Two hundred three were benign, including reactive and reparative conditions. Tumors with cartilaginous differentiation were the largest single category of neoplasms. Enhondromas and chondrosarcomas were the most common. Noncartilaginous malignant tumors were uncommon. These masses showed typical radiologic and pathologic features. A larger proportion of lesions in the hand and foot bones than in other skeletal sites were florid reactive periostitis, bizarre parosteal osteochondromatous proliferations, and giant cell reparative granulomas (Tables 1 and 2).

Conclusion.—Florid reactive periostitis, bizarre parosteal osteochondromatous proliferations, giant cell reparative granulomas, and cartilaginous lesions (except for osteochondromas) commonly occur in the bones of the hands and feet. Many radiologic and microscopic features are useful for distinguishing between benign and malignant cartilaginous neoplasms.

▶ More than half of the skeletal bones are located in the hands and feet, and a wide variety of bone lesions can occur in these sites with some

TABLE 1.—Benign Lesions of the Bones of the Hands and Feet

Bone-forming tumors	
Osteoid osteoma	9
Osteoblastoma	3
Cartilage-forming tumors	
Enchondroma	29
Periosteal chondroma	12
Osteochondroma*	7
Chondroblastoma	5
Chondromyxoid fibroma	4
Giant cell tumor	2
Vascular tumors	
Hemangioma	3
Glomus tumor	1
Other connective tissue tumors	
Desmoplastic fibroma	1
Lipoma	1
Tumor-like lesions	
Florid reactive periostitis	16
Solitary bone cyst	5
Aneurysmal bone cyst	3
Intraosseous ganglion	3
Myositis ossificans	3
Hyperparathyroidism	1
Other lesions	
Reaction to injury	40
Giant cell reparative granuloma	24
Nora tumor	9
Fracture	7
Osteomyelitis	5
Epidermal inclusion cyst	3
Ischemic necrosis	2
Calcium pyrophosphate deposition disease	1
Gout	1
Skeletal angiomatosis	1
Tuberculosis	1
Vascular malformation	1
Total	203

*Includes 1 case of Dupuytren's (subungual) exostosis.
(Courtesy of Ostrowski ML, Spjut HJ: Lesions of the bones of the hands and feet. *Am J Surg Pathol* 21:676–690, 1997.)

TABLE 2.—Malignant Lesions of the Bones of the Hands and Feet

Chondrosarcoma	15
Osteosarcoma	5
Ewing's sarcoma	5
Fibrosarcoma	4
Angiosarcoma*	3
Malignant fibrous histiocytoma	2
Multiple myeloma	1
Adamantinoma	1
Metastatic squamous cell carcinoma	1
Total	37

*Includes 1 case of an epithelioid hemangioendothelioma.
(Courtesy of Ostrowski ML, Spjut HJ: Lesions of the bones of the hands and feet. *Am J Surg Pathol* 21:676–690, 1997.)

conditions having a certain predilection for the hand or foot. This paper nicely groups under "1 roof" benign and malignant bone lesions of the hand and foot. The amount of page flipping from 1 bone pathology reference book chapter to another when examining an unusual bone lesion of the hand or foot will, accordingly, be markedly reduced if this paper is kept conveniently close to the microscope. The problem is not trivial; as mentioned in this article, lesions of the hand and foot are commonly submitted to biopsy or treated at hospitals without large orthopedic tumor services. Therefore, it becomes very important to the general surgical pathologist to be familiar with the morphologic characteristics of lesions that may occur in these sites.

K.E. Sirgi, M.D.

Cytology of Typical and Atypical Ewing's Sarcoma/PNET

Renshaw AA, Perez-Atayde AR, Fletcher JA, et al (Harvard Med School, Boston; Brigham and Women's Hosp, Boston; Children's Hosp, Boston)
Am J Clin Pathol 106:620–624, 1996   10–3

Introduction.—The typical and atypical cytologic features of Ewing's sarcoma/peripheral neuroectodermal tumor (ES/PNET) have been reported. However, most previous series have been small. Two reliable ancillary tests for the identification of ES/PNET have recently become available: reactivity for CD99 and a characteristic cytogenetic finding, t(11;22)(q24;q12). The cytologic findings in 22 cases of confirmed ES/PNET were presented.

Findings.—All cases had histologic confirmation as well as confirmation by either immunohistochemical reactivity for CD99 or cytogenetic characterization. Nine of 9 cases characterized cytogenetically showed the characteristic t(11;22)(q24;q12). The typical cytologic features were found in 15 cases: small round cells, scant cytoplasm, round nuclei, fine chromatin, and conspicuous but distinct basophilic nucleoli. Two atypical large cell variants showed abundant eosinophilic cytoplasm, large irregular nuclei, vesicular chromatin, and prominent eosinophilic nucleoli. The immunophenotypic findings of ES/PNET, including CD99 reactivity, were found in both of these cases. In the remaining 5 cases, the cytologic findings fell between those of typical and atypical ES/PNET. In these cases, the pattern included abundant cytoplasm, intranuclear grooves, and pale vesicular nuclei.

Conclusions.—There is a spectrum of cytologic findings in ES/PNET, ranging from typical to atypical. The results may fall somewhere in between typical and atypical in up to one fifth of cases. If these tumors are found in unusual locations, e.g., the adrenal, they may be easily misdiagnosed. Ancillary studies can help to provide the correct diagnosis.

Fine-Needle Aspiration Biopsy of Synovial Sarcoma: A Cytomorphologic Analysis of Primary, Recurrent, and Metastatic Tumors
Kilpatrick SE, Teot LA, Stanley MW, et al (Wake Forest Univ, Winston-Salem, NC; Univ of Rochester, NY; Univ of Arkansas, Little Rock)
Am J Clin Pathol 106:769–775, 1996
10–4

Objective.—Synovial sarcoma is an uncommon tumor, usually affecting the extremities in young adults, that is potentially lethal. The histologic picture of synovial sarcoma has been well described, but not so the cytologic findings. The fine-needle aspiration biopsy findings of 10 patients with synovial sarcoma were reported.

Methods.—A total of 13 aspiration specimens were analyzed. Five specimens came from a primary tumor, 4 from a locally recurrent tumor, 3 from pulmonary metastases, and 1 from mediastinal metastasis. The patients were 6 men and 4 women aged 22–65 years. The diagnosis was confirmed by a biopsy and/or resection specimen in every case.

Results.—Histologic evaluation revealed monophasic fibrous disease in 5 patients, monophasic epithelial disease in 1, biphasic disease in 3, and poorly differentiated disease in 1. Most aspiration specimens showed moderate-to-marked smear cellularity. There were clusters of spindle-shaped cells, showing ovoid hyperchromatic nuclei and scanty tapering cytoplasm. The specimens did not show prominent nuclei. The case with monophasic epithelial disease showed epithelial tumor cells with ovoid-to-round, mostly regular nuclei with scant-to-abundant cytoplasm. These were found along with spindle cells in 1 of the patients with biphasic disease. None of the tumors showed multinucleated tumor giant cells. In the biphasic cases, the neoplastic spindle cells predominated over the epithelial cells. This made it difficult to distinguish biphasic tumors from monophasic synovial sarcoma or other spindle-cell soft tissue tumors.

Conclusions.—It is possible to make the diagnosis of synovial sarcoma by cytologic study. However, correct classification depends on clinical correlation, particularly for the monophasic-type tumors.

▶ My comment on the 2 preceding articles (Abstracts 10–3 and 10–4) is borrowed from an excellent editorial article[1] that reviewed the growing role of fine-needle aspiration in mesenchymal pathology:

"Fine-needle aspiration over the past few decades has become wildly successful in the realm of epithelial pathology, but still remains relatively unproven for mesenchymal lesions… Proving the utility of cytology for mesenchymal lesions will be no small task. An inability to accurately assess features including mitotic activity, encapsulation, infiltrative growth, size, and subtle architecture leave the cytopathologist seemingly impotent against many mesenchymal lesions. This is not to suggest we scrap the burgeoning practice of mesenchymal cytopathology, but instead acknowledge, accept, and perhaps even promote its current limitations. Doing so will likely free us from unreasonable expectations and ultimately grant us an uncluttered platform from which we may promote the strengths of mesenchymal cytopathology."

K.E. Sirgi, M.D.

Reference

1. Ryan M: Cytology and mesenchymal pathology: How far will we go? *Am J Clin Pathol* 106:561–564, 1996.

Mixed Tumors and Myoepitheliomas of Soft Tissue: A Clinicopathologic Study of 19 Cases With a Unifying Concept
Kilpatrick SE, Hitchcock MG, Kraus MD, et al (Bowman Gray School of Medicine, Winston-Salem, NC; Brigham and Women's Hosp, Boston; St Thomas's Hosp, London)
Am J Surg Pathol 21:13–22, 1997   10–5

Introduction.—Tumors of the parotid gland with epithelial and mesenchymal features are known as a mixed tumor. A mixed tumor of the salivary gland is often referred to as pleomorphic adenoma, and a mixed tumor of the skin is known as chondroid syringoma. In soft tissues and salivary glands, mixed tumors are characterized as well-circumscribed lesions exhibiting epithelial or myoepithelial elements within a hyalinized to chondromyxoid stroma. Although there have been many reports generated regarding salivary gland myoepitheliomas, little is known about mixed tumors or myoepitheliomas involving deep subcutaneous and subfascial soft tissues. Nineteen unusual cases of myoepitheliomas and mixed tumors in soft tissues were reported.

Methods.—A review found 12 males and 7 females with neoplasms in the soft tissues. The patients ranged in age from 2 to 83 years. Sections were examined immunohistochemically. Positive and negative controls were used throughout the procedures. The patients' medical records were reviewed for clinical data. Ten patients were followed from 6 months to 20 years.

Results.—The upper limb was the site of 8 tumors; the lower limb, of 6 tumors; the trunk, of 3 tumors; and the head and neck region, of 2 tumors. Dermis and subcutis were involved in 3 patients; 13 had subcutaneous involvement and 3 had deep subfascial soft-tissue involvement. Painless swelling, lasting from 2 weeks to 1 year, was the most common complaint. Microscopically, the tumors were circumscribed and lobulated. A focally infiltrative margin was seen in 6 tumors. Nests, cords, and ductules of epithelioid cells and/or nests of spindled cells within a hyalinized to chondromyxoid stroma were the cardinal morphologic features. One tumor was devoid of epithelial differentiation and dominated by myoepithelial cells Two tumors had cytoplasmic hyaline inclusions, and 1 had squamous differentiation. In 3 tumors, osteoid production and/or metaplastic bone were found. Chondroid differentiation was seen in 4 cases. Two tumors had adipocytic differentiation. Immunohistochemistry showed pan-keratin to be expressed in 16 of 16 tumors. S-100 protein was expressed in 16 of 17 tumors, alpha smooth muscle actin in 6 of 15, muscle specific actin in 2 of 10, desmin in 2 of 10, glial fibrillary acidic protein in 3 of 11, and epithelial membrane antigen in 3 of 16. Follow-up revealed that 2 patients had local recurrences and 2 had metastasis to lung and lymph nodes; the latter 2 patients died.

Conclusion.—Neoplasms composed predominantly of myoepithelial cells seem to characterize cutaneous mixed tumors; the term should also include tumors in deeper subcutaneous and/or subfascial tissues. These tumors are most often benign; however, a minority metastasize. Criteria used in comparable salivary gland tumors should apply to their treatment until larger studies with longer follow-up are conducted.

"Proximal-Type" Epithelioid Sarcoma, a Distinctive Aggressive Neoplasm Showing Rhabdoid Features: Clinicopathologic, Immunohistochemical, and Ultrastructural Study of a Series
Guillou L, Wadden C, Coindre J-M, et al (Institut Universitaire de Pathologie, Lausanne, Switzerland; Brigham and Women's Hosp, Boston; Institut Bergonié, Bordeaux, France; et al)
Am J Surg Pathol 21:130–146, 1997   10–6

Introduction.—In the classic form, epithelioid sarcoma occurs in the hand and around the wrist of young adults as a slow-growing, solitary or multiple, deep or superficial soft tissue neoplasm. Commonly seen as a multinodular proliferation of eosinophilic epithelioid-appearing and spindle-shaped cells with minimal cytologic atypia, epithelioid sarcoma cells may occasionally have a rhabdoid appearance. Eighteen young–to–middle-aged adults with aggressive, malignant soft-tissue neoplasms found in the pelvic, perineal, and genital tract areas were described. The tumors share the ultrastructural, morphologic, and immunohistochemical features of epithelioid sarcoma, extrarenal rhabdoid tumor, and undifferentiated carcinoma, and they may represent distinctive "proximal-type" epithelioid sarcoma.

Methods.—The retrospective review showed that the median age of the 11 males and 7 females was 35.5 years. The main presenting symptom was development of a mass. Referring pathologists provided the clinical data and follow-up information. The samples were examined with a light microscope, and all were examined immunohistochemically. Seven samples were examined with an electron microscope.

Results.—The pelvis and perineal regions were the site of 6 tumors; the pubic region and vulva were the site of 4 tumors; the buttocks were the site of 1 tumor; and then deep soft tissues of the left hip, the penis, the left forearm, the left axilla, and the occiput were each the site of 1 tumor. Ranging in size from 1 to 20 cm, the tumors invaded the subcutaneous or deep soft tissues and had rhabdoid or prominent epithelioid features. Areas of necrosis were often seen; half the tumors grew in a multinodular pattern. Two tumors had a granuloma-like pattern similar to that of the classic epithelioid sarcoma. In all but 1 patient, positivity for cytokeratin, epithelial membrane, antigen, and vimentin was found immunohistochemically. Ten of 16 tumors reacted with desmin and 8 of 16 reacted with CD34. Five of 15 reacted focally with smooth-muscle actin; 3 of 13 reacted for HMB-15; and 1 of 10 reacted for carcinoembryonic antigen. Four of 7 tumors examined at the ultrastructural level showed prominent intracytoplasmic intermediate filament aggregates which accumulated into paranuclear whorls, which is in keeping with the rhabdoid phenotype. Epithelial differentiation was seen in 5 tumors. Conventional epithelioid sarcoma, extrarenal malignant rhabdoid tumor, epithelioid malignant peripheral nerve sheath, undifferentiated carcinoma, melanoma, and rhabdomyosarcoma were the differential diagnoses. Follow-up revealed local recurrence in 1 patient and metastatic dissemination in 6 patients.

Conclusion.—This is a "proximal-type" of epithelioid sarcoma that is characterized by larger cell size, marked cytologic atypia, frequent occurrence of rhabdoid features, and lack of granuloma-like pattern. This type seems to be more aggressive than usual epithelioid sarcoma and seems to metastasize earlier.

▶ Open any issue of the *American Journal of Surgical Pathology* and you will find *at least 2* articles from Dr. Fletcher and his colleagues masterfully describing a new soft tissue lesion, or expertly modifying the criteria for another one. If you do not find an article from this author, you can bet your hospital administrator's gold Rolex watch that some clerk at the AJSP headquarters has misplaced the Fletcher monthly batch of approved articles.

On a more serious note (not that I was not dead serious in the paragraph above), these 2 articles (Abstracts 10–5 and 10–6) emphasize the dynamic evolution of soft-tissue pathology. With the help of immunohistochemistry, our understanding of soft-tissue neoplasms is continuously expanding. Believe it or not, the next wave of even more detailed tumor classification has already started with the addition of molecular techniques for routine surgical pathology. Please stay tuned!

K.E. Sirgi, M.D.

The Molecular Pathology of Small Round-Cell Tumours: Relevance to Diagnosis, Prognosis, and Classification
McManus AP, Gusterson BA, Pinkerton CR, et al (Inst of Cancer Research, Sutton, England)
J Pathol 178:116–121, 1996   10–7

Introduction.—A precise histologic diagnosis was not crucial when treatment of small round-cell tumors (SRCTs) only involved resection and radiotherapy. With the continued development of disease-specific therapeutic strategies and concomitant improvement in prognosis, accurate tumor diagnosis and classification are critical. The SRCTs include neuroblastoma, the Ewing family of tumors, and rhabdomyosarcoma. These tumors constitute about 15% of all childhood cancers. Detection strategies have been enhanced with the recent molecular genetic characterization of the chromosomal abnormalities characteristic of the SRCTs. These recent advances and their impact on the diagnosis, prognosis, and classification of SRCTs were described.

The Ewing Family of Tumors.—Ewing's sarcoma is typified by t(11;22)(q24;q12), a highly recurrent chromosome translocation and the expression of the glycoprotein p30/32, encoded by the *MIC2* gene. The translocation causes production of a chimeric gene between *EWS*, a novel putative RNA-binding gene located at 22q12 and *FLI1*, a member of the ETS family located at 11q24. The resulting fusion transcript has transforming activity and is believed to be involved in pathogenesis. This discovery has aided diagnosis and strengthened the theory that these tumors are part of a disease spectrum forming a Ewing family of tumors. Interphase fluorescence in situ hybridization (FISH) and reverse transcription polymerase chain reaction (RT-PCR) have been useful in obtaining this valuable information.

Neuroblastoma.—Cytogenetic investigation has shown that neuroblastoma involves characteristic chromosome changes that support the diagnosis, correlate with disease stage, and help predict tumor behavior. These changes include: deletions of the short arm of chromosome 1 (at 1p36.2-3), amplification of the proto-oncogene *MYCN*, and abnormalities of ploidy. Again, interphase FISH and RT-PCR have been used in these determinations.

Desmoplastic SRCT.—Few investigations have been performed on desmoplastic SRCT, a recently recognized clinicopathologic entity that is a rare, highly aggressive polyphenotypic malignancy. No interphase FISH investigations have been reported, but RT-PCR has been used diagnostically. t(11;22)(p13;q12) has been observed and molecular characterization of the breakpoint regions has shown the creation of a fusion gene between the *EWS* gene and the Wilm's tumor 1 gene.

Rhabdomyosarcoma.—Interphase FISH and RT-PCR have revealed translocation t(2;13)(q35;q14) in the alveolar form and loss of heterozygosity on the short arm of chromosome 11 at 11p15.5 in rhabdomyosarcoma.

Conclusion.—The increased emphasis on precise histologic diagnosis has resulted in substantial improvements in the treatment and survival in children with SRCT. The goal of tumor classification is to determine disease entities that are biologically distinct and whose recognition is of clinical value. Findings indicate that the SRCTs are genotypically and phenotypically distinct tumor types and that the genetic abnormalities depict key alterations that influence the morphology and clinical behavior of the tumor.

Common and Variant Gene Fusions Predict Distinct Clinical Phenotypes in Rhabdomyosarcoma
Kelly KM, Womer RB, Sorensen PHB, et al (Children's Hosp of Philadelphia; Univ of Pennsylvania, Philadelphia; British Columbia's Children's Hosp, Vancouver)
J Clin Oncol 15:1831–1836, 1997   10–8

Introduction.—Rhabdomyosarcoma is usually characterized as 2 separate diseases because of the embryonal and alveolar histology. Molecular assays using reverse-transcriptase polymerase chain reaction (RT-PCR) are capable of detecting both chromosomal translocations associated with rhabdomyosarcoma. The role of fusion gene status as a biologic marker was analyzed in 34 patients with rhabdomyosarcoma.

Methods.—Gene fusions in 34 patients were determined using RT-PCR assays. Eighteen of the patients had rhabdomyosarcoma with PAX3-FKHR fusions, 16 had rhabdomyosarcoma with PAX7-FKHR fusions. These data were compared retrospectively with molecular results.

Results.—Extremity lesion, younger age, and localized tumors were observed significantly more often in the group with PAX7-FKHR than the group with PAX3-FKHR (82% versus 22%). In patients with metastatic disease, PAX7-FKHR was more frequently involved in only bone or only distant nodes, compared to PAX3-FKHR in which multiple sites, such as bone, marrow, lungs, distant nodes, skin, and brain were involved. There were no significant between-group differences in relapse rate. Overall survival tended to be better and event-free survival was significantly better in the PAX7-FKHR group than the PAX3-FKHR group.

Conclusion.—It may be that the PAX3-FKHR and the variant PAX7-FKHR fusions are correlated with distinct clinical phenotypes. It may be helpful diagnostically to identify fusion gene status in patients with rhabdomyosarcoma.

Amplification of the t(2;13) and the t(1;13) Translocations of Alveolar Rhabdomyosarcoma in Small Formalin-Fixed Biopsies Using a Modified Reverse Transcriptase Polymerase Chain Reaction
Anderson J, Renshaw J, McManus A, et al (Inst of Cancer Research, Sutton, England; John Radcliffe Hosp, Oxford, England)
Am J Pathol 150:477–482, 1997   10–9

Introduction.—Detection of chromosomal translocations in pediatric solid tumors is difficult because adequate amounts of fresh viable tumor tissue may not be available and it is often hard to obtain a karyotype from a solid tumor. Reverse transcriptase polymerase chain reaction (RT-PCR) may be used to amplify the characteristic chimeric ribonucleic acid (RNA) products of translocations. With this method, only small amounts of tumor tissue are needed and formalin-fixed tissue may be used. Described is a modified RT-PCR technique used for the rapid and specific detection of characteristic chromosomal translocations of alveolar rhabdomyosarcoma using small amounts of formalin-fixed tissue as the starting material.

Method.—Four 5-μm sections from tissue blocks were dewaxed and RNA was extracted. One μg of RNA was reverse transcribed and a single-stranded nucleic acid binding protein was added. The presence of the t(2;13) and t(1;13) translocations were tested using semi-nested PCR. After amplification, the PCR products were separated and viewed under ultraviolet light. Original histologic reports of the tumors were reviewed. When there were discrepancies, the original sections were reexamined.

Results.—Alveolar rhabdomyosarcoma sections were used to develop a highly sensitive RT-PCR assay for detection of tumor-specific translocations of formalin-fixed tumors. Five embryonal rhabdomyosarcoma sections were used for control. Of 27 samples evaluated using the modified RT-PCR technique, there were 4 samples for which the detection of translocations cast doubt on the original histopathologic diagnosis.

Conclusion.—The modified RT-PCR technique can be appropriately used in prospective and retrospective investigations of the prognostic significance of translocations in rhabdomyosarcoma tumors.

Chromosomal Rearrangement t(11;22) in Extraskeletal Ewing's Sarcoma and Primitive Neuroectodermal Tumour Analysed by Flourescence *In Situ* Hybridization Using Paraffin-embedded Tissue
Nagao K, Ito H, Yoshida H, et al (Tottori Univ, Japan; Natl Yonago Hosp, Japan; Jikei Univ, Tokyo)
J Pathol 181:62–66, 1997   10–10

Introduction.—Recent findings have uncovered translocations (ranging from 20% to 96%) specific for each tumor type of soft tissue sarcomas. The cytogenetic abnormality specific for Ewing's sarcoma (ES) of bone and soft tissue origin has been revealed as a balanced chromosomal t(11;22) (q24;q12) by karotypic analysis. Immunohistological analysis of MIC 2 expression and fluorescence *in situ* hybridization (FISH) analysis was done using formalin-fixed, paraffin-embedded tissues. Nine round cell sarcomas originally diagnosed as extraskeletal ES (2); primitive neuroectodermal tumor, including Askin's tumor (4); and neuroblastoma (3) were analyzed by immunostaining for MIC 2 and were used to find t(11;22) by FISH analysis.

Methods.—Immunostaining was completed after use of a monoclonal antibody against the human MIC 2 gene. The FISH technique was done on formalin-fixed, paraffin-embedded tissue with *a*-satellite DNA probe for chromosome 11, a chromosome 22 marker probe for the q13.3 region, and whole chromosome painting probes for chromosomes 11 and 22.

Results.—Both ES and all 4 primitive neuroectodermal tumor specimens were immunoreactive for MIC 2. The tumor-specific t(11;22) was contained in both ES, 3 of 4 PNET, and 0 of 3 neuroblastomas.

Conclusion.—Ewing's sarcoma may be closely related to primitive neuroectodermal tumor, as determined by cytogenetic results and immunohistological investigation of MIC 2 expression. The FISH technique is useful in detecting chromosomal translocation and determining tumor type of soft tissue sarcomas, using only paraffin-embedded tissue.

Intra-Abdominal Polyphenotypic Tumor
Thorner P (Univ of Toronto)
Pediatr Pathol Lab Med 16:161–169, 1996   10–11

Introduction.—The diagnosis of Ewing's sarcoma and peripheral primitive neuroectodermal tumor (pPNET) is considered when t(11;22) (q24;12) is detected. Described is an intra-abdominal polyphenotypic tumor that possessed this translocation.

> *Case Report.*—Child, 37 months, was seen for sudden onset of abdominal pain and shock. He had a large abdominal mass and free fluid in the abdomen. A large, nonhomogeneous retroperitoneal mass contiguous with the liver was observed on computed tomography (CT) scan. A friable mass was found on laparotomy and a biopsy was performed. The boy was treated with a modified Ewing sarcoma protocol and the mass decreased markedly. The mass was resected and a small amount of residual tumor was left at the porta hepatis. The whole abdomen was irradiated. A CT scan at 4 months showed recurrence at the site of known residual tumor. This was resected using involved surgical margins. At 12 months from diagnosis, he had no detectable disease.

Findings.—A diagnosis of polyphenotypic tumor was given. The tumor was not similar to any pediatric malignancy at the histologic level. Other diagnoses considered and rejected included Ewing sarcoma, pPNET, ectomesenchymoma, and intra-abdominal small cell desmoplastic tumor. Genetic studies were conducted to better define the nature of this tumor. A translocation at t(11;22)(q24;q12) and 100 copies of the MDM2 gene were detected.

Conclusion.—The presence of the t(11;22)(q24;q12) translocation should not be diagnostic of Ewing sarcoma and pPNET without supporting histologic evidence. Treatment for tumors should probably be based on phenotype rather than genotype when these 2 profiles are not in agreement.

▶ Small "round cell" or "blue-cell" tumors of childhood (primitive / peripheral neuroectodermal tumor / PNET [Ewing's tumor]; neuroblastoma; desmoplastic small round-cell tumor; rhabdomyosarcoma; leukemia / lymphoma) have proved to be strongly associated with reproducible chromosomal abnormalities. Definitive diagnosis is moving away from morphologic criteria; genetic studies are becoming the standard. The review by McManus et al. (Abstract 10–7) provides a birdwatcher's guide and emphasizes the need to handle tissues at biopsy or resection in a manner that will permit specialty centers to undertake molecular-pathology diagnosis. Look through this article with your procedure manual in hand: Are you up to date?

We can expect pressure toward more detailed cytogenetic and molecular analysis from our clinical colleagues. It is well known that alveolar rhabdomyosarcoma has a worse prognosis than does embryonal, and that certain translocations characterize alveolar rhabdomyosarcoma. Kelly et al. (Abstract 10–8) now provide evidence that different classes of translocation within alveolar rhabdomyosarcoma are associated with different clinical behaviors. As tumor biology is more finely dissected, we will have to process tissue specimens more painstakingly, and for good clinical reasons.

But there is hope. Perhaps soon it will no longer be necessary to send tissue for cytogenetic studies, to freeze tissue for mRNA extraction, reverse transcriptase treatment, and PCR across gene fusion sites, or to do touch preparations that will permit FISH assays for translocations. Anderson et al. (Abstract 10–9) report extracting mRNA from small (is there any other kind from children?), formalin-fixed tumor biopsies. The mRNA successfully underwent reverse transcriptase and PCR treatment, and the results matched those from usual mRNA extraction or karyotypic studies in parallel samples from the same patients. Until this result is reproduced elsewhere and becomes more widely available, however, we should handle tumor tissue to enable a variety of studies: The belt-and-suspenders approach.

Is all lost if only formalin-fixed, paraffin-embedded tissue is available, and, for some reason, immunohistochemistry fails to be of use in separating—for example—small-cell osteosarcoma from PNET / Ewing's tumor? Maybe not. FISH assays to document chromosomal rearrangements can perhaps pull the chestnuts out of the fire, as reported by Nagao et al. (Abstract 10–10) Still, how much better to handle the tissue appropriately in the first place! Bear in mind, finally, that the genetics-ueber-alles approach has its pitfalls. A cautionary report from Thorner (Abstract 10–11) describes an unusual malignancy that had none of the usual light-microscopic features of PNET / Ewing's-group tumors but on molecular-biology analysis had evidence of the chromosomal translocation characteristic of this set of neoplasms. He proposes that acquired karyotypic lesions may not represent biologic behavior, and that therapy may sometimes be more effectively guided by phenotypic data (although the presence of a small alveolar-rhabdomyosarcoma component in a largely embryonal tumor may be detectable only by molecular analysis, and may confer a worse prognosis; see Abstract 10–10). As always, consider all the evidence and remember: the paraffin sections still have something to tell us.

A.S. Knisely, M.D.

11 Neuropathology

Improving Diagnostic Accuracy and Interobserver Concordance in the Classification and Grading of Primary Gliomas
Coons SW, Johnson PC, Scheithauer BW, et al (Barrow Neurological Inst, Phoenix, Ariz; Mayo Clinic and Found, Rochester, Minn; Ohio State Univ, Columbus)
Cancer 79:1381–1393, 1997 11–1

Introduction.—The management and study of glioma depend on accurate histologic diagnosis. However, current histologic criteria for the classification and grading of glioma are subjective, leading to potential problems in diagnostic accuracy and reproducibility. Standardized definitions of histologic subtype and grade were used in an effort to reduce interobserver variation in the diagnosis of glioma.

Methods.—Four independent neuropathologists reviewed the histologic findings of 4 sets of supratentorial and infratentorial gliomas, for a total of 244 cases. The results were then reviewed to identify the most common sources of disagreement regarding classification or grade. Criteria to enhance consistency in classification were then developed. Concordance among the neuropathologists was evaluated not only for diagnosis and grade but also for the histologic criteria. Two of the pathologists used the new criteria to review a different set of 315 gliomas. The value of the new criteria was validated through known long-term survival data.

Results.—Concordance rates for the first review were 52% for all 4 reviewers, 60% for any 3 reviewers, and 70% for 2 reviewers. By the fourth review, these rates had improved to 69%, 75%, and 80%, respectively. There were some problems with features important in grading, especially microvascular proliferation. However, most of the disagreements stemmed from tumor classification. With the new criteria, much of the improvement in agreement arose from refinements in distinguishing diffuse astrocytomas from oligodendromas or oligoastrocytomas and pilocytic astrocytomas. The new criteria stipulated that the finding of any typical oligodendroma was enough to remove a tumor from the astrocytoma category. In the validation series, "grade 3/anaplastic astrocytomas" reclassified as mixed tumors or oligodendromas showed significantly better survival than did those confirmed as being astrocytomas. The final review suggested that as many as one fourth of gliomas were oligodendroglial tumors, a significantly higher proportion than previously reported.

Conclusions.—The findings point out ongoing problems with reproducibility and interobserver variability in the classification and grading of primary gliomas. More work is needed to refine the definition of microvascular proliferations, especially in oligodendroglial tumors. Also, more research is needed to establish the best measure of proliferative activity in these tumors. Progress in differentiation between oligodendroglioma and oligoastrocytoma requires new insight into the histogenesis of these tumors.

▶ This highly important study deals with the fundamental issue of observer subjectivity in the neuropathologic diagnosis of gliomas. Multiple diagnostic points are addressed and discussed in this multistep endeavor: determining initial rates of concordance between multiple neuropathologists in diagnosis of gliomas, identifying major components of diagnostic disagreement, generating standardized definitions of histologic subtype and grade, and reevaluating diagnostic concordance rates after application of the new, standardized definitions.

I believe that the most compelling aspect of this study involves the findings regarding diagnoses of oligodendrogliomas. Patients receive specific treatments and are placed in specific prognostic categories according to both the histologic type and grade of glial tumors. Although an objective, biologic, measurable marker (such as proliferation index!) has been avidly sought to explain the apparent heterogeneity in clinical outcome for patients with intermediate grade astrocytomas, these are convincing data supporting the argument that at least part of this clinical heterogeneity has been caused by misdiagnosis of some oligodendrogliomas as astrocytomas. Use of these liberal diagnostic criteria for classification of oligodendrogliomas does result in separation of this large group of patients into much more homogeneous prognostic groups, and patients carrying diagnoses of oligodendrogliomas exhibit significantly longer mean survival times than do those with intermediate grade astrocytomas. It also results in a significant increase in the percentage of oligodendrogliomas among all patients with primary gliomas, to approximately 25%. Although the distinction between oligodendroglioma and oligoastrocytoma was a continuous diagnostic problem in this group, the authors make a good point in stating that the clinical significance of this distinction is minimal at present because patients with these tumors receive similar treatment.

Although these authors' criteria and conclusions are controversial, their honest consideration of the fundamental issue of subjectivity in pathologic diagnosis and its potential effects on patient management is extremely valuable.

D. Grzybicki, M.D., Ph.D.

Frozen Section Evaluation of Stereotactic Brain Biopsies: Diagnostic Yield at the Stereotactic Target Position in 188 Cases

Brainard JA, Prayson RA, Barnett GH (Cleveland Clinic Found, Ohio)
Arch Pathol Lab Med 121:481–484, 1997   11–2

Background.—Image-guided stereotactic brain biopsy can safely and reliably diagnose intracranial lesions that were previously inaccessible. Frozen-section evaluation permits immediate assessment of the adequacy of the biopsy specimen, with prompt feedback to the neurosurgeon. However, there is little information on the diagnostic yield of frozen-section evaluation of the initial stereotactic target (FS-0). This issue was addressed in a retrospective study of stereotactic brain biopsy samples from 185 patients.

Methods.—A total of 188 stereotactic brain biopsy samples were obtained during a 5-year period. There were 107 male patients and 68 female patients, mean age 48. All specimens were obtained with a stereotactic frame under CT or MRI guidance. The diagnostic yield of FS-0 was reviewed.

Findings.—A diagnosis was reached at FS-0 in 67% of cases. A neoplastic condition was diagnosed in 73% of 131 cases (Table 1) and a nonneoplastic condition was diagnosed in 50% of 46 cases (Table 2); the biopsy was nondiagnostic in 6% of cases. In 16% of cases—including 16% of neoplasms and 15% of nonneoplastic conditions—the correct diagnosis was made on subsequent frozen-section evaluation. The correct diagnosis was made on the second frozen-section in 54% of cases and by the fourth frozen section in 89%. Sampling error led to an inaccurate diagnosis at FS-0 in 11% of neoplastic cases. Significant diagnostic errors occurred in 1.7% of cases. If only 1 biopsy specimen had been taken from FS-0, one third of the cases diagnosed would have been misdiagnosed.

Conclusions.—In patients undergoing stereotactic brain biopsy, frozen-section or cytologic evaluation of material obtained at surgery must be performed to make sure that the tissue obtained is adequate for diagnostic purposes. The diagnostic yield is significantly increased by obtaining as many as 4 biopsy samples. At FS-0, definitive diagnosis is more likely for neoplastic lesions than for nonneoplastic lesions. Optimal diagnostic accuracy relies on communication between the neurosurgeon and pathologist.

► This report provides a valuable, concise assessment of the diagnostic yield of stereotactic brain biopsy samples, with the results well summarized in Tables 1 and 2. The major conclusions of the study are as follows. (1) Stereotactic brain biopsy is useful for diagnosis of neoplastic lesions but not useful at all for nonneoplastic lesions. (2) A diagnostic biopsy will only occur approximately two thirds of the time on the first pass. (3) The neoplastic lesion that is most often not diagnosed on the first pass, requiring multiple biopsies, is glioblastoma multiforme. These findings are most likely not surprising to pathologists interpreting frozen sections of stereotactic brain

TABLE 1.—Summary of Stereotactic Biopsy Results of Neoplastic Cases

Diagnosis	No. of Cases	FS-0 Diagnostic	Subsequent FS Diagnostic	FS Nondiagnostic*	Sampling Error†	Error in Diagnosis
Low-grade astrocytoma	20	15	4	1	0	0
Anaplastic astrocytoma	14	10	1	3	3	0
GBM	43	30	8	5	9	0
Recurrent astrocytoma‡	15	12	2	1	0	0
Brainstem glioma	2	2	0	0	0	0
Mixed glioma	3	1	0	2	2	0
Oligodendroglioma	4	4	0	0	0	0
Anaplastic oligodendroglioma	2	2	0	0	0	0
Meningioma	2	1	1	0	0	0
PNET	1	0	0	1	0	1
Lymphoma	11	7	3	1	0	0
Metastasis	13	11	2	0	0	0
Infiltrating glioma	1	1	0	0	0	0
Total, n (%)	131	96 (73)	21 (16)	14 (11)	14 (11)	1 (0.8)

Abbreviations: GBM, Glioblastoma multiforme; *PNET*, primitive neuroectodermal tumor; *FS*, frozen section.
*Although frozen sections performed at the time of surgery were not diagnostic, permanent sections were diagnostic in all cases.
†Sampling errors resulted when biopsy material was taken from within the lesion but was not sufficiently representative to accurately diagnose the lesion.
‡Recurrent/residual tumors after radiation therapy were not graded.
(Courtesy of Brainard JA, Prayson RA, Barnett GH: Frozen section evaluation of stereotactic brain biopsies: Diagnostic yield at the stereotactic target position in 188 cases. *Arch Pathol Lab Med* 121:481–484, 1997.)

TABLE 2.—Summary of Stereotactic Biopsy Results of Nonneoplastic Cases

Diagnosis	No. of Cases	FS-0 Diagnostic	Subsequent FS Diagnostic	FS Nondiagnostic*	Error in Diagnosis
Vasculitis	3	0	1	0	2
Demyelinating disease	11	6	0	5	0
Radiation effect	11	8	2	1	0
Sclerosing vasculopathy	3	0	1	2	0
Infections	10	4	2	4	0
Other	8	5	1	2	0
Total, n (%)	46	23 (50)	7 (15)	14 (31)	2 (4)

Abbreviation: FS, frozen section.
*Although frozen sections performed at the time of surgery were not diagnostic, permanent sections were diagnostic in all cases.
(Courtesy of Brainard JA, Prayson RA, Barnett GH: Frozen section evaluation of stereotactic brain biopsies: Diagnostic yield at the stereotactic target position in 188 cases. *Arch Pathol Lab Med* 121:481–484, 1997)

biopsy samples, particularly the 33% misdiagnosis rate on a single pass! However, in my experience, neurosurgeons have been surprised by these data, emphasizing the need for good pathologist-surgeon communication in this setting. Burger and Nelson[1] stress good communication and provide additional information regarding stereotactic brain biopsy sample preparation and evaluation in their article, which precedes this study in the May 1997 issue of *Archives of Pathology and Laboratory Medicine.*

D. Grzybicki, M.D., Ph.D.

Reference

1. Burger PC, Nelson JS: Stereotactic brain biopsies. *Arch Pathol Lab Med* 121:477–480, 1997.

Analysis of Proliferation Markers and p53 Expression in Gliomas of Astrocytic Origin: Relationships and Prognostic Value
Cunningham JM, Kimmel DW, Scheithauer BW, et al (Mayo Clinic and Found, Rochester, Minn)
J Neurosurg 86:121–130, 1997   11–3

Background.—The p53 gene is altered in about half of all astrocytomas. This alteration is generally accompanied by overexpression of the protein product. The prognostic value of p53 expression and the proliferation markers MIB-1 and proliferating cell nuclear antigen (PCNA) was studied in patients with newly diagnosed cerebral astrocytomas.

Methods.—Consecutive paraffin sections of 105 astrocytomas and 15 oligoastrocytomas were examined. Previously, these tumors had been evaluated for genetic abnormalities and by flow cytometry.

Findings.—Expression of p53 was noted in 40% of the tumors, regardless of tumor stage and grade and patient age and sex. Expression of p53 was associated with a loss on chromosome 17p and was more common in aneuploid tumors. However, it was unrelated to survival time. The MIB-1 and PCNA labeling indices rose with increasing tumor grade but were unassociated with other clinicopathologic parameters. Concordance among MIB-1, PCNA, and p53 was poor in individual tumors. Findings for p53 and MIB-1 for astrocytomas and oligoastrocytomas were similar. Values of MIB-1 and PCNA seemed to have prognostic value in a univariate analysis but not after adjustment for tumor grade and patient age.

Conclusions.—Patient age and tumor grade were the strongest predictors of survival in this group of patients with infiltrative gliomas. Overexpression of p53 was unassociated with survival. Also, PCNA and MIB-1 were not related to survival in multivariate analysis. Because of the poor concordance of these 2 proliferation markers, clinicians should use them cautiously, if at all, in clinical settings.

▶ This recent paper describes an excellent study investigating the prognostic value of p53 expression and expression of 2 proliferation markers in a large group of patients with astrocytomas. A huge body of literature has recently been generated looking at expression of these biological markers in many types of brain tumors, including astrocytomas. The vast majority of these studies have yielded contradictory results, stemming from several basic study weaknesses, including use of small numbers of cases, use of variable and nonstandardized quantitation methods, and most importantly, use of univariate statistical analysis, rather than multivariate analysis.

This present study of 120 gliomas (astrocytomas or oligoastrocytomas) does a good job of illustrating the importance of multivariate analysis in assessing the independent prognostic value of these biological markers. Although both MIB-1 and PCNA positivity (but not p53) appeared to have prognostic utility in univariate analysis (similar to many other reports in the literature describing astrocytomas, oligodendrogliomas, and meningiomas), these proliferation markers were not independent prognostic factors in a multivariate analysis with patient age and tumor grade taken into account. This means that performing proliferation marker immunohistochemistry and semiquantitative assessment of proliferation index on astrocytic tumors will not provide any additional prognostic information beyond that already provided by the patient's age and tumor histologic grading.

Additionally, this study provides evidence supporting the idea that MIB-1 and PCNA indices may not correlate in a given individual tumor, therefore leaving open to question conclusions about the "proliferative potential" of a tumor based on data from immunostaining for just one marker.

Although these authors present essentially negative results, their findings are important in exposing the potential pitfalls of univariate analysis in these sorts of studies, and contributing to our knowledge regarding the probable lack of usefulness of proliferation indices and p53 expression with regards to predicting clinical outcome in patients with primary cerebral astrocytic tumors.

D. Grzybicki, M.D., Ph.D.

Atypical Central Neurocytoma

Söylemezoglu F, Scheithauer BW, Esteve J, et al (Inst of Neuropathology, Zürich, Switzerland; Mayo Clinic, Rochester, Minn; Internatl Agency for Research on Cancer, Lyon, France)
J Neuropathol Exp Neurol 56:551–556, 1997   11–4

Purpose.—Central neurocytoma, an intraventricular tumor composed of uniform round cells with neuronal differentiation, is designated as a grade I tumor. However, there have been reports of mitotic activity, vascular proliferation, and focal necrosis in some neurocytomas. The proliferative potential of central neurocytomas was studied and correlated with their clinical behavior.

Methods.—The study included 41 central neurocytomas in 36 patients. The diagnosis was based on the tumors' location in the lateral ventricles, the histopathologic findings, and the immunohistochemical detection of

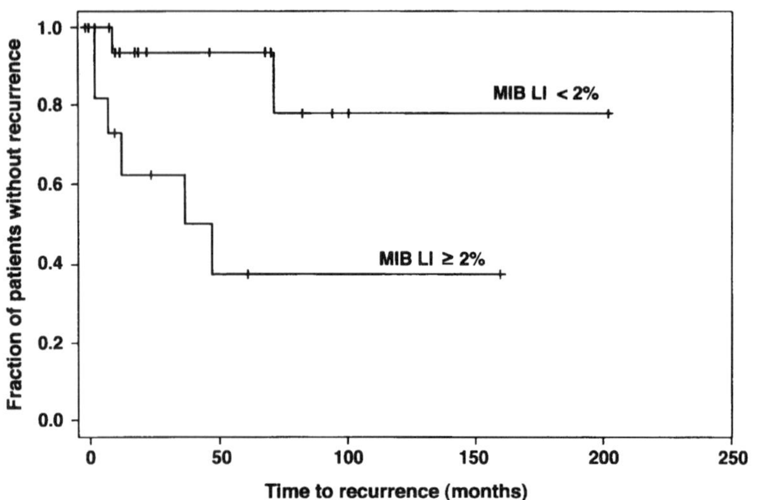

FIGURE 3.—Kaplan-Meier analysis of the recurrence of central neurocytomas. Tumors with MIB-1 LI greater than 2% are associated with a significantly less favorable clinical course. (Courtesy of Söylemezoglu F, Scheithauer BW, Esteve J, et al: Atypical central neurocytoma. *J Neuropathol Exp Neurol* 56:551–556, 1997. Reproduced with permission from the *Journal of Neuropathology and Experimental Neurology*.)

synaptophysin. Immunostaining studies with the monoclonal antibody MIB-1, and the MIB-1 labeling index (LI) was calculated to assess the mean size of the growth fraction.

Findings.—The mean MIB-1 LI was 3.4% ± 3.7% with a wide range of 0.1% to 8.6%. Thirty-nine percent of neurocytomas had an MIB-1 LI of greater than 2%, which was closely associated with the presence of vascular proliferation. On Kaplan-Meier analysis, disease-free survival was significantly related to MIB-1 LI. At follow-up of 150 months, the relapse rate was 22% for patients with an MIB-1 LI less than 2% versus 63% for those with an MIB-LI greater than 2% (Fig 3).

Conclusions.—Proliferative potential varies among central neurocytomas. Since tumors with an MIB-1 LI of 2% or greater, vascular proliferation, or both have a relatively unfavorable clinical course, the authors propose using these criteria to designate. Designation of such tumors as *atypical central neurocytomas* is proposed. Further study is needed to clarify the biologic behavior of this variant of central neurocytoma and to assess the need for modifications of treatment, such as postoperative radiotherapy.

► Since the recent original report of central neurocytoma by Hassoun et al.[1] in 1982, most descriptions of this entity are of a histologically and biologically benign tumor, with most patients having a good prognosis after surgical resection. However, case reports of "atypical" central neurocytomas have appeared in the literature, describing tumors exhibiting such features as histologic anaplasia and poor clinical outcome. This study addresses the question of whether there is a correlation between proliferative activity and clinical outcome in a representative group of central neurocytomas, thereby addressing the question of whether a higher grade central neurocytoma can and should be identified. It is a good representative of the many recent studies attempting to prognostically subdivide tumors within a histologic group on the basis of proliferative activity, as measured by semiquantitative analysis of MIB-1 immunohistochemistry.

This study convincingly illustrates that all central neurocytomas do not look and act the same, and an atypical group therefore exists. A biphasic distribution of the MIB-1 LI was demonstrated for this group of central neurocytomas that on univariate statistical analysis appears to correlate with the clinical course (see Fig 3). However, tumors with an MIB-1 LI >2% usually contained mitoses (>3/10 high-power fields), and they do not demonstrate an independent correlation with multivariate analysis for proliferative activity and outcome. Perhaps identifying central neurocytomas with atypical histologic features (such as increased mitotic activity) would be enough information alone to predict a poorer clinical prognosis. This study does not actually provide the information to answer this question but nevertheless implies that a measurement of proliferative activity is needed.

A true test of the value of an MIB-1 LI index cutoff of >2% would be to apply this cutoff to a *new* set of central neurocytomas and determine whether it predicts prognosis with statistical significance.

D. Grzybicki, M.D., Ph.D.

Reference

1. Hassoun J, Gambarelli D, Grisoli F: Central neurocytoma: An electron-microscopic study of two cases. *Acta Neuropathol* 56:151–156, 1982.

Telomerase Activity in Ordinary Meningiomas Predicts Poor Outcome
Langford LA, Piatyszek MA, Xu R, et al (Univ of Texas, Houston; Univ of Texas, Dallas; Geron Corp, Menlo Park, Calif)
Hum Pathol 28:416–420, 1997   11–5

Introduction.—The biological behavior of meningiomas is highly variable and its correlation with histologic features has been imprecise. Therefore, the ability to identify meningiomas with malignant potential could improve the clinical management of patients with meningiomas. Telomerase is an enzyme that stabilizes the length of telomeres, long stretches of repetitive DNA sequences that prevent the chromosome ends from being recognized as broken DNA molecules in need of repair. Nearly all types of cancer are associated with telomerase reactivation, which may be essential for unlimited cell proliferation. In this study, telomerase activity was compared with clinical behavior in ordinary meningiomas.

Methods.—The study included 52 patients undergoing surgery for meningioma. Each tumor was evaluated for telomerase activity by means of the telomeric repeat amplification protocol, a highly sensitive assay. Neoplasms with and without detectable telomerase activity were identified, and the patients in these 2 groups were compared for freedom from recurrence.

Results.—Half of the tumors had detectable telomerase activity. Twenty-two tumors were classified as malignant or atypical—all but 1 of these had detectable telomerase activity. Most patients with such tumors had poor outcome. The remaining 30 tumors were ordinary (morphologically benign) meningiomas. Seventeen percent of these tumors had detectable telomerase activity. Three of 5 patients with telomerase-active ordinary meningiomas had rapid tumor regrowth after gross total resection; the other 2 patients had other primary cancers. The presence of telomerase activity in an ordinary meningioma was highly significantly correlated with poor prognosis.

Conclusions.—Assessment of telomerase activity may be relevant in benign meningiomas. The finding of telomerase activity suggests that the apparently benign tumors may have a population of immortal cells. Studies of telomerase activity may be useful in identifying benign meningiomas that are likely to recur after complete surgical resection. New treatments could be aimed at blocking telomerase.

▶ This is a good example of recent studies investigating the possible correlation between brain tumor telomerase activity and clinical outcome. Overall, the huge body of literature that has been generated regarding a possible correlation between outcome and proliferative activity in brain tumors has been disappointing. Therefore, telomerase activity has become the next possible new prognostic tumor marker.

This particular study examines 52 patients with meningiomas, reporting a general correlation between histologic grade and telomerase activity. Among the histologically benign group of meningiomas (which did not significantly differ morphologically from one another), 5 of 30 (17%) also showed telomerase activity and, most significantly according to these authors, 3 of these 5 patients have had rapid recurrences. The authors perform a univariate statistical analysis, showing that the difference between the prognosis for patients with telomerase-active ordinary meningiomas and those with non–telomerase-active ordinary meningiomas is highly significant.

These are preliminary data on a small number of tumors. As with proliferative activity, there may be a general correlation between histologic grade and telomerase activity, but other factors need to be studied in parallel with multivariate analysis to verify that telomerase activity independently correlates with outcome. Specifically, in the case of meningiomas degree of excision of the lesion is known to to be important for prognosis, and in fact it may be the most significant factor. In this study, degree of excision was not addressed.

These studies are interesting, but they are preliminary and in no way justify performing telomerase activity studies in the diagnostic workup of meningiomas.

D. Grzybicki, M.D., Ph.D.

Primary Intracranial Germ Cell Tumors: A Clinical Analysis of 153 Histologically Verified Cases
Matsutani M, Sano K, Takakura K, et al (Univ of Tokyo; Saitama Med School, Japan; Teikyo Univ, Tokyo; et al)
J Neurosurg 86:446–455, 1997   11–6

Objective.—It is difficult to study the pathology and treatment of intracranial germ-cell tumors because of their low incidence and the lack of histologic diagnosis in patients initially treated with radiation therapy alone. Debate continues as to the nomenclature of these tumors, their diagnostic evaluation, their treatment by surgery, and the appropriate treatment for various histologic subtypes. The clinical findings of 153 patients with histologically verified intracranial germ-cell tumors are reported.

Patients.—One hundred twenty-two male and 31 female patients were treated for intracranial germ-cell tumors during a 31-year period. According to hospital policy, treatment was surgery followed by radiation therapy, with or without chemotherapy. The histologic diagnosis was verified in 147 patients: 41% had germinoma, 20% had teratoma, and 39% had other tumor types, usually mixed tumor. These groups were similar in terms of age, tumor location, and sex.

Outcomes.—Patients with pure germinoma had survivals of 93% at 10 years and 81% at 20 years. Ten-year survival was 93% for patients with mature teratoma and 71% for those with malignant teratoma. However, 3-year survival was only 27% for patients with pure malignant germ-cell tumors: embryonal carcinoma, yolk-sac tumor, and choriocarcinoma. The patients with mixed tumors could be classified into 3 subgroups with varying 3-year survivals. Survival was 94% for patients with mixed germinoma and teratoma; 70% for those whose tumors were predominantly germinoma or teratoma, combined with some elements of pure malignant tumors; and 9% for those whose tumors had predominantly pure malignant elements (Table 7). For patients with malignant tumors, combination chemotherapy including cisplatin or carboplatin, with or without radiation, gave no better results than did radiation therapy alone.

Conclusions.—This is the largest group of patients with primary intracranial germ-cell tumors ever reported. Analysis suggests that such patients can be divided into 3 treatment groups with good, intermediate, and poor prognoses. Treatment should begin with surgery for histologic verification, perhaps followed by extensive mass reduction. Patients with germinomatous malignant tumors will not achieve local control with local radiation therapy only; they need systemic chemotherapy followed by radiation therapy. Carboplatin or cisplatin chemotherapy controls tumor growth for

TABLE 7.—Survival Rates in 134 Patients

Histology	No. of Cases	Patient Survival Rates (%)				
		1 Yr	3 Yrs	5 Yrs	10 Yrs	15 Yrs
germinoma	50	100.0	95.4	95.4	92.7	87.9
germinoma w/STGCs	7	100.0	100.0	83.3	83.3	—
mature teratoma	16	100.0	92.9	92.9	92.9	—
MT	11	100.0	70.7	70.7	70.7	—
PM	11	45.5	27.3	27.3	—	—
mixed tumors	39	87.2	61.0	57.1	40.1	—
MGT	17	94.1	94.1	84.7	70.6	—
MXB	10	80.0	70.0	52.5	35.0	—
MXM	12	83.3	9.3	9.3	—	—

Abbreviations: MGT, mixed germinoma and teratoma; *MT*, immature teratoma and teratoma with malignant elements; *MXB*, mixed tumor mainly conisting of germinoma or teratoma with a small portion of malignant tumors; *MXM*, mixed tumor mainly consisting of PM; *PM*, pure type of choriocarcinoma, embryonal carcinoma, and yolk sac tumor; data could not be calculated because the follow-up period was too short or because there were too few survivors.

(Courtesy of Matsutani M, Sano K, Takakura K, et al: Primary intracranial germ cell tumors: A clinical analysis of 153 histologically verified cases. *J Neurosurg* 86:446–455, 1997.)

patients in the intermediate group; those in the group with poor prognosis need more aggressive chemotherapy.

▶ This is the largest single-group study published to date examining primary intracranial germ-cell tumors. The authors provide a dense, extremely informative report on these tumors, which have been difficult to statistically analyze because of their relatively low incidence. On the basis of their analysis of 153 cases, interesting and important conclusions are offered, the most important being that prognosis is dependent on specific tumor histology (Table 7) and that a therapeutic classification of these tumors can be constructed based on specific histology.

For the practicing pathologist, these conclusions mean that subdivision of germ-cell tumors into histologic types—specifically, recognition of subtypes of mixed tumors—is important. This need for specific diagnoses may necessitate specific requests for adequate tissue to identify possible minor histologic components. This point illuminates a possible source of diagnostic error in this study, which is that a percentage of all tumor types were diagnosed by biopsy rather than subtotal or gross total removal, leaving open the question of whether some mixed tumors were called pure tumors because of sampling error.

Two additional significant clinical conclusions reported in this study are as follows: (1) For pure malignant and mixed tumors in the pineal region, extensive surgical removal results in a better survival rate (vs. partial removal or biopsy). (2) Overall, the combination of chemotherapy and radiation is not significantly more effective than is radiation alone for those patients with malignant tumors.

Although intracranial germ-cell tumors are relatively rare, this article provides important data useful for the pathologic diagnosis and management of the young patients we do see with these tumors.

D. Grzybicki, M.D., Ph.D.

Pleomorphic Xanthoastrocytoma: Report of Six Cases With Special Consideration of Diagnostic and Therapeutic Pitfalls
Tonn JC, Paulus W, Warmuth-Metz M, et al (Univ of Würzburg, Germany; Univ of Giessen, Germany)
Surg Neurol 47:162–169, 1997   11–7

Introduction.—There is no uniform consensus regarding the management of patients with pleomorphic xanthoastrocytoma (PXA). Initially classified as a fibrous xanthoma of the meninges, this was changed when glial fibrillary acidic protein was detected immunohistochemically in PXA. PXA was recently classified by the World Health Organization as a variant of astrocytoma. Diagnostic and therapeutic pitfalls of this rare tumor are described using data from 6 patients with PXA.

Findings.—Mean patient age was 14.3 years. A seizure initiated diagnostic workup in all 6 patients. Five of 6 tumors were located in the temporal lobe. Of these, 2 extended to either the parietal lobe or the occipital lobe. The site of the remaining tumor was parietaloccipital with extensive infiltration of the tentorial dura. The MRI pattern was similar in most patients: isointensity of the solid tumor component to gray matter on the T_1-weighted images and more or less hyperintensity on T_2-weighted scans. With gadolinium application, solid tumor nodules at the margin of a cystic formation were always enhanced.

Discussion/Conclusion.—A uniform prognosis for PXA is not possible. Prognosis is favorable for most patients, but there are reports of malignant recurrences with fatal courses. Two patients in this series had progression into a malignant glioma. One patient had primary anaplastic PXA and the other patient had increased mitotic activity, which seemed indicative of a worse clinical course. Malignant transformation did not seem to occur with local infiltration of the brain. The treatment of choice in patients with PXA is surgical removal. Close follow-up is imperative for detection and treatment of potential malignant recurrence.

▶ This article provides important basic clinico-pathologic information about the relatively rare tumor, pleomorphic xanthoastrocytoma (PXA). These cases nicely illustrate that: 1) although PXA is relatively rare it is probably underdiagnosed, 2) certain histopathologic features correlate with poor outcome, and 3) regardless of the histopathologic features of a given tumor, patients with this tumor need to be closely followed after surgery due to a significant variability in biologic behavior and therefore possible clinical outcome.

D. Grzybicki, M.D., Ph.D.

Diagnostic Criteria for Sporadic Creutzfeldt-Jakob Disease

Kretzschmar HA, Ironside JW, DeArmond SJ, et al (Univ of Göttingen, Germany; Univ of Edinburgh, Scotland; Univ of California, San Francisco; et al)

Arch Neurol 53:913–920, 1996

11–8

Purpose.—The clinical diagnosis of Creutzfeldt-Jakob disease (CJD) is based on neurologic signs, including rapidly progressive dementia, ataxia, myoclonus, and electroencephalographic changes. However, the definitive diagnosis is made only through neuropathologic evaluation. Thus, reliable techniques are needed for the neuropathologic evaluation and diagnosis of CJD. The diagnostic and neuropathologic techniques used by laboratories experienced in the study of CJD are discussed.

Methods.—The investigators evaluated the morphologic techniques used by German, British, Japanese, and U.S. laboratories experienced in the investigation of CJD, emphasizing the immunohistochemical techniques. The laboratory diagnostic techniques were also evaluated. The goal was to achieve a consensus as to the definition of "definite CJD."

Findings.—The classic neuropathologic changes of CJD include spongiform degeneration, neuronal loss, and astrocytic gliosis, though spongiform degeneration is the only one of these with any specificity. Identified with immunohistochemical techniques, the protease-resistant form of the prion protein (PrP) provides the most reliable available marker for transmissible spongiform encephalopathies. Several techniques have been developed for the detection of PrP in tissue sections outside of plaques, all involving denaturing of tissue sections followed by immunohistochemistry with antibodies against PrP. Though intracellular positive reaction is rare, perineuronal and synaptic positivity are sometimes observed. Histoblotting technique has been widely used in experimental prion research. It is a sensitive technique that can be used in human biopsy and autopsy specimens, though it must be performed in fresh, unfixed material. Electron microscopy can identify viruslike particles in thin sections of infected brains, but this technique is rarely used for diagnostic purposes.

With refinements in Western blotting technique, positive results can be achieved with small biopsy samples. Unfixed brain tissue is needed. Hereditary cases of CJD feature mutations in the open reading frame of the PrP gene, so the diagnosis can be confirmed through polymerase chain reaction amplification of the open reading frame and identification of mutations. With recent advances, animal transmission studies may provide a useful diagnostic approach. Scrapie-associated fibrils and prion rods can be found as specific evidence for scrapie in animals and CJD in humans. However, unfixed, fresh tissue and electron microscopy are required. No specific cerebrospinal fluid markers of CJD have been found.

Discussion.—Evaluation of the morphologic and diagnostic techniques used to define CJD lead to a recommended diagnostic approach. A probable diagnosis can be established on clinical grounds, as outlined in published criteria. Light microscopy of samples from various brain regions may lead to a definitive diagnosis. Immunohistochemical studies with antibodies against PrP should be performed whenever CJD is suspected and are essential if the results of histologic study are equivocal. Additional special techniques are available if needed.

▶ This useful article discusses a consensus opinion regarding diagnostic criteria for a "definite" diagnosis of sporadic CJD. The impetus of this report was at least partially a recent description by Will et al.[1] of a new variant of CJD in the United Kingdom, possibly associated with consumption of beef from animals with bovine spongiform encephalopathy ("mad cow disease").

On the basis of considerations of test sensitivity, specificity, and practicality, these authors recommend that a diagnosis of "definite" CJD be rendered after a probable or possible CJD clinical diagnosis with the presence of one or more light microscopic changes associated with CJD or demonstration of the presence of PrP by immunohistochemistry. Use of other techniques to demonstrate PrP, such as Western blotting, should be considered if light microscopic and PrP immunohistochemistry results are equivocal. Cases in which PrP cannot be demonstrated should be worked up for other causes of dementia, such as Lewy body disease.

These criteria are reasonable and are most likely already being used by most institutions, with most variability among institutions probably being in whether "classic" histologic cases or cases completely *without* typical spongiform change are analyzed for PrP. I think it is important to perform PrP studies in all clinically suspected cases of CJD because, as these authors point out, in some cases PrP has been demonstrated in anatomic areas not exhibiting the most typical histologic changes of spongiform encephalopathy. Also, the specificity of the PrP immunohistochemical technique is high; false-positive results in control brains with other neurologic diseases are essentially nonexistent. Therefore, performance of PrP studies is probably always worthwhile on biopsy samples, regardless of histology, in the face of high clinical suspicion.

Collection of meaningful epidemiologic data on human cases of spongiform encephalopathies in this and other countries to help sort out possible sources of infection and to continue work on mechanisms of disease requires an attempt at standardization of neuropathologic diagnostic criteria. This article is an excellent reference for this purpose.

D. Grzybicki, M.D., Ph.D.

Reference

1. Will RG, Ironside JW, Zeidler M, et al: A new variant of Creutzfeldt-Jakob disease in the UK. *Lancet* 347:921–925, 1996.

Cerebral Amyloid Deposition and Diffuse Plaques in "Normal" Aging: Evidence For Presymptomatic and Very Mild Alzheimer's Disease

Morris JC, Storandt M, McKeel DW, et al (Washington Univ, St Louis, Mo)
Neurology 46:710–719, 1996   11–9

Background.—Senile plaques in the neocortex of apparently nondemented elderly patients are often considered part of normal aging. However, the finding of β-amyloid–containing plaques may indicate very early Alzheimer's disease (AD). The relationships of cognitively normal aging, very mild dementia of the Alzheimer type, and the presence of neocortical senile plaques were investigated.

Methods and Findings.—Clinicopathologic correlations were performed in 21 healthy elderly individuals, studied longitudinally until they died at a mean age of 84.5 years. Nine had markedly high-plaque densities in the neocortex. Two of these individuals died of head injury, exhibiting no signs of cognitive impairment before their death. The other 7 had clinical evidence of very mild cognitive impairment at some time and mildly impaired psychometric performance at the last assessment before their death. The remaining 12 individuals showed no impairment clinically or psychometrically and had few or no neocortical AD lesions.

Conclusions.—Senile plaques may not be part of normal aging. They may instead represent presymptomatic or unrecognized early symptomatic AD. The high density of senile plaques, mainly of the diffuse subtype, in the cortex of individuals at the threshold of detectable dementia supports the hypothesis that β-amyloid deposition is an initial pathogenetic event in AD development.

▶ This paper investigates the following important question: What is the relationship between the presence of neocortical senile plaques and cognition? The current diagnostic criteria for AD are based on quantification of neocortical senile plaques, with more emphasis generally placed on neocortical neuritic plaques vs. diffuse plaques. This would imply that the presence of neocortical senile plaques is believed to have some relationship to the presence of clinical dementia. However, the presence of a significant number of neocortical senile plaques, particularly diffuse plaques, has been reported frequently in patients with no clinical history of dementia. This observation has supported the idea that the presence of neocortical diffuse plaques, even in significant numbers, may be simply part of the normal aging process, despite evidence that diffuse plaques contain β-amyloid and may be precursor lesions of neuritic plaques.

These authors have done an interesting prospective clinical and pathologic study of 21 cognitively normal elderly individuals. They present a very detailed report, demonstrating that 7 of the 9 patients shown at autopsy to meet neuropathologic criteria for AD also exhibited minimal-to-mild clinical evidence of dementia. This clinical evidence was based on relatively rigorous questioning of family members as well as on cognitive and psychometric testing. None of the 12 patients without neuropathologic AD exhibited similar clinical evidence of dementia. The most prevalent distinguishing feature in brains from minimal-mild AD patients vs. the nondemented elderly patients was the large number of diffuse plaques distributed widely in the neocortex. Although the numbers of patients in this study is small, I believe these authors' data support their conclusion that samples of apparently nondemented elderly subjects (most likely based on relatively nonrigorous cognitive assessment) are contaminated by cases of unrecognized mild AD.

These findings may justify a shift in thinking about the clinical relevance of senile plaques. In those patients without clinical evidence of dementia but with autopsy evidence for significant numbers of neocortical senile plaques, diffuse or neuritic, a possible diagnosis of minimal-to-mild AD (perhaps only detectable by rigorous cognitive testing) may be suggested.

D. Grzybicki M.D., Ph.D.

Dementia With Lewy Bodies Versus Pure Alzheimer Disease: Differences in Cognition, Neuropathology, Cholinergic Dysfunction, and Synapse Density
Samuel W, Alford M, Hofstetter CR, et al (Univ of California, San Diego; VA Med Ctr, San Diego, Calif)
J Neuropathol Exp Neurol 56:499–508, 1997   11–10

Background.—About 20% of demented elderly patients are found to have brainstem and cortical Lewy bodies (LBs) at autopsy. Most of these patients had received a clinical diagnosis of Alzheimer's disease (AD) and would also meet neuropathologic criteria for AD. Patients with findings of LBs and AD can be classified as having the Lewy body variant of AD (LBV); those with LBs but no evidence of AD pathology are considered to have diffuse Lewy body disease (DLBD). Dementia is less severe in DLBD than in LBV, but both groups typically exhibit some features of idiopathic Parkinson's disease. Autopsy tissue from demented patients with LBV, DLBD, or AD and from normal controls was examined to determine which neuropathologic abnormalities correlated with cognitive impairment in the 3 patient subgroups.

Methods.—Tissue examined was from 12 cases of LBV, 5 of DLBD, 12 of pure AD, and 5 age-matched normal controls. All autopsies were performed within 24 hours post mortem. Included in the analysis were (1) counts of midfrontal neocortical LBs, neocortical neuritic plaques (NPs), and neocortical neurofibrillary tangles (NFTs); (2) quantification of synapse density and choline acetyltransferase (ChAT); (3) modified Braak staging of AD-type neurofibrillary pathology; and (4) gross brain weight.

Results.—The patient and control groups were similar in mean age, and the 3 patient groups were comparable in mean estimated duration of disease. The LBV and AD groups were equally demented; the DLBD group scored significantly higher on the Mini-Mental State Examination and significantly lower on the Information-Memory-Concentration test, indicating less severe impairment. Among the cases of dementia with LBs, correlations were observed between dementia severity and neocortical LB counts, modified Braak stages of NFT burden in the entorhinal cortex, neocortical NP counts, and loss of ChAT activity. In contrast to AD, neocortical NFTs and antisynaptophysin activity showed no correlation with dementia with LBs. And despite significantly less severe dementia in the DLBD patients, their LB counts and ChAT loss were similar to those in LBV patients. Brain weight was significantly greater for both controls and DLBD patients compared with AD and LBV patients.

Discussion.—The physical basis of cognitive impairment in dementia with LBs is complex and multiply determined. In both LBV and DLBD, neocortical LB counts, NPs, modified Braak stages of AD neurofibrillary pathology, and depletion of neocortical ChAT are all correlated with dementia. The moderate dementia observed in DLBD may result from LB accumulation and ChAT depletion. More profound dementia—as seen in advanced severe AD—may occur with the addition of neocortical NPs and more advanced Braak stages of neurofibrillary pathology. Synapse loss appears to be a dominant factor in AD, whereas damage to the cholinergic neurotransmitter system may be more important in dementia with LBs.

Diffuse Lewy Body Disease: Clinical Features in Nine Cases Without Coexistent Alzheimer's Disease

Hely MA, Reid WGJ, Halliday GM, et al (Westmead Hosp, Sydney, Australia; Prince of Wales Med Research Inst, Australia; Royal Prince Alfred Hosp, Australia, et al)
J Neurol Neurosurg Psychiatry 60:531–538, 1996   11–11

Introduction.—Diffuse Lewy body disease (DLBD) has yet to be fully defined, but it has clinical and pathologic features that overlap with both Alzheimer's disease (AD) and Parkinson's disease. A study of 9 cases of pure DLBD was designed to examine its relationship with Parkinson's disease.

Methods.—The patients, 7 men and 2 women, ranged in age from 54 to 69 years at disease onset; age at the time of death ranged from 61 to 75 years. All patients were thought to have Parkinson's disease or AD. Brains were collected at postmortem examination and prepared for examination. A diagnosis of DLBD was based upon the finding of cortical Lewy bodies (LBs) (at least 3/200 × field in 4 of 10 successive fields along cortical layers 5/6). All patients were studied by neurologists or psychiatrists from disease onset until death, and detailed records of history and of physical and mental examinations were available.

Results.—Initial symptoms were bradykinesia in 5 patients, memory loss in 3, and dysphasia in 1. Six patients had rest tremor. Bradykinesia was classified as moderate in 7 patients and mild in 2. Degree of rigidity (mild or moderate) was correlated with degree of bradykinesia. Initial clinical features in 5 patients were indistinguishable from idiopathic Parkinson's disease, and all 5 of these patients subsequently became demented (at a mean of 3 years after presentation). Two patients had parkinsonism and dementia when first examined, and 2 first exhibited dementia and later showed signs of parkinsonism. Hallucinations appeared as a first sign of disease in 1 patient; 6 others experienced hallucinations from 2.5 to 9 years after symptom onset. During the course of their disease, all patients had a rapid and generalized decline in cognitive functioning. In addition to the finding of diffuse cortical LBs at pathologic examination, all patients had the midbrain changes required to meet the pathologic criteria of idiopathic Parkinson's disease.

Conclusion.—Pure DLBD, first reported in 1961, may initially be indistinguishable from levodopa-responsive idiopathic Parkinson's disease. Although dementia coexisting with early parkinsonian features should suggest DLBD, this entity is difficult to distinguish clinically from AD and coexistent idiopathic Parkinson's disease. Initial symptoms of DLBD depend upon whether the pathology begins in the midbrain, the cortex, or both.

▶ Diffuse Lewy Body disease is a neurodegenerative disease which is currently being looked for and, therefore, recognized with increasing frequency by neuropathologists; however, the clinical and pathologic features of this process are not entirely clear and are still being defined. These 2 studies (Abstracts 11–10 and 11–11) provide extremely helpful and interesting information regarding this entity, the paper by Hely et al. focusing on "pure" DLBD (cases without concomitant AD features) and the paper by Samuel et al. investigating a larger group of patients with dementia including subgroups with overlapping AD features.

Both studies provide good descriptive correlative information. The paper by Samuel et al. also provides interesting conclusions about the possible anatomical determinates of the cognitive impairments seen in the "pure" form vs. those cases also exhibiting AD changes. Any patient with clinical symptoms consistent with Parkinson's disease and/or dementia (especially dementia with extrapyramidal signs) should be considered a candidate for dementia with LBs and worked up accordingly at autopsy.

D. Grzybicki M.D., Ph.D.

Clinical and Genetic Abnormalities in Patients With Friedreich's Ataxia
Dürr A, Cossee M, Agid Y, et al (Hôpital de la Salpêtrière, Paris; Institut de Génétique et de Biologie Moléculaire et Cellulaire, Strasbourg, France; Centre Hospitalier Général de Saint-Pierre, Ile de La Réunion, France)
N Engl J Med 335:1169–1175, 1996   11–12

Background.—Friedreich's ataxia, the most common hereditary ataxia, usually appears before age 20 and is characterized by ataxia of all 4 limbs. The locus of the genetic defect responsible for the disorder has been mapped to chromosome 9. More recently, Friedreich's ataxia was found to be associated with a mutation that consists of an unstable expansion of GAA repeats in the first intron of the *frataxin* gene on chromosome 9. The finding of patients with autosomal recessive cerebellar ataxia and linkage to chromosome 9q13, but with intact tendon reflexes or late-onset disease, suggests that the clinical spectrum is broader than previously thought. A group of 187 patients with progressive ataxia was studied for GAA expansion in the *frataxin* gene and for the relationship between clinical manifestations, number of GAA repeats, and disease duration.

Methods.—The patients represented 147 families. Diagnostic criteria for typical Friedreich's ataxia were met by 103 patients; an additional 10 patients had a disease duration of less than 5 years but met remaining criteria and were classified in the typical disease group. The remaining 74 patients failed to meet at least 1 of the essential criteria after 5 years of disease. GAA repeats in the 187 patients were analyzed by Southern blotting.

Results.—Expanded GAA repeats were found on both alleles of the *frataxin* gene in 140 patients representing 114 families. Age at disease onset in the patients homozygous for the GAA expansion ranged from 2 to 51 years (mean, 15.5 years). About 25% of patients who were homozygous had atypical Friedreich's ataxia, with older age at disease onset, intact tendon reflexes, and/or an absence of extensor plantar response; these patients represented 46% of the 74 patients with atypical disease. Correlations were observed between larger GAA expansions (overall range was 120 to 1700 repeats) and both earlier age at onset and shorter times to loss of ambulation. The size of GAA expansions was associated with the frequency of cardiomyopathy and loss of reflexes in the upper limbs.

Conclusion.—Current diagnostic criteria for Friedreich's ataxia appear to lack sensitivity, for about one-fourth of patients in this series who were homozygous for the GAA expansion failed to meet at least one of the criteria. The size of the expansion also varied considerably, both among patients and within and among families. Because the spectrum of Friedreich's ataxia is broader than previously thought, patients with recessive or sporadic cerebellar ataxias should be evaluated with the direct molecular test for the GAA expansion on chromosome 9.

▶ Multiple neurologic disorders are now known to be associated with abnormal expansions of trinucleotides within particular genes. Most of the papers reporting the continuously evolving molecular information regarding these disorders (including this one) do not deal directly with the associated neuropathology; however, they do reveal important information about the molecular mechanisms underlying the characteristic neuropathologic changes. Additionally, papers such as this one touch on the issue of redefining diagnostic criteria for diseases based on newly discovered molecular information.

The major point of this paper is well supported by the data presented, i.e., that approximately 50% of patients with clinically "atypical" Friedreich's ataxia (FA) also exhibit either a homozygous or heterozygous repeat expansion and, therefore, should be included in the same diagnostic category as those with classic FA. However, the authors do not discuss in detail the patients with atypical clinical FA who exhibit neither a homozygous nor a heterozygous repeat expansion (approximately 50%).

One explanation of these findings is that the patients have an undiscovered mutation in both alleles, resulting in a similar loss of function. Another explanation is that they have a disease that clinically looks like FA (by the new expanded definition) but really is not. Should the diagnosis of FA in atypical patients be based on molecular genetic studies, and those patients without the expanded repeat be given an alternative diagnosis and perhaps counseled differently? Filla et al., who present esentially the same findings in an earlier paper but in a smaller number of patients, present a slightly broader discussion of this question in their report.[1] These findings have also been confirmed by Montermini et al.[2]

D. Grzybicki M.D., Ph.D.

References

1. Filla A, De Michele G, Cavalcanti F, et al: The relationship between trinucleotide (GAA) repeat length and clinical features in Friedreich ataxia. *Am J Hum Genet* 59:554–560, 1996.
2. Montermini L, Richter A, Morgan K, et al: Phenotypic variability in Friedreich ataxia: Role of the associated GAA triplet repeat expansion. *Ann Neurol* 41:675–682, 1997.

Mutations in the Sarcoglycan Genes in Patients With Myopathy
Duggan DJ, Gorospe JR, Fanin M, et al (Univ of Pittsburgh, Pa; Univ of Padua, Italy)
N Engl J Med 336:618–624, 1997   11–13

Background.—Mutations of the genes coding for the sarcoglycan protein are present in some patients with autosomal recessive limb-girdle muscular dystrophy. Mutations in 1 sarcoglycan gene can lead to secondary deficiencies of the other sarcoglycan proteins, so it should be possible to detect a genetic defect in any component of the protein complex by using antibodies against any of the sarcoglycan proteins. The frequency of sarcoglycan gene mutations and their impact on the clinical findings were investigated in a large group of patients with myopathy.

Methods.—The study included muscle biopsy specimens from 556 patients with myopathy. All had normal dystrophin genes, which are often deleted in X-linked muscular dystrophy. Each specimen was stained with antibody against α-sarcoglycan. If this protein was deficient on immunostaining, mutations of the α-, β-, and γ-sarcoglycan genes were sought by reverse transcription of muscle RNA, with single-strand conformation polymorphism analysis and DNA sequencing.

Results.—Ten percent of patients had reduced levels of α-sarcoglycan on immunostaining of muscle biopsy specimens. Twenty-five of these 54 patients had no detectable α-sarcoglycan. Fifty patients underwent DNA studies for sarcoglycan gene mutations. Twenty-nine patients had such mutations, including 29 with mutations of the α-sarcoglycan gene, 8 with mutations of the β-sarcoglycan gene, and 4 with mutations of the γ-sarcoglycan gene. The other 21 patients with reduced levels of α-sarcoglycan had no sarcoglycan gene mutations. Eighty-three percent of patients with severe, Duchenne-like muscular dystrophy beginning in childhood had sarcoglycan gene mutations, as did 6% of patients with proximal, limb-girdle muscular dystrophy of later onset. The finding of complete deficiency of α-sarcoglycan on immunostaining was more specific for mutations of the α-sarcoglycan gene than those of the β- and γ-sarcoglycan gene.

Conclusions.—Patients with Duchenne-like and limb-girdle muscular dystrophy who have normal dystrophin may have mutations of the genes coding for the sarcoglycan proteins. The frequency of this finding is about 11% in such patients. Patients with primary sarcoglycanopathy cannot be clinically distinguished from those with either Duchenne's or Becker's muscular dystrophy.

▶ This report is a good example of recent articles dealing with the molecular diagnosis of muscular dystrophies. It significantly adds to the current knowledge of a subset of autosomal recessive dystophies by describing sarcoglycan protein and gene abnormalities in a large group of patients with myopathy and normal dystrophin.

This large study of 1556 patients follows from an earlier report by this group (Duggan et al.,[1] 1996) describing primary and secondary α-sarcoglycan (adhalin) deficiency in a smaller group of 30 patients with normal dystrophin. Some important conclusions from the present study are as follows: (1) patients with primary sarcoglycanopathies are clinically indistinguishable from patients with Duchenne's or Becker's muscular dystophy; (2) 10% of patients with myopathy and normal dystrophin show a deficiency of adhalin protein, and this percentage doubles in the smaller subset of patients with Duchenne-like or limb-girdle muscular dystrophies; (3) only 58% of these adhalin-deficient patients have mutations in one of the sarcoglycan genes, thus not accounting for all cases of adhalin deficiency; and (4) a complete deficiency of adhalin is more specific for a mutation in the α-sarcoglycan gene than is a partial deficiency (as suggested in an earlier article).[1]

The title of the editorial by Dubowitz[2] accompanying this article is "The Muscular Dystrophies—Clarity or Chaos?" Although the myriad unfolding molecular details may seem chaotic, Dubowitz makes the important point that only from the continuing clarity provided by knowledge of specific gene defects can we hope to develop effective replacement therapies for this group of disorders.

D. Grzybicki, M.D., Ph.D.

References

1. Duggan DJ, Fanin M, Pegoraro E, et al: alpha-Sarcoglycan (adhalin) deficiency: complete deficiency patients are 5% of childhood-onset dystrophin-normal muscular dystrophy and most partial deficiency patients do not have gene mutations. *J Neurol Sci* 140:30–39, 1996.
2. Dubowitz V: The muscular dystrophies: Clarity or chaos? *N Engl J Med* 336:650–651, 1997.

12 Endocrine System

Thyroid Paraganglioma: A Clinicopathologic and Immunohistochemical Study of Three Cases
LaGuette J, Matias-Guiu X, Rosai J (Mem Sloan-Kettering Cancer Ctr, New York; Hosp de la Santa Cruz y San Pablo, Barcelona)
Am J Surg Pathol 21:748–753, 1997   12–1

Background.—Primary thyroid neuroendocrine tumors (other than nonmedullary carcinoma) are very rare. Paragangliomas (PGs), neuroendocrine neoplasms of paraganglia, may be found exceptionally in the thyroid gland. The clinical and pathologic characteristics of thyroid PGs were described.

Methods and Findings.—The 3 cases of intrathyroidal PG occurred in 3 women, aged 55, 56, and 64 years, initially seeking medical attention for an asymptomatic thyroid nodule. None had a significant personal or family history. The tumors were single, well-circumscribed solid masses in 1 thyroid lobe and measured 2 cm in greatest diameter. Microscopic examination showed that they were encapsulated with the typical nesting pattern of PG in other sites. Two tumors were made up of small–to–medium-sized cells with granular amphophilic cytoplasm. The third tumor was composed of relatively large cells with a similar staining quality. On immunohistochemical assessment, all tumors were positive for neuron-specific enolase, chromogranin A, and synaptophysin. All 3 cases had S-100 protein-positive sustentacular cells. Other tumors considered in the differential diagnosis (medullary carcinoma, hyalinizing trabecular adenoma, atypical follicular adenoma, Hurthle-cell neoplasm, and metastatic carcinoid tumor) were excluded by negative staining for epithelial markers, thyroglobulin, carcinoembryonic antigen, calcitonin, calcitonin gene–related peptide, serotonin, vimentin, and Congo red. At the last follow-up assessment, all 3 patients were alive and well, with no evidence of recurrent disease.

Conclusion.—Although exceptionally rare, intrathyroidal PGs do exist. These tumors can be distinguished from other thyroid neoplasms with similar appearances.

Metastatic Neuroendocrine Tumors to the Thyroid Gland Mimicking Medullary Carcinoma: A Pathologic and Immunohistochemical Study of Six Cases

Matias-Guiu X, LaGuette J, Puras-Gil AM, et al (Hosp de la Santa Cruz y San Pablo, Barcelona; Mem Sloan-Kettering Cancer Ctr, New York; Hosp Virgen del Camino, Pamplona, Spain)
Am J Surg Pathol 21:754–762, 1997   12–2

Background.—Medullary thyroid carcinoma (MTC) may not be distinguishable morphologically from other neuroendocrine carcinomas, including carcinoid tumors. The pathologic and immunohistochemical features of 6 cases of metastatic neuroendocrine neoplasms to the thyroid, initially interpreted as MTC, were reported.

Patients and Findings.—The patients, aged 24 to 70 years, were all women with a single mass or multiple thyroid nodules but no symptoms or significant medical history. The primary source of the tumor was found only on follow-up. In 2 women, the neoplasms were classical carcinoid tumors; in 1, a carcinoid primarily made of large cells; in 1, a prominent oval to spindle cell component; and in 2, atypical carcinoid/high-grade neuroendocrine carcinomas. All lesions were negative for calcitonin and only 2 were focally positive for carcinoembryonic antigen (CEA), which is not consistent with the immunohistochemical profile of MTC. The tumors showed a variable pattern of staining for other neuroendocrine and epithelial markers.

Conclusion.—Distinguishing between MTC and metastatic neuroendocrine carcinoma to the thyroid is important, as treatment and prognosis differ greatly. Despite morphologic and immunohistochemical similarities to MTC, a diagnosis of metastatic neuroendocrine tumor to the thyroid should be made when there are a predominantly interstitial pattern of spread, multiple tumor foci, folliculotropism, rosette formations with lumen and cuticular borders, and lack of immunoreactivity to calcitonin and CEA.

▶ These 2 articles (Abstracts 12–1 and 12–2) were published in the same issue of the *American Journal of Surgical Pathology* and originated from the same institution. All cases described in both articles were gathered from the personal consultation files of Dr. Juan Rosai. This, by itself, speaks for the extremely rare occurrence of these lesions in the thyroid gland. As indicated by Dr. Rosai and his colleagues, it is important to make the correct diagnosis regarding both entities because their confusion with other, more common epithelial neoplasms of the thyroid gland (neuroendocrine or not) would significantly alter treatment and final clinical outcome. The morphologic and immunohistochemical criteria beautifully described in both articles would certainly be of great assistance if providence decided to present us with such a case during our professional lifetime.

K.E. Sirgi, M.D.

Multinucleate Giant Cells in Papillary Thyroid Carcinoma: A Morphologic and Immunohistochemical Study

Guiter GE, DeLellis RA (New England Med Ctr, Boston; Tufts Univ, Boston)
Am J Clin Pathol 106:765–768, 1996   12–3

Introduction.—Multinucleate giant cells (MGCs) are seen in a variety of inflammatory, hyperplastic, and neoplastic thyroid disorders and have been detected in fine-needle aspiration biopsies (FNABs) of papillary thyroid carcinoma (PTC). The frequency and origin of MGCs have not been established. The frequency of MGCs in routine histologic sections and cytologic preparations of PTCs were analyzed. The origin of MGCs was

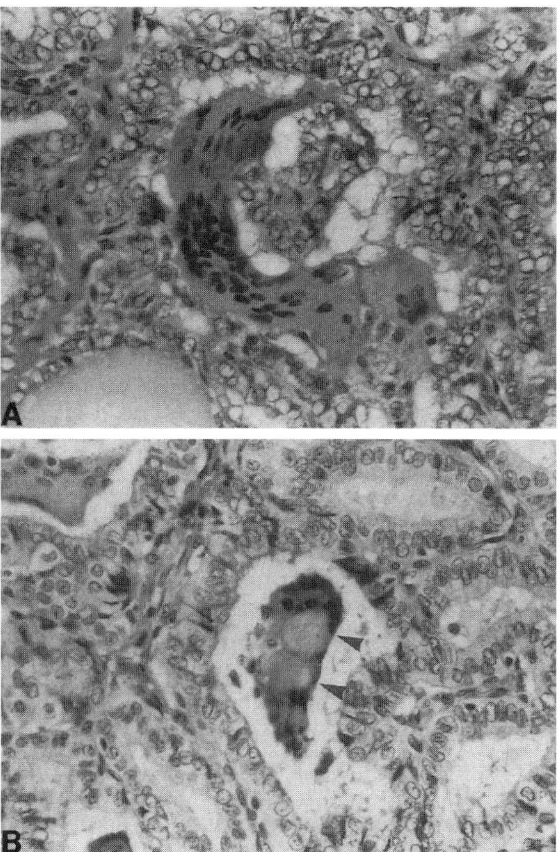

FIGURE 2.—**A,** papillary thyroid carcinoma. A multinucleate giant cell is present in the center adjacent to a small pailla; hematoxylin-eosin; original magnification, ×400. **B,** papillary thyroid carcinoma. The central follicle contains a multinucleate giant cell and is devoid of colloid. The giant cell contains 2 cytoplasmic deposits of colloid (colloidophagy) (*arrows*); hematoxylin-eosin, original magnification, ×400. (Courtesy of Guiter GE, DeLellis RA: Multinucleate giant cells in papillary thyroid carcinoma: A morphologic and immunohistochemical study. *Am J Clin Pathol* 106:765–768, 1996.)

investigated using immunohistochemical markers of epithelial and histocytic differentiation.

Methods.—The histologic sections from 76 patients with PTC were reviewed. Epithelial and histiocytic markers underwent immunohistochemical analysis. An additional 22 FNAB specimens of PTC were examined for the presence of MGCs.

Results.—Thirty-five of 76 PTC specimens had histologically-identified MGCs. Of these, MGCs were numerous in 10 specimens. In specimens with MGCs, 43% were papillary in type and 57% were mixed papillary/follicular variants or pure follicular variants. Twenty of the 35 patients (57%) whose tumors contained MGCs had undergone previous FNAB. At follow-up, 95% of patients with PTC without MGCs and all patients with PTC with MGCs were disease free. Twelve of 22 additional patients (55%) undergoing FNAB had MGCs in biopsy specimens. The MGCs were observed most frequently with follicular lumens or adjacent to papillae. They were often associated with partial or complete resorption of colloid (colloidophagy). In some specimens, intracytoplasmic deposits of colloid were observed within the cytoplasm of MGCs (Fig 2). Immunohistochemical analysis revealed that MGCs were of histiocytic, not epithelial, origin.

Conclusion.—The appearance of MGCs in FNABs of PTCs is well-known. These findings show that MGCs occur with comparable frequency in histologic sections of these tumors. They occur most frequently in areas of colloid resorption with evidence of colloid deposition within their cytoplasm. Their presence should prompt a careful assessment of associated PTC.

▶ The presence of MGCs in thyroid FNAB specimens has already been described as a subtle clue, although not pathognomonic, to the possible presence of a PTC. If you intuitively thought that these MGCs were of histiocytic origin, you now have the irrefutable immunohistochemical proof that you were right. Their scavenger of colloid material function (colloidophagy), as demonstrated in this study by their cytoplasmic and surface reactivity to the immunostain thyroglobulin, has not been proven in another, similar study.[1]

K.E. Sirgi, M.D.

Reference

1. Tabbara SO, Acoury N, Sidawy MK: Multinucleated giant cells in thyroid neoplasms: A cytologic, histologic and immunohistochemical study. *Acta Cytol* 40:1184–1188, 1996.

Solitary Fibrous Tumor of the Adrenal Gland

Prévot S, Penna C, Imbert J-C; et al (Saint-Antoine Hosp, Paris)
Mod Pathol 9:1170–1174, 1996   12–4

Background.—Solitary fibrous tumors (SFTs), rare neoplasms that usually involve the pleura, have recently been reported in various other locations. An SFT arising from the adrenal gland was reported for the first time.

Methods and Findings.—The tumor occurred in the right adrenal gland in a 42–year-old woman. It was found incidentally during abdominopelvic ultrasound examination. The pathologic and immunohistologic characteristics of the SFT were identical to those of other SFTs. Three fourths of this unencapsulated infiltrating tumoral mass had foci of hemorrhage, composed of small, round, epithelioid-like cells expressing the CD34 antigen more weakly than the typical spindle cells often seen in SFTs. Despite

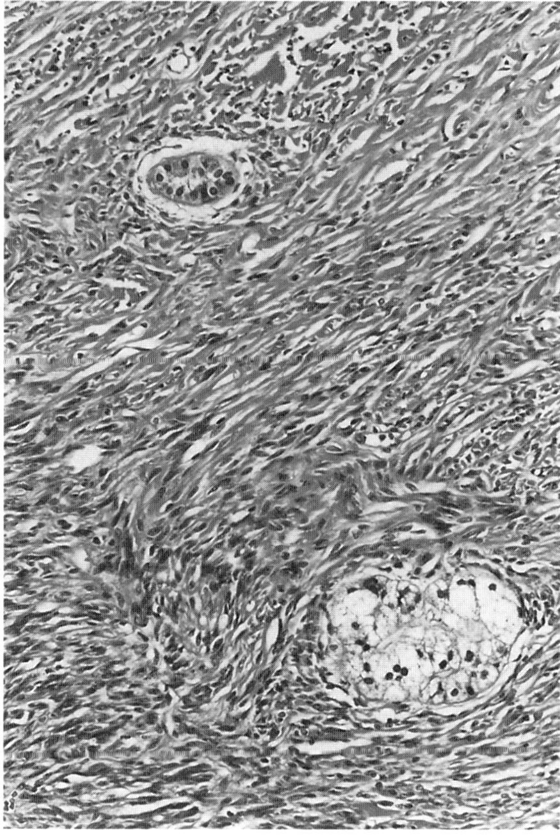

FIGURE 2.—Spindle cells arranged in small interlacing fascicles separated by bundles of collagen. Adrenal gland elements are embedded in the tumor. (Courtesy of Prévot S, Penna C, Imbert J-C, et al: Solitary fibrous tumor of the adrenal gland. *Mod Pathol* 9[12]:1170–1174, 1996.)

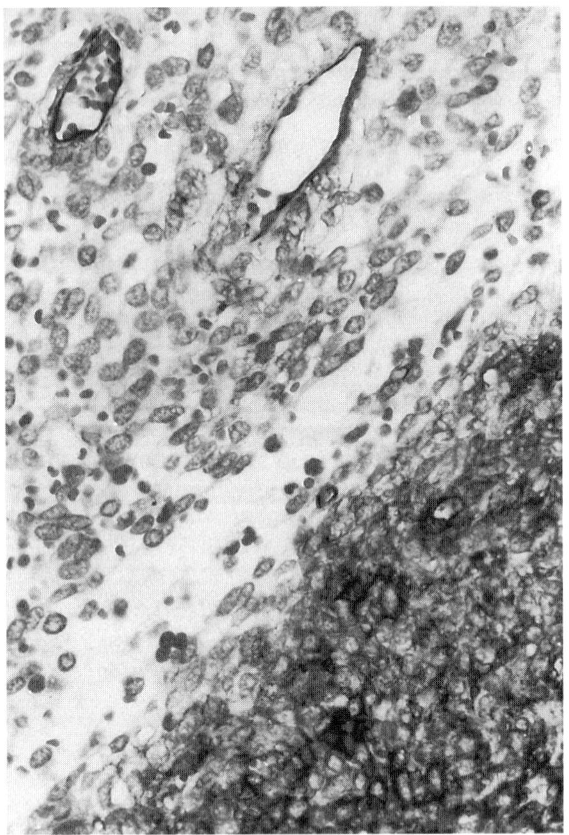

FIGURE 3.—The labeling with the anti-CD34 antibody is stronger and more uniform in the spindle cells (*lower right*) than in the round cells scattered in a myxoid background (*upper left*). (Courtesy of Prévot S, Penna C, Imbert J-C, et al: Solitary fibrous tumor of the adrenal gland. *Mod Pathol* 9[12]:1170–1174, 1996.)

bleeding and poor limitation, the behavior of the tumor was innocuous. The lesion remained unchanged for more than 5 years before the patient agreed to surgery, which was recommended when the mass suddenly became enlarged (Figs 2 and 3).

Conclusion.—Solitary fibrous tumors are not necessarily confined to serosal surfaces. This is the first report of an SFT arising in the adrenal gland.

Adenomatoid Tumor of the Adrenal Gland: A Report of Four New Cases and a Review of the Literature

Raaf HN, Grant LD, Santoscoy C, et al (Cuyahoga County Coroner's Office, Cleveland, Ohio; United Pathology, Sierra Vista, Ariz; Cleveland Clinc Found, Ohio; et al)

Mod Pathol 9:1046–1051, 1996

12–5

Background.—Adenomatoid tumors of the adrenal gland are rare, benign, and asymptomatic. They have usually been found incidentally, always in men, and always on the left side. Four additional patients with adenomatoid tumor of the adrenal gland were reported, including 1 woman; 2 of the lesions were in the right adrenal gland.

Patients and Findings.—The cases were identified from the authors' autopsy and surgical files between 1990 and 1994. The mean patient age was 49 years, compared with the average age of 34 years reported previously. The adrenal masses were described, on gross pathologic evaluation, as discrete, white, smooth, solid, and firm in the autopsy files of 3 of the patients. In the surgical patient, the mass measured $6 \times 4 \times 3.4$ cm and had a variegated external surface which was purple-tan, smooth, and glistening. The cut surface mainly showed a unilocular cyst with a thin rim of yellow tissue in the cyst wall (Fig 2). On light microscopic examination, the histopathologic features in all 4 specimens were characteristic of adenomatoid tumor. The autopsy files showed variably arranged tumor cells with solid nests, dilated "empty" tubular channels, and irregularly shaped glandlike spaces lined by flattened or cuboidal cells (Fig 4).

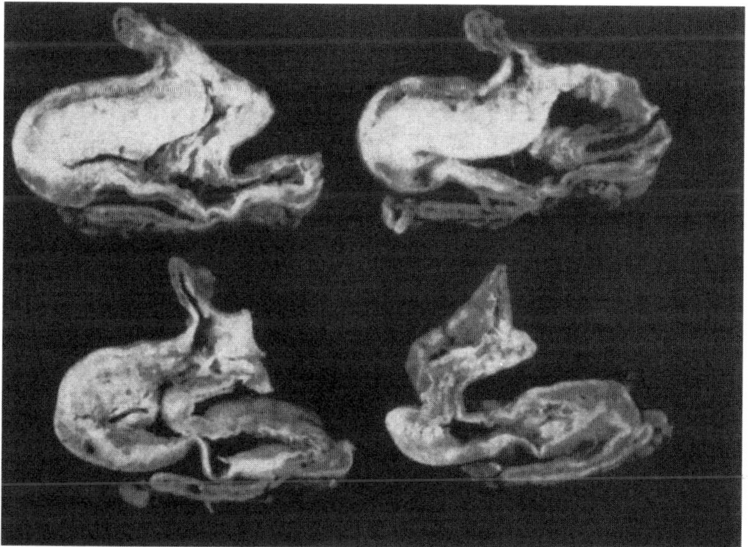

FIGURE 2.—Cut surface of cystic and solid adenomatoid tumor of adrenal gland. (Courtesy of Raaf HN, Grant LD, Santoscoy C, et al: Adenomatoid tumor of the adrenal gland: A report of four new cases and a review of the literature. *Mod Pathol* 9[11]:1046–1051, 1996.)

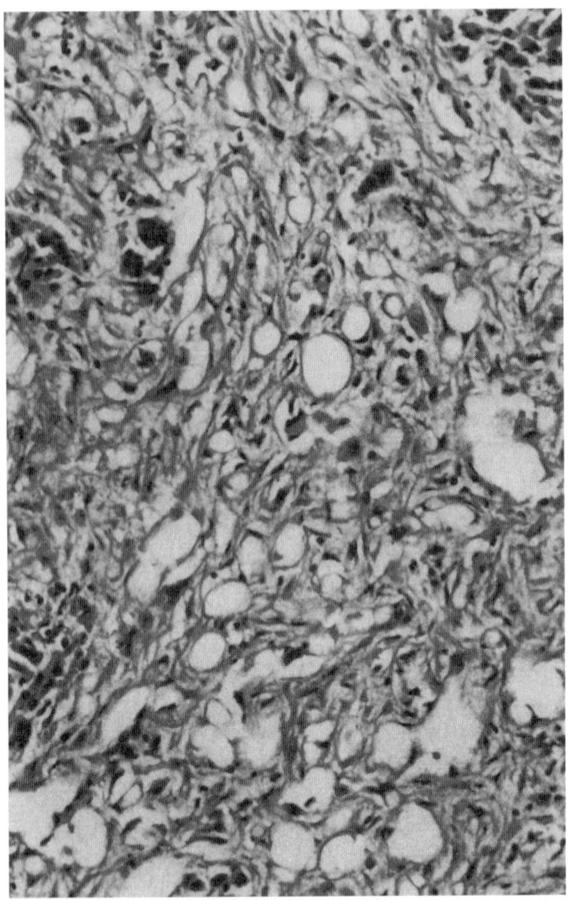

FIGURE 4.—Cells of adenomatoid tumor have large, clear vacuoles. Adrenal cortical cells are at the *left* and *upper right*. (Courtesy of Raaf HN, Grant LD, Santoscoy C, et al: Adenomatoid tumor of the adrenal gland: A report of four new cases and a review of the literature. *Mod Pathol* 9[11]:1046–1051, 1996.)

Discussion.—Electron microscopic and immunohistochemical analysis in these 4 patients support the notion of a mesothelial derivation for adenomatoid tumors of the adrenal gland. The differential diagnosis includes a variety of solid and cystic tumors. The ability to recognize these rare tumors is important so that they are not misclassified as metastatic or primary malignant vascular tumors.

▶ Intra-abdominal organs that, in the recent past, were only accessible by open surgery or at autopsy are today routinely sampled by radiographically guided needle biopsy techniques. These two articles (Abstracts 12–4 and 12–5) show that the adrenal gland, for example, is a known target for metastatic lung carcinoma, among other neoplasms. The radiographic detection of a mass in the adrenal gland during the staging of a lung neoplasm

Subscribe to the related journal in your field!

Yes! Begin my one-year subscription to *The Journal of Laboratory and Clinical Medicine* (12 issues).

Name _______________________________

Institution _______________________________

Address _______________________________

City _______________________ State _________

ZIP/PC __________ Country _______________

Specialty _______________________________
(Students/residents, please list Institution)

Method of payment

Enclose payment (check or credit card number) and we'll send an extra issue FREE!

❑ Check (in U.S. dollars, drawn on a U.S. bank, and payable to *The Journal of Laboratory and Clinical Medicine*)

❑ VISA ❑ MasterCard ❑ Discover

❑ AmEx ❑ Bill me Exp. date__________

Card #_______________________________

Signature _______________________________

*Includes Canadian GST

Individual/student subscriptions must be in the name of, billed to, and paid for by the individual.

Airmail rates available upon request.
Prices subject to change without notice.

Subscription prices (through 9/30/98)

		USA	Canada*	Int'l
Individuals	❑	$135.00	$170.13	$159.00
Institutions	❑	282.00	327.42	306.00
Students, residents	❑	56.00	85.60	80.00

J005983YA

Reservation Card for the Year Book

Yes! I would like my own copy of *Year Book of Pathology and Laboratory Medicine®* at the price of **$83.00** plus sales tax, postage, and handling. Please begin my subscription with the current edition according to the terms described below.* I understand that I will have 30 days to examine each annual edition.

Name _______________________________

Address _______________________________

City _______________________ State __________ ZIP__________

Method of Payment

Check (in U.S. dollars, drawn on a U.S. bank, payable to *Year Book of Pathology and Laboratory Medicine®*)

❑ VISA ❑ MasterCard ❑ Discover ❑ AmEx ❑ Bill me

Card number _______________________________ Exp. date: __________

Signature _______________________________

Prices are subject to change without notice.

PMC-027

---

*Your Year Book service guarantee:

When you subscribe to the *Year Book*, you will receive advance notice of future annual volumes about two months before publication. To receive the new edition, you need do nothing—we'll send you the new volume as soon as it is available. If you want to discontinue, the advance notice allows you time to notify us of your decision. If you are not completely satisfied, you have 30 days to return any *Year Book*.

BUSINESS REPLY MAIL
FIRST-CLASS MAIL   PERMIT NO 135   ST LOUIS MO

POSTAGE WILL BE PAID BY ADDRESSEE

SUBSCRIPTION SERVICES
MOSBY–YEAR BOOK, INC.
11830 WESTLINE INDUSTRIAL DRIVE
ST. LOUIS   MO 63146-9988

BUSINESS REPLY MAIL
FIRST-CLASS MAIL   PERMIT NO 135   ST LOUIS MO

POSTAGE WILL BE PAID BY ADDRESSEE

Mosby

PAT NEWMAN
11830 WESTLINE INDUSTRIAL DRIVE
PO BOX 46908
ST. LOUIS   MO 63146-9934

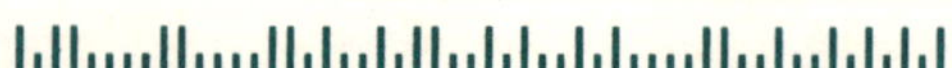

Want to speed up the process?

**To order the *Year Book*,
you also may call 1-800-426-4545**

**To subscribe to the journal today,
call toll-free in the U.S.:
1-800-453-4351
or fax 314-432-1158**

Outside the U.S., call: 314-453-4351

Visit us at:
www.mosby.com/Mosby/Periodicals

Mosby–Year Book, Inc.
Subscription Services
11830 Westline Industrial Drive
St. Louis, MO   63146 U.S.A.

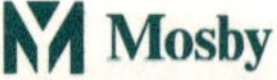 **Mosby**

will almost certainly be followed, in a modern institution, by a radiographically guided needle biopsy (fine-needle aspiration or needle core biopsy) to confirm the metastatic nature of the adrenal mass. This has increased the pathologist's familiarity with the different lesions that may occur in that organ and has enriched the pathology literature with newly discovered lesions in that location.

K.E. Sirgi, M.D.

Adrenocortical Neoplasms: Role of Prognostic Markers MIB-1, P53, and RB

Vargas MP, Vargas HI, Kleiner DE, et al (Natl Cancer Inst, Bethesda, Md)
Am J Surg Pathol 21:556–562, 1997   12–6

Background.—Diagnostic criteria for adrenocortical carcinoma include weight loss, urinary 17–ketosteroid excretion, response to adrenocorticotropic hormone stimulation, and a tumor mass greater than 100g, as well as the established histologic criteria. Even with all these parameters, it can be difficult to distinguish between benign and malignant adrenocortical neoplasms. The antibody MiB-1 and the retinoblastoma susceptibility (RB) and p53 genes were studied for correlation with the histologic diagnosis and clinical outcome of adrenocortical neoplasms.

Methods.—The analysis included 40 adrenocortical lesions obtained from pathology files: 10 hyperplasias, 10 adenomas, 12 carcinomas, and 8 metastatic or recurrent adrenocortical carcinomas. Immunohistochemical studies for MiB-1, p53, and RB gene product were performed. The tumor proliferating fraction (TPF) was calculated as the number of MiB-1–positive nuclei per 1,000 tumor cells. The findings were correlated with the clinical data.

Results.—Mean TPF was 15 in adenomas, 31.5 in hyperplasias, 208 in carcinomas, and 166 in recurrent or metastatic cancers. For benign lesions, the TPF was always less than 80; for malignancies, the TPF was always greater than 80. Forty-five percent of malignancies were positive for p53, compared with none of the benign lesions. All interpretable specimens were positive for RB. The disease-free interval was short for patients with a TPF of greater than 200 and positive p53 staining. It was not possible to evaluate survival.

Conclusions.—A high TPF on MiB-1 staining and positivity for p53 are strongly correlated with malignancy in adrenocortical neoplasms. Immunohistochemical studies for MiB-1 and p53 may therefore be useful in differentiating between benign and malignant adrenal lesions. These 2 parameters may be predictive of prognosis. Immunohistochemical staining for RB does not help to distinguish between benign and malignant lesions.

▶ Based on the results of this study, is it conceivable that it will soon be possible to establish a diagnosis of adrenocortical carcinoma on fine-needle aspiration specimens of adrenal cortical masses by evaluating the tumor cell nuclear reactivity for the MIB-1 and p53 antibodies? I imagine that some of you are already working on such a project.

K.E. Sirgi, M.D.

Microglandular Carcinoma of the Pancreas: Immunohistochemical and Ultrastructural Study of an Unusual Variant of Pancreatic Carcinoma That May Closely Resemble a Neuroendocrine Neoplasm
Berho M, Blaustein A, Willis I, et al (Univ of Miami, Fla)
Am J Clin Pathol 105:727–732, 1996   12–7

Introduction.—Microglandular carcinoma of the pancreas is rare and literature describing it is scarce. Reported are 2 patients with microglandular carcinoma of the pancreas. Immunohistochemical and ultrastructural analyses are presented.

Case Report 1.—Male, 56, was seen for abdominal pain and 40 lb weight loss. He had a 9-month history of recurrent pancreatitis. Computed tomography showed a cystic mass at the head of the pancreas. A large pancreatic mass was found on laparotomy and the liver was of normal size and consistency. The mesenteric and retroperitoneal lymph nodes were normal size. A Whipple's procedure was performed and he underwent chemotherapy and radiation therapy.

Case Report 2.—Man, 78, was seen for an incidental mass in the head of the pancreas that was detected on a scan of the abdomen performed as part of his yearly metastatic melanoma workup. Liver function tests were normal. He underwent extensive resection; peripancreatic lymph nodes were normal. He was given chemotherapy and radiotherapy.

Results.—Histologic findings were similar in both patients. Scanning magnification revealed that the lesions were composed of solid areas with scattered small gland-like spaces. There was scant cytoplasm with distinct cell borders and round to oval nuclei with irregular clumping of chromatin and small, inconspicuous nucleoli in the tumor cells. On immunohistochemical examination, both patients had positivity of the neoplastic cells with CAM 5.2 antibodies and negative staining with a battery of neuroendocrine-related markers. A cohesive population of cells forming abortive glandular lumens lined by imperfectly formed microvilli with well-developed junctional complexes were observed on ultrastructural examination. A ductal type of differentiation was given for these tumors in the absence of dense core neurosecretory granules or zymogen granules.

Conclusion.—This rare variant needs to be recognized to avoid misdiagnosis. Immunohistochemical and ultrastructural examinations are valuable here.

▶ This is an unusual form of pancreatic adenocarcinoma which is easy to confuse morphologically with a neuroendocrine neoplasm. Establishing the correct diagnosis with the help of immunohistochemistry and electron microscopy will be important because of the different natural history and treatment of neuroendocrine neoplasms.

K.E. Sirgi, M.D.

13 Dermatopathology

Hypermelanotic Nevus: Clinical, Histopathologic, and Ultrastructural Features in 316 Cases
Cohen LM, Bennion SD, Johnson TW, et al (Univ of Colorado, Denver; Fitzsimmons Army Med Ctr, Aurora, Colo)
Am J Dermatopathol 19:23–30, 1997   13–1

Background.—Acquired melanocytic nevi often develop in childhood, increase in number for 20 or 30 years, then slowly regress. Nevi can range from 2 mm to more than 2 cm, but most are smaller than 1 cm. They can be pink or peach, tan, brown, or black. The majority are well-circumscribed, smooth, and symmetrical. Clinically, it may not be possible to distinguish small, darkly pigmented junctional nevi from lentigines. A series of benign melanocytic nevi with unique features was described.

Findings.—The clinical, histopathologic, and ultrastructural features of 316 hypermelanotic nevi were analyzed. Patients included slightly more

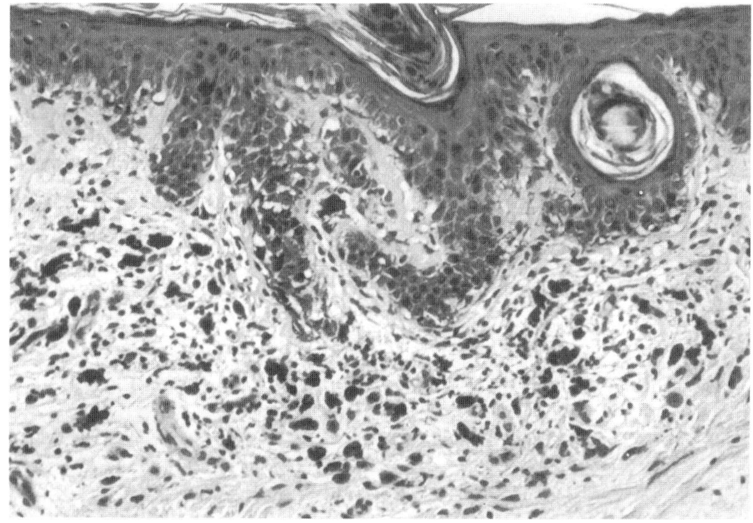

FIGURE 6.—These lesions typically develop in a dermal infiltrate composed of lymphocytes and numerous melanophages; hematoxylin-eosin. (Courtesy of Cohen LM, Bennion SD, Johnson TW, et al: Hypermelanotic nevus: Clinical, histopathologic, and ultrastructural features in 316 cases. *Am J Dermatopathol* 19:23–30, 1997.)

females than males, and the mean patient age was 40 years. The lesions ranged from dark brown to black macules or papules. Most were located on the back. These hypermelanotic nevi can be distinguished histopathologically by (1) melanin within a compact stratum corneum, (2) small nests of nevus cells at the dermal-epidermal junction and nests within the papillary dermis, (3) heavy melanin within keratinocytes in the lower epidermis, (4) a sparse or moderate lymphocytic infiltrate and melanophages in the superficial dermis (Fig 6), and (5) a lack of cytologic atypia. Electron microscopic examination showed abundant melanin in melanosome complexes within keratinocytes. Well-developed dendritic processes and golgi were noted in less pigmented melanocytes.

Discussion.—The name "hypermelanotic nevus" is proposed to describe this benign lesion. The literature showed that patients with this lesion were more often older and male than patients with ordinary nevi. Hypermelanotic nevi tended to be junctional nevi more often than control nevi. They were also smaller, dark brown or black, and had a worrisome clinical appearance.

▶ The authors describe a large series of highly pigmented but benign nevi. Obviously, the key lesion to distinguish, both clinically and histologically, is malignant melanoma. The key morphologic features are included in the abstract (see also Fig 6). One important aspect lacking in this study is clinical follow-up, and, therefore, the possibility of a misdiagnosed melanoma cannot be entirely excluded.

M.B. Cohen, M.D.

Melanoma In Situ Versus Melanocytic Hyperplasia in Sun-damaged Skin: Assessment of the Significance of Histopathologic Criteria for Differential Diagnosis

Weyers W, Bonczkowitz M, Weyers I, et al (Justus-Liebig Univ, Giessen, Germany; Philipps Univ, Marburg, Germany)
Am J Dermatopathol 18:560–566, 1996   13–2

Background.—Several criteria have been proposed for differentiating melanoma in situ (MIS) from melanocytic hyperplasia (MH) in sun-damaged skin. The sensitivity and specificity of those criteria were assessed in the current study.

Methods and Findings.—The epidermis adjacent to 50 consecutive basal cell carcinomas and 50 MIS in skin with significant solar elastosis was examined histopathologically. The following criteria were the most useful for distinguishing MIS from MH: (1) presence of nests of melanocytes, (2) irregular distribution of melanocytes, (3) descent of melanocytes far down adnexal epithelial structures, (4) irregular distribution of pigment, (5) presence of melanocytes above the junction, (6) a high number of melanocytes, (7) pleomorphism of melanocytes, and (8) atypical nuclei of melanocytes. Criteria of low or no value for differential diagnosis included the following: (1) collapse of cytoplasm around the nuclei of melanocytes; (2) flattening of rete ridges; (3) difference in the area, shape, and contour of melanocyte nuclei, as determined by nuclear morphometry; and (4) the presence of melanocytes stained by HMB-45 and Ki-67/MIB-1 monoclonal antibodies.

Conclusions.—Differentiating MIS from MH histopathologically in sun-damaged skin may be difficult but is usually possible using established criteria. Diagnosis should be based on a combination of findings rather than on only one.

▶ The authors have tried to identify useful morphological criteria in separating MIS from MH in a difficult setting; that of sun-damaged skin. Importantly, ancillary studies [morphometry and immunohistochemistry for HMB-45 and the proliferation marker MIB-1 (Ki-67 analogue)] were of little value. Hopefully these criteria will be useful prospectively in distinguishing these two lesions.

M.B. Cohen, M.D.

Silhouette Symmetry: An Unsupportable Histologic Criterion for Distinguishing Spitz Nevi and Compound Nevi From Malignant Melanoma
Okun MR (Dermatopathology Found, Canton, Mass)
Arch Pathol Lab Med 121:48–53, 1997   13–3

Background.—Several years ago Ackerman suggested that pattern analysis can be more accurate than nuclear morphologic assessment in the evaluation of neoplasms. He reported that malignant melanomas tend to be asymmetrical, whereas benign melanocytic neoplasms tend to be symmetrical. The validity of this contention was investigated.

Methods.—Standard sections of 55 Spitz nevi, 44 compound nevi, and 75 malignant melanomas randomly selected from the files at 1 center were examined. A loupe and higher magnifications were used.

Results.—The ratio of symmetrical to asymmetrical lesions, as observed in histologic sections, was about the same in malignant melanomas and in Spitz and compound nevi. The configuration noted in sections did not always reflect the 3-dimensional configuration of the lesion. Lesions with 3-dimensional reflective symmetry could not be identified as having this property in sections unless cuts were made perpendicular to the place of symmetry, which is impossible.

Conclusions.—The presence or absence of symmetry in sections of neoplasms is coincidental or focal. Both empirically and theoretically, symmetry is not a valid criterion for distinguishing malignant melanomas from Spitz and compound nevi.

▶ The differential diagnosis between compound nevi and Spitz nevi and malignant melanoma is well known to pathologists. In this study, the author attempted to verify Ackerman's pattern analysis of neoplasms. The results are summarized below:

Lesion	No. cases	Incidence of symmetry (%)
Compound nevus	44	32
Spitz nevus	55	57
Malignant melanomas	75	42

The author concludes that: "the proposal that histologic symmetry favors benignity in a melanocytic neoplasm and that histologic asymmetry favors malignancy, is without validity." On the basis of the results of this study, it is difficult to argue with this notion, albeit somewhat emphatically stated.

M.B. Cohen, M.D.

Desmoplastic and Spindle-cell Malignant Melanoma: An Immunohistochemical Study

Longacre TA, Egbert BM, Rouse RV (Standford Univ, Calif; Veterans Affairs Med Ctr, Palo Alto, Calif)
Am J Surg Pathol 20:1489–1500, 1996   13–4

Background.—In 1971, the term "desmoplastic malignant melanoma" was introduced to describe a morphologic subtype of malignant melanoma with spindle cells with pronounced desmoplasia often seen in pigmented skin lesions of the head and neck. A neurotropic variant of desmoplastic malignant melanoma was later described; it was distinguished by neuroma-like features and invasion of nerve fascicles by neoplastic spindle cells, but not always by a recognizable melanocytic proliferation at the dermal-epidermal junction.

Subjects.—The clinical, histologic, and immunologic features of 22 desmoplastic malignant melanomas, 10 mixed desmoplastic and spindle cell melanomas (DMM/SMM), and 2 cellular spindle cell melanomas were examined. There were 34 patients (mean age, 67 years); 23 patients were men. There were 17 cases occurring in sun-damaged skin of the head and neck, 11 on extremities, and 6 on the trunk. All but 2 cases were Clark's level IV or V.

Results.—Of the 34 cases, 22 were associated with a recognizable overlying pigmented lesion. Of the 32 cases of desmoplastic malignant melanoma and DMM/SMM, 30 were positive for S100. In 2 cases of DMM/SMM, S100 staining was seen in less than 5% of spindle cells. All cases of desmoplastic malignant melanoma were negative for HMB45. Immunoreactivity to HMB45 was seen in 3 cases of DMM/SMM and both cases of cellular spindle cell melanoma. CD68 staining was seen in less than 5% of spindle cells in 2 of the 32 cases of desmoplastic malignant melanoma and DMM/SMM, and in 20% of cells in 1 of 2 cellular spindle cell melanomas. In 9 cases of desmoplastic malignant melanoma and DMM/SMM, significant numbers of spindle cells were immunoreactive for SMA, but not desmin. In 5 cases, the number of actin-positive spindle cells was equal to or greater than the number of spindle cells positive for S100. Two color stains for SMA and S100 showed that smooth-muscle actin-positive cells made up a separate spindle cell population.

Discussion.—These findings suggest that the immunohistologic features of desmoplastic malignant melanoma and of conventional melanoma are different. HMB45 will generally not confirm a diagnosis of desmoplastic malignant melanoma in problematic spindle cell skin lesions with suspected melanocytic process. S100 expression is also variable, and the absence of S100 staining cannot reliably exclude desmoplastic malignant melanoma if the clinical and histological features suggest it. Because desmoplastic malignant melanoma can have significant numbers of actin-positive spindle cells, the presence of these cells without other confirming data should be interpreted with caution.

▶ This study, concerning yet another difficult diagnosis, highlights the fact that immunohistochemistry is generally not useful: 0 of 22 desmoplastic malignant melanomas, 3 of 10 DMM/SMM, and 2/2 spindle cell melanomas were HMB-45 positive, and CD68 staining was identifiable in only 3 of 34 cases. S-100 protein staining, however, was usually positive (1+–4+), but 2 of 10 DMM/SMM revealed less than 5% of cells staining. In addition, staining for smooth muscle specific action indicated that these spindled cells were a separate, presumably reactive, component. Taken together, these observations indicate that the diagnosis of spindled melanomas is difficult and remains one based on histologic criteria, as put forth by Conley and others.[1-3]

M.B. Cohen, M.D.

References

1. Conley J, Lattes R, Orr W: Desmoplastic malignant melanoma (a rare variant of spindle cell melanoma). *Cancer* 28:914–936, 1971.
2. Egbert B, Kempson R, Sagebiel R: Desmoplastic malignant melanoma: A clinico-histopathologic study of 25 cases. *Cancer* 62:2033–2041, 1988.
3. Reed RJ, Leonard DD: Neurotropic melanoma: A variant of desmoplastic melanoma. *Am J Surg Pathol* 3:301–311, 1979.

Clinical and Histological Features of Poor Prognosis in Cutaneous Metastatic Melanomas

Hofmann-Wellenhof R, Woltsche-Kahr I, Smolle J, et al (Univ of Graz, Austria)
J Cutan Pathol 23:199–204, 1996

13–5

Introduction.—Formation of distant metastases is the crucial step from local growth to fatal disseminated disease in solid tumors. In patients suffering from primary melanoma of the skin, cutaneous melanoma metastases are known as a poor prognostic sign. There are few relevant prognostic parameters in cutaneous metastases. The clinical and histologic features of melanoma metastatic to the skin were investigated to determine which of these corresponded with poor outcome.

Methods.—Samples were taken of 59 cutaneous and subcutaneous melanoma metastases from 16 patients who died of metastatic melanoma to other anatomical sites within 1 year after removal of the lesion. A comparison was made with 285 metastases removed from 68 patients who survived longer than 1 year after resection of the cutaneous metastases. Recordings were taken of clinical and histologic data of the primary tumor, such as the age of onset, anatomical location, maximum vertical tumor thickness and Clark's level of invasion.

Results.—Men had metastases associated with death within 1 year more often than women (54.2% versus 34.7%). Younger patients had metastases associated with death within 1 year more often than older patients (51.1 ± 14.1 years versus 58.8 ± 15.3 years). Metastases that developed earlier after the primary tumor were more often associated with death within 1 year (mean time 21.7 ± 19.9 months). They also were found more often in the subcutis (74.5% versus 56.1%) and were found more often in distant sites than they were in regional sites (45.7% versus 30.5%). Histologic samples showed a prevalence of simple invasion between collagen of reticular dermis and preservation of preexistent collagen in patients with poor outcomes. For patients with lesion with subcutaneous growth, poor outcome was more frequently associated with subcutis and fatty tissue, where capsule formation was seen less frequently.

Conclusion.—Certain clinical and histologic features were associated with metastatic melanomas of the skin, with particularly poor outcomes which differed from other cutaneous melanoma metastases. Future design of clinical trials should take these factors into account.

▶ This study is intriguing. Cutaneous melanoma metastases are not uncommon, and it is important to report the histologic features in cutaneous metastases that correlate with prognosis. In follow-up to previous work on primary melanomas,[1] the authors attempted to correlate histologic features with good (greater than 1 year survival) and poor (less than 1 year survival) metastases. They claim that retention of pre-existing collagen and simple invasion into the dermis correlate with poor outcome in the subset of metastases with dermal involvement. Similarly, in lesions with subcutaneous involvement, the findings of pre-existing fat in the tumor and simple invasion into the subcutaneous tissue correlated with poor prognosis. A drawback of the study is that the actual statistics were not presented for us to make our own judgments. Also, these correlations were determined by univariate analysis, not multivariate, and multivariate analysis is a much stronger predictor. Using multivariate analysis, only the histologic finding of fat cells within the tumor bulk correlated with prognosis. Also, interobserver concordance data regarding the presence or absence of these criteria were not well presented (one criteria had remarkably low interobserver agreement), and I believe, the wrong statistical measure (interobserver agreement instead of kappa) was used. To me, this indicates that there are considerable weaknesses in this work, and I am not convinced that pathologists should examine for the select criteria that the authors have found. The work does show that certain features (e.g., mitotic count, mean tumor area) are not important and probably can be excluded in a pathology report. I think the most important feature to report is if the tumor is subcutaneous or dermal. The other criteria will have to wait for further study.

S. Raab, M.D.

Reference

1. Smolle J, Woltsche I, Hofmann-Wellenhof R, et al: Pathology of tumor-stroma interaction in melanoma metastatic to the skin. *Hum Pathol* 26:8561, 1995.

Cutaneous Pilar Leiomyoma: Clinicopathologic Analysis of 53 Lesions in 45 Patients
Raj S, Calonje E, Kraus M, et al (St. Thomas's Hosp, London; Darlington Mem Hosp, England; Brigham and Women's Hosp, Boston)
Am J Dermatopathol 19:2–9, 1997   13–6

Introduction.—Cutaneous pilar leiomyomas are smooth muscle tumors commonly located on the extremities. The lesions are often multiple and appear as firm dermal papules, with a skin-colored, pink or reddish-brown surface. Because relatively few studies have been devoted to cutaneous pilar leiomyomas, investigators analyzed the clinicopathologic features of 53 lesions from 45 patients.

Methods.—Case reports were retrieved from hospital files. A total of 62 lesions from 54 patients were diagnosed microscopically as dermal leiomyoma. Reassessment of histologic features resulted in the exclusion of 9 cases. The remaining case records were reviewed for patient characteristics, involved areas, clinical descriptions of the lesions, symptoms, and histologic criteria for diagnosis.

Results.—Men and women were equally represented in the patient group. Twenty-one (12 women) had multiple lesions and 18 (11 men) had solitary lesions. The age range of the patients at diagnosis was 17 to 74 years. The most frequently involved areas were the extremities and trunk, but solitary lesions occurred predominantly on the limbs. Multiple lesions had an average size of 0.7 cm; the largest solitary lesion was 1.5 cm in diameter. Pain was present in 17 patients, including 48% of those with multiple lesions and 40% of those with solitary lesions. Clinical features led to an accurate diagnosis in only 3 of 53 lesions. Follow-up, ranging from 9 months to 9 years, was available in 15 patients.

Histologic examination showed ill-defined bundles of well-differentiated smooth muscle cells in the reticular dermis in all cases. A more nodular pattern was observed in 9 lesions. More than half of the cases (54.7%) showed overlying epidermal hyperplasia. Immunohistochemical examination indicated the presence of an increased number of nerve fibers within and surrounding the tumors. Fifteen lesions exhibited mitotic activity; 13 had less than 1 mitosis per 10 HPF and 2 had 1 to 2 mitoses per 10 HPF. There were no recurrences in the 10 mitotically active tumors that had follow up.

Conclusion.—In contrast to some previous studies, the distribution of cutaneous pilar leiomyomas was similar in men and women, and there was an almost equal prevalence of solitary and multiple lesions. The mechanism of pain is uncertain, but a neural origin is probable. Although some lesions may exhibit a low mitotic activity of less than 1 per 10 HPF, this finding does not indicate an adverse prognosis.

▶ Raj et al. provide a good review, particularly in terms of the controversy regarding the mitotic rate of cutaneous smooth muscle tumors. Unfortunately, the number and type of mitoses needed to classify a lesion as a leiomyoma or a leiomyosarcoma is not settled. Raj et al. argue that if the lesion has less than 1 mitosis per 10 HPF, the lesion can safely be called a leiomyoma, and I agree with this assumption. Interestingly, subcutaneous leiomyomas may be infiltrative and, in this study, in a number of cases, the neoplastic cells infiltrated underlying fat or skeletal muscle or overlying papillary dermis. Although it would seem that the diagnosis of a subcutaneous leiomyoma should not be problematic, difficulties in correctly classifying these lesions are not rare. Raj et al. report that 9 cases were excluded from the analysis because of misclassification. They also report that immunohistochemistry was performed in some cases, although the reasons why are uncertain.

S. Raab, M.D.

CD34 and Factor-XIIIa Immunoreactivity in Dermatofibrosarcoma Protuberans and Dermatofibroma
Goldblum JR, Tuthill RJ (Cleveland Clinic Found, Ohio)
Am J Dermatopathol 19:147–153, 1997   13–7

Objective.—It can be difficult to distinguish between dermatofibrosarcoma protuberans (DFSP) and the fibrous type of benign fibrous histiocytoma, or dermatofibroma. Previous reports have suggested that immunoreactivity for CD34 and factor XIIIa may help to make the distinction. These 2 markers were studied for their ability to differentiate between DFSP and dermatofibroma.

Methods.—Published criteria were used to classify 30 cases as dermatofibroma and 24 as DFSP. These diagnoses were independently evaluated and agreed on by the authors. The specimens were then stained with antibodies to CD34 and factor XIIIa, with immunopositivity scored on a scale of 0 to 5. The markers were evaluated for their ability to distinguish between dermatofibroma and DFSP.

Results.—Ninety-two percent of DFSPs were immunoreactive to CD34, compared with just 40% of dermatofibromas. Mean CD34 scores were 4.6 and 0.6, respectively. Factor XIIIa immunoreactivity was noted in 97% of dermatofibromas and 75% of DFSPs; however, in the latter group, the factor XIIIa-reactive cells were believed to be entrapped nonneoplastic dermal dendrocytes. Mean factor XIIIa scores were 4.1 in the dermatofibroma group and 1.3 in the DFSP group.

Conclusions.—Immunostaining studies for CD34 and factor XIIIa can usually distinguish between DFSP and the fibrous type of dermatofibroma. However, it is important to remember that some CD34-reactive cells are found in dermatofibromas and some factor XIIIa-reactive cells are found in DFSPs. The immunostaining results can be used in addition to, not instead of, histologic analysis.

▶ It is important to make the separation of a dermatofibroma from a DFSP, because DFSPs have a greater probability of local recurrence. The literature indicates that DFSPs are generally immunoreactive for CD34 antigen and that fibrous dermatofibromas are immunoreactive for factor VIIIA antigen.[1, 2] Goldblum and Tuthill studied whether these immunostains could effectively be used to differentiate DFSP from fibrous dermatofibroma. They found that when cases are scored quantitatively by cell count, most DFSPs are immunoreactive for CD34 (and dermatofibromas are not), whereas most dermatofibromas are immunoreactive for factor VIIIA (and DFSPs are not). I believe that these results show a trend, but they do not convince me that I should use these stains to separate these tumors in my practice. There are several flaws in the study. First, included tumors did not necessarily reflect diagnostic problems. Many DFSPs are easily separated from fibrous dermatofibromas histologically, and the authors should have studied whether locally recurring tumors can be separated from nonrecurring tumors by these stains. Second, a true gold standard is lacking. The authors used their ability to separate these tumors by light microscopy as the gold standard for diagnosis, but this is hardly convincing; if we can separate these tumors by light microscopy, then we hardly need immunostains. Third, the authors excluded 6 (12%) of the cases because of lack of observer agreement as to how these cases actually should be diagnosed. Aren't these the very cases that should have been studied, because these represent the diagnostic problems? Fourth, the sensitivity and specificity are less than perfect to separate DFSP and dermatofibroma with these immunostains. A negative CD34 stain result does not mean that dermatofibrosarcoma can be excluded, and a positive CD34 stain result does not mean that dermatofibroma is excluded. In your practice, on a difficult case, immunohistochemical results might help to sway you one way or another, but these stains are less than definitive.

S. Raab, M.D.

References

1. Kamino H, Jacobson M: Dermatofibroma extending into subcutaneous tissue: Differential diagnosis from dermatofibrosarcoma protuberans. *Am J Surg Pathol* 14:1156–1164, 1990.

2. Abenoza P, Lillemoe T: CD34 and factor XIIIa in the differential diagnosis of dermatofibroma and dermatofibrosarcoma protuberans. *Am J Dermatopathol* 15:429–434, 1993.

Differential Expression of CD44 in Malignant Cutaneous Epithelial Neoplasms

Prieto VG, Reed JA, McNutt NS, et al (New York Hosp—Cornell Med Ctr)
Am J Dermatopathol 17:447–451, 1995   13–8

Background.—The CD44 antigen is a highly glycosylated cell-surface polypeptide. Various CD44 isoforms are involved in cellular functions, such as cell adhesion, hyaluran binding and internalization, chemotaxis of lymphocytes to mesenteric lymphoid tissue, and activation of T lymphocytes. CD44 is also expressed by astrocytomas, meningiomas, and colonic adenocarcinomas. CD44 gives cell lines derived from certain adenocarcinomas the potential to metastasize. In the skin, CD44 is normally found in epidermal keratinocytes and hair follicular, sebaceous, and eccrine epithelial cells. There is little information regarding the expression of CD44 in primary cutaneous neoplasms, or differential expression of CD44 in primary or metastatic tumors in the skin.

Findings.—Immunohistochemistry was used to analyze the expression of CD44 in cutaneous invasive and metastatic squamous cell carcinomas, metastatic adenocarcinomas, and basal cell carcinomas. Strong expression of CD44 was seen in all invasive and metastatic squamous cell carcinomas and in metastatic adenocarcinomas. Basal cell carcinomas were nonreactive or had focal, minimal reactivity. CD44 expression was seen in adjacent normal skin throughout the epidermis, including the basal layer, and in hair follicles and sebaceous, and eccrine glands.

Discussion.—This is the first confirmation of a differential expression of CD44 in various epithelial neoplasms in the skin. These findings indicate that expression of CD44 in these tumors may be related to tumor progression and ability to metastasize, rather then to malignant transformation.

▶ CD44 is an intriguing group of cellular adhesion molecules that has received increasing attention in the pathology literature, in part as a prognostic marker for identifying metastatic behavior. This immunohistochemical study involved a series of primary carcinomas (basal cell and squamous) and secondary carcinomas (metastatic squamous and adenocarcinomas). Normal epidermis was CD44-positive at all levels. Squamous cell carcinomas were also positive, as were the adenocarcinomas. The basal cell carcinomas however, were negative with this antibody (Clone A1G3 from Oncogene Science Inc).

It is unclear as to why the authors used cytoplasmic staining because CD44 is a transmembrane molecule. In addition, it is somewhat difficult to understand the stated conclusion that "expression of CD44... may be related to tumor progression and the ability to metastasize." Lastly, more intriguing results have been obtained with melanocytic lesions.

M.B. Cohen, M.D.

Monoclonal Origin of Multicentric Kaposi's Sarcoma Lesions

Rabkin CS, Janz S, Lash A, et al (Natl Cancer Inst, Bethesda, Md; Univ Teaching Hosp, Lusaka, Zambia)
N Engl J Med 336:988–993, 1997
13–9

Background.—Patients with Kaposi's sarcoma can have multiple lesions, appearing synchronously in widely dispersed areas. Proliferating spindle cells, which most likely originate from endothelial cells, are a characteristic component of the lesions. The neoplastic or hyperplastic nature of spindle cells has been a subject of debate, but the demonstration that individual Kaposi's sarcoma lesions are clonal proliferations supports classifying the lesions as neoplastic. A study of patients with multiple nodular Kaposi's sarcoma lesions tested the hypothesis that the lesions originate from a single clone of precursor cells.

Methods.—Ten patients, all women, were recruited from a clinic of the University Teaching Hospital in Lusaka, Zambia. Eight had serologic confirmation of HIV infection and 2 were diagnosed clinically. Only 2 patients had been treated for Kaposi's sarcoma, having received a single dose of IV vincristine 2 to 5 months before study entry. Biopsy specimens were obtained from normal skin and from 5 widely separated superficial cutaneous nodular tumors in each patient. Clonal relatedness in the cells was assessed by studying patterns of X-chromosome methylation. The marker gene used was the X-linked androgen-receptor gene *(HUMARA)*. About half the copies of each *HUMARA* allele are methylated in polyclonal tissues, in contrast to cells derived from a single clone in which all the copies of only 1 allele are methylated.

Results.—Two patients were homozygous for the *HUMARA* gene and were excluded from further analysis. Thirty-two of the 40 tumors from the remaining 8 patients could be studied for clonality. A total of 27 tumors from the 6 women who had balanced methylation patterns in normal dermis could be evaluated. Unbalanced methylation, the predominance of 1 *HUMARA* allele, was found in 23 of these tumors, whereas the remaining 4 had balanced methylation. In each patient, the same *HUMARA* allele was methylated in all tumors showing unbalanced methylation.

Conclusion.—The finding of concordance among the patterns of methylation of the X-linked *HUMARA* alleles in different Kaposi's sarcoma lesions from a given patient indicates that a single clone of cells is the origin of multiple lesions in the same patient. Kaposi's sarcoma thus appears to be a disseminated monoclonal cancer. Changes that allow the clonal outgrowth of spindle cells occur before spread of the disease.

▶ This important and interesting paper addresses the long-standing controversy regarding the pathogenesis of Kaposi's sarcoma. Should it be regarded as a multicentric hyperplastic, multicentric neoplastic, or metastatic neoplastic process? These authors use an elegant clonality assay to try to answer this question, based on looking at patterns of X-chromosome methylation. Although this study is limited by a small number of patients (10) and by investigation of AIDS-associated Kaposi's lesions only, the data convincingly support a monoclonal origin for these lesions, leading to the conclusion that this form of Kaposi's sarcoma is a true metastatic sarcoma. This information will likely impact therapy strategies for this neoplasm, particularly in patients with AIDS who also commonly manifest significant visceral involvement.

D. Grzybicki, M.D., Ph.D.

Lymphangioma-like Variant of Kaposi's Sarcoma: Clinicopathologic Study of Seven Cases With Review of the Literature
Cossu S, Satta R, Cottoni F, et al (Univ of Sassari, Italy)
Am J Dermatopathol 19:16–22, 1997   13–10

Background.—Kaposi's sarcoma is a multifocal vascular disease characterized by clinical and histologic polymorphism. A lymphangioma-like variant was first reported in 1957. Harawi included the lymphangioma-like variant in his classification in a recent study of Kaposi's sarcoma in patients with HIV infection. There is little information on the incidence, clinical features, histologic pattern, and biological behavior of this lymphangioma-like variant of Kaposi's sarcoma.

Findings.—The clinical and histopathologic features of 7 cases of this variant of Kaposi's sarcoma were examined. The variant is more common in men 59 to 80 years of age; 6 of the 7 patients in this study were men. The clinical appearance has some of the classic features of Kaposi's sarcoma, but a bullalike appearance is considered a clinical hallmark of this variant. A few cases have been aggressive, but more often the disease progresses slowly, with localized or diffuse involvement of the lower limbs. Histologically, a permeation of dermal collagen by labyrinthine vascular channels lined by a flattened endothelium was seen. These channels were closely applied to the dermal collagen bundles and had a narrow lumen with several slender papillary projections (Fig 3). The endothelial cells were larger and more crowded than in normal lymphatic vessels. There were no nuclear atypia or mitoses. Erythrocytes were absent from most of the vascular spaces.

Discussion.—The histologic pattern of the lymphangioma-like variant of Kaposi's sarcoma must be distinguished from spindle cell hemangioendothelioma, low-grade angiosarcoma, targetoid hemosiderotic hemangioma, and benign lymphangioendothelioma. Some authors believe that this

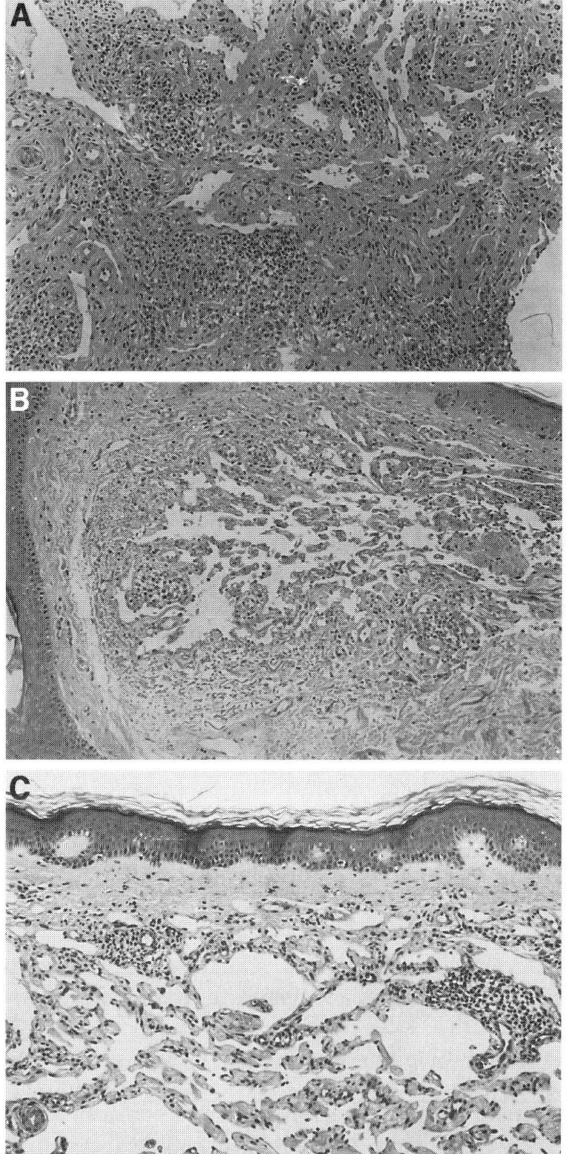

FIGURE 3.—As shown in microscopic studies in 3 patients, a constant feature of lymphangioma-like Kaposi's sarcoma is a wild lymphoplasmacytic infiltrate among the vascular spaces. (Courtesy of Cossu S, Satta R, Cottoni F, et al: Lymphangioma-like variant of Kaposi's sarcoma: Clinicopathologic study of seven cases with review of the literature. *Am J Dermatopathol* 19:16–22, 1997.)

variant is actually Kaposi's sarcoma in its initial stages, but because lesions were observed lasting for different periods of time, it was concluded that there is no association with any disease stage. This study was conducted in an area with a high prevalence of endemic Kaposi's sarcoma. The small number of cases of this lymphangioma-like variant examined in 15 years confirms its rarity.

▶ The histopathologic diagnosis of Kaposi's sarcoma is difficult, in part because of its varied presentation. In this article, the authors describe another, albeit rare, variant of Kaposi's sarcoma. The main reason for recognizing this variant is not to confuse it with other benign and malignant vascular neoplasms. It is important to emphasize that this study is based on so-called classic Kaposi's sarcoma, although a report by Harawi[1] indicates that this pattern may also be seen in HIV-associated Kaposi's sarcoma.

M.B. Cohen, M.D.

Reference

1. Harawi SJ: Kaposi's sarcoma, in Harawi SJ, O'Hara CJ (eds): *Pathology and Pathophysiology of AIDS and HIV-Related Disease.* St Louis, Mosby, 1989, pp 83–131.

Cytokeratin 20 Immunoreactivity Distinguishes Merkel Cell (Primary Cutaneous Neuroendocrine) Carcinomas and Salivary Gland Small Cell Carcinomas From Small Cell Carcinomas of Various Sites
Chan JKC, Suster S, Wenig BM, et al (Queen Elizabeth Hosp, Hong Kong; Univ of Miami, Fla; Armed Forces Inst of Pathology, Washington, DC)
Am J Surg Pathol 21:226–234, 1997   13–11

Background.—Cytokeratin 20 (CK20) is a low–molecular-weight cytokeratin with limited expression in the gastrointestinal epithelium, urothelium, and Merkel cell. It has been suggested that the consistent CK20 positivity of Merkel cell carcinoma may distinguish it from pulmonary small-cell carcinoma. Only a small number of these tumors have been examined, and the pattern of CK20 expression in other small cell carcinomas has not been defined.

Methods.—Expression of CK20 was analyzed in small-cell carcinomas from various sites. Immunohistochemical studies were carried out on paraffin sections with CK20 antibody after antigen retrieval by pressure cooking in citrate buffer. There were 34 Merkel cell carcinomas and 89 small-cell carcinomas from various sites. Immunostaining with pan-CK and low–molecular-weight CK antibodies was performed.

Results.—All but 1 Merkel cell carcinoma showed positivity for CK20, and 30 of 33 had a punctate pattern. Nearly all tumor cells tested positive; in 2 cases, there was 10% and 30% staining of tumor cells. Only 5 of the other small-cell carcinomas were positive for CK20 (1 of 37 pulmonary, 1 of 11 cervical, and 3 of 5 salivary gland).

Discussion.—Positivity for CK20 in small-cell carcinoma of unknown origin is a strong predictor of Merkel cell carcinoma, especially if most tumor cells test positive. Negativity for CK20 can usually exclude Merkel cell carcinoma if an effective antigen retrieval technique is used and if appropriate staining with other CK antibodies is obtained. In this study, the CK20 positivity in salivary gland small-cell carcinoma indicates that some of these carcinomas may be closer biologically to Merkel cell carcinoma than to pulmonary-type small-cell carcinoma, and may explain why these carcinomas are less aggressive than other small-cell carcinomas.

▶ This study focuses on the difficult, and perhaps uncommon, differential diagnosis that includes Merkel cell carcinoma and small-cell carcinomas of various sites, including, most notably, the salivary glands. The staining was performed on formalin-fixed, paraffin-embedded sections, using a commercial antibody, CK20 (clone K$_s$20.8 from Dako). It is worth emphasizing that the pattern of staining, i.e., punctate, is important.

M.B. Cohen, M.D.

Induction of Cutaneous Hyperplasias by Altered Stroma
Requena L, Sánchez E, Simón P, et al (Universidad Autónoma, Madrid; Universidad Complutense, Madrid)
Am J Dermatopathol 18:248–268, 1996   13–12

Introduction.—In studying neoplastic change, pathology has historically devoted attention to the parenchymal influences of stroma, rather than vice versa. However, the stromal influences of parenchyma may play the more important role in the biologic behavior of tumors. Cutaneous hyperplasias may result from an inductive effect on the altered dermis on epidermis and adnexal epithelia. Though inductive changes are known to be present in dermatofibroma, they have been interpreted in differing ways. An experience with induction of cutaneous hyperplasias by altered stroma is reviewed, focusing on the disease's processes in which these changes occur most frequently.

Methods and Results.—The study included cutaneous biopsy specimens with epidermal hyperplasia or hyperplasia of the adnexal epithelium in the area of a highly vascularized dermis with numerous fibrocytes and abundant ground substance. The induced epithelial hyperplasias were classified as epidermal hyperplasia, pseudocarcinomatous hyperplasia (PCH), adnexal hyperplasia with follicular differentiation, adnexal hyperplasia with sebaceous differentiation, and adnexal hyperplasia with ductal differentiation. Induced follicular differentiation was further subclassified as primitive, infundibular, or anagen follicular differentiation. In each category, many different types of epithelial hyperplasia and neoplasms were thought to result from induction (Table 1).

Conclusions.—A broad range of types of epithelial hyperplasia and neoplasms may result from induction of pluripotent germinative cells by stromal stimuli. Some lesions generally regarded as neoplasms may be alternatively interpreted as hyperplasias caused by stromal induction. The findings in each category of stroma-induced hyperplasias—epidermal hy-

TABLE 1.—Cutaneous Hyperplasias That Can Be Considered the Result of Induction by Altered Stroma and Their Associated Primary Disease

Epidermal hyperplasia
  Dermatofibroma
  Angioma
  Granular cell tumor
  Keratoacanthoma
  Squamous cell carcinoma
  Basal cell carcinoma
  Scar
  Fibrosis surrounding ruptured infundibular cysts
Pseudocarcinomatous hyperplasia (adnexal hyperplasia with squamous
  differentiation)
    Deep fungal infections
    Halogen eruptions
    Lupus vulgaris
    Spitz nevi
    Granular cell tumors
Adnexal hyperplasias with
  Follicular differentiation
    Dermatofibroma
    Focal mucinosis
    Nevus sebaceus of Jadassohn
    Seborrheic keratosis
    Wart
    Neurofibroma
    Scar
    Angioma
    Anetodermic pilomatricoma
    Chronic lymphedema
    Dermatofibrosarcoma protuberans
  Sebaceous differentiation
    Dermatofibroma
    Neurofibroma
    Melanocytic nevus
    Tag
  Ductal differentiation
    Scarring alopecia
    Nevus sebaceus of Jadassohn
    Chronic lymphedema
    Focal mucinosis
    Keratoacanthoma
    Squamous cell carcinoma

(Courtesy of Requena L, Sánchez E, Simón P, et al: Induction of cutaneous hyperplasias by altered stroma. *Am J Dermatopathol* 18:248–268, 1996.)

perplasias, pseudocarcinomatous hyperplasias, and adnexal hyperplasias with follicular, sebaceous, and ductal differentiation—are detailed.

▶ The meat of this article lies in Table 1, which is reproduced here. As is well known, one can see a variety of epithelial hyperplasias related to either stromal tumors, inflammatory conditions, or other diseases. This article breaks down different types of epithelial hyperplasias and provides a list, which is not inclusive, of the entities that cause these hyperplasias. Such a list can be helpful with either superficial or small biopsy procedures, but may not actually excise the lesion of interest. For example, Requena et al. suggest that a superficial biopsy sample of a dermatofibroma may show epidermal hyperplasia, adnexal hyperplasia with follicular differentiation, or adnexal hyperplasia with sebaceous differentiation. Some types of hyperplasia may resemble a tumor. We should be strict on our criteria to classify a tumor; if we fall into the trap of misclassifying a hyperplasia as an epithelial tumor, we may miss the underlying lesion.

S. Raab, M.D.

Mitotic Granuloma Annulare: A Clinicopathologic Study of 20 Cases

Trotter MJ, Crawford RI, O'Connell JX, et al (Vancouver Hosp and Health Sciences Centre, BC; Univ of British Columbia, Vancouver)
J Cutan Pathol 23:537–545, 1996
13–13

Background.—Granuloma annulare is a benign idiopathic inflammatory dermatosis. Clinically, it appears as localized or generalized papules and plaques, often in an annular pattern. Histologically, it is characterized by a dispersed or aggregated dermal histiocytic infiltrate, often in a palisaded pattern. Typically, palisaded histiocytes surround a central area of collagen degeneration and mucin deposition. Rare cases of a granulomatous pattern resembling sarcoidosis have been reported, as well as deep granuloma annulare and perforating granuloma annulare.

Findings.—The histologic and pathologic features of 20 cases of a cellular, mitotically active variant of granuloma annulare were analyzed. Patients had at least 1 mitosis per 10 HPF (Table 1). The patients were 9

TABLE 1.—Summary of Results

#	Age and sex	Site	Clinical diagnosis	Histologic pattern	Mitoses per 10 hpf	MIB-1 index
1	53F	Hand	Fungal infection	Classic	2.9	0.18
2	68M	Elbow	GA	Classic	1.5	0.09
3	48F	Arm	GA	Classic	1.6	0.11
4	70F	Palm	None given	Classic	3.8	0.18
5	39F	Finger	GA	Classic	1.0	0.05
6	71F	Finger	GA vs molluscum	Classic	1.3	ND
7	32F	Ankle	GA	Classic	3.0	0.12
8	50F	Thigh	?RA-related	Classic	2.3	0.17
9	50M	Neck	GA	Classic	2.5	0.08
10	27M	Neck	GA	Interstitial	4.0	0.13
11	48F	Hand	GA	Classic	2.0	0.16
12	10M	Arm	GA	Classic	3.3	0.14
13	45M	Finger	GA	Classic	1.8	0.15
14	49M	Neck	Not given	Classic	3.7	0.18
15	66F	Thigh	GA	Interstitial	3.3	0.16
16	49M	Elbow	Papular eczema	Classic	3.1	0.12
17	49F	Elbow	GA	Classic	2.8	0.10
18	64F	Neck	Inclusion cyst	Classic	5.5	0.29
19	45M	Ear	CNH	Classic	7.2	0.25
20	59M	Neck	None given	Classic	2.6	0.25

Abbreviations: CNH, chondrodermatitis nodularis helicis; *GA,* granuloma annulare; *ND,* not done; *RA,* rheumatoid arthritis.
(Courtesy of Trotter MJ, Crawford RI, O'Connell JX, et al: Mitotic granuloma annulare: A clinicopathologic study of 20 cases. *J Cutan Pathol* 23:537–545. Copyright 1996, Munksgaard International Publishers Ltd., Copenhagen, Denmark.)

men and 11 women; the average patient age was 49 years. A control group of 60 patients was also examined. The clinical appearance of these lesions was indistinguishable from typical localized granuloma annulare. Histologically, a classic palisading granuloma pattern was seen in 18 of 20 cases. The lesions were more cellular than typical granuloma annulare and were located in the mid-dermis. Histiocytes had enlarged nuclei and prominent nucleoli. In the study group, there was a mean of 3.0 mitoses per 10 HPF. In the control group, there was a mean of 0.3 mitoses per 10 HPF. The lesions had occasional atypical mitotic figures. MIB-1 staining confirmed the proliferative nature of these lesions. Positivity for MIB-1 was seen in 5% to 29% of cells.

Discussion.—Histologically, mitotic granuloma annulare must be differentiated from neoplastic processes, especially epithelioid sarcoma. Histiocytes in typical granuloma annulare can have a high mitotic rate. It is important to recognize this variant of granuloma annulare to avoid overdiagnosing of malignant conditions.

▶ The thrust of this article is to bring to attention the fact that granuloma annulare can have mitotic figures in the macrophages present in this lesion. The numbers of mitotic figures varied between 1.0 and 7.2 per HPF in the 20 cases studied; a few cases, not further defined, had atypical mitotic figures. Importantly, 18 of 20 cases had a classic histologic pattern; 2 of 20 had an interstitial pattern. Although it is pointed out that mitoses could lead to confusion with other, malignant lesions—e.g., epithelioid sarcoma—this is generally unlikely.

M.B. Cohen, M.D.

Idiopathic Perniosis and Its Mimics: A Clinical and Histological Study of 38 Cases

Crowson AN, Magro CM (Misericordia Gen Hosp, Winnipeg, Man; Harvard Med School, Cambridge, Mass)
Hum Pathol 28:478–484, 1997   13–14

Background.—The histopathology of perniosis is described as a lymphocytic vascular reaction with variable papillary dermal edema. It has been suggested that it originates as an abnormal response to cold, with resulting ischemia of vessel walls. Systemic lupus erythematosus, Behçet's disease, and other connective tissue diseases may cause acral perniotic lesions that mimic perniosis.

Methods.—Skin biopsies from 38 patients with acral purpuric lesions were examined. The 39 lesions were diagnosed clinically or pathologically as perniosis.

Findings.—In 17 patients, a systemic or extracutaneous disease was established, including systemic lupus erythematosus, antiphospholipid antibodies, viral hepatitis, rheumatoid arthritis, cryofibrinogenemia, hypergammaglobulinemia, iritis, and Crohn's disease. In the other 21 patients,

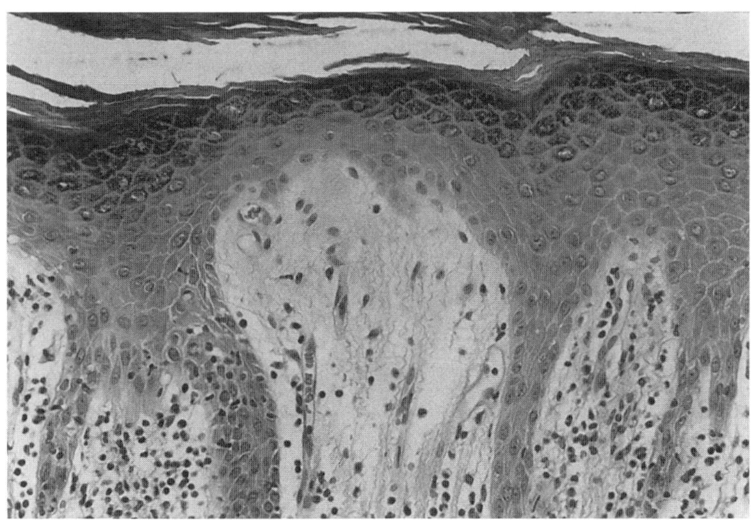

FIGURE 3.—Idiopathic perniosis. Exocytosis of lymphocytes with localization to the retia and acrosyringia with only minimal accompanying epidermal injury. (Courtesy of Crowson AN, Magro CM: Idiopathic perniosis and its mimics: A clinical and histological study of 38 cases. *Hum Pathol* 28:478–484, 1997.)

further studies were done in 12 patients, and a positive antinuclear antibody was detected in 10. In these 21 patients, idiopathic perniosis was diagnosed based on the absence of other serologic markers or signs of a specific systemic disease. Many of these patients had Raynaud's phenomenon, small joint arthralgia, atopy, or a family history of connective tissue disease or Raynaud's disease. Histopathology showed a superficial and deep angiocentric lymphocytic infiltrate with papillary dermal edema and lymphocytic exocytosis into the retia and acrosyringia (Fig 3). In a few cases, a mild vacuolopathic or lichenoid interface dermatitis, adventitial dermal mucinosis, lymphocytic eccrine hidradenitis, vascular ectasia, and thrombosis of dermal papillary capillaries were seen. In patients with iritis, rheumatoid arthritis, or Crohn's disease, biopsy specimens showed a granulomatous vasculitis and a granuloma annulare–like tissue reaction. In patients with systemic lupus erythematosus, cryofibrinogenemia, antiphospholipid antibodies, or hypergammaglobulinemia, biopsy specimens showed an interface dermatitis, superficial and deep angiocentric and eccrinotropic lymphocytic infiltrates, vascular ectasia, and dermal mucinosis with prominent involvement of the eccrine coil.

Discussion.—Among these patients, many did not have features of idiopathic perniosis, for example, those with papillary dermal edema, thrombosis of dermal papillary capillaries, and lymphocytic exocytosis into the retia and acrosyringia. Vascular fibrin deposition involving reticular dermal vessels was seen; it was a significant discriminator of idiopathic perniosis and perniotic lesions with underlying systemic disease. Some of the latter cases were associated with cold exposure and were designated secondary perniosis; other cases were not associated with cold exposure and were designated perniotic mimics based on gross and microscopic lesion morphology.

▶ Perniosis is a cutaneous inflammatory lesion that is associated with cold exposure. Morphologically, there is a superficial and deep lymphocytic infiltrate often associated with dermal edema. In the majority of cases, a systemic underlying disease process—most notably rheumatologic diseases—can be identified. In this study of 38 patients no such disease could be identified, and the term "idiopathic" perniosis has therefore been suggested. Two features thought to be relatively selective for idiopathic perniosis (as opposed to "secondary" perniosis and other mimics of perniosis) were lymphocytic exocytosis to retia and acrosyringia, and the absence of vascular fibrin deposition in reticular dermal vessels. Experience of others will, hopefully, help to confirm these features.

M.B. Cohen, M.D.

Cutaneous Vasculitis in Behçet's Disease: A Clinical and Histopathologic Study of 20 Patients
Chen K-R, Kawahara Y, Miyakawa S, et al (Kawasaki City Hosp, Japan; Keio Univ, Tokyo)
J Am Acad Dermatol 36:689–696, 1997   13–15

Background.—Although small vessel vasculitis is frequent in skin lesions of Behçet's disease (BD), BD is considered a neutrophilic dermatosis. Whether the various cutaneous manifestations of BD are secondary to cutaneous vasculitis was determined.

Methods.—Forty-eight skin biopsy specimens from 42 patients with BD collected between 1980 and 1995 were reviewed. Twenty-three specimens with histologically proved necrotizing vasculitis from 20 patients were further examined.

Findings.—The cutaneous vasculitic manifestations appeared as erythema nodosum-like eruptions, palpable purpura, hemorrhagic blisters, infiltrated erythema, Sweet's syndrome–like eruptions, papulopustular lesions, and extragenital ulcerations. It was common for a patient to have combinations of various skin lesions. Venous vessels were affected in the entire dermis to the subcutis, with sparing of arterial vessels from middermis to subcutis. Histologically, leukocytoclastic vasculitis was seen in 7 patients and lymphocytic vasculitis in 13, with extensive to focal localized fibrinoid necrosis of vessel walls.

Conclusions.—Cutaneous vasculitis associated with BD is mainly venulitis or phlebitis. In the current series, 48% of patients with BD and cutaneous lesions had lymphocytic or leukocytoclastic vasculitis. Behçet's disease should be considered a vasculitis-associated disease separate from the neutrophilic dermatoses.

▶ Behçet's disease is a systemic inflammatory disease process with a propensity for (1) oral and genital ulcerations (and other sites of involvement as well), and (2) Japanese and Middle Eastern men and women. The criteria for diagnosis have been well described.[1, 2] The cutaneous manifestations are quite diverse, and typically this disease is categorized with the neutrophilic dermatoses. This study found that a significant percentage of patients had lymphocytic vasculitis, typically involving the venous system, or leukocytoclastic vasculitis. Consequently, the authors have made a reasonable claim that BD should be considered as a vasculitis-associated disease process and that, in fact, this may be the initiating lesion in cutaneous manifestations of this disease.

M.B. Cohen, M.D.

References

1. International Study Group for Behçet's disease: Criteria for diagnosis of Behçet's disease. *Lancet* 335:1078–1080, 1990.
2. Behçet's Disease Research Committee of Japan: Behçet's disease: Guide to diagnosis of Behçet's disease. *Jpn J Ophthalmol* 18:291–294, 1974.

Histology of Hidradenitis Suppurativa

Jemec GBE, Hansen U (Bispebjerg Hosp, Copenhagen; Univ of Copenhagen)
J Am Acad Dermatol 34:994–999, 1996   13–16

Introduction.—Hidradenitis is sometimes described as an inflammation of the apocrine gland. However, other reports have regarded it as a type of acne inversa involving the pilosebaceous unit, not the apocrine gland. The histologic findings of 60 cases of hiradenitis suppurativa are reported.

Methods.—The analysis included 60 consecutive biopsy specimens from patients with hidradenitis. There were 28 women and 8 men, mean age 33. Thirty-two of the specimens were taken from the groin, 24 from the axilla, 3 from the breast, and 1 from the buttocks. The histologic findings were classified according to predefined criteria and compared with those of control specimens of clinically uninvolved skin from the same regions.

Results.—The histologic classification was poral occlusion in 28% of specimens, simple folliculitis without poral occlusion in 28%, sinus tracts in 15%, epithelial cyst in 10%, abscess in 8%, apocrinitis in 5%, diffuse dermal inflammation in 3%, and pyogenic granuloma and scarring in 2%. Twelve percent of specimens showed secondary involvement of the apocrine glands, whereas 25% showed secondary involvement of the eccrine glands. Sinus tracts were more likely to be present in specimens with poral occlusion or epithelial cysts. Many of the control specimens showed changes similar to those expected in the early stages of follicular involvement. Apocrine glands were more likely to be found in axillary specimens than in groin specimens.

Conclusions.—Lesions with clinical evidence of hidradenitis show a broad range of histologic findings. This heterogeneity may account for the difficulty of treating hidradenitis. It is mainly a follicular disease. Primary involvement of the apocrine glands is found in a minority of cases with axillary involvement. Controls often show low-grade poral occlusion in the regions where hidradenitis typically occurs.

▶ Hidradenitis suppurativa is a disease with many histologic faces, and numerous histologic findings are documented in this study. Jemec and Hansen show that apocrine units are primarily involved in only a minority of lesions and that most cases of hidradenitis suppurativa show predominantly follicular disease. This means you do not need to see apocrine inflammation to make a diagnosis of hidradenitis suppurativa. This work is not without flaws. Hidradenitis suppurativa was classified as having a single predominant disease component (why must this always be the case?), and the component was chosen by flowchart analysis. For the authors, first on the flowchart was the presence of poral occlusion; if a case had this finding, no further dominant classification was made. Lower in the flowchart was appocrinitis. Thus, if a case showed poral occlusion, this feature would be chosen as the dominant component and, naturally, appocrinitis would not be listed as the dominant finding. This bias may have led to fewer cases being classified as appocrinitis. In addition, the authors should have compared clinical duration with histologic findings. The length of time the disease has been present may correlate with the "dominant" histologic finding.

S. Raab, M.D.

Diagnostic Screening of Systemic Amyloidosis by Abdominal Fat Aspiration: An Analysis of 100 Cases
Masouyé I (Univ Hosp, Geneva)
Am J Dermatopathol 19:41–45, 1997   13–17

Background.—Fine-needle aspiration of subcutaneous abdominal fat is a reliable method for the diagnosis of systemic amyloidosis, yielding a sensitivity comparable to that of rectal biopsy, widely considered the method of choice. Although cutaneous lesions are common in patients with systemic amyloidosis, the fine-needle fat aspiration technique has not been reported in dermatologic literature. This study of 100 patients reports results of screening for the disease by fine-needle aspiration of subcutaneous fat and compares results obtained by this technique with those of standard histologic examination of skin biopsies.

Methods.—Congo red staining of abdominal fat aspirates was used for screening the patients, all of whom had symptoms suggestive of systemic amyloidosis. Small fragments of subcutaneous fat obtained by fine-needle aspiration were prepared for staining and interpretation. All samples were analyzed by a dermatopathologist unaware of the patients' disease status. Sixteen of the 100 patients underwent both fat aspiration and cutaneous biopsy within a period of 2 months.

Results.—The patient group of 57 women and 43 men had a mean age of 69 years. Forty-nine patients had a predisposing disease for secondary amyloidosis; other reasons for screening included multiple myeloma or benign monoclonal gammopathy, cardiopathy, and peripheral neuropathy. Subcutaneous aspirates from 9 patients showed a clear, green birefringence of congophilic material at microscopic examination and were considered positive for amyloid. Connective tissue surrounding the fat cells showed amyloid deposits. All 9 patients had clinical features suggestive of amyloid disease. Two patients with negative fat aspirates had biopsy specimens positive for amyloidosis. Results of Congo red staining were concordant in all 16 patients who underwent both abdominal fat aspiration and cutaneous biopsy.

Discussion.—Abdominal fat aspiration had a sensitivity of 82%, a specificity of 100%, and a positive predictive value of 100% in the diagnostic screening for systemic amyloidosis. Because fat aspirates can be inadequate for analysis (as were 5 in this series), the sample should be examined immediately to determine whether the procedure needs to be repeated. The method is recommended for diagnosing primary and secondary amyloidosis and familial amyloid polyneuropathy.

▶ I presume that cytopathologists are well aware that abdominal fat pad aspirations can be used to diagnose amyolidosis. In some centers, dermatopathologists also may obtain aspirates, and if your forte is in cytopathology, you still may have to examine these specimens. This article by Masouyé isn't super, but it does describe the appropriate staining techniques. I believe the performance data (e.g., sensitivity and specificity) reported by Masouyé are biased and, therefore, are probably too high.[1, 2] For example, the sensitivity is reported as 82%, but good follow up data were lacking in 66% of the cases. Also, the histology was used as the gold standard but, as Masouyé readily admits, histologic specimens lacked perfect sensitivity and specificity. Masouyé does review some of the literature relating to the previously described sensitivity of abdominal fine-needle aspiration for different types of amyloidosis, and this review is helpful.

One problem that I think is relatively common, and which was not addressed in this study, was that abdominal fine-needle aspiration for amyloid often does not yield binary (positive or negative) results. Frequently, we see cases that are "suspicious" for amyloidosis. What should be done in these cases? This difficulty should be better addressed.

S. Raab, M.D.

References

1. Klemi PJ, Sorsa S, Happonen RP: Fine needle aspiration biopsy from subcutaneous fat: An easy way to diagnose secondary amyloidosis. *Scand J Rheumatol* 16:429–431, 1987.
2. Duston MA, Skinner M, Meenan RF, et al: Sensitivity, specificity and predictive value of abdominal fat aspiration for the diagnosis of amyloidosis. *Arthritis Rheum* 32:82–85, 1989.

14 Cardiovascular System

A Histopathologic Grading System of Hyperacute (Humoral, Antibody-mediated) Cardiac Xenograft and Allograft Rejection
Rose AG, Cooper DKC (Univ of Minnesota, St Paul, Minn; Baptist Med Ctr, Oklahoma City, Okla)
J Heart Lung Transplant 15:804–817, 1996   14–1

Background.—There are many grading systems for histologic evaluation of acute cellular rejection in cardiac allografts. There is no formal grading system for hyperacute rejection based on a review of experimental and clinical data. If xenografting becomes feasible in clinical practice, it will be imperative to have a grading system of hyperacute rejection that is clinically relevant and reproducible.

Methods.—The histologic sections from 112 hearts were examined. Of the 109 experimental and 3 clinical xenografts, 44 were discordant xenografts, 41 were concordant xenografts, and 27 were allografts. The histopathologic features and clinical data were documented and analyzed.

TABLE 3.—Histologic Grading of Hyperacute Rejection of the Heart

Grade A
  Stage 1: Initial (mild)
    Myocardium appears normal apart from:
      Venular thrombi
      Swelling of capillary endothelial cells
  Stage 2: Intermediate (moderate)
    All of the above plus:
      Interstitial edema
      Congestion, sludging of erythrocytes in capillaries
      Scanty capillary thrombi
  Stage 3: Late (severe)
    All of the above plus:
      Disruption of capillaries subtended by thrombosed venules: interstitial hemorrhage*
      Areas of myocyte necrosis†
      Intravascular thrombi are more evident, including the small arteries‡
      Acute neutrophilic vasculitis of small arteries and arterioles may rarely occur
Grade B: Mixed hyperacute and acute cellular rejection
  Focal aggregates of lymphocytes are present within the edematous, hemorrhagic interstitium

*Neutrophils in interstitium are in proportion to the extravasated erythrocytes.
†Coagulative and/or myocytolytic necrosis and/or contraction banding of myocytes.
‡Some thrombi may show signs of organization in delayed vascular rejection.
(Courtesy of Rose AG, Cooper DKC: A histologic grading system of hyperacute [humoral, antibody-mediated] cardiac xenograft and allograft rejection. *J Heart Lung Tranplant* 15:804–817, 1996.)

Results.—A grading system was developed that allowed each sample to be placed in 1 of 2 categories: grade A, unmodified hyperacute rejection, or grade B, mixed hyperacute and acute cellular rejection. Grades A and B were subdivided into 3 stages of mild (initial), moderate (intermediate), and severe (late) rejection (Table 3).

Discussion.—Hyperacute and delayed hyperacute rejection have the same basic pathologic features, but differ in rapidity of onset. Mixed acute cellular and hyperacute rejection is pathologically separate and is produced when 2 pathologic forms of rejection overlap. Although histologic grading systems evolve with new knowledge and therapy, it is unlikely that the main histopathologic features would change in the short term once xenografting is feasible in clinical practice. This histologic grading system is proposed as a basis for meaningful pathologic evaluation of hyperacute rejection.

▶ The goal of this study was to develop a grading scheme for humoral/antibody-mediated/vascular cardiac rejection. Most of the work was based on experimental studies of xenografts, both concordant (e.g., monkey to baboon) and discordant (e.g., pig to baboon); 2 clinical allografts and 2 clinical xenografts were also included. The proposed grading system (Table 3) provides a pathologic basis for evaluation of hyperacute rejection.

M.B. Cohen, M.D.

Influence of Acute or Chronic Rejection on Myocardial Collagen Density in Serial Endomyocardial Biopsy Specimens From Cardiac Allografts

Fornes P, Heudes D, Simon D, et al (Broussais Hôpital, Paris; Univ. of California, San Francisco)
J Heart Lung Transplant 15:796–803, 1996   14–2

Background.—More than 60% of patients who have heart transplantation can expect to live at least 5 years, but the long-term changes that can occur in the transplanted heart are not entirely known. Myocardial fibrosis is a major structural change that can adversely affect long-term cardiac function. It is unclear if myocardial fibrosis is caused by cyclosporine, prolonged donor heart ischemic time, or acute or chronic rejection. Myocardial collagen content in multiple biopsy specimens has not been investigated in studies with a long-term follow-up.

Methods.—Light microscopic computer-assisted morphometry was used to examine collagen density in 200 right ventricular endomyocardial biopsy specimens from 21 patients who had heart transplantation. The patients were divided into 2 groups: group 1 had 11 patients with no chronic rejection and group 2 had 10 patients with chronic rejection. The groups were divided into subgroups according to the highest grade of acute rejection during follow-up. The mean follow-up was 36 months.

Results.—Relatively little variation in serial determinations of myocardial collagen density was seen in patients with no chronic rejection. In patients with chronic rejection, there was no increase in myocardial collagen density during prechronic or chronic phases. No consistent relationship was seen between myocardial collagen density and severity of acute rejection in either group. In both groups, occasional highly elevated values for myocardial collagen density were seen. These values were significantly higher than the serial determinations and generally resulted from scars; interstitial or perivascular fibrosis was not detected.

Discussion.—These findings showed no consistent relationship between acute or chronic rejection and myocardial collagen density. Some specimens had occasional high collagen density resulting from scar fibrosis, indicating previous myocyte damage. It is unclear if acute or chronic rejection or prolonged donor heart ischemic time is responsible. It is recommended that at least 4 separate biopsy specimens be obtained because of the small size and sparse distribution of scars. It is also recommended that multiple sections from each specimen be examined so that focal lesions are not missed.

▶ As more patients undergo cardiac transplantation, the evaluation of right ventricular endomyocardial biopsies will not remain in the "ivory tower"; currently, the 5-year survival rate is about 60%. In this study, 21 patients, most of whom had cardiomyopathies, were studied for an average of 3 years, and the 200 corresponding specimens were examined for collagen density. Collagen deposition may result from a number of causes, including drug therapy and rejection. The 2 important conclusions from this study are: (1) the severity of acute rejection episodes did not correlate with myocardial fibrosis, and (2) patients with chronic rejection were no more likely to have myocardial fibrosis (than those without chronic rejection). These results should help the pathologist evaluate such biopsies from long-term heart transplant patients.

M.B. Cohen, M.D.

Calcified Amorphous Tumor of the Heart (Cardiac CAT)

Reynolds C, Tazelaar HD, Edwards WD (Mayo Clinic, Rochester, Minn)
Hum Pathol 26:601–606, 1997   14–3

Background.—Nonneoplastic cardiac masses are rare and have generally been reported as "pseudotumors." These masses can mimic common forms of heart disease and true neoplasms. Most of the reported pseudotumors have represented organized thrombi. In a few reports of cardiac lesions with marked calcification, the masses were assumed to be thrombi.

Methods.—Eleven cases of intracardiac masses initially diagnosed as pseudotumor were reviewed. Each mass was considered neoplastic because of its clinical characteristics. Each patient's clinical history was reviewed and follow-up information was obtained.

Results.—The masses occurred in 7 women and 4 men who had a mean age of 52 years. The patients had a variety of symptoms and underlying diseases. In 6 of 8 patients who had echocardiography, the lesions were diagnosed as a primary cardiac neoplasm. Ten patients had surgical excision and 1 patient died of noncardiac causes 30 days after the mass was detected. On gross examination, the lesions were firm, yellow-white, partially calcified, and occurred in any of the 4 chambers. On microscopic examination, the lesions were characterized by nodular calcium in a background of degenerating blood elements and chronic inflammation. These lesions were benign in all patients. Two patients had repeat echocardiography that showed residual calcium in the region of the initial tumor.

Discussion.—These lesions may represent calcified thrombi, but their clinical characteristics do not suggest thrombosis. The name "calcified amorphous tumors" (cardiac CAT) is proposed to describe these nonneoplastic cardiac masses based on their clinical presentation and microscopic appearance.

▶ This article describes a very unusual cardiac tumor, calcified amorphous tumor (CAT), which is best viewed as a pseudotumor because it appears to be nonneoplastic. Its origin remains enigmatic. In this series of 11 cases, the histopathologic findings are well outlined. The findings, noted in the abstract, were quite uniform among all the cases. These tumors have also been termed rocks, thrombus, and mimics of myxoma. Although the tumor is rare, pathologists should be aware of this entity.

M.B. Cohen, M.D.

Apoptosis in Myocytes in End-Stage Heart Failure
Narula J, Haider N, Virmani R, et al (Harvard Med School, Boston; Northeastern Univ, Boston; Armed Forces Inst of Pathology, Washington, DC)
N Engl J Med 335:1182–1189, 1996   14–4

Background.—Heart failure can result from a variety of causes. However, the cellular mechanisms responsible for the progressive deterioration of myocardial function are unclear. Heart failure may involve apoptosis, or programmed cell death.

Methods.—Seven explanted hearts were obtained from patients with severe chronic heart failure undergoing heart transplantation and examined for evidence of apoptosis. Four had idiopathic dilated cardiomyopathy, and 3 had ischemic cardiomyopathy. DNA fragmentation, an indicator of apoptosis, was identified histochemically by in situ end-labeling and agarose-gel electrophoresis of end-labeled DNA. Myocardial tissue from 4 patients who had had a myocardial infarction 1–2 days earlier served as positive controls for the end-labeling assessments. Heart tissue from 4 patients who died in motor vehicle accidents was used as negative controls.

Findings.—Histochemical evidence of DNA fragmentation was found in all 4 hearts from patients with idiopathic dilated cardiomyopathy and from 1 heart with ischemic cardiomyopathy. All 4 samples from the patients with dilated cardiomyopathy also showed DNA laddering, a feature of apoptosis, which was not present in any of the tissue from patients with ischemic cardiomyopathy. Apoptosis was evident in the central necrotic zone of acute myocardial infarcts but not in myocardium that was remote from the infarcted zone. Rare isolated apoptotic myocytes were noted in myocardium from the persons who had died in accidents.

Conclusions.—These findings support the hypothesis that apoptosis is one mechanism leading to end-stage heart disease. Additional research is needed to establish the prevalence of apoptosis and its role in the progression of myocardial hypertrophy to overt heart failure. Though apoptosis appears to be irreversible, it may be modulated by growth factors or cytokines.

▶ Since the original recognition of apoptosis (programmed cell death) as a unique form of cell death in the early 1970s, interest has increased exponentially into its molecular mechanisms and its clinical importance in development and disease. In this report, 7 explanted hearts were examined to determine if apoptosis played a role in the failing heart. Using several techniques to assay apoptosis, including DNA laddering, the authors found that 4 of 4 hearts with idiopathic dilated cardiomyopathy and 1 of 3 hearts with ischemic cardiomyopathy show evidence of apoptosis. Their conclusion, which is eminently reasonable, is that myocyte loss may be due to apoptosis and contribute to progressive heart failure. Thus, ischemic necrosis may not be the only mechanism.

M.B. Cohen, M.D.

Secondary Pericardial Malignancies: A Critical Appraisal of the Role of Cytology, Pericardial Biopsy, and DNA Ploidy Analysis
Bardales RH, Stanley MW, Schaefer RF, et al (John L. McClellan Mem Veterans Hosp, Little Rock, Ark; Univ of Arkansas, Little Rock; Montefiore Med Ctr, Bronx, NY)
Am J Clin Pathol 106:29–34, 1996   14–5

Background.—The value of pericardial fluid cytology has been noted. With few exceptions, series are affected by the small number of malignant cases studied, lack of histologic correlation, or lack of detailed statistical interpretation. Further, it is difficult to determine the role of ploidy analysis in pericardial effusions because there are few reported cases.

Methods.—There were 112 pericardial fluid specimens from 63 men and 33 women. The patients were between 14 and 82 years old. Of the 112 specimens, 45 were malignant and 67 were benign. Cytologic analysis was done in 112 specimens, histologic analysis was done in 61 specimens, and ploidy analysis was done in 34 specimens.

Results.—In 41 patients with malignancy, the primary site was known in 34 patients, but unknown in 3 patients. The initial diagnosis was obtained by pericardial cytology in 4 patients. All cytologic and histologic specimens were reviewed, and 7 cases of true discrepancy were detected; 6 of these had positive cytologic findings. These discrepancies resulted from tissue biopsy sampling error. There was a correlation between DNA diploidy obtained by flow cytometry and benign cytology. In 32 of 34 cases, aneuploidy correlated with malignant cytology. Diploid DNA was seen in cytologic malignant effusions in 2 of 10 cases.

Discussion.—The most important parameter in evaluating secondary pericardial malignancy is cytology, which should be considered the diagnostic gold standard. Because false negative cytologic diagnoses can result from scant cellularity and obscuring blood, careful screening is critical. Routine use of flow cytometric DNA analysis is not recommended because of its low sensitivity.

▶ This article culls the experience of 2 institutions for analyzing both histologic and cytologic pericardial specimens. Sixty-one paired specimens were included in the study, but cytology was superior to biopsy for establishing a diagnosis of malignancy, most of which were metastatic lung carcinomas. Cytology did "miss" some of the cases and these were most often attributable to scant cellularity (6 cases) and obscuring blood (5). The authors also included DNA ploidy analysis in their study. This I believe is more of academic interest and is not in routine use in most laboratories, including our own, particularly given the financial challenges facing contemporary health care delivery. The authors' conclusion about this was: "Flow cytometric DNA ploidy analysis of pericardial fluid for detecting carcinoma does not meet high expectations."

M.B. Cohen, M.D.

Spiraled Collagen in the Major Blood Vessels
Ishii T, Asuwa N (Toho Univ, Tokyo; Tokyo Med College)
Mod Pathol 9:843–848, 1996   14–6

Background.—Spiraled collagen is a morphological form of collagen fibril and has been detected in mesenchymal tissues. It has also been detected in the vascular system in vasculopathies caused by atherosclerosis, aneurysm in Marfan's syndrome, arteritis, Buerger's disease, diabetic angiopathy, and varix of various blood vessels, and in major blood vessels under normal conditions. The morphogenesis of spiraled collagen has not been determined and is complicated by a lack of comprehensive data of spiraled collagen under normal and pathologic conditions in various blood vessels.

Methods.—In 45 autopsies, vascular spiraled collagen was examined by electron microscope and immunohistochemical methods in anatomically corresponding pairs of the major arteries and veins under normal and pathologic conditions. The frequency and extent of spiraled collagen in the arteries and veins were compared.

Results.—Spiraled collagen was noted especially in the left anterior descending coronary artery under a myocardial bridge free from atherosclerosis. This contrasted with sites in the nonbridged vessel, which is always involved in atherosclerosis. Spiraled collagen was evident in the normal great saphenous vein compared to the phlebosclerotic vessel. The diameter of spiraled collagen increased with age. The cellular components around the spiraled collagen were often contractile-type smooth muscle cells with a round or oval nucleus, abundant myofibril, and few organelles (Fig 3). There was significant expression of matrix metalloproteinase-1 in smooth muscle cells of vascular wall with abundant spiraled collagen. Tissue inhibitor of matrix metalloproteinase-1 was not seen in smooth muscle cells regardless of presence of spiraled collagen.

Discussion.—These findings and the common association of spiraled collagen with degraded elastic fibers and contractile-type smooth muscle cells suggest that normal collagen fibrils are degraded at extracellular spaces by interstitial enzymes, but that cellular activities of contractile-type smooth muscle cells remain stationary during aging. Spiraled collagen is

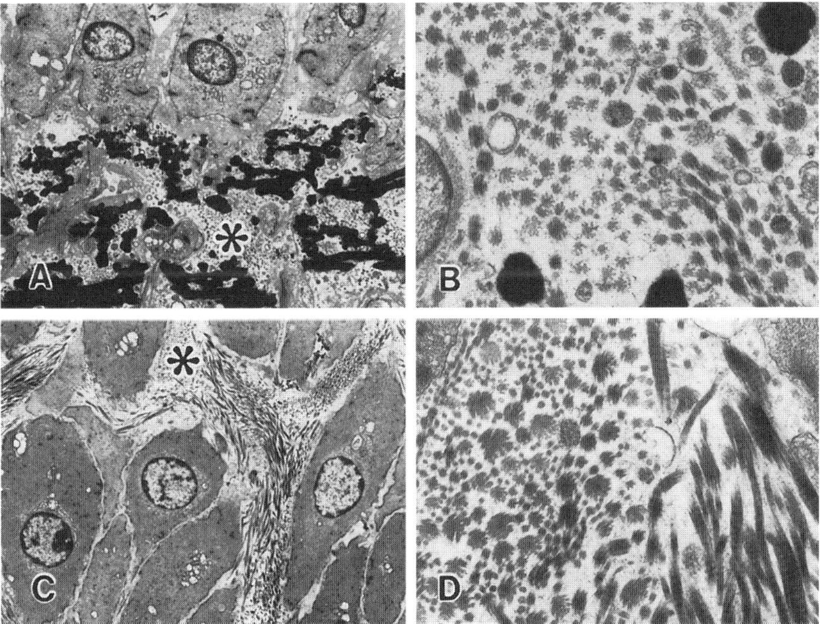

FIGURE 3.—A, bridged left anterior descending coronary artery. All smooth muscle cells in the intima adjacent to internal elastic lamina exhibit contractile-type features; original magnification, ×3,000. **B,** higher magnification of a part marked with an *asterisk* in **A**. Numerous typical spiraled collagens are shown within internal elastic lamina; original magnification, ×25,000. **C,** great saphenous vein. Contractile-type smooth muscle cells are also shown in the media of the great saphenous vein; original magnification, ×3000. **D,** higher magnification of a part marked with an *asterisk*. Cross-sections and longitudinal sections of spiraled collagen are abundantly demonstrated; original magnification, ×25,000. (Courtesy of Ishii T, Asuwa N: Spiraled collagen in the major blood vessels. *Mod Pathol* 9[8]:843–848, 1996.)

formed preferentially in normal blood vessels by degradation of normal collagen fibrils.

▶ Spiraled collagen, which is recognized at the ultrastructural level, is a form of collagen fibril with a unique appearance that has been associated with a number of disease entities. This report adds to that literature by examining a number of paired vessels from 45 patients (age range, 1–88 years). Spiraled collagen was more prevalent in veins, principally located in the media and adventitia, associated with matrix metalloproteinases, and probably part of a normal physiologic process.

M.B. Cohen, M.D.

15 Hematolymphoid System

A Clinical Evaluation of the International Lymphoma Study Group Classification of Non-Hodgkin's Lymphoma
Armitage JO, for the Non-Hodgkin's Lymphoma Classification Project (Univ of Nebraska, Omaha)
Blood 89:3909–3918, 1997
15–1

Purpose.—Advances in immunology and genetics have permitted the identification of several previously unrecognized varieties of lymphoma, including mantle cell lymphoma, monocytoid B-cell lymphoma, extranodal lymphoma of mucosa-associated lymphoid tissue, splenic marginal zone lymphoma, primary mediastinal large B-cell lymphoma, and anaplastic large-cell lymphoma and other T-cell lymphomas. These discoveries have led to proposed modifications of lymphoma classification by the International Lymphoma Study Group (ILSG) (Table 1). However, the clinical relevance of the new classification is so far unknown. A clinical evaluation of the ILSG classification of non-Hodgkin's lymphoma (NHL) is reported.

Methods.—The analysis included 1,403 cases of NHL collected at 9 sites worldwide. All patients were consecutively seen and previously untreated. Each patient underwent a standardized clinical and histologic analysis, along with immunophenotyping. Classification according to the proposed ILSG system was by consensus of a team of expert hematopathologists. The classification results were then rereviewed and compared with the clinical data.

Results.—Of the "new" lymphoma types, the ones most frequently recognized were marginal zone B-cell lymphoma of the mucosa-associated lymphoid tissue (MALT) type, with a frequency of 7.6%; mantle cell lymphoma, 6.0%; primary mediastinal large B-cell lymphoma, 2.4%; and anaplastic large T/null-cell lymphoma, 2.4% (Table 3). Approximately 97% of cases were specifically classified with the new system. Percent agreement among the experts varied. For example, agreement was just 53% for high-grade B-cell Burkitt-like tumors, and 86% for marginal zone B-cell lymphomas of MALT. When the cases were rereviewed by the

TABLE 1.—International Lymphoma Study Group Classification (Including Provisional Categories)

B-Cell Lymphoma	T/NK-Cell Lymphoma	Others
Precursor B-lymphoblastic	Precursor T-lymphoblastic	Composite lymphoma (types specified)†
Small lymphocytic (CLL)	T-cell chronic lymphocytic leukemia	Malignant lymphoma, unclassifiable low grade
Lymphoplasmacytic	Large granular lymphocyte leukemia	Malignant lymphoma unclassifiable high grade
Mantle cell	Mycosis fungoides	Malignant lymphoma, unclassifiable
Follicle center, follicular	Peripheral T cell, unspecified	
*Grade 1**	*Medium-sized*	Hodgkin's disease
*Grade 2**	*Mixed medium and large cell*	Diagnosis other than lymphoma
*Grade 3**	*Large cell*	Case unclassifiable
Follicle center diffuse, small cell	*Lymphoepithelioid*	
Marginal zone B-cell, MALT type	*Hepatosplenic*	
Marginal zone B-cell, nodal	*Subcutaneous panniculitic*	
Marginal zone B-cell, splenic	Angioimmunoblastic	
Hairy cell leukemia	Angiocentric, nasal	
Plasmacytoma	Intestinal	
Diffuse large B-cell	Adult T-cell lymphoma/leukemia	
Diffuse mediastinal large B-cell	Anaplastic large cell (including null phenotype)	
Burkitt's	*Anaplastic large cell, Hodgkin's-like*	
High grade B-cell, Burkitt-like	Unclassifiable low grade	
Unclassifiable low grade	Unclassifiable high grade	
Unclassifiable high grade		

Note: Provisional categories are indicated in italic type.

*Follicular lymphomas are designated as such and were graded according to the Berard method.[90]

†Composite lymphomas consisted of two distinctly different cytologic subtypes of lymphoma. Data from Harris et al.[84]

Abbreviations: CLL, chronic lymphocytic leukemia; *MALT,* mucosal-associated lymphoid tissue.

(Courtesy of Armitage JO, for the Non-Hodgkin's Lymphoma Classification Project: A clinical evaluation of the international lymphoma study group classification of non-Hodgkin's lymphoma. *Blood* 89:3909–3918, 1997.)

TABLE 3.—Distribution of NHL Cases by the Consensus Diagnosis

Consensus Diagnosis	No. of Cases	% of Total Cases
Diffuse large B-cell	422	30.6
Follicular	304	22.1
Grade 1	131	9.5
Grade 2	85	6.2
Grade 3	88	6.4
Marginal zone B-cell, MALT	105	7.6
Peripheral T-cell	96	7.0
Medium-sized, mixed, and large	51	3.7
Angiocentric, nasal	19	1.4
Angioimmunoblastic	17	1.2
Intestinal	5	<1
Lymphoepithelioid	2	<1
Hepatosplenic	1	<1
Adult T-cell leukemia/lymphoma	1	<1
Small B-lymphocytic (CLL)	93	6.7
Mantle cell	83	6.0
Primary mediastinal large B-cell	33	2.4
Anaplastic large T/null-cell	33	2.4
High grade B-cell, Burkitt-like	29	2.1
Marginal zone B-cell, nodal	25	1.8
Precursor T-lymphoblastic	23	1.7
Lymphoplasmacytoid	16	1.2
Marginal zone B-cell, splenic	11	<1
Mycosis fungoides	11	<1
Burkitt's	10	<1
All other types	84	6.1

Abbreviation: CLL, chronic lymphocytic leukemia.

(Courtesy of Armitage JO, for the Non-Hodgkin's Lymphoma Classification Project: A clinical evaluation of the international lymphoma study group classification of non-Hodgkin's lymphoma. *Blood* 89:3909–3918, 1997.)

experts, only 6% were classified differently than in the original classification.

Clinically, marginal zone B-cell lymphoma of MALT type showed a high frequency of localized extranodal disease and prolonged survival rate. In contrast, nodal marginal zone B-cell lymphoma at an advanced stage had poor survival rate. Mantle cell lymphoma affected mostly men, often in an advanced stage with bone marrow involvement, and had poor 5-year survival. Young women were more likely to have primary mediastinal large B-cell lymphoma, which was often of low stage but did not have any better survival rate than other diffuse large B-cell lymphomas. Young patients were most likely to have anaplastic large T/null-cell lymphoma, with surprisingly good 5-year survival. Average 5-year survival was better than 70% for follicular lymphoma, marginal zone B-cell lymphoma of MALT type, and anaplastic large T/null-cell lymphoma; between 50% and 75% for small lymphocytic, lymphoplasmacytoid, and nodal marginal zone B-cell lymphoma; 30% to 49% for diffuse large B-cell, primary mediastinal large B-cell, and high-grade B-cell Burkitt-like and Burkitt lymphomas; and less than 30% for peripheral T-cell, precursor T-lymphoblastic, and mantle cell lymphoma.

Conclusions.—This clinical evaluation shows that the new ILSG classification identifies clinically relevant subtypes of NHL. For purposes of clinical decision making, the histologic diagnosis of NHL must be compared with the prognostic factors of the International Prognostic Factor index. For some major lymphoma types, immunophenotyping makes an important contribution to the accuracy of diagnosis.

▶ The usefulness of the International Lymphoma Study Group Classification of non-Hodgkin's lymphoma (revised European-American Classification of Lymphoid Neoplasms) is examined in this study and received passing marks, living up to its intention of defining distinct clinicopathologic entities. The study demonstrates how immunophenotyping studies allow better recognition of categories such as mantle cell lymphoma, precursor T-lymphoblastic lymphoma, anaplastic large-cell lymphomas, and peripheral T-cell lymphomas. In these days of cost containment, the study demonstrates which entities may be reliably diagnosed on morphology alone, such as follicular lymphoma and most small lymphocytic lymphomas. The study also highlights the disorders that are difficult to classify with the current definitions, such as lymphoplasmacytoid lymphoma and high-grade B-cell Burkitt-like lymphoma. The grading of follicular lymphomas also remains problematic.

Importantly, the study shows the usefulness of subclassifying the new categories of lymphoma with regard to clinical outcome and in some categories showed surprising information. For example, anaplastic large-cell lymphoma had an overall 5-year survival greater than other large cell lymphomas or other types of peripheral T-cell lymphomas. The study provides clinicians with useful information gathered by comparing the International Prognostic Index[1] with the specific types of lymphoma.

J.F. Turner, Jr., M.D.

Reference

1. The International Non-Hodgkin's Lymphoma Prognostic Factors Project: A predictive model for aggressive non-Hodgkin's lymphoma. *N Engl J Med* 329:987–994, 1993.

Subclassification of Diffuse Large B-Cell Lymphomas According to the Kiel Classification: Distinction of Centroblastic and Immunoblastic Lymphomas Is a Significant Prognostic Risk Factor
Engelhard M, Brittinger G, Huhn D, et al (Universitätsklinikum Essen, Germany; Humboldt-Universität, Berlin, Germany; Städtische Kliniken, Duisburg, Germany, et al)
Blood 89:2291–2297, 1997

15–2

Background.—The updated Kiel classification identified 3 major subtypes of diffuse large B-cell lymphomas: centroblastic (CB), B-immunoblastic (B-IB), and B large-cell anaplastic or anaplastic large cell (B-ALC). However, the International Lymphoma Study Group combines these 3 subtypes into a single category of diffuse large B-cell lymphomas, partially because of problems with reproducibility. The clinical relevance of the 3 subtypes of large B-cell lymphomas was investigated.

Methods.—The analysis was based on a prospective, randomized, multicenter trial in 219 adult patients with untreated Ann Arbor stage II to IV high-grade malignant non-Hodgkin's lymphomas. In each case, the diagnosis was confirmed by histomorphologic evaluation with Giemsa stain and by immunohistochemistry. Treatment was with the COP-BLAM/ IMVP-16 regimen in combination, with or without adjuvant radiotherapy, for complete responders. The patients were classified according to the updated Kiel classification, the prognostic relevance of which was assessed. The CB tumors were composed of sheets of typical centroblasts; the B-IB lymphomas consisted of sheets of large immunoblasts; and the B-ALC lymphomas had larger and more irregular tumor cells with less basophilic cytoplasm. Median follow-up in survivors was 3.5 years.

Results.—The subtype diagnosis was CB in 75% of cases, B-IB in 15%, and B-ALC in 10%. Patients with CB lymphoma had a better prognosis than patients with B-ALC, who had a better prognosis than those with B-IB. There was a similar pattern of relapse-free survival. Multivariate analyses—including the risk factors of the International Index—confirmed the differences in prognosis between CB and B-IB. Patients with B-IB tended to be men with lower performance status, more advanced and active disease, and a higher incidence of skin or skeleton infiltration. Bone marrow involvement was more frequent with CB lymphomas. The pattern of differences was similar for B-ALC lymphomas, except for the male predominance.

Conclusions.—The subtypes of diffuse large B-cell lymphomas defined in the updated Kiel classification are of clinical prognostic relevance. The differences suggest inherent biologic differences between these entities, possibly genetically determined. Placing all subtypes into one common category will miss patients who might benefit from early intensified therapy.

▶ A brief translating statement is in order. In the Kiel classification, centroblasts are the equivalent to large, noncleaved cells in the Working Formulation. Immunoblasts are described similarly in both classifications, with the exception of the cytoplasm being described as deeply basophilic in the Kiel classification. This is from the routine use of the Giemsa stain by European hematopathologists. On H and E stained sections, the cytoplasm appears eosinophilic or amphophilic.

This paper lends support for separating immunoblastic lymphoma from other diffuse, large B-cell lymphomas. However, this distinction may be difficult, as authors of the revised European-American classification of lymphoid neoplasms have demonstrated in a small reproducibility study. Lack of reproducibility in distinguishing these neoplasms may be from the lack of a precise definition of what constitutes a majority of immunoblasts. Is it >50%, or should it be >90%, as is being proposed in the upcoming World Health Organization classification of neoplastic diseases of hematopoietic and lymphoid tissues? The 90% figure will certainly eliminate many borderline cases and make the diagnosis of immunoblastic lymphoma a less frequent diagnosis. Finding sheets of immunoblasts, as reported in this paper, seems a helpful feature for defining immunoblastic lymphoma.

Separation of anaplastic large-cell lymphomas of B-cell lineage from immunoblastic lymphoma also can be difficult. However, recognition of the often sinusoidal growth pattern of the pleomorphic cells in anaplastic large-cell lymphoma helps distinguish these categories of lymphoma. The anaplastic cells should be CD30 positive. However, CD30 staining cannot be used alone in making the diagnosis of anaplastic large-cell lymphoma because other types of large B-cell lymphomas with nonanaplastic morphology may be positive.

J.F. Turner, Jr., M.D.

Suggested Reading

Harris NL, Jaffe ES, Stein H, et al: A revised European-American classification of lymphoid neoplasms: A proposal from the International Lymphoma Study Group. *Blood* 84:1361, 1994.

Jaffe ES, Berard CW, Dibold J, et al: Proposed World Health Organization classification of neoplastic diseases of hematopoietic and lymphoid tissues. *Am J Surg Pathol* 21:114–121, 1997.

Lennert K, Feller AC: Histopathology of non-Hodgkin's lymphomas (based on the updated Kiel classification), ed 2. New York, Springer-Verlag, 1990.

Marginal Zone Lymphoma (Low-grade B-cell Lymphoma of Mucosa-Associated Lymphoid Tissue Type) of Skin and Subcutaneous Tissue: A Study of 15 Patients
Bailey EM, Ferry JA, Harris NL, et al (Massachusetts Gen Hosp, Boston; Albany Med Ctr, NY; Brigham and Women's Hosp, Boston, et al)
Am J Surg Pathol 20:1011–1023, 1996   15–3

Purpose.—Low-grade B-cell lymphoma of mucosa-associated lymphoid tissue (MALT) has been reported in various extranodal locations, including the stomach, salivary gland, thyroid, orbit, lung and trachea, breast, kidney, prostate, gallbladder, and cervix. The MALT-type lymphomas tend to respond to local therapy and remain localized; when they spread, other mucosal sites are often involved. Although low-grade B-cell MALT-type lymphoma is relatively rare among cutaneous lymphomas, it accounts for as many as one fourth of primary cutaneous B-cell lymphomas. Fifteen cases of low-grade B-cell MALT-type lymphoma involving the skin and subcutaneous tissue are described.

Patients.—All patients had a histologic diagnosis of MALT-type lymphoma that involved the skin or subcutaneous tissue at some time. There were 7 patients with primary MALT-type lymphoma of the skin or subcutaneous tissues; all had cutaneous or subcutaneous nodules of the trunk or head and neck. The 5 men and 2 women in this group had a median age of 53 years; the skin was involved in 6 cases and the subcutaneous tissue in 1. At a median follow-up of 36 months, 6 patients were disease free and 1 was alive with disease.

Three patients had concurrent MALT-type lymphoma of both the subcutaneous tissue and extracutaneous sites. There were 2 women and 1 man, median age 57 years. The extracutaneous sites included the lung, breast, orbit, lymph node, and bone marrow. All patients in this group had relapsed or recurrent disease.

Secondary involvement of the skin or subcutaneous tissue by MALT-type lymphoma was identified in 5 patients. This group included 4 women and 1 man, median age 63 years. The primary tumor was of the ocular adnexa in 3 patients and the parotid gland in 2. All patients in this group had relapses involving the skin or subcutaneous tissue, parotid gland, lacrimal gland, breast, and lymph nodes. All patients were alive at follow-up of at least 5 years—2 with disease and 3 without.

Findings.—Regardless of type, each case showed the histologic characteristics of low-grade B-cell lymphoma of MALT type. Marginal zone cells (centrocyte-like or monocytoid B-cells) were found in all 15 cases, and plasmacytic differentiation in 10 of 15. Ten cases showed reactive germinal centers, and 3 had Dutcher bodies. Pan B-cell antigens and monotypic immunoglobulin were expressed in all cases.

Conclusions.—Primary or secondary low-grade B-cell lymphomas of the MALT type may involve the skin or subcutaneous tissue. These tumors, found most frequently in middle-aged to older women, generally permit extended survival despite multiple extranodal relapses. Among patients with primary skin or subcutaneous B-cell MALT-type lymphomas, prolonged disease-free survival is more likely for those without extracutaneous spread at presentation. Differentiation of these tumors from reactive lymphoid infiltrate or "pseudolymphoma" is aided by immunohistochemical stains showing light-chain restriction.

▶ Although this study is based on a small series of patients, it is one of the first to describe the clinicopathologic findings of patients with cutaneous MALT-type lymphomas as defined in the revised European-American Lymphoma Classification of Lymphoid Neoplasms. The lymphoma shares morphologic and clinical features with MALT-type lymphomas of other sites.

The equivalent of lymphoepithelial lesions in the more common gastric MALT-type lymphoma were "epithelial-infiltrating lymphocytes" of the pilosebaceous units. Rather than a lymphocytic infiltrate of the epidermis, a Grenz zone was noted. Interestingly, when the lymphocytic infiltrate was concentrated in the subcutaneous tissue, these patients had other extranodal sites of MALT-type lymphoma.

Differentiation of MALT-type lymphomas from lymphoid hyperplasia (pseudolymphomas) may be difficult. However, finding sheets of monocytoid B-cells is the most helpful morphologic feature in suggesting the diagnosis of MALT-type lymphoma. In many cases, demonstration of monoclonality is ultimately needed for the diagnosis of MALT-type lymphoma.

J.F. Turner, Jr., M.D.

Suggested Reading

LeBoit PE, McNutt NS, Reed JA, et al: Primary cutaneous immunocytoma: A B-cell lymphoma that can easily be mistaken for cutaneous lymphoid hyperplasia. *Am J Surg Pathol* 18:969–978, 1994.

Willemze R, Kerl H, Sterry W, et al: EORTC classification for primary cutaneous lymphomas: A proposal from the cutaneous lymphoma study group of the European Organization for Research and Treatment of Cancer. *Blood* 90:354–371, 1997.

Lymphocyte-Predominant Hodgkin's Disease: An Immunohistochemical Analysis of 208 Reviewed Hodgkin's Disease Cases From the German Hodgkin Study Group
von Wasielewski R, Werner M, Fischer R, et al (Pathologische Institute der Medizinische Hochschule Hannover, Germany; Universität Köln, Germany; Universität Frankfurt, Germany; et al)
Am J Pathol 150:793–803, 1997   15–4

Introduction.—Lymphocyte predominance Hodgkin's disease (LPHD) is generally considered a distinct entity of B-cell origin. However, previous studies of LPHD have yielded inconsistent immunophenotyping results and low confirmation rates. These findings raise questions about whether LPHD is an entity with varying marker profiles or a mixture of morphologically similar entities. This study evaluated whether the diagnosis of LPHD should be reserved for cases meeting both the morphologic and immunophenotypic criteria.

Methods.—Two thousand eight hundred thirty-six biopsies diagnosed as Hodgkin's disease (HD) were reviewed. Two groups of specimens were subjected to immunophenotyping: 104 cases morphologically classified as being LPHD (group A) and 104 cases morphologically classified as classic HD (group B). The immunohistochemical findings of the 2 groups were compared. The major immunophenotypic divisions were: LPHD-like (CD20$^+$, CD45$^\pm$, CD15$^-$, CD30$^-$, CD3$^-$) and classic HD-like (CD20$^-$, CD45$^-$, CD15$^+$, CD30$^+$, CD3$^-$). For each antibody used, cases with specific staining of a majority of cells were scored positive. A CD57 score was calculated based on the number of positive cells within 1 high-power field in the area with the highest number of positive cells under low magnification.

Results.—In group A, the immunohistochemical classification of LPHD was confirmed in 76% of specimens. The remaining cases had an immunophenotype similar to that of classic HD. In group B, 88% of cases were classified as classic HD. On classification according to immunohistochemi-

TABLE 3.—Results of Immunophenotyping According to the Two Histological Groups

Immunophenotyping categories		Total number	GHSG classification	
			LPHD, group A	cHD, group B
LPHD-like				
1)	High CD57	73	62	11
	Ig light chain mRNA	25/28	16/19	9/9
	EBV	0/45	0/33	0/11
2)	Low CD57	6	5	1
	Ig light chain mRNA	3/5	2/4	1/1
	EBV	0/5	0/4	0/1
cHD-like				
3)	High CD57	2	2	0
	Ig light chain mRNA	0/1	0/1	–/–
	EBV	0/2	0/2	–/–
4)	Low CD57	100	22	78
	Ig light chain mRNA	0/25	0/10	0/15
	EBV	21/46	5/19	16/27
Not fully consistent				
5)	See Table 4	27	13	14
	Ig light chain mRNA	7/16	7/8	0/8
	EBV	8/25	1/12	7/13
Total number		208	104	104

(Courtesy of von Wasielewski R, Werner M, Fischer R, et al: Lymphocyte-predominant Hodgkin's disease: An immuno-histochemical analysis of 208 reviewed Hodgkin's disease cases from the German Hodgkin Study Group. *Am J Pathol* 150:793–803, 1996. Permission granted: copyright American Society for Investigative Pathology.)

cal categories, none of the cases with an LPHD-like marker pattern was positive for Epstein-Barr virus (EBV). However, 85% of these specimens were positive for light chain RNA. No case was positive for both Ig light chain mRNA and EBV, and no case with a high CD57 score was positive for EBV. None of the classic HD-like cases were positive for light chain mRNA. However, 72% of classic HD cases that had been classified as mixed cellularity HD were positive for EBV. Even though the marker profiles did not completely match the LPHD or classic HD patterns, the immunophenotypic findings supported the histologic results in 93% of cases (Table 3). Although few cases of LPHD had a pure diffuse architecture, most had at least a partly nodular growth pattern. Positivity for CD45 was 0% among classic HD-like cases compared with 58% among LPHD-like cases.

Conclusions.—About two thirds of cases of HD histologically confirmed as LPHD show an LPHD-like immunophenotype. Thus this diagnosis is more an immunohistochemical one than a strictly morphologic one. If a treatment other than that for classic HD is being considered, immunophenotyping of the biopsy specimen must be performed. The CD57 score used in this study was often helpful in distinguishing LPHD from classic HD.

▶ By studying a large number of patients with HD, the authors make some important observations. They confirm that LPHD represents a minority of the total cases of Hodgkin's disease (<5% of 2,836 cases in the study). They confirm that the presence of CD57⁺ T-lymphocytes surrounding L and H

Reed-Sternberg cells is a useful feature in distinguishing between LPHD and classic HD. In addition, they show that the presence of mRNA Ig light chain detected by in situ hybridization and the lack of Epstein-Barr virus–positive Reed-Sternberg cells correlates with the immunophenotype of LPHD. These 2 additional techniques may prove useful in distinguishing between LPHD and classic HD. Further studies will be needed to demonstrate the diagnostic use. Surprisingly, 25% of the cases designated as LPHD by the expert panel had the immunophenotype of classic HD with CD15+ Reed-Sternberg cells. This differs from the commonly held belief that CD15 is typically negative in LPHD. As the authors suggest, this may indicate that LPHD is an entity with a nonuniform immunophenotype or that the current morphologic definition of LPHD is not precise. Alternatively, one can speculate that these cases are similar to the cellular phase of nodular sclerosis HD.[1] The authors raise the question of what the criteria are for diagnosis of LPHD. Should this be reserved for cases fulfilling both morphologic and immunophenotypic criteria? The answer to this question remains to be determined; however, in this study the LPHD-like immunophenotype correlates with a better survival than the classic HD-like immunophenotype.

J.F. Turner, Jr., M.D.

Reference

1. Colby TV, Hoppe RT, Warnke RA: Hodgkin's disease: A clinicopathologic study of 659 cases. *Cancer* 49:1848–1858, 1981.

Suggested Reading

Hollowood K, Fletcher CDM: Malignant fibrous histiocytoma: Morphologic pattern or pathologic entity? *Semin Diagn Pathol* 12:210–220, 1995.

Fascin, a Sensitive New Marker for Reed-Sternberg Cells of Hodgkin's Disease: Evidence for a Dendritic or B Cell Derivation?
Pinkus GS, Pinkus JL, Langhoff E, et al (Harvard Med School, Boston; Rutger's Univ, Piscataway, NJ; Univ of California, Los Angeles)
Am J Pathol 150:543–562, 1997   15–5

Introduction.—The origin of the Reed-Sternberg cell, the hallmark of Hodgkin's disease, remains controversial despite the discovery of this disease more than 150 years ago. A localization pattern that appeared highly restricted to dendritic cells was demonstrated by human peripheral blood cells, using a monoclonal antibody to human fascin, a 55-kd actin-bundling protein initially isolated from HeLa cells. A comprehensive staining profile for fascin in normal and neoplastic lymphoid tissues was defined. To determine whether reactivity for fascin may provide insights into the pathogenesis of Hodgkin's disease, a large series of cases of Hodgkin's disease of various histologic types and a variety of non-Hodgkin's lymphomas were evaluated.

Methods.—There were 187 cases of Hodgkin's disease retrieved with 132 having nodular sclerosis, 34 having mixed cellularity, 14 having lymphocyte predominance, 2 having lymphocyte depletion, and 5 that were unclassified. These were compared with neoplastic tissues of 14 reactive lymph nodes, 4 thymuses, and 3 spleens. The comparison also included 156 specimens that involved B- or T-cell neoplasms. Fixed tissues were used to perform all the studies.

Results.—Reactivity was highly selective and localized predominantly in dendritic cells in nonneoplastic tissues. Fascin was localized to medullary dendritic cells in the thymus. In reactive lymph nodes, fascin strongly reacted with the interdigitating reticulum cells of T-zones; other reticular network cells and follicular dendritic cells reacted less intensely or were non-reactive. Only dendritic cells were reactive for fascin in the peripheral blood. In the non-lymphocyte predominance Hodgkin's disease cases, all or nearly all Reed-Sternberg cells and variants were immunoreactive for fascin. Strong diffuse cytoplasmic staining and frequently assumed dendritic shapes, producing an interdigitating meshwork or syncytial network of cells, were found in the neoplastic cells. L&H variants were nonreactive in all 14 patients with the nodular lymphocyte–predominance type. By contrast, reactivity for fascin was demonstrated in 24 of 156 other lymphoid neoplasms (15%), and this evaluation included 127 B-cell, 27 T-cell, and 2 null-cell neoplasms (Table 2).

Conclusion.—Fascin represent a highly effective marker for detection of certain dendritic cells in normal and neoplastic tissues. Fascin is also extremely consistent as a marker for Reed-Sternberg cells (Table 1) and variants of Hodgkin's disease (except L&H types), and, in difficult cases, fascin may help distinguish between Hodgkin's disease and non-Hodgkin's disease. The Epstein-Barr virus may induce fascin expression. Thus, in patients with Epstein-Barr virus, the role of viral induction of fascin in lymphoid or other cells types must be considered.

▶ Although current studies support the B-cell lineage of L&H Reed-Sternberg cells of nodular lymphocyte–predominant Hodgkin's disease, we have not yet agreed on the lineage of classic Reed-Sternberg cells in nodular sclerosis, mixed cellularity, or lymphocyte depletion subtypes of Hodgkin's disease. Currently, polymerase chain reaction assays of micro-dissected Reed-Sternberg cells suggest a possible B-cell lineage.[1, 2] These molecular findings are congruent with the immunophenotypic findings of rare cases of Hodgkin's disease with Reed-Sternberg cells that are both CD15 and CD20 positive. However, the reactivity of fascin in both normal dendritic cells and classic Reed-Sternberg cells certainly allows for continued speculation on the cell of origin of classic Reed-Sternberg cells.

J.F. Turner, Jr., M.D.

TABLE 2.—Immunoreactivity for Fascin in Neoplastic Cells of Various Lymphoid Malignancies

Diagnosis	Number of cases reactive/number of cases evaluated
SL/CLL	0/1
SC/mixed FCC	0/4
LC/LNCFCC	1/53*(weak)
Small non-cleaved	0/10
T cell-rich/histiocyte-rich B cell	0/11
Immunoblastic	
B cell	6/32†
T cell	1/4‡
Anaplastic large cell	
T cell	7/10 (weak)
B cell	1/3§
Null	2/2 (weak)
Other peripheral T cell	
lymphomas	0/9
Lymphoblastic	3/5‖
Post-transplant EBV-associated	3/8¶
Hairy cell leukemia (spleen)	0/2
Plasmacytomas	0/2
Total	24/156 (15%)

Note: All lymphomas were diffuse, except for 5 cases (2 SC and 3 LC/LNC cell types) that revealed a follicular growth pattern The series includes 13 lymphomas (12 B immunoblastic, 1 LNC in HIV[+] patients, with 3/8 (*EBV*)[+] cases (all B immunoblastic) reactive for fascin.

*Approximately 50% of neoplastic cells showed weak cytoplasmic staining.

†In most cases, < 5% of cells were reactive. A variable pattern was seen, from weak cytoplasmic staining to occasional strongly reactive large polyploid cells. Included are 3 of 8 EBV[+] cases in HIV[+] patients.

‡Weak reactivity in approximately 50% of cells.

§Less than 5% of neoplastic cells showed variable cytoplasmic reactivity.

‖Two of 4 T cells (weak); 1 pre-B cell.

¶Reactivity in 5%, 30%, or 50% of cells, respectively

Abbreviations: SL/CLL, small lymphocytic lympoma/chronic lymphocytic leukemia; *SC/mixed FCC,* small cleaved/mixed small and large cell follicular center cell lymphoma; *LC/LNCFCC,* large cleaved/large noncleaved follicular center cell lymphoma; *EBV,* Epstein-Barr virus.

(Courtesy of Pinkus GS, Pinkus JL, Langhoff E, et al: Fascin, a sensitive new marker for Reed-Sternberg cells of Hodgkin's disease: Evidence for a dendritic or B cell derivation? *Am J Pathol* 150:543–562. Copyright 1997, American Society for Investigative Pathology.)

TABLE 1.—Immunoreactivity for Fascin in Reed-Sternberg Cells and Variants of Hodgkin's Disease

Histological type	Number of cases reactive/number of cases evaluated
Nodular sclerosis	132/132
Mixed cellularity	34/34
Lymphocyte depletion	2/2
Unclassified	5/5
Lymphocyte predominance,	
nodular	0/14

Note: In the majority of reactive cases, essentially all Reed-Sternberg cells and variants were stained.

(Courtesy of Pinkus GS, Pinkus JL, Langhoff E, et al: Fascin, a sensitive new marker for Reed-Sternberg cells of Hodgkin's disease: Evidence for a dendritic or B cell derivation? *Am J Pathol* 150:543–562. Copyright 1997, American Society for Investigative Pathology.)

References

1. Hummel M, Marafioti T, Ziemann K, et al: Ig rearrangements in isolated Reed-Sternberg cells: Conclusions from four different studies. *Ann Oncol* 7:S31–S33. 1996.
2. Chan WC, Delabie J: Single cell analysis of H/RS cells. *Ann Oncol* 7:S41–S43, 1996.

Follicular Dendritic Cell Tumor: Report of 13 Additional Cases of Distinctive Entity

Perez-Ordonez B, Erlandson RA, Rosai J (Mem Sloan-Kettering Cancer Ctr, New York)

Am J Surg Pathol 20:944–955, 1996   15–6

Objective.—To describe the clinicopathologic characteristics of 13 cases of follicular dendritic cell tumor.

Background.—Follicular dendritic cells are among several nonlymphoid, nonphagocytic elements, which are termed *accessory cells* of the lymphoid system. Their function is to capture and present antigens and immune complexes. They are located in germinal centers, have a dendritic form, can be multinucleated, and have surface complement receptors and HLA-DR. In 1986, primary neoplasms of the lymph nodes with features of follicular dendritic cell differentiation were first reported. These tumors are very rare, and there are only 17 other well-documented cases.

Methods.—Clinical and follow-up data were collected on 13 cases of follicular dendritic cell tumor. Immunohistochemical stains were performed. The tumors were resected from 7 men and 6 women between 27 and 62 years of age.

Results.—There was involvement of the cervical lymph nodes in 6 cases and of the mediastinum in 3 cases. In one case each, there was involvement of the axilla, tonsil, spleen, and peripancreatic soft tissues. The tumors were between 1 cm and 13 cm and were gray or tan. They were made up of oval or spindle cells with eosinophilic cytoplasm arranged in sheets and fascicles, with a focal storiform pattern and whorls, as seen in meningioma. The nuclei were oval or elongated and had thin nuclear membranes, small eosinophilic nucleoli, and clear or dispersed chromatin. The cells typically were mixed with small lymphocytes with a conspicuous perivascular cuffing. In 7 cases, multinucleated tumor cells were noted. In 7 cases, necrosis, significant cellular atypia, a high mitotic rate, or abnormal mitoses was observed. Tumor cells tested positive for CD21, CD35, Ki-M4p, Ki-FDC1p, vimentin, and S-100 protein (Table 3). Common muscle actin was present in 1 case. In situ hybridization was performed in 6 cases, but did not show Epstein-Barr virus RNA. Eight cases had long, complex, and sometimes interdigitating cytoplasmic processes connected by desmosomes. The behavior of these tumors resembled that of low-grade soft tissue sarcoma rather than that of malignant lymphoma. These neoplasms are characterized by local recurrence and metastases. At the last follow-up

TABLE 3.—Immunohistochemical Features of Follicular Dendritic Cell Tumors

Case no.	CD21	CD35	Ki-M4p	Ki-FDC1p	CD1a	CAM 5.2	AE1/AE3	EMA	HMB-45	S-100	Vimentin	CMA	MSA	CD45	CD20
1						−	−		−	−	+			−	−
2	++	+	+++	++	−					+	+++	−	−	−	−
3	+++	++	+++	++	−	−			−	+	+++	−	−	−	
4	++	+	+++	++	−	−	−	−	−	−	+++			−	
5	+++	++			−		−		−	++				−	
6	−	++	−	−	−	−	−	−	−	−	+				−
7	++	++				−	−	−		++				−	−
8	+	+	+++	++						−	−			−	−
9	+	+	+++							−					
10	+++	+	+++	++	−	−					−			−	
11	+++	++			−	−		−	−	−	++			−	−
12	+	−	++	++	−					−		−	++	−	
13															

Note: −, no staining; +, weak; ++, moderate; +++, strong; *CD21*, C3d receptor; *CD35*, C3b receptor
Abbreviations: CMA, common muscle actin; *MSA*, muscle-specific actin.
(Courtesy of Perez-Ordonez B, Erlandson RA, Rosai J: Follicular dendritic cell tumor: Report of 13 additional cases of a distinctive entity. *Am J Surg Pathol* 63:450–454, 1997.)

examination, 8 patients were alive without tumor, 2 were alive with recurrence or metastasis, 2 died of the tumor, and 1 patient was lost to follow-up.

Discussion.—In 50% of cases of follicular dendritic cell tumor, the most common clinical feature is a painless, slow-growing cervical lymphadenopathy. Diagnosis can be confirmed with immunohistochemistry or electron microscopy. Complete resection is the preferred treatment for primary or recurrent tumors. Radiotherapy may benefit patients with residual or locally recurrent tumors.

Follicular Dendritic Cell Sarcoma: Clinicopathologic Analysis of 17 Cases Suggesting a Malignant Potential Higher Than Currently Recognized

Chan JKC, Fletcher CDM, Nayler SJ, et al (Queen Elizabeth Hosp, Hong Kong; Brigham and Women's Hosp, Boston; Univ of the Witwatersrand, Johannesburg, South Africa)

Cancer 79:294–313, 1997   15–7

Objective.—Follicular dendritic cells (FDC) are an essential component of B-cell follicles that can proliferate under various reactive and neoplastic conditions. Over the last decade, several reports have described FDC tumors, but usually only 1 or a few cases at a time. Seventeen cases of FDC sarcoma are reported, including the clinical findings, morphologic findings, response to treatment, and immunophenotypic findings.

Patients.—The 17 cases included 8 previously unreported patients. There were 10 women and 7 men, mean age 38 years. Fifteen patients sought medical attention for a mass lesion; lymph nodes were involved in 7 cases and various extranodal sites in 10 (including the tonsil in 3 cases). Ten patients had associated hyaline-vascular Castleman's disease. The average maximal dimension of the tumors was 6.7 cm. Treatment consisted of surgical excision, often with adjuvant radiotherapy or chemotherapy, after protocols used for aggressive lymphomas. Thirteen patients were followed up for a median of 3 years. Six had local recurrence and 6 had metastasis; 3 died of disease.

Findings.—The major histologic finding was spindle, ovoid, or polygonal cells arranged in a storiform or fascicular pattern. The cells had oval nuclei, a delicate nuclear membrane, vesicular or granular chromatin, and distinct nucleoli with indistinct cell borders. Fibrillary cytoplasm was a frequent finding. Scattered multinucleated forms were sometimes seen. Tumor cells could be found in sheets, whorls, follicle-like structures, trabeculae, or pseudovascular spaces (Fig 3). Small lymphocytes were sometimes seen with or without cuffing around blood vessels. In every case, the neoplastic cells were immunoreactive to CD21 and CD35. They were positive for desmoplakin in 59% of cases, epithelial membrane antigen in 88%, S-100 protein in 35%, and CD68 in 12%. No case was positive for

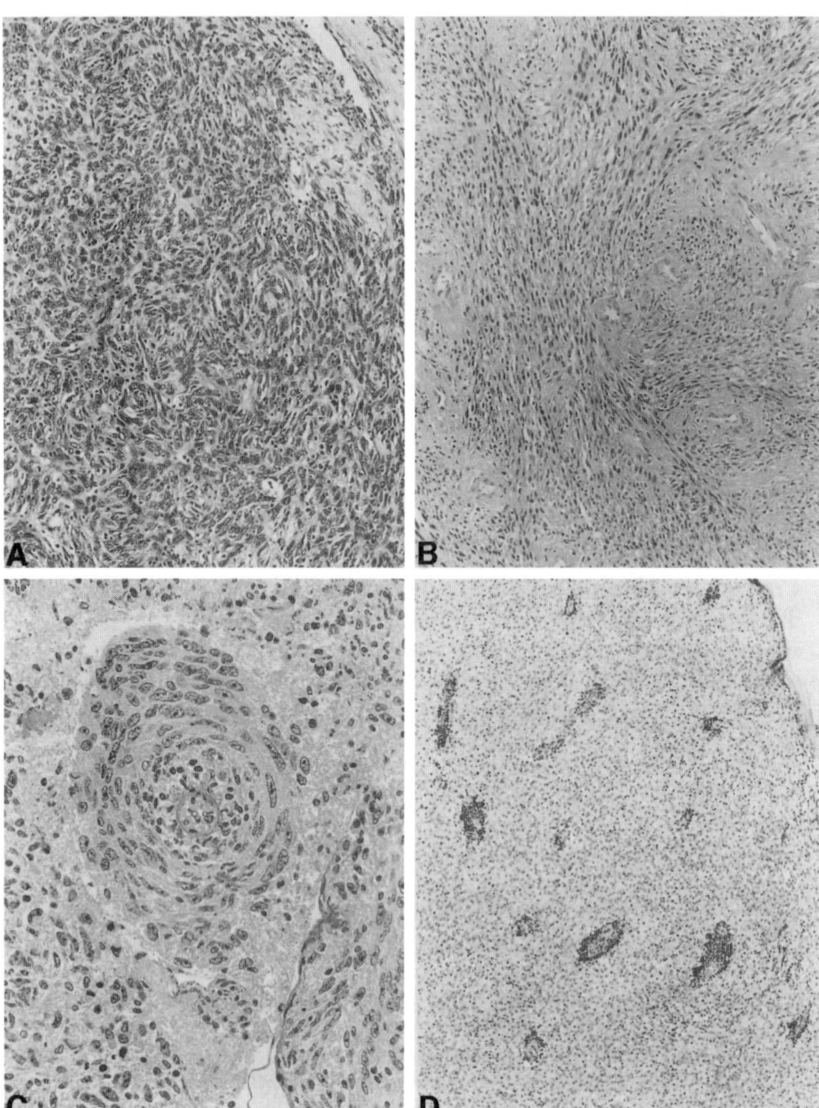

FIGURE 3.—Growth patterns of follicular dendritic cell sarcoma. Note also the characteristic sprinkling of small lymphocytes. **A,** Storiform pattern (case 2). **B,** Interlacing fascicles (case 10). This case also exhibits rich vascularity and perivascular sclerosis. **C,** Circular whorls (case 15). This whorl is centered on a blood vessel. **D,** Diffuse sheets (case 14); note the perivascular cuffing of small lymphocytes. (Courtesy of Chan JKC, Fletcher CDM, Nayler SJ, et al: Follicular dendritic cell sarcoma: Clinicopathologic analysis of 17 cases suggesting a malignant potential higher than currently recognized. *Cancer* 79:294–313, 1997. ©1997 American Cancer Society. Reprinted by permission of Wiley-Liss, Inc., a subsidiary of John Wiley & Sons, Inc.)

cytokeratin. Villous processes connected by desmosomes were discovered on ultrastructural studies.

Conclusions.—A large series of cases of FDC sarcoma was reviewed. Although this tumor has distinctive histologic characteristics, it must be confirmed with special diagnostic studies. The pattern of recurrences and metastases encountered in this study suggests that FDC sarcoma is an intermediate-grade malignancy. Patients with intraabdominal FDC may have a particularly aggressive clinical course.

▶ These articles (Abstracts 15–6 and 15–7) serve as an excellent morphologic reference for this rare tumor. Once this neoplasm is considered in the differential diagnosis of spindled neoplasms (or less commonly epithelioid neoplasms), the distinctive morphologic features will facilitate its diagnosis. However, ultimately the diagnosis rests on demonstration of follicular dendritic cell origin with immunohistochemical stains such as CD21. Fortunately, this marker works quite well on routine paraffin embedded tissue.

The architectural pattern is most commonly composed of cells arranged in fascicles or sheets. However, Chan et al. (Abstract 15–7) report a trabecular and nodular pattern that was not previously emphasized. Regardless of the growth pattern, the admixed small lymphocytes and perivascular cuffing are very helpful morphologic features. The tumor may occur in various sites. However, if this neoplasm occurs in the mediastinum, differentiation from thymoma may be particularly difficult on morphologic grounds. Using cytokeratin AE1/AE3 in the immunohistochemical staining panel will solve this dilemma, with thymomas being positive. The clinical behavior of this tumor is variable. However, both groups of authors note that features of nuclear atypia, mitotic rate (5/10 mitotic figures per high-powered field) and necrosis seem to correlate with a higher recurrence rate and metastatic spread.

J.F. Turner, Jr., M.D.

Suggested Reading

Histiocytic and dendritic cell proliferations, in Rosai J, Sobin LH (eds): *Tumors of the lymph nodes and spleen*, ed 3. Washington, DC, Armed Forces of Pathology, 1994, pp 341–384.

Mantle Cell Lymphoma: Correlation of Clinical Outcome and Biologic Features With Three Histologic Variants

Majlis A, Pugh WC, Rodriguez MA, et al (Univ of Texas, Houston)
J Clin Oncol 15:1664–1671, 1997   15–8

Background.—Mantle cell lymphoma comprises a range of non-Hodgkin's lymphomas classified as intermediate or intermediately differentiated lymphocytic lymphoma. Although recent studies have offered insight into the biologic nature of these tumors, there is uncertainty as to their clinical biologic behavior and therefore the appropriate clinical response. The clinical response patterns of mantle cell lymphoma were analyzed in a review of 46 previously untreated cases.

Methods.—Histologic, immunophenotypic, and molecular studies on each case were reviewed by an expert hematopathologist. The growth pattern of each case was classified as mantle zone, with neoplastic cells proliferating as wide collars around reactive or atrophic germinal centers; nodular, an intermediate pattern with frankly nodular growth resulting from centripetal and centrifugal expansion of the follicular mantle zone; and diffuse, with confluent growth obliterating the lymph node architecture and residual nodularity.

Results.—The growth pattern was diffuse in 61% of cases, mantle zone in 26%, and nodular in 13%. Sixty-nine percent of patients had bone marrow infiltration, which was most frequent in patients with the diffuse growth pattern. Half of the patients had other sites of extranodal involvement. Ninety-two percent of cases studied showed nuclear positivity on cyclin-D1 staining, and 33% showed rearrangement at the *bcl*-1 major translocation cluster.

Growth pattern was closely related to response to doxorubicin-based chemotherapy. None of the patients with the mantle zone growth pattern had an unfavorable tumor score. Complete response rate was 73% in patients with the mantle zone pattern versus 25% in those with the nodular pattern and 19% in those with the diffuse pattern. Three-year survival was 100% versus 50% and 55%, respectively.

Conclusions.—The clinical behavior of mantle cell lymphoma is closely related to the histologic growth pattern. Treatment response and prognosis are good for patients with the mantle zone variant, which acts like a low-grade lymphoma, and less favorable for those with the diffuse and nodular variants, which behave more like intermediate-grade lymphomas. Mantle cell lymphomas are not curable by current treatment regimens, analysis of the treatment failure data suggests. The authors note that their criterion of at least 90% nodules to show a loss of mantle zone configuration for inclusion in the nodular category is an arbitrary one.

Mantle Cell Lymphoma: A Clinicopathologic Study of 80 Cases
Argatoff LH, Connors JM, Klasa RJ, et al (Univ of British Columbia, Vancouver)
Blood 89:2067–2078, 1997   15–9

Introduction.—Mantle cell lymphoma (MCL) accounts for approximately 5% of cases of malignant lymphoma. Although it is recognized as a distinct entity, there are limited data on the clinical and pathologic characteristics of this tumor. A 7-year clinicopathologic review of MCL is presented.

Methods.—The retrospective study included 80 cases of MCL seen at 1 Canadian cancer referral center. The clinical and histologic findings were reviewed to identify prognostically significant factors.

Findings.—Seventy percent of patients were men and 88% had advanced disease; mean age was 63 years. The patients survived for a median of 43 months. The only clinical factor with a significant effect on prognosis was performance status.

On histologic examination, none of the tumors showed proliferation centers. A few cases with diffuse architecture had occasional compressed germinal centers, but these lacked a normal mantle zone (MZ). The architecture was classified as diffuse in 78% of cases, "nodular" in 16%, and MZ zone in 6%. The nodular cases were those with well-defined nodularity but no significant MZ pattern. If the pattern was mixed, the case was assigned to the pattern occupying more than 50% of the cross-sectional area of all sections available for review (Fig 3). Five cases had so many blastic cells that it was difficult do distinguish MCL from lymphoblastic lymphoma. Survival was not significantly different for cases that had some degree of transformation but were not truly blastic. However, outcome was poor for patients with more than 20 mitotic figures per high-powered field. Twenty-seven of 69 cases analyzed had peripheral blc d (PB) involvement by lymphoma cells. The typical pattern was a polymorphous mixture of small, medium, and large lymphocytes. The major cell

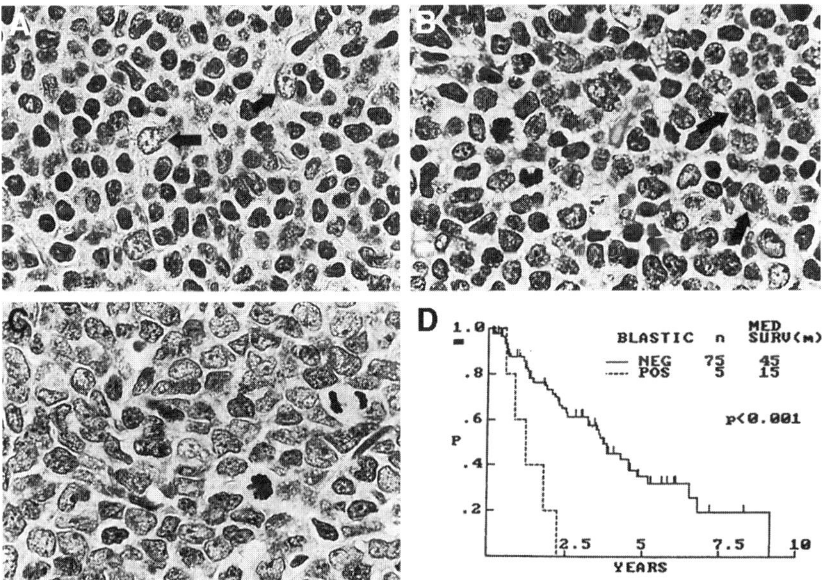

FIGURE 3.—Composite photograph showing the cytologic features of MCL. **A,** Typical cytology of MCL characterized by cells with small, slightly irregular nuclei, inconspicuous nucleoli, and minimal cytoplasm. Note the frequent epithelioid histiocytes (*arrows*). **B,** MCL with prominent features of transformation but not clearly blastic. Increased numbers of larger cells with fine chromatin and inconspicuous nucleoli are shown (*arrows*). **C,** Blastic MCL. Note the cytologic resemblance to lymphoblastic lymphoma. **D,** Overall survival of 80 patients with MCL based on the presence of blastic features. The 5 cases designated as blastic MCL were associated with a significantly shorter survival when compared with that of all others (n = 75), including those with features of transformation as shown in **B**. (Courtesy of Argatoff LH, Connors JM, Klasa RJ, et al: Mantle cell lymphoma: a clinicopathologic study of 80 cases. *Blood* 89:2067–2078, 1997.)

TABLE 5.—Results of Immunophenotyping in 44 Cases of MCL

Antigen	Positive	No. of Cases Negative	Not Analyzed
CD5	42	1	1
CD10	1	41	1
CD19/20	44	0	0
CD23	1(dim)	14	29
FMC-7	11	0	33
χ^*	18	—	0
λ^*	26	—	0

*Surface IG brightness was moderate to strong in those cases (11) in which it was documented.
(Courtesy of Argatoff LH, Connors JM, Klasa RJ, et al: Mantle cell lymphoma: A clinicopathologic study of 80 cases. *Blood* 89:2067–2078, 1997.)

type had a slightly irregular nucleus with fine chromatin, a small nucleolus, and a thin rim of gray-blue cytoplasm. There were also some cells with a morphologic picture similar to that of small cleaved cells or chronic lymphocytic leukemia cells, and immature cells with L1 and L2 lympho-blast-like morphologic characteristics. Some cases with PB involvement did not have an elevated lymphocyte count. Patients with leukemic pre-sentation had significantly reduced survival.

On bone marrow biopsy, lymphomatous infiltration was found mainly in an interstitial or intertrabecular location. This infiltrate could be ar-ranged in nodular aggregates and/or diffuse infiltrates. The cellular mor-phologic findings were very close to those of MCL in lymph nodes, without large transformed cells and proliferation centers. Bone marrow involvement was positive in 50 cases, not evident in 25 cases, and un-known in 5. There were no significant differences in outcome between these groups. Overall survival tended to be shorter for patients with heavy MCL involvement. Immunophenotyping by flow cytometry disclosed a characteristic pattern (Table 5).

Conclusions.—In this clinicopathologic review of MCL, factors associ-ated with a poor prognosis include increased mitotic activity, blastic mor-phologic features, and PB involvement at presentation. The criteria for a true MZ pattern in this tumor are undefined and variable between observ-ers. This study permits no conclusions about the effectiveness of different treatments because none of the treatment groups did well.

▶ Although these articles (Abstracts 15–8 and 15–9) are published in jour-nals targeted for clinicians, they provide pathologists with useful informa-tion. These articles alert us to the morphologic observations the clinicians may be asking of us in our pathology reports. Architectural pattern, mitotic rate, and blastic morphology in mantle cell lymphoma are histologic features that may have an impact on prognosis.

As the articles point out, there are not uniform definitions of these mor-phologic variants. For example, the definition of the mantle zone variant that Majlis et al. (Abstract 15–8) used in their study may have included some of the cases of the nodular variant in the study by Argatoff et al. (Abstract 15–9)

This difference in criteria for the mantle zone variant may have given Majlis et al. a larger enough group of patients with the mantle zone variant to show a significant increase in survival advantage for patients with the mantle zone pattern.

Both articles recognize a blastic variant of mantle cell lymphoma that has a poor prognosis. However, a uniform definition of this blastic variant of mantle cell lymphoma is lacking. A practical definition may be a lymphoma that morphologically resembles lymphoblastic lymphoma yet is immunophenotypically consistent with mantle cell lymphoma. The studies of Argatoff et al. and others have demonstrated that the number of cells with blastic morphology and the mitotic rate increase in sequential biopsies from the same patient. However, when cases have less than 20 mitotic figures/10 high-powered field, there is not a negative correlation with median overall survival.

Mantle cell lymphoma is emerging as a distinct entity. The diffuse variant clearly has a median survival similar to other intermediate-grade lymphomas in the Working Formulation. The nodular variant also seems to have a similar decrease in median survival. Whether the mantle zone variant should be considered low grade remains unclear. Future studies are needed to better define the mantle zone variant and to clarify its significance.

J.F. Turner, Jr., M.D.

Suggested Reading

Banks PM, Chan J, Cleary ML, et al: Mantle cell lymphoma: A proposal for unification of morphologic, immunologic, and molecular data. *Am J Surg Pathol* 16:637, 1992.

Duggan MJ, Weisenburger DD, Ye YL, et al: Mantle zone lymphoma: A clinicopathologic study of 22 cases. *Cancer* 66:522–529, 1990.

Lardelli P, Bookman MA, Sundeen J, et al: Lymphocytic lymphoma of intermediate differentiation: Morphologic and immunophenotypic spectrum and clinical correlations. *Am J Surg Pathol* 14:752, 1990.

Pittaluga S, Wlodarska I, Stul MS, et al: Mantle cell lymphoma: A clinicopathological study of 55 cases. *Histopathology* 26:17–24, 1995.

Weisenburger DD, Armitage JO: Mantle cell lymphoma: An entity comes of age. *Blood* 87:4483, 1996.

Use of CD23 (BU38) on Paraffin Sections in the Diagnosis of Small Lymphocytic Lymphoma and Mantle Cell Lymphoma
Kumar S, Green GA, Teruya-Feldstein J, et al (NIH, Bethesda, Md)
Mod Pathol 9:925–929, 1996   15–10

Introduction.—The histologic findings are usually sufficient for the diagnosis of small lymphocytic lymphoma/chronic lymphocytic leukemia

(SLL/CLL) and mantle cell lymphoma (MCL). However, when there is morphologic overlap, the distinction can be difficult to make. Both SLL and MCL are positive for CD20 and CD5; however, on CD23 staining, SLL is usually positive and MCL is usually negative. However, CD23 studies generally require fresh tissues. A method of staining for CD23 in fixed tissues was evaluated for use in distinguishing between SLL and MCL.

Methods.—The study included formalin- or B5–fixed paraffin-embedded blocks of 44 cases of SLL/CLL, 3 cases of lymphoplasmacytoid lymphoma (LPL), and 39 cases of MCL. According to published criteria, SLL/CLL was characterized by diffuse small lymphocytes with scant cytoplasm and round nuclei. Specimens showing proliferation of plasmacytoid lymphocytes and plasma cells, plus Dutcher bodies and without the typical features of SLL/CLL, were classified as LPL. Findings characteristic of MCL were a vaguely nodular or diffuse, monotonous infiltrate of small lymphocytes, with irregular nuclei and no larger transformed cells. The specimens were stained with the BU38 antibody, which detects a fixation-resistant epitope of the CD23 antigen.

Results.—Ninety-three percent of cases of SLL stained positively for CD23. The staining followed a membranous pattern, with about three fourths of the neoplastic cells staining positive. Most CD23-positive SLLs showed moderately intense staining, though not as intense as in the follicular dendritic cells. The other 4 positive cases showed weak but positive staining in most cells. One case of LPL and 1 of MCL stained positive for CD23.

Conclusions.—In certain situations it can be difficult to morphologically distinguish between SLL/CLL and MCL. When fresh tissue is unavailable, the BU38 antibody is useful in demonstrating CD23 on the cells of SLLs in paraffin sections.

▶ Distinction of mantle cell lymphoma from small lymphocytic lymphoma is important for therapeutic decisions and prognosis. Morphologic features allow distinction between these entities in the majority of cases. CD23 has been demonstrated to be a discriminatory marker between these entities. However, this analysis has been previously limited to flow cytometric techniques and frozen immunohistochemistry. This study demonstrates the usefulness of adding CD23 to a panel of immunohistochemical stains that are currently available for use in either formalin-fixed or B5-fixed paraffin embedded tissue. Except for one case of mantle cell lymphoma that was positive for CD23, the remainder of the mantle cell cases were CD23 negative. This aberrant case was the blastoid variant of mantle cell lymphoma, and distinction from small lymphocytic lymphoma would not have been a problem. Instead, distinction from lymphoblastic lymphoma would have required ancillary studies.

When the morphologic distinction between small lymphocytic lymphoma and mantle cell lymphoma is not possible and CD23 is negative, there are several additional ancillary studies that help in separating these lymphomas. Cyclin-D1 is expressed by mantle cell lymphoma and not small lymphocytic lymphoma. Cyclin-D1 may be evaluated on paraffin tissue by immunohistochemical techniques. Analysis for the *Bcl*-1 gene rearrangement may be attempted from paraffin-embedded tissue or fresh tissue; however, a negative result does not exclude mantle cell lymphoma. Alternatively, fresh tissue could be analyzed by flow cytometry, looking for comparison of surface light chain intensity as well as CD23 coexpression on the B-lymphocytes.

J.F. Turner, Jr., M.D.

Suggested Reading

Dorfman DM, Pinkus GS: Distinction between small lymphocytic and mantle cell lymphoma by immunoreactivity for CD23. *Mod Pathol* 7:326, 1994.

Lim LC, Segal GH, Wittwer CT: Detection of *bcl*-1 gene rearrangement and B-cell clonality in mantle cell lymphoma using formalin-fixed, paraffin-embedded tissues. *Am J Clin Pathol* 104:689–695, 1995.

Medeiros LJ, Van Krieken JH, Jaffe ES, et al: Association of *bcl*-1 rearrangements with lymphocytic lymphoma of intermediate differentiation. *Blood* 76:2086, 1990.

Inflammatory Pseudotumor of Lymph Nodes: A Study of 25 Cases With Emphasis on Morphological Heterogeneity
Moran CA, Suster S, Abbondanzo SL (Armed Forces Inst of Pathology, Washington, DC; Mount Sinai Med Ctr, Miami, Fla; Univ of Miami, Fla)
Hum Pathol 28:332–338, 1997   15–11

Objective.—Inflammatory pseudotumor (IPT) is an inflammatory/fibrosing tumoral process that may occur in various organ systems. Although IPT can resemble a neoplasm, its clinical behavior is benign. The cause is unknown, but IPT may occur as an unusual response to tissue injury. Twenty-five cases of IPT involving the lymph nodes are reported.

Methods.—The patients were 13 women and 12 men, ranging in age from 8 to 81 years. Clinical findings included previous infection, fatigue, abdominal pain, weight loss, fever, pelvic inflammatory disease, nausea, and night sweats. The disease was classified as stage I in 3 cases, stage II in 17 cases, and stage III in 5 cases.

Histologic Findings.—On histopathologic examination, the stage I lesions had small, sharply circumscribed, discrete nodules of the lymph node parenchyma. These cases showed very focalized findings, although with a cellular infiltrate similar to that seen in stage II lesions.

In stage II lesions, scanning magnification revealed extensive replacement of the lymph node by inflammatory cells combined with a spindle cell fibroblastic/myofibroblastic proliferation. This proliferation extended along the subscapular and trabecular sinuses in radial fashion, sometimes involving the capsule. The inflammatory infiltrate consisted of small lymphocytes with scattered immunoblasts, plasma cells, histiocytes, and occasional polymorphonuclear leukocytes or eosinophils. Sometimes plasma

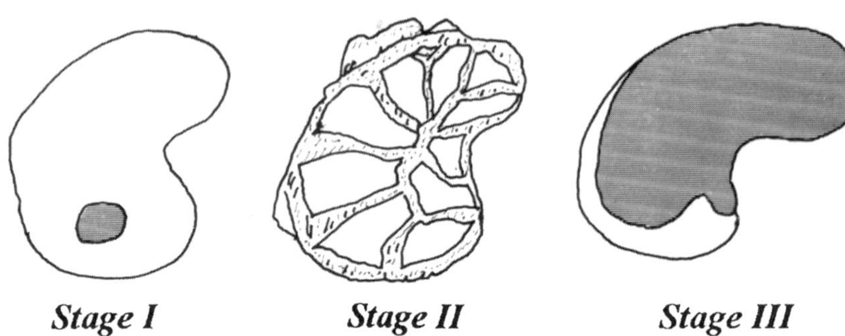

FIGURE 8.—Diagrammatic picture of the histological stages of inflammatory pseudotumor of lymph node. (Courtesy of Moran CA, Suster S, Abbondanzo SL: Inflammatory pseudotumor of lymph nodes: A study of 25 cases with emphasis on morphological heterogeneity. *Hum Pathol* 28:332–338, 1997.)

cells were the major component of the inflammatory response. The spindle cells were characterized by elongated nuclei with irregularly distributed chromatin and small chromocenters, sometimes occurring in longitudinal fascicles and sometimes beside short collagen strands. None of the stage II cases were necrotic. Outside the capsule, there was destruction of small and medium-sized vessels, constriction and fibrous obliteration of the vascular walls, and sometimes areas of vasculitis. No organisms were detected on special stains. In the uninvolved lymph tissue, there was reactive follicular hyperplasia with some progressive transformation of germinal centers and areas of paracortical hyperplasia.

Stage III lesions showed extensive, dense sclerosis with a minor inflammatory cell response and small areas of lymphoid tissue. As in stage II cases, there was no evidence of necrosis or infarction.

Immunohistochemical Findings.—On immunostaining, T-lymphocytes were predominant. There were isolated mononuclear cells positive for Leu M1, with many plasma cells positive for Ber-H2. Three stage I cases showed vimentin-positive fibroblastic spindle cells. Most spindle cells showed evidence of a myofibroblastic phenotype. In stage III lesions, spindle cells in areas of fibrosis were rarely positive for actin and even more rarely positive for vimentin.

Conclusions.—The findings of IPT involving the lymph nodes are reviewed. These lesions appear to be an evolving, dynamic process whose morphologic appearance may depend on its stage of evolution. The pathologist must be able to recognize these stages to differentiate IPT from other fibrosing or inflammatory conditions of the lymph nodes (Fig 8).

▶ The authors provide histologic and immunophenotypic evidence for various stages of inflammatory pseudotumor. The stages may be likened to a normal reparative process such as granulation tissue. With each different stage, there is a varying differential diagnosis of other benign as well as some malignant processes. The stage II architectural pattern of an inflammatory and fibrosing process extending along the trabecular and subcapsular sinuses is distinctive. Recognition of the pattern is helpful in distinguishing inflammatory pseudotumor from Hodgkin's disease, which has a similar polymorphic inflammatory background. There was no mention of Reed-Sternberg–like or other cytologically atypical cells in inflammatory pseudo-tumor. This is important because the authors mention occasional mononu-clear cells staining positive for CD15 (Leu M1). The classic membranous and Golgi staining pattern of Reed-Sternberg cells was not described.

J.F. Turner, Jr., M.D.

Suggested Reading

Davis RE, Warnke RA, Dorfman RF: Inflammatory pseudotumor lymph nodes. *Am J Surg Pathol* 15:744–756, 1991.

Perrone T, De Wolf-Peeters C, Frizzera G: Inflammatory pseudotumor of lymph nodes: a distinctive pattern of nodal reaction. *Am J Surg Pathol* 12:351–361, 1988.

Inflammatory Malignant Fibrous Histiocytoma: Distinction From Hodgkin's Disease and Non-Hodgkin's Lymphoma by a Panel of Leuko-cyte Markers
Khalidi HS, Singleton TP, Weiss SW (Univ of Michigan, Ann Arbor)
Mod Pathol 10:438–442, 1997   15–12

Background.—The uncommon entity inflammatory malignant fibrous histiocytoma (IMFH) most often occurs as a large intraabdominal mass. The patient sometimes has systemic symptoms such as fever, leukocytosis, and peripheral eosinophilia. The diagnosis of IMFH is easy to make in large resection specimens, but not so in small biopsy specimens. Such difficulties will become more common as more patients undergo computed tomographic–guided biopsy in the outpatient setting. A panel of leukocyte markers was tested for ability to identify IMFH.

Methods and Results.—Eight histologically typical examples of IMFH were stained with various leukocyte markers, including CD30, CD15, CD45/CD45RB, CD43, CD45RO, CD20, and CD68. Each case had at least focal areas resembling conventional malignant fibrous histiocytoma. These areas showed spindled tumor cells in a haphazard pattern, with less abundant inflammatory cells and benign xanthoma cells within. Nearly all anaplastic histiocyte-like cells—including the xanthomatous cells and those resembling Reed-Sternberg cells—were negative for all leukocyte markers studied. The exception was focal cytoplasmic staining for CD68 in 1 case. In contrast, the benign-appearing histiocyte was diffusely posi-tive for CD68 in all cases. Six cases were focally positive for CD15, and 2 were occasionally and focally positive for CD45/CD45RB and CD43. Scattered small T cells expressed CD43 and CD45RO. There were some small B lymphocytes expressing CD20, particularly in lymphoid aggre-gates. CD15 and CD45/CD45RB were expressed by granulocytes. Lyso-zyme was found in tumor cells in 5 of 5 cases, apparently the result of phagocytosis of neutrophils. One case was positive for desmin, and all were negative for cytokeratin, actin, and S-100 protein.

Conclusions.—Immunophenotypic study of the anaplastic cells in IMFH gives results different from those obtained in most cases of Hodgkin's disease and Ki-1 anaplastic large-cell lymphoma. Such studies are a useful aid to diagnosis as long as benign histiocytes and inflammatory cells are excluded from the analysis. Classic Reed-Sternberg cells are a rare finding in IMFH.

▶ This study demonstrates that the cytologically malignant cells in inflammatory malignant fibrous histiocytoma do not react with the immunohistochemical stains commonly used in the differential diagnosis of classic Hodgkin's disease (mixed cellularity, nodular sclerosis, and lymphocyte depletion) and anaplastic large-cell lymphoma. Because the panel of immunohistochemical stains is used to exclude Hodgkin's disease and anaplastic large-cell lymphoma, it is important to note positive staining of inflammatory cells that serve as an internal control. As the authors mentioned, other nonhematopoietic neoplasms such as anaplastic carcinoma may have a similar morphologic appearance. Therefore the diagnosis of inflammatory malignant fibrous histiocytoma on small biopsy specimens may require an extensive immunohistochemical panel at least including AE1/AE3. It is comforting to note that areas of typical malignant fibrous histiocytoma were focally observed in the biopsy specimens of this study.

J.F. Turner, Jr., M.D.

Posttransplantation Lymphoproliferative Disorders in Bone Marrow Transplant Recipients Are Aggressive Diseases With a High Incidence of Adverse Histologic and Immunobiologic Features
Orazi A, Hromas RA, Neiman RS, et al (Indiana Univ, Indianapolis; Univ of Nebraska, Omaha)
Am J Clin Pathol 107:419–429, 1997   15–13

Introduction.—In organ transplant recipients receiving immunosuppressive therapies, posttransplantation lymphoproliferative disorders (PT-LPDs) are a well-documented complication. Reports focusing on the characteristics of these disorders following allogeneic bone marrow transplantation are few. The overall incidence of PT-LPDs varies from 0.6% to 7.4% with a higher incidence (16% to 20%) in transplants from unrelated or mismatched donors. Bone marrow transplant patients have a high incidence of extensive dissemination of this disorder at presentation, an aggressive course, and a high fatality rate when compared with solid organ recipients. A group of patients receiving bone marrow transplants were examined for the clinical characteristics, the histologic and immunohistologic features, the proliferative fraction, and the genotypic status of their PT-LPDs.

Methods.—Ten patients with PT-LPDs were studied after T-cell–depleted allogeneic bone marrow transplantation. The morphology of the lesions and their clonality based on immunoglobulin heavy-chain gene rearrangement by polymerase chain reaction analysis and immunohistochemistry were studied. The proliferative activity of the lesions was measured by immunoperoxidase staining for the proliferating cell nuclear antigen (PCNA) and p53 gene product overexpression was studied. Epstein-Barr virus (EBV) was evaluated by anti-EBV latent membrane protein and by polymerase chain reaction analysis for the EBV genome.

Results.—Seven patients had polymorphic B-cell lymphoma and 3 had malignant immunoblastic lymphoma. Four of the patients with polymorphic B-cell lymphoma had B-cell monoclonality by immunologic or genotypic criteria or both. All 3 of the patients with malignant immunoblastic lymphoma had B-cell clonality by genotypic analysis, but 2 were polyclonal by immunologic analysis. All 10 patients had the EBV genome, the expression of EBV-LMP, or both. The patients with polymorphic B-cell lymphoma averaged PCNA expression of 58%, and the patients with malignant immunoblastic lymphoma averaged PCNA expression of 84%. Five patients tested positive for p53. With the administration of donor leukocytes, 2 of 4 cases of polymorphic B-cell lymphoma resolved; the rest of the patients died of PT-LPD within a short time of diagnosis.

Conclusion.—A high frequency of high-grade histologic subtypes, high proliferative activity, frequent monoclonality, frequent overexpression of p53 gene product, and poor prognosis are the characteristics of PT-LPDs after T-cell–depleted bone marrow transplantation.

▶ This is one of a few reports detailing the clinical and pathologic features of posttransplantation lymphoproliferative disorders occurring in patients who have received bone marrow transplants. It is worth sharing this report with our clinical colleagues who are struggling with treatment decisions for these patients.

J.F. Turner, Jr., M.D.

Suggested Reading

Davey DD, Kamat D, Laszewski M, et al: Epstein-Barr virus–related lymphoproliferative disorders following bone marrow transplantation: An immunologic and genotypic analysis. *Mod Pathol* 2:27–34, 1989.

Shapiro RS, McClain K, Frizzera G, et al: Epstein-Barr virus–associated B cell lymphoproliferative disorders following bone marrow transplantation. *Blood* 71:1234–1243, 1988.

Zutter MM, Martin PJ, Sale G, et al: Epstein-Barr virus lymphoproliferation after bone marrow transplantation. *Blood* 72:520–529, 1988.

Clinical Features and Treatment Outcome of Childhood T-Lineage Acute Lymphoblastic Leukemia According to the Apparent Maturational Stage of T-Lineage Leukemic Blasts: A Children's Cancer Group Study
Uckman FM, Gaynon PS, Sensel MG, et al (Hughs Inst, St Paul, Minn; Children's Health Care—Minneapolis; Univ of Wisconsin, Madison; et al)
J Clin Oncol 15:2214–2221, 1997   15–14

Introduction.—Before their migration into the thymus, CD7 is the earliest differentiation antigen acquired by T-cell precursors. At least 3 distinct stages of T-cell ontogeny can be defined based on the surface expression of CD7, CD2, CD5, and CD3: stage I T-cell precursors, or pro-thymocytes; stage II T-cell precursors, or immature thymocytes; and stage III T-cell precursors, or mature thymocytes. About 15% of all pediatric acute lymphoblastic leukemia patients have T-lineage leukemia. It is unclear what the clinical significance of interpatient differences are in the apparent maturational stage of leukemic T-cell precursors. In children with T-lineage acute lymphoblastic leukemia, the influence of leukemic cell apparent maturational stage on treatment outcomes was determined.

Methods.—Two sequential series of risk-adjusted treatment protocols were designed for 407 children with T-lineage acute lymphoblastic leukemia over a 10-year period. In this series, the children were immunophenotypically classified according to $CD7^+CD2^-CD5^-$ pro-thymocyte leukemia, $CD7^+(CD2$ or $CD5)^+CD3^-$ immature thymocyte leukemia, and $CD7^+CD2^+CD5^+CD3^+$ mature thymocyte leukemia.

Results.—The pro-thymocyte group had an induction outcome of 91.4%, the immature thymocyte group had an induction outcome of 97.1%, and the mature thymocyte group had an induction outcome of 98.3%. For pro-thymocyte leukemia patients, 4-year event-free survival was lower (57.1%) than for immature thymocyte (68.5%) and mature thymocyte (88.1%) patients. The prognostic influence of the ontogeny group was independent of that of other prognostic factors according to multivariate analysis.

Conclusion.—A small subgroup of T-lineage acute lymphoblastic leukemia children who have a significantly worse event-free survival outcome than those whose cells are of a more mature stage of development were identified by leukemic cells of the pro-thymocyte leukemia maturation.

▶ The prognostic significance of immunologic subtypes of T-lineage acute lymphoblastic leukemia remains controversial. This is in part due to the varying immunologic definitions used in different studies. However, this large study does demonstrate a subgroup (pro–T-lineage) which has a worse prognosis than other T-lineage acute lymphoblastic leukemias.

J.F. Turner, Jr., M.D.

Suggested Reading

Head DR, Behm FG: Acute lymphoblastic leukemia and the lymphoblastic lymphomas of childhood. *Semin Diagn Pathol* 12:325–334, 1995.

Pui C-H, Behm FG, Crist WM: Clinical and biologic relevance of immunologic marker studies in childhood acute lymphoblastic leukemia. *Blood* 82:343–362, 1993.

Useful Panel of Antibodies for the Classification of Acute Leukemia by Immunohistochemical Methods in Bone Marrow Trephine Biopsy Specimens

Chuang S-S, Li C-Y (Mayo Clinic and Found, Rochester, Minn)
Am J Clin Pathol 107:410–418, 1997   15–15

Introduction.—In some patients of acute leukemia, smears of peripheral blood or marrow aspirate are inadequate and pathologists may need to rely on paraffin blocks of bone marrow for diagnosing and classifying this disease. During the last few years, cell lineage-specific antibodies have become available to be applied to paraffin sections. There are few reports on the use of these newly developed, commercially available cell lineage-specific antibodies to study the entire subset of acute leukemia immunohistochemically. Paraffin sections in immunohistochemical studies were evaluated in their ability to accurately subtype acute leukemia. To diagnose the spectrum of acute leukemia, a practical cost-effective immunohistochemical study was established.

Methods.—There were 72 patients with previously established acute leukemia (covering the spectrum of 17 known subtypes) with routinely processed bone marrow biopsy specimens studied immunohistochemically.

TABLE 3.—Sensitivity and Specificity of the Antibodies Tested for Acute Leukemias

Antibody	CD No.	Leukemia	Sensitivity*	Specificity†
Group 1				
AntiHb		M6 & M6v	6/6 (100)	66/66 + 0 (100)
Anti-CD3	CD3	T ALL	8/8 (100)	64/64 + 0 (100)
HM57	CD79a	B-lineage ALL	19/19 (100)	53/53 + 0 (100)
Group 2				
PG-M1	CD68	M4, M5	11/12 (92)	60/60 + 0 (100)
Anti-TGF-β1		M6 & M6v	4/6 (67)	66/66 + 0 (100)
Anti-F8RA		M7	3/4 (75)	68/68 + 0 (100)
Y2/5	CD61	M7	3/4 (75)	68/68 + 0 (100)
Group 3				
Anti-MPO		Neutrophilic myeloblast	16/19 (84)	53/53 + 4‡ (93)
L26	CD20	B-lineage ALL	7/19 (37)	53/53 + 0 (100)
Group 4				
LCA	CD45	Acute leukemia	31/72 (43)	NA
HPCA-1	CD34	Acute leukemia	8/72 (11)	NA

*Number of positive cases/number of study cases in the particular lineage of leukemia (%).
†True number of negative cases/true number of negative cases plus the number of false-positive cases (%).
‡All 4 cases of acute eosinophilic leukemia were positive for myeloperoxidase.
Abbreviations: Hb, hemoglobin; *ALL,* acute lymphoblastic leukemia; *TGF,* transforming growth factor; *F8RA,* factor VIII-related antigen; *MPO,* myeloperoxidase; *NA,* not applicable.
(Courtesy of Chuang S-S, Li C-Y: Useful panel of antibodies for the classification of acute leukemia by immunohistochemical methods in bone marrow trephine biopsy specimens. *Am J Clin Pathol* 107:410–418, 1997.)

Twelve commercially available antibodies were tested on these subtypes of leukemia, which were classified into 4 groups (Table 3).

Results.—In 16 of 19 patients (84%), the leukemic myeloblasts were positive for myeloperoxidase, M1–M4, and M6. In 11 of 12 M4 and M5 patients, most leukemic cells were positive for CD68 (PG-M1). Hemoglobin resulted in staining for all 6 M6 patients. Three of 4 M7 patients had leukemic megakaryoblasts that were positive for factor VIII-related antigen. Eight T-lineage acute lymphoblastic leukemia patients had almost all of their leukemic cells positive for CD3 and 19 B-lineage acute lymphoblastic leukemia patients were positive for CD79a (HM58). In the more differentiated B-lineage acute lymphoblastic leukemia patients, staining with CD20 (L26) was positive and strongest in L3.

Conclusion.—This panel of cell lineage-specific antibodies can be used for most types of acute leukemia for immunohistochemical typing. For T-lineage acute lymphoblastic leukemia, the most sensitive and specific cell lineage marker was anti-CD3; for B-lineage acute lymphoblastic leukemia, the most sensitive and specific marker was anti-CD79a, and for erythroblasts, the most sensitive and specific marker was anti-Hb.

▶ Cytochemical stains and, if necessary, flow cytometric analysis are the preferred methods for determining cell lineage in acute leukemias. However, this report demonstrates the potential utility of immunohistochemical stains in determining cell lineage among blastic hematopoietic malignancies.

J.F. Turner, Jr., M.D.

Nonnasal Lymphoma Expressing the Natural Killer Cell Marker CD56: A Clinicopathologic Study of 49 Cases of an Uncommon Aggressive Neoplasm

Chan JKC, Sin VC, Wong KF, et al (Queen Elizabeth Hosp, Hong Kong; Caritas Med Ctr, Hong Kong)
Blood 89:4501–4513, 1997   15–16

Introduction.—The neuronal cell adhesion molecule is recognized by CD56 antibody, a natural killer marker, and is rarely expressed in leukemias and lymphomas. A previous study found that most CD56[+] lymphomas occurred in the nasal or nasopharyngeal region, which soon became classified as a distinctive clinicopathologic entity referred to as nasal Natural Killer/T-cell lymphoma. These lymphomas are more common among South Americans, Mexicans, and Asians than Western populations and appears as dramatic midfacial destruction. Another study discovered nonnasal lymphomas that were immunophenotypically and morphologically similar to the nasal/nasopharyngeal Natural Killer/T-cell lymphomas, but information on this group of neoplasms is limited. To characterize the clinicopathologic spectrum of these rare neoplasms, patients with nonnasal CD56[+] lymphomas were analyzed.

TABLE 4.—Summary of the Major Types of Nonnasal CD56+ Lymphomas, Based on Information From Current Series and Cases Reported in the Literature

	Nasal-Type NK/T-Cell Lymphoma	Aggressive NK Cell Leukemia/Lymphoma	Blastoid NK Cell Lymphoma	Other Specific Lymphoma Types With CD56 Expression
Age	Usually adults	Usually young or middle-aged adults	Adults	Variable
Sex	M > F	M ≥ F	?	Variable
Clinical presentation	Presenting with extranodal disease, often involving multiple sites (high stage disease at presentation). Skin, upper aerodigestive tract, soft tissues, testis and gastrointestinal tract are commonest sites of involvement.	Presenting with fever and systemic symptoms. Often have hepatosplenomegaly and sometimes lymphadenopathy.	Presenting with extranodal disease, especially skin	Variable; either nodal or extranodal presentation. Distinctive features may be seen in some specific lymphoma types, such as hepatosplenic γδ T-cell lymphomas.
Histologic features	Lymphoma cells often show irregular nuclear foldings and granular chromatin. They can be small, medium-sized or large; either a single cell type predominates, or a mixture of cell types. May be variably admixed with inflammatory cells. Necrosis common. Angiocentric growth may be identified.	Diffuse, monotonous infiltrate of medium-sized cells with condensed chromatin. Nuclei often appear round. May show angiocentric growth and necrosis.	Diffuse, monotonous infiltrate of medium-sized cells with fine chromatin and frequent mitoses. Resembling lymphoblastic lymphoma or granulocytic sarcoma.	Variable, corresponding to the specific lymphoma types.

(*Continued*)

TABLE 4 (cont.)

	Nasal-Type NK/T-Cell Lymphoma	Aggressive NK Cell Leukemia/Lymphoma	Blastoid NK Cell Lymphoma	Other Specific Lymphoma Types With CD50 Expression
Commonest immunophenotype	CD2$^-$, CD3/Leu4$^-$, CD3ϵ^+, CD56$^+$, CD16$^-$, CD57$^-$	CD2$^-$, CD3/Leu4$^-$, CD3ϵ^+, CD56$^+$, CD16, CD57$^-$	CD2$^{-/-}$, CD3/Leu4$^-$, CD3ϵ^+, CD56$^+$, TdT$^-$	CD2$^-$, CD3/Leu4$^-$, CD3ϵ^+, CD56$^+$, other T-lineage markers$^-$
T-cell receptor genes	Germline	Germline	Germline	Rearranged
Association with EBV	>90%	>90%	0%	Variable, usually negative
Clinical behavior	Aggressive, with early dissemination. Relapse is very common despite initial response to chemotherapy.	Fulminant course	Aggressive	Aggressive

(Courtesy of Chan JKC, Sin VC, Wong KF, et al: Nonnasal lymphoma expressing the natural killer cell marker CD56: A clinicopathologic study of 49 cases of an uncommon aggressive neoplasm. *Blood* 89:4501–4513, 1997.)

Methods.—Frozen sections or cell smears using the antibody NKH1 or paraffin sections using the antibody 123C3 were used to identify the CD56 status immunohistochemically. There were 49 Chinese patients identified and their clinical data and follow-up information were collected. Nonisotopic in situ hybridization for identifying Epstein-Barr virus was used.

Results.—Among the 49 patients, 4 categories (Table 4) were delineated. In the first group, 34 patients had nasal-type Natural Killer/T cell lymphoma with extranodal disease, usually in multiple sites. The skin, testis, soft tissue, gastrointestinal tract, spleen, and upper aerodigestive tract were the most common sites. Pleomorphic with irregular nuclei and granular chromatin, the neoplastic cells often had angiocentric growth. Epstein-Barr virus was found in 32 of these patients, and the characteristic immunophenotype was $CD2^+CD3/Leu4^-CD3\epsilon^+CD56+CD16^-CD57^-$. In 29 patients, in which follow-up information was available, 24 died at a median of 3.5 months, 2 were alive at 3 and 5 years, respectively, and 3 were alive with relapse at 4 months to 2.5 years.

In the second category, 5 patients had aggressive Natural Killer cell leukemia/lymphoma with hepatomegaly and blood/marrow involvement, sometimes with splenomegaly or lymphadenopathy. Within 6 weeks all of these patients died. They all had Epstein-Barr virus and an immunophenotype of $CD2^+CD3/Leu4^-CD56^+CD16^-CD57^-$.

The third category consisted of 2 patients with blastoid Natural Killer cell lymphoma, in which the lymphoma cells resembled lymphoblastic or myeloid leukemia.

In the fourth group, 8 patients had other specific lymphoma types with CD56 expression, including hepatosplenic $\gamma\delta$T-cell lymphoma and S100 protein$^+$ T-cell lymphoproliferative disease, T-chronic lymphocytic/prolymphocytic leukemia, true histiocytic lymphoma, and lymphoblastic lymphoma. At a median of 6.5 months, 6 patients died.

Conclusion.—All nonnasal $CD56^+$ lymphomas pursue a highly aggressive clinical course and are heterogeneous. Distinctive clinicopathological features and a very strong association with Epstein-Barr virus are shown with the nasal-type NK-T-cell lymphoma and aggressive NK cell leukemia/lymphoma.

▶ This report summarizes the current understanding of CD56$^+$ lymphomas occurring outside of the nasopharynx. Although these neoplasms are rare, they are important to recognize because of the associated aggressive clinical course.

J.F. Turner, Jr., M.D.

Suggested Reading

Jaffe ES, Chan JKC, Su I-J, et al: Report of the workshop on nasal and related extranodal angiocentric T/natural killer cell lymphomas, definitions, differential diagnosis, and epidemiology. *Am J Surg Pathol* 20:103–111, 1996.

Neural Cell Adhesion Molecule (CD56)-Positve Acute Myelogenous Leukemia and Myelodysplastic and Myeloproliferative Syndromes

Mann KP, DeCastro CM, Liu J, et al (Duke Univ, Durham, NC)
Am J Clin Pathol 107:653–660, 1997

15–17

Introduction.—Unique features in some types of myeloid leukemia have been identified by molecular biologic studies, and their assessment has provided information on more precise diagnosis, more accurate prognostication, and altered therapeutic approaches. The CD56 antigen is characteristically expressed on normal lymphoid cells with natural-killer function, but its aberrant expression has been detected in a variety of unrelated hematopoietic neoplasms. Expression of CD56 in patients with increased myeloblasts and a diagnosis of acute myelogenous leukemia, myelodysplastic syndromes, or myeloproliferative syndromes were studied to determine the significance of CD56 expression in myeloid neoplasia. These findings were correlated with response to therapy, cytogenetic findings, clinical outcome, and status of the mixed lineage leukemia gene.

Methods.—Multiparameter flow cytometry was used to analyze 114 clinical samples with increased myeloblasts from a 16-month period to determine anomalous expression of CD56. Morphologic review was performed on CD56+ blast cells from 23 patients, including those with acute myelogenous leukemia, myelodysplastic syndromes, and chronic myelogenous leukemia in blast crisis. A review was conducted of clinical information and cytogenetic data. When possible, detection of rearrangement of the mixed lineage leukemia gene was performed with Southern blot analysis.

Results.—At least partial monocytic differentiation was demonstrated on the samples from 10 of 15 patients with CD56⁺ acute myelogenous leukemia. The samples of 12 patients had dysplastic features. There was no correlation with specific cytogenetic abnormalities. In 5 of 18 patients, the mixed lineage leukemia gene was rearranged. There was median survival of 4.6 months for patients with acute myelogenous leukemia, and 17 patients died. Complete remission was sustained by 3 patients. High-grade myelodysplastic syndrome was found on 1 patient.

Conclusion.—In 20% of patients with increased myeloblasts, expression of CD56 was found. Dysplasia, monocytic differentiation, and rearrangement of the mixed lineage leukemia gene was associated with this phenotype, which is also associated with early death and difficulty in achieving remission. Patients with mixed lineage leukemia gene died of their disease within 1 year of diagnosis, and are probably a poor prognostic group.

► CD56 is an isoform of the neural cell adhesion molecule (NCAM) which participates in cellular adhesion interactions.[1] It is expressed in neural tissue and muscle, as well as in hematopoietic cells. Due to alternative RNA splicing and post-translational glycosylation, the forms of CD56 expressed in these different tissues are highly variable.[1] The normal hematopoietic cells that are CD56 positive include natural-killer cells, a small percentage of cytotoxic T-cells, and a small percentage of peripheral blood monocytes.[2] CD56 is expressed on hematopoietic neoplasms of disparate lineage including large granular lymphocyte leukemia, aggressive T-cell lymphomas, multiple myeloma, and acute myeloid leukemias (AML).

Neoplasms with CD56 expression have been the subject of at least 45 articles within the last 2 years. These articles mainly discussed CD56 positivity in multiple myeloma and lymphoid neoplasms. This report expands the list of CD56 positive hematopoietic neoplasms to include myelodysplastic syndromes. The article also confirms that CD56 is expressed in a variety of AML subtypes (as formalized in the French-American-British classification system), as well as in the myeloid blasts noted in blast crisis of chronic myelogenous leukemia. Interestingly, a high incidence of monocytic differentiation (10 of 15 cases) was noted in the CD56 positive cases of AML. In addition, the mixed lineage leukemia (MLL) gene was frequently noted in these cases with monocytic differentiation. As the authors suggest, because the MLL gene is associated with a poor prognosis, CD56 positivity may serve as a screening tool to indicate which cases require investigation of rearrangement of the MLL gene. However, before evaluation of CD56 is advocated for a routine practice, the correlation between CD56 positivity and the presence of the MLL gene needs confirmation.

J.F. Turner, Jr., M.D.

References

1. Lanier LL, Testi Ri, Bindl J, et al: Identity of Leu-19 (CD56) leukocyte differentiation antigen and neural cell adhesion molecule. *J Exp Med* 169:2233, 1989.
2. Robertson MJ, Ritz J: Biology and clinical relevance of human natural killer cells. *Blood* 76:2421, 1990.

Suggested Reading

Hurwitz CA, Raimondi SC, Head D, et al: Distinctive immunophenotypic features of t(8;21) (q22;q22) acute myeloblastic leukemia in children. *Blood* 80:3182–3188, 1992.

Reuss-Borst MA, Steinke B, Waller HD, et al: Phenotype and clinical heterogeneity of CD56-positive acute nonlymphoblastic leukemia. *Ann Hematol* 64:78–82, 1992.

Scott AA, Head DR, Kopecky KJ, et al: HLA-DR$^-$, CD33$^+$, CD56$^+$, CD16$^-$ myeloid/natural killer cell acute leukemia: A previously unrecognized form of acute leukemia potentially misdiagnosed as French-American-British acute myeloid leukemia-M3. *Blood* 84:244–255, 1994.

11q23 Rearrangements in Acute Leukemia

Rubnitz JE, Behm FG, Downing JR (St Jude Children's Res Hosp, Memphis, Tenn; Univ of Tennessee, Memphis)
Leukemia 10:74–82, 1996　　　　　　　　　　　　　　　　　　　15–18

Background.—Alterations of chromosome 11, band q23, occur in about 10% of cases of acute lymphoblastic leukemia (ALL) and 5% of cases of acute myeloblastic leukemia (AML). These cytogenetic abnormalities are also observed in about 85% of secondary leukemias occurring in patients treated with topoisomerase II inhibitors. Twenty different reciprocal chromosomal loci have been shown to take part in 11q23 translocations. The gene that is disrupted by these various translocations was recently cloned and designated MLL. The clinical and biologic features of leukemias associated with 11q23 rearrangements are reviewed, along with the molecular biology of MLL translocations.

Features of 11q23 Leukemias.—The various chromosomal lesions of 11q23 are associated with specific clinical, pathological, and biological characteristics in ALL as well as AML. 11q23 translocations are also associated with a distinct subtype of secondary AML. Standard cytogenetic studies can detect 11q23 translocations in the leukemic blasts of more than 50% of infants with ALL. In contrast, translocations are found in less than 5% of adult cases of ALL. The 11q23 abnormalities are now recognized as a heterogeneous group of gene rearrangements. The MLL gene is affected in most but not all 11q23 translocations; it is unaffected in most 11q23 deletions and inversions. The molecular rearrangements of MLL are more clinically specific and predictive than the structural abnormalities of 11q23.

Detection of MLL Rearrangements.—Several studies have used molecular genetics to characterize the 11q23 leukemias. Up to 81% of cases of infant ALL have shown MLL rearrangements, including many cases that lack detectable 11q23 abnormalities. These rearrangements are also common in children aged 13- to 18-months-old. Even on aggressive chemotherapy protocols, infants with ALL and MLL rearrangements do poorly, with a long-term survival rate of less than 20%. It is essential to identify these high-risk patients at diagnosis so that they can be targeted for bone marrow transplantation or other new treatments. The prognostic relevance of MLL rearrangements in older ALL children is unknown. However, the most recent evidence suggests that they too do poorly with current treatments. Children with balanced translocations of 11q23 who lack MLL rearrangements appear to have a favorable prognosis. Secondary AMLs associated with topoisomerase II inhibitor treatment are associated with MLL rearrangements similar to those noted in ALL.

Discussion.—Current knowledge of 11q23 rearrangements in acute leukemia are reviewed, with an emphasis on MLL gene rearrangements. Reverse transcriptase-polymerase chain reaction can be used to screen for fusion transcripts resulting from the most common translocations. The Southern blot technique can then be performed to identify other MLL alterations. Patients with MLL gene rearrangements must be identified and targeted for aggressive therapies. Further study of the MLL gene and its role in the development of leukemia should lead to specific treatments for these high-risk patients.

▶ This review provides an overview of the importance of identifying mixed lineage leukemia (MLL) gene rearrangements in leukemia. As indicated in this review, the analysis of MLL gene rearrangements by the molecular techniques of reverse transcriptase-polymerase chain reaction and Southern blot may potentially be used for stratifying acute leukemia into different prognostic groups. Since routine cytogenetic analysis may not detect rearrangements of genes such as MLL and not all translocations at a particular breakpoint are indicative of the rearranged gene, these molecular techniques will prove useful in the future.

J.F. Turner, Jr., M.D.

16 Pathology Outcomes Analysis

The Cost of Production in Cervical Cytology: Comparison of Conventional and Automated Primary Screening Systems
Bishop JW (Creighton Univ, Omaha, NE)
Am J Clin Pathol 107:445–450, 1997   16–1

Introduction.—Because costs often exceed the potential reimbursement, the cost of production is an important issue for cervical cytology in the current setting of managed care and capitation and with the advent of automated cytology. A method for the calculation of the cost of production in cervical cytology was described and compared with the cost of conventional and automated interpretation of a cervical sample.

Methods.—Cost components were observed in a university practice setting during the parallel processing and evaluation of 2,106 thin-layer preparations and conventional slides using a robotic batch processor. Cost analysis was based on 6 elements: technologist screening cost (wages and benefits) per slide, material (disposables) cost per slide, processing cost (wages and benefits) per slide, pathologist review cost (average per slide), facilities cost (lease and utilities) per slide, and instrument cost (capital equipment) depreciated per slide. Some costs, such as courier services and billing, are not included in the formula. Calculations are presented for a conventional cervical smear, a thin-layer smear read by computer-assisted technology, and the proposed conventional smear–thin-layer combination.

Results.—For the laboratory at the study institution and its annual cytology volume of 20,000 cases, the production cost for a conventional smear is $9.75. If approved for primary screening, the comparable production cost by a primary screening automated method would be $12.07. A capital investment of $250,000 was used for the CytoRich device (CytoRich, Autocyte, Elon College, NC).

Discussion.—The difference between the conventional and automated methods ($9.75 vs. $12.07) is striking, particularly given the usual Medicare-allowed reimbursement in the study institution's region ($7.15). The cost of production is 24% higher for the automated system, but the difference would be lowered to 14% at an annual value of 40,000 specimens. Combinations of conventional and automated examinations would not be cost-effective without passing the additional production expense through to the payers. As for the status quo, convential cervical smear reports are loss leaders when they no longer serve the purpose of gaining other business.

▶ The value of this article is twofold. The first is of introducing us to the concept of cost analysis, a necessity in an era of managed care and cost-driven competition. The second is of working through a specific example of cost analysis, that of comparing the cost of production of conventional and automated primary cervical vaginal screening systems. Bishop does a wonderful job of simplifying particular aspects of the cost of production, which, to be honest, has rarely been done before in anatomical pathology. Others have attempted "cost analysis" before but have left out important aspects of cost, such as material and overhead costs.[1-3]

It is interesting that Bishop showed that the cost of production of conventional screening was lower than that of automated screening. However, this does not mean that conventional screening is more cost-effective, because cost-effectiveness depends on weighing both the costs and utilities, and the utilities (e.g., sensitivity) of the 2 systems were never compared. A myriad of questions may be asked after the reading of this article. These include what is the cost of production of other surgical pathology tests; how can costs be effectively reduced; how do costs compare with utilities; what is the relation between costs, charges, and reimbursements; should we perform tests that lose money; and what other costs should be entered into a cost analysis (e.g., malpractice costs)? This whole area is one that will guide pathology research in the rest of this century and the beginning of the next.

S. Raab, M.D.

References

1. National Committee for Clinical Laboratory Standards: *Cost Accounting in the Clinical Laboratory: Tentative Guideline.* Villanova, Pa, National Committee for Clinical Laboratory Standards, 1993. NCCLS document GP11–T.
2. Hutchinson ML: Assessing the costs and benefits of alternative rescreening strategies. *Acta Cytol* 40:4–8, 1996.
3. Castleberry BM, Yablonsky T, Wargelin L: 1994 wage and vacancy survey of medical laboratories. *Lab Med* 26:106–112, 1995.

Consequences of Neural Network Technology for Cervical Screening: Increase in Diagnostic Consistency and Positive Scores
Kok MR, Boon ME (Leiden Cytology and Pathology Lab, The Netherlands)
Cancer 78:112–117, 1996   16–2

Introduction.—False negative diagnoses are a problem with human screening of cervical smears. Most of these false negative results are related to the relatively small numbers of abnormal cells in the specimen, rather than to unfamiliarity with the diagnostic criteria. Available neural network technology may offer 1 way to help the cytotechnologist in identifying the abnormal cells that are present. One such network, the PAPNET system, was studied for use in a cervical smear screening program.

Methods.—Seven cytotechnologists involved in daily cervical smear screening participated in the study. The results of 91,294 smears screened over a 3-year period were analyzed—25,767 screened conventionally and 65,527 with the aid of PAPNET. Scores for atypias of undetermined significance, squamous or glandular (positive I); low-grade squamous precursor lesions (positive II); and high-grade squamous lesions and invasive carcinoma (positive III) were calculated for each cytotechnologist and by both screening methods. Histologic scores were calculated as well.

Results.—All 7 cytotechnologists had higher mean positive scores using PAPNET than with conventional screening. Coefficients of variability were lower with PAPNET as well. Screening consistency for positive III smears was significantly better with PAPNET. The sensitivity of screening increased, as indicated by higher histologically positive scores for carcinoma in situ and invasive carcinoma.

Conclusions.—The PAPNET neural network can enhance diagnostic consistency and screening efficacy of cytotechnologists involved in daily cervical smear screening. The PAPNET system complements human screening.

▶ I think that this article on automated cytology screening is important not so much because of its content but because it was published in *Cancer*, rather than in a primary pathology journal. For a number of reasons, information on automated cytology screening has circumvented pathologists, and often, clinicians know more than pathologists about the accuracy of automated screening systems. I write this not to complain about information flow, but to encourage all of us to keep abreast of the automated cytology screening literature.[1-4]

Automated instruments may be used for primary screening or secondary screening (rescreening), although at the time of writing this comment, in the United States, only secondary screening is approved by the Food and Drug Administration for some instruments. Europe is a different ballpark. Kok and Boon examined side-by-side primary screening using the conventional method and PAPNET. It is critical to note that this study did not compare false negative rates, although the data indicated that PAPNET detected more atypias of undetermined significance, squamous or glandular, low-grade squamous epithelial lesions, and high-grade squamous epithelial lesions than conventional screening. Even assuming that the additional cases detected by PAPNET were "missed" by conventional screening (which again, is not a valid assumption!), PAPNET would have detected 2.2 additional cases of high-grade squamous epithelial lesions per 1,000 patients. The PAPNET system also would have detected 6.6 more cases of atypias of undetermined significance, squamous or glandular.

Does this mean we should use automated screening? Not necessarily, because I do not think that the appropriate cost-benefit studies, evaluating the utility of detecting more high-grade squamous epithelial lesions, have been done. Remember that there have not been studies examining the potential harmful impact of false negatives in a population that undergoes yearly routine screening. In addition, in the United States system, where some patients with squamous atypias of undetermined significance, are treated, the cost-benefit of detecting more squamous atypias of undetermined significance has not been assessed. Of course, others may interpret this article as supporting the utility of automated rescreening, so be prepared. I think that there are not enough data to draw this conclusion.

S. Raab, M.D.

References

1. Rosenthal DL, Acosta DA, Peters RK: Computer-assisted rescreening of clinically important false-negative cervical smears using the PAPNET testing system. *Acta Cytol* 40:120–126, 1996.
2. Mango LJ, for Neuromedical Systems, Inc: Industrial developments in automated cytology. *Acta Cytol* 40:53–59, 1996.
3. Boon ME, Kok LP, Beck S: Histologic validation of neural network-assisted cervical screening: Comparison with the conventional procedure. *Cell Vision* 2:23–27, 1995.
4. Mango LJ, Herriman JM: The PAPNET cytological screening system: Compendium on the computerized cytology and histology laboratory, in Wied GL, Bartels PH, Rosenthal DL, et al (eds): Tutorials of Cytology. Chicago, Wied Publications, pp 320–334, 1994.

Comparison of the Costs of Fine-needle Aspiration and Open Surgical Biopsy as Methods for Obtaining a Pathologic Diagnosis
Rimm DL, Stastny JF, Rimm EB, et al (Yale Univ, New Haven, Conn; Virginia Commonwealth Univ, Richmond; Harvard School of Public Health, Boston)
Cancer 81:51–56, 1997   16–3

Background.—Fine-needle aspiration biopsy was first performed more than 60 years ago, gaining popularity in Europe 20–30 years later and in North America 10–15 years after that. It is considered a less expensive alternative to surgical biopsy. It has been difficult to analyze the actual savings of this procedure. Use of fine-needle aspiration biopsy is often higher in countries with a lower per capita health care expenditure. Savings resulting from the use of this procedure were evaluated.

Methods.—Data collected by the cytopathology service at a medical college during a 20-year period were obtained. Of 12,452 cases, 9,810 cases of palpable lesions were selected. Cost savings were estimated in dollars and as relative value units using the 1995 *Physicians' Fee Reference* or Medicare participant fees. Charges for fine-needle aspiration and open surgical biopsy were compared, omitting other biopsy-related costs.

Results.—A sufficient pathologic diagnosis was obtained by fine-needle aspiration biopsy to avoid surgical biopsy in 63% to 85% of cases. The cost savings based on distribution of cases and indications for surgery were estimated to be $250,000–$750,000 per 1,000 fine-needle aspiration biopsies performed, or 5,500 relative value units.

Summary.—Use of fine-needle aspiration biopsy results in significant cost savings over use of open surgical biopsy. This estimate of savings is conservative and may be substantially lower than actual savings because of the omission of biopsy-related costs.

▶ Wow! Here are the data you've been waiting for. This is a detailed, conservative estimate of how much can be saved by doing fine-needle aspirations (FNAs) very well. We should keep in mind that doing them well requires a certain minimum volume, and that doing more only makes us more skilled. But what do we tell the chairperson or the administration? It is very easy to reward the staff for doing something that makes money. However, as medicine moves away from this type of reimbursement, our role becomes more important as we facilitate the saving of money by allowing the system to omit a procedure that would otherwise be performed. Not spending is the most direct way to save. We need a macro-economic view that places this information in the context of the institution or system as a whole. Just looking at the department's billing for FNA services tells only a small part of a much larger story. The approach and the information in this paper should be useful to those whose departments or institution have FNA services.

M.W. Stanley, M.D.

Suggested Reading

Layfield LJ, Chrischilles EA, Cohen MB, et al: The palpable breast nodule: A cost-effectiveness analysis of alternate diagnostic approaches. *Cancer* 72:1642–1651, 1993.

Vetto J, Pommier R, Schmidt W, et al: Use of the "triple test" for palpable breast lesions yields high diagnostic accuracy and cost savings. *Am J Surg* 169:519–522, 1995.

College of American Pathologists Conference XXX on Quality and Liability Issues With the Papanicolaou Smear: Summation
Austin RM (Univ of South Carolina, Charleston)
Arch Pathol Lab Med 121:341–342, 1997   16–4

Purpose.—The Papanicolaou (Pap) smear is the most successful cancer screening test in history. However, there is increasing attention to the limitations of this test. The public and plaintiffs' attorneys insist on elimination of false-negative results; however, the available data suggest that this is not possible. Enhanced Pap smears have been developed, but their greater expense raises difficult questions at a time of increased emphasis on cost control. Current quality and liability issues related to the Pap smear were reviewed.

Discussion.—There are professional standards governing the performance of Pap smears, and quantitative measures have been developed to reduce error to the greatest extent possible. However, even laboratories that adhere to professional standards and achieve near-minimum error rates may be held, retrospectively, to unachieveably low standards of error. This has led some hospitals to "outsource" their Pap tests to large regional laboratories. The outsourcing trend reduces the likelihood the cytologic-histologic correlation will be performed, when indicated. Laboratory reviews must maintain their educational and quality improvement benefits without leading to liability problems. If biased, retrospective review was to become the new standard, the price of Pap smears would increase, with negative public health implications.

In medicolegal cases, the rights of injured defendants must be balanced against reasonable, scientifically grounded standards for professionals performing Pap smears. However, law firms have even solicited the families of patients with cervical cancer to file suits. Cytologists must be educated as to the legal meaning of the reasonable prudent practitioner standard, because the courts rely on expert witnesses. The practitioner is required to use "average reasonable care," not to be perfect. Patients and professionals alike should understand the limitations of Pap smears, with more contextual information provided along with smear reports when the results are normal, negative, or benign. Informed consent forms for patients in gynecologic practices are being tested, but more for their educational value than for legal protection. Guidelines for the review of Pap smears will encourage a rational approach to case review, and in assessing the expert witness's concept of the reasonable practitioner standard. Guidelines should be aimed toward an achievable standard and peer accountability for accurate scientific statements.

Conclusions.—The quality and liability issues that surround Pap smears are a societal problem. These issues may not be resolved until society perceives that public access to affordable cervical cancer screening is threatened. The coming years will have an important influence on the ultimate fate of this highly successful public health intervention.

▶ The published proceedings of this important conference need to be considered as a whole. This brief commentary can only point out what seem to be some of the highlights from comments offered by a wide range of speakers. Interpretive problems are clearly discussed and effectively illustrated by Dr. DeMay. Legal issues, quality assurance, review of smears by experts, automation in cytology, and accreditation are discussed. The false-negative fraction is gaining acceptance as a quality/accuracy measure for evaluation of screening; it is described in detail by Dr. Naryshkin. In one of the most fascinating essays, Dr. Derman likens quality issues in cytology to the science of error prevention in industry. The difficult area of amended reports after retrospective slide review is discussed clearly. Many points emerged from the conference and are crystallized in these articles. The Pap smear is not perfect and will always have a failure rate because not all abnormal cells will be detected. Furthermore, we will never achieve complete agreement about the significance of some abnormal cells. High practice standards and education of the public seem to be common themes in the "what is to be done" portion of these essays. Problems with unreasonable testimony by "rogue experts" from our own profession were mentioned by several speakers; no effective means for addressing these difficulties were forthcoming. In my mind, the most noteworthy commentary on this conference, and on these publications is that at the time of this writing about 1½ years later, not much seems to be happening, and absolutely nothing seems to be changing. The energy seems to have dissipated.

M.W. Stanley, M.D.

Malpractice Protection: Communication of Diagnostic Uncertainty
Skoumal SM, Florell SR, Bydalek MK, et al (Creighton Univ, Omaha, Neb; Univ of Utah, Salt Lake City)
Diagn Cytopathol 14:385–389, 1996   16–5

Objective.—The number of malpractice claims filed against pathologists for misdiagnosis, particularly for cervical smears and fine-needle aspirates of breast lumps (BFNAs), is increasing. Improved communication between pathologist and clinician is critical in preventing malpractice actions. Qualitative anatomic reporting methods, diagnostic inaccuracies associated with certain cytologic areas that carry high litigation risk, malpractice liability concepts, and suggestions to improve report communication are discussed.

Qualitative Anatomic Reporting.—Although a specific binary diagnosis is often not possible, qualitative information is not clinically useful. A conditional probability report would provide information to clinicians about the degree of the pathologist's certainty.

Diagnostic Inaccuracies and Binary Diagnoses.—The false-negative rate for BFNA is 8.0%, which includes a 7% sampling error and a 1% interpretation error, and the false-positive rate is 1%, according to an interinstitutional study (BFNA's Q Probe). Diagnostic sensitivity for ±75% of pathology groups was 100%. A group with a false-negative BFNA result should not, however, necessarily settle a malpractice claim.

Malpractice and the Application of Res Ipsa Loquitur.—Previously, negligence had to be proved by the plaintiff for malpractice to be established. Recently, there has been a trend toward application of the principle of "res ipsa loquitur," which examines whether an action would have occurred under ordinary circumstances. If not, negligence is presumed, and the defendant has the burden of rebuttal. To lower their liability profile, pathologists should communicate the limitations of their anatomic reports and include known error rates.

Reports on BFNAs.—Performance practice norms from BFNA's Q Probe study should be available to clinicians, so that they have up-to-date information.

Cervical (Pap) Cytology Reports.—A recent study of errors in simultaneously sampled cervical smears and biopsy samples found that 64% were caused by sampling, 29% were interpretive, and 7% were both. On rescreening negative cervical smears, a recent interinstitutional comparison program found an 8% false-negative incidence, with 6.3% of these cases resulting from screening errors, interpretive errors, or a combination of the two, and 85.2% resulting from sampling errors. A statement of limitation should include a false-negative rate of 8% and recommend clinical correlation.

Conclusion.—Improving communication between pathologist and clinician by changing the language of the cytology report and including limitations should lower pathologists' liability profile.

▶ These authors suggest the use of disclaimers about diagnostic limitations in pathology reports. Others have said that this would have little effect on one's fate should a lawsuit be filed. Regardless of any potential effect on a legal action, however, report disclaimers can have considerable educational value for clinicians, and, through clinicians (as "learned intermediaries") for patients. It is amazing how many doctors (and their office staffs, who actually spend a great deal of time speaking with patients) have no idea that a patient with disease may have a negative Pap smear result (or any other nondiagnostic laboratory test result, for that matter).

M.W. Stanley, M.D.

Suggested Reading

Robb J: The Pap smear is a cancer screening test: Why not put the screening error rate in the report? *Diagn Cytopathol* 9:485–486, 1993.

Troxel DB, Sabella JD: Problem areas in pathology practice uncovered by a review of malpractice claims. *Am J Surg Pathol* 18:821–831, 1994.

Interinstitutional Comparison of Frozen Section Consultation in Small Hospitals
Novis DA, Gephardt GN, Zarbo RJ (Wentworth Douglass Hosp, Dover, NH; Kennestone Hosp, Marietta, Ga; Henry Ford Hosp, Detroit)
Arch Pathol Lab Med 120:1087–1093, 1996   16–6

Introduction.—The Q-Probes program of the College of American Pathologists has created multi-institutional reference databases of quality attributes of intraoperative consultation. Out of concern that Q-Probes better serve larger than smaller hospitals, a series of 3 Q-Probes investigations were initiated to examine the diagnostic accuracy of frozen sections (FS) performed exclusively in small hospitals with occupied bed capacities of less than 330. Reported are findings of the third Q-Probes investigation.

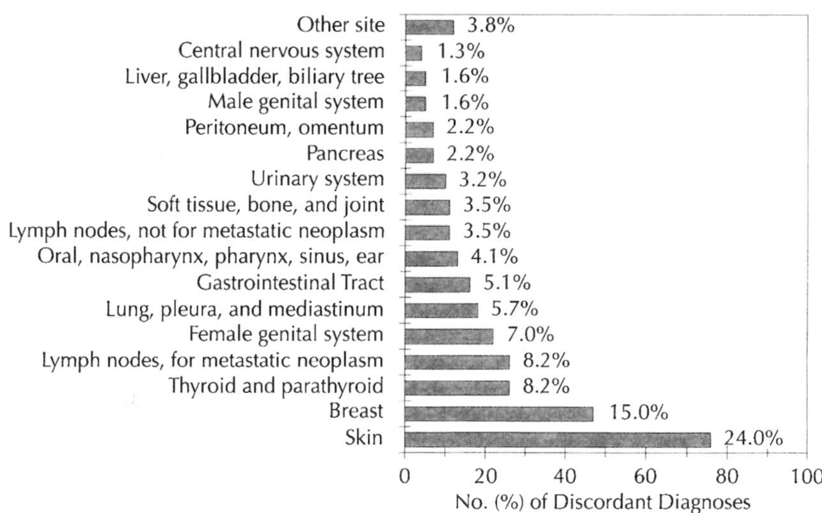

FIGURE 1.—Breakdown of discordant frozen-section diagnoses (n = 316) by anatomical site. (Courtesy of Novis DA, Gephardt GN, Zarbo RJ: Interinstitutional comparison of frozen section consultation in small hospitals. *Arch Pathol Lab Med* 120:1087–1093, 1996.)

Methods.—In 1994, 232 institutions in North America and 1 institution in New Zealand completed questionnaires regarding workload and pathology practices. Data were prospectively collected on up to 20 FS procedures performed over a 5–month period. Discordance and deferral rates of FS diagnoses and reasons for FS discordance relative to corresponding diagnoses made on paraffin sections were recorded.

Results.—Of 18,532 frozen section diagnoses from 327,884 surgical patients, 859 (4.6%) diagnoses were deferred until availability of permanent sections. Of nondeferred diagnoses, 17,357 (98.2%) were in agreement and 316 (1.8%) (Fig 1) disagreed with diagnoses rendered on permanent sections. The most frequent cause of discordance was underdiagnosis of neoplasia, usually because of block- or tissue-sampling errors.

Conclusion.—The median FS discordance rate of this Q-Probe investigation of small hospitals is similar to that of larger institutions. It is recommended that laboratories routinely monitor FS discordance, cut additional sections deeper into the frozen block, and/or sample additional tissue in the presence of negative or nonproductive initial FS. All discordant FS diagnoses should be reconciled in the final report. It is important to analyze the value of performing FS periodically.

▶ Anyone who routinely browses through *Archives of Pathology and Laboratory Medicine* is familiar with the Q-Probe study, which presents a plethora of data that may seem mind-boggling. Other Q-Probe studies published in the past year, which I recommend reading, are concerned with "extraneous" surgical pathology tissue, autopsy turnaround time, and laboratory computer availability.[1-3] Q-probes serve as a quality improvement monitor that reaches across hospitals. The work by Novis, et al. is third in a series of

Q-Probes examining frozen sections. For the practicing pathologist in the small hospital, this study is important because one can compare one's practice of frozen section with the practice of others. A drawback to this study was that the mean percentage of frozen section by site was not presented. It would be nice to know whether the percentage by site of frozen sections done in one hospital is the same as at another hospital, because error rate depends on specimen site. Novis, et al. reported a 4.6% mean deferral rate and a 1.8% mean discordant rate, with almost 40% of all discordancies arising from frozen section of skin or breast. These rates are similar to those presented in previous Q-Probes, indicating that pathologists at smaller hospitals perform similarly in regards to frozen-section accuracy as pathologists at larger hospitals.

To me a drawback of these frozen-section Q-Probes is that, in some aspects, not enough data are presented. For example, I would like to see more quantification about the types of errors made, so that I will not make these errors in the future. The information of all Q-Probe studies should be pooled and the specific errors in each organ system should be presented. Other data I would like to know are: do these institutions section through an entire block if there is a negative diagnosis; are touch preparations done; what percentage of frozen sections do the pathologists think are unnecessary; and what is done about these errors? I think that unless your institution is an outlier on the deferral or discordant rate, this other information will be more important.

S. Raab, M.D.

References

1. Gephardt GN, Zarbo RJ: Extraneous tissue in surgical pathology: A College of American Pathologists Q-probes study of 275 laboratories. *Arch Pathol Lab Med* 120:1009–1014, 1996.
2. Baker PB, Zarbo RJ, Howanitz PJ: Quality assurance of autopsy face sheet reporting, final autopsy report turnaround time, and autopsy rates: A College of American Pathologists Q-probes study of 10,003 autopsies from 418 institutions. *Arch Pathol Lab Med* 120:1003–1008, 1996.
3. Valenstein P, Aller RD: Laboratory computer availability: A College of American Pathologists Q-probe study of computer downtime in 422 institutions. *Arch Pathol Lab Med* 120:626–632, 1996.

Diagnostic Accuracy of an International Static-imaging Telepathology Consultation Service

Halliday BE, Bhattacharyya AK, Graham AR, et al (Univ of Arizona, Tucson)
Hum Pathol 28:17–21, 1997
16–7

Introduction.—The diagnostic accuracy of telepathology has rarely been evaluated in actual clinical practice. The Arizona-International Telemedicine Network (AITN) offers static-imaging telepathology services to rural and metropolitan hospitals and to pathologists in solo and group practices. Reported are AITN results of the accuracy of static-image diagnoses in 171 patients.

Methods.—Digital images were sent by pathologists from 6 participating institutions from Arizona, Mexico, and China. Representative glass slides (GS) from individual patients were mailed for GS review for quality assurance purposes. Glass slides were reviewed by 1 of 3 triage pathologists who either gave a telepathology diagnosis; showed the video images to a subspecialty pathologist, then rendered a telepathology diagnosis; or deferred rendering the final diagnosis until evaluating the GS. A review panel of 2 staff pathologists retrospectively reviewed GS from each patient. Their consensual diagnosis was considered the "truth" diagnosis.

Results.—Of 171 patients, a telepathology diagnosis (TP) was rendered for 144 and diagnosis was deferred in 27 (to review GS for conventional light microscopy in 14 patients [8.1%] and for results of immunohistochemistry in 13 patients [7.6%]). The concordance between TP and GS diagnoses was 88.2% (127 of 144 patients). For clinically important diagnoses, the concordance was 96.5% (139 of 144 patients).

Conclusion.—The correct diagnoses were provided by static-image telepathology in 127 of 171 patients (74.9%) at the time of telepathology diagnostic sessions. Factors that may decrease the value of consultations based on the viewing of static images include inappropriate field selection and sampling biases of referring pathologists and tendency of static-image telepathologists to underestimate the complexity of static-images they are evaluating.

▶ Telepathology is one of the "hot" areas in pathology and is currently undergoing technologic assessment. *Human Pathology* recently devoted a large portion of one issue to this subject, and this article was one of the more intriguing; the other articles are listed as references at the end of this comment.[1-6] Three potential uses of telepathology are: (1) frozen-section diagnosis; (2) expert consultation; and (3) evaluation of "routine" specimens at small hospitals with low volumes. Most previous studies have focused on the performance evaluation of telepathologic frozen-section diagnosis or the evaluation of routine specimens. Halliday, et al. studied expert consultation and showed that a "correct" diagnosis was rendered by static-image telepathology in only 74.3% of cases, and a deferral was made in 15.7% of cases. For some specimen types, particularly those that might need immunohistochemistry or other special studies, telepathology would appear to be unwarranted, because these cases probably would be deferred and sent to the expert consultant anyway. "Incorrect," clinically significant diagnoses were made in 5 (3%) cases. This 3% incorrect rate is not an insignificant figure, but more studies are needed to determine whether this accuracy can be improved using a static or a real time system. For evaluation of frozen sections and routine specimens, other studies have shown diagnostic accuracies in the range of 80% to 95%. Are these figures sufficiently high that we should use telepathology? I think that eventually we may, but not, at least for most pathology groups, while telepathology is still an infant. Particularly we must wait for the studies demonstrating the cost-effectiveness of telepathology.

S. Raab, M.D.

References

1. Weinstein RS, Bhattacharyya AK, Graham AR, et al: Telepathology: A ten-year progress report. *Hum Pathol* 28:1–7, 1997.
2. Dunn BE, Almagro UA, Choi H, et al: Dynamic-robotic telepathology: Department of Veterans Affairs feasibility study. *Hum Pathol* 28:8–12, 1997.
3. Eusebi V, Foschini L, Erde S, et al: Transcontinental consults in surgical pathology via the internet. *Hum Pathol* 28:13–16, 1997.
4. Weinstein MH, Epstein JI: Telepathology diagnosis of prostate needle biopsies. *Hum Pathol* 28:22–29, 1997.
5. Weinstein LJ, Epstein JI, Edlow D, et al: Static image analysis of skin specimens: The application of telepathology to frozen section evaluation. *Hum Pathol* 28:30–35, 1997.
6. Doolittle MH, Doolittle KW, Winkelman Z, et al: Color images in telepathology: How many colors do we need? *Hum Pathol* 28:36–41, 1997.

The Need for Specialist Review of Pathology in Paediatric Cancer

Parkes SE, Muir KR, Cameron AH, et al (Birmingham Children's Hosp, England; Queen's Med Centre, Nottingham, England; Univ of Birmingham, England; et al)

Br J Cancer 75:1156–1159, 1997

16–8

Background.—Although rare, pediatric cancer demands an accurate diagnosis and treatment to avoid long-term consequences. In this retrospective review, the authors evaluated inter-rater agreement in diagnosing solid cancer tumors in pediatric patients.

Methods.—Between 1957 and 1992, 4,592 cases of pediatric cancer were reported. Leukemias were excluded from the current analysis, and the only cases included were those for which at least 3 sections of material were available. Thus specimens from 2,104 cases of pediatric cancer were reexamined by three specialist pathologists blinded to the original diagnosis. The Birch-Marsden classification system was used to classify childhood tumors, and consensus was reached when at least 2 of the 3 reviewing pathologists agreed.

Findings.—Inter-rater agreement averaged 90% (range 78% for lymphoma to 100% for retinoblastoma). When current raters' diagnoses were compared with the original diagnoses, in 16.5% of cases there was a difference; agreement here averaged 85% (range 65% for hepatic tumors to 100% for retinoblastoma). When the latter data were reexamined, agreement with the current raters' opinions was greater when the original diagnosis had been made by a pediatric pathologist rather than a general pathologist (89% vs. 78%).

Conclusions.—Even among experts, tumor identification differed substantially. Furthermore, pediatric pathologists were better at identifying cancerous tumors in children than were the general pathologists. Thus specialist review by a pediatric pathologist seems justified in most cases of childhood solid tumors.

▶ Parkes et al. showed that the interobserver agreement between expert pediatric pathologists and general pathologists is far from perfect and conclude that there is a need for specialist review for most pediatric pathology diagnoses. I do not find that this conclusion is a necessary one and think that these data should be used in other ways. First, there was far from perfect agreement among expert pediatric pathologists. Are some experts better than others? Interobserver disagreement does not necessarily mean that one pathologist is wrong and another is right; it could just mean a difference in opinion. Patient follow up data, which are lacking in this study, are needed to show that one side is more accurate, for how do we know that the less experienced are not the more "right" than the experts, who seemingly were chosen as the gold standard? In addition, might any specimen type, when sent to an expert in that field, result in a change in diagnosis? If so, does this mean that every specimen should be sent to an expert in a particular field? Taking this to the extreme, no specimens would be left for the general pathologist to interpret. I think the matter of choice of sending or not sending a pathology case to an expert should take precedence and should depend on the judgment of the practicing pathologist. These data should be used to stress that interobserver diagnostic variability is inherent in the system. This has practical and legal implications. For example, just because there is a difference in diagnostic opinion does not indicate that one diagnosis is a misdiagnosis and is an invitation for a lawsuit.[1] As pathologists, we should join together to stress that differences are inherent, rather than that one group of pathologists is better than another group.

S. Raab, M.D.

Reference

1. Machin D, Parmar MKB: Pathology review and the diagnosis of cancer. *Lancet* 343:55, 1994.

Accuracy of Admission and Clinical Diagnosis of Tumours as Revealed by 2000 Autopsies
Szende B, Kendrey G, Lapis K, et al (Semmelweis Med Univ, Budapest, Hungary; Imre Haynal Univ, Budapest, Hungary; PN Lee Statistics and Computing Ltd, Sutton, England)
Eur J Cancer 32A:1102–1108, 1996   16–9

Background.—Many researchers have reported marked discrepancies between clinical diagnoses and autopsy diagnoses. Because autopsy rates are decreasing in most countries, the probability of diagnostic error is rising. Diagnostic discrepancies among patients for whom neoplasms were reported at admission and at autopsy were determined.

Methods and Findings.—The diagnoses of 2,000 consecutive patients, aged 30 to 80 years, made in 2 pathology departments in Budapest, Hungary, were analyzed. The rates of false negative diagnoses of tumor, regardless of site, as the underlying cause of death were 37.4% at admission and 8.8% clinically. The false positive rates were 8.4% and 9.1%, respectively. General practitioners correctly diagnosing a tumor as the cause of terminal disease did not correctly identify the primary site in 20.6% of the patients. Hospital clinicians wrongly identified the primary tumor site in 20.4%. Twenty-seven percent of the site-specific tumors judged to be the cause of death at autopsy were incorrectly diagnosed clinically, and 50.4% were incorrectly diagnosed at admission. Diagnostic errors were especially common in patients with lung, liver, ovary, and gallbladder cancer.

Conclusions.—Statistical data from autopsy diagnoses may be useful for graduate and postgraduate education, health care planning, and quality of cancer care. Further research is needed on the consequences of clinical misdiagnosis of cancer.

▶ This European article presents data again confirming the utility of the autopsy, this time in determing the cause of death in patients with tumors. What else is new? Well, *Archives of Pathology and Laboratory Medicine* had a whole issue on autopsy-related topics, and some of these articles are referenced below.[1–10] In a nutshell, these articles reported the state of affairs of the autopsy in the United States. Unless you have been hiding under some rock, you know that autopsy rates in the United States are tiny and continue to dwindle and that the autopsy serves as an invaluable outcomes-related measure.

Again and again, articles such as this one by Szende et al. have shown that the autopsy has corrected a major clinical diagnosis in a sufficient percentage of cases (over 35%). So why are more not done? There are multiple reasons, including lack of clinician understanding, lack of pathologist desire, and lack of reimbursement. Haque et al. showed that some institutions perform autopsies at a much higher rate and listed ways to increase autopsy rates. Unfortunately, I think that most of the cry to bring back the autopsy falls on deaf ears. I also was guilty of autopsy apathy, until I read these articles showing the utility of autopsy.

What is the solution? I probably have too much of a Big Brother paranoia, but I see medicine, including pathology, becoming increasingly under the influence of outside forces (e.g., government, insurance companies), which are sometimes aggressive and sometimes benevolent. To me, if we smarten up we can use these influences to our advantage, particularly for the autopsy. If we were to hard-sell the autopsy as a quality-control measure that actually, in the long term, reduces costs (as well as improves medical care), we possibly could be reimbursed sufficiently to want to do them. Of course, this scenario greatly oversimplifies the situation, and I am uncertain whether anyone truly knows the fate of the autopsy.

S. Raab, M.D.

References

1. AMA Council on Scientific Affairs: Autopsy: A comprehensive review of current issues. *JAMA* 258:364–369, 1987.
2. Kaufman SR: Autopsy: A crucial component of human clinical investigation. *Arch Pathol Lab Med* 120:767–770, 1996.
3. Moore GW, Berman JJ, Hanzlick RL, et al: A prototype internet autopsy database: 1,625 consecutive fetal and neonatal autopsy facesheets spanning 20 years. *Arch Pathol Lab Med* 120:782–785, 1996.
4. Setlow VP: The need for a national autopsy policy. *Arch Pathol Lab Med* 773–777, 1996.
5. Haque AK, Patterson RC, Grafe JR: High autopsy rates at a university medical center: What has gone right? *Arch Pathol Lab Med* 120:727–732, 1996.
6. Hill RB: College of American Pathologists Conference XXIX on restructuring autopsy practice for health care reform: Summary. *Arch Pathol Lab Med* 120:778–781, 1996.
7. Trelstad RL, Amenta PS, Foran DJ, et al: The role for regional autopsy centers in the evaluation of covered deaths: Survey of opinions of US and Canadian chairs of pathology and major health insurers in the United States. *Arch Pathol Lab Med* 120:753–758, 1996.
8. Botega NJ, Metze K, Marques E, et al: Attitudes of medical students to necropsy. *J Clin Pathol* 50:64–66, 1997.
9. Huston BM, Malouf NN, Azar HA: Percutaneous needle autopsy sampling. *Mod Pathol* 9:1101–1107, 1996.
10. Bierig JR: A potpourri of legal issues relating to the autopsy. *Arch Pathol Lab Med* 120:759–762, 1996.

Postmortem Fetal MR Imaging: Comparison With Findings at Autopsy

Woodward PJ, Sohaey R, Harris DP, et al (Univ of Utah, Salt Lake City)
AJR 168:41–46, 1997
16–10

Introduction.—For documenting fetal malformations and determining the cause of death, an autopsy provides vital information and can determine risks for future pregnancies. Some parents, however, may refuse autopsy because of the devastating and highly traumatic experience of fetal death. In postmortem evaluation, MRI may be of value; however, a large spectrum of fetal anomalies has not been prospectively evaluated to assess the usefulness of MRI as an alternative to autopsy. The efficacy of 3-dimensional fast spin-echo MRI was examined.

Methods.—On a 1.5-T MRI scanner using 2-dimensional and high-resolution 3-dimensional fast spin-echo techniques, 26 fetuses were imaged immediately before autopsy. Three radiologists reviewed the MR images independently and evaluated them for major and minor malformations. The findings were compared with those found on autopsy.

Results.—There were 47 major and 11 minor malformations in the 26 fetuses. On the MR images, all 3 radiologists identified 37 of the major malformations, a detection rate of 79%. One of the 3 reviewers identified 43 of the abnormalities, a detection rate of 91%. The reviewers found only 1 of the 11 minor anomalies. There were 6 false positive diagnoses. Magnetic resonance imaging was superior to autopsy in defining in situ relationships, particularly in 2 fetuses, both of which had major CNS malformations. In cardiac anomalies, MRI did not do well. For microscopic evaluation, MRI cannot replace autopsy.

Conclusion.—When autopsy is refused, MRI is an excellent alternative, and it can be a valuable adjunct to autopsy for fetuses with CNS anomalies. Even in fetuses as young as 13 weeks' gestation, all major organs can be identified with MR images. A limited charge that is less than half that of an autopsy is suggested for MRI when autopsy is refused.

▶ If your perinatal autopsy rates are falling, is it because your colleagues in Diagnostic Imaging have begun to propose postmortem MRI as an alternative? Don't worry too much. This interesting study of congenital malformations in 26 fetuses, comparing interpretations on postmortem MRI with evaluations at autopsy, demonstrates that pathologists can—at this writing—identify both major and minor anomalies, particularly in the cardiovascular system, more effectively than can radiologists. (The exception may lie in the CNS, which is so easy to disrupt at dissection. Perhaps rare and unusual [CNS] malformations will warrant an MRI consultation.)

A.S. Knisely, M.D.

The Hidden Increase in Histopathologists' Workload
Parham DM (Royal Bournemouth Hosp, England)
J Clin Pathol 49:689–690, 1996

16–11

Introduction.—The increasing complexity of the workload of histopathologists in interpreting and reporting specimens is recognized, but has not been quantified. The increase in the amount of information contained in histopathologic reports over the last decade was evaluated to determine how it has affected the workload of histopathologists.

Methods.—Information from histopathologic reports was quantified for 2-week periods in select years between 1985 and 1995. Reports were evaluated for number of items of information recorded, including details of the nature of the specimen, measurement, histologic description, diagnosis, grade, individual prognostic factors, and excision margins.

Results.—Over a 5-year period from 1990 to 1995, there was an average increase of 7% in the amount of information per report. The increase in information per report, compounded by the increasing number of specimens received, has resulted in an exponential rise in the amount of information generated by histopathologists per year.

Conclusion.—The 7% increase in information output by pathologists has significant resource implications. The increasing complexity of the histopathology workload has been recognized by the Royal College of Pathologists, but recommendations regarding upper limits of specimens per year are made without regard to the types of specimens submitted or clinical demands for examining specimens.

▶ I find this article almost too simple, but fascinating, particularly in regard to the attempt to quantify specific aspects of pathology work. Pathologists, like the rest of health care providers, work in a cost driven system, but yet must provide high quality care. The output of a pathology department is a pathology report, which not only provides a diagnosis, but also a host of other information that is used in a variety of ways. Parham showed that the average amount of information contained in a pathology report at the Royal Bournemouth Hospital increased exponentially from 1984 to 1996. I believe that the same probably holds true in the North American pathology laboratories. This study would have been improved if the type of information included in pathology reports had been subclassified to reflect that some information is more important than others. In addition, it would have been better to show how this information actually affected patient care, and if excluding this information negatively affected clinician perception or patient management. Parham explained that medical information doubles every 7–10 years, and I think we are supposed to infer that much of this information needs to be presented by pathologists. This implies that we must know and report more. To handle this information, we need efficient technology (e.g., computers) and personnel. Increased information also suggests that synoptic reports that standardize this information are a good idea. Although there may be increased "hidden" work, the data would indicate that clinicians are also more dependent on us to provide this information. This dependence may not be a bad thing insofar as it provides continued business.

S. Raab, M.D.

The Relationships Among Performance Measures in the Selection of Diagnostic Tests
Einstein AJ, Bodian CA, Gil J (Mount Sinai School of Medicine, New York)
Arch Pathol Lab Med 121:110–117, 1997   16–12

Introduction.—Medical practice has moved away from subjective judgments and toward objective tests. The main performance criteria by which such tests are measured are sensitivity, specificity, positive and negative predictive value, accuracy, and likelihood ratio. These values are of differing importance in different diagnostic situations. Many studies will report the values of some but not all of the measures. In some situations, the unreported values may be useful in deciding whether to perform a test. The relationships between the different performance measures and how the unreported measures can often be calculated from the reported ones are discussed.

Calculating Performance Measures. If 3 of 5 measures are known— the 5 being sensitivity, specificity, positive and negative predictive value, and accuracy—it is usually possible to calculate the other 2. Formulas for the calculation of sensitivity, specificity, and positive and negative predictive value are reported. Once the 4th measure is known, accuracy can be calculated as well. There are some exceptions to the reported equations, such as when 1 or more of the measures is equal to 0% or 100%. Likelihood ratios can also be calculated when sensitivity and specificity are known. Although the likelihood ratio does not offer any new information, it may be useful for presenting information. Decisions about which measure is most important depend on the diagnostic situation: sensitivity may be the important value in a screening test, whereas specificity may be more important in a confirmatory test. Sensitivity is important for serious, treatable diseases in which a false-positive result is not harmful to the patient; specificity is more important for diseases that are serious but not curable, in which false-positive results may have harmful ramifications. The positive predictive value becomes key when a false-positive result would be disastrous. Accuracy is the most important for diseases that are serious and treatable and for which false-positive and false-negative results would be equally deleterious. Decisions about testing in a particular laboratory should consider the performance expected under the existing conditions not the test's performance under a range of operating conditions. It is important to remember that performance measures are affected by both disease prevalence and the choice of a cutoff point.

Discussion.—The interrelationships among various measures of diagnostic performance are reviewed. The article includes discussion of the applicability of published performance measures and illustrates the concepts using the diagnostic example of acute myocardial infarction. Using the published equations, it is possible to use limited information to estimate performance measures relevant to the given situation. This aids in such problems as selecting the most appropriate test and deciding on cutoff values.

▶ Alright, I admit it. This article is best suited for the geeks, who like statistical analysis. For those who never want to see another mathematical equation, feel free to bypass this article with a wide excisional margin. However, for those who at least have a modicum of interest in the performance characteristics of tests, I think this article is excellent for showing the interrelation of these characteristics. Although perhaps designed more for the clinical laboratory, these performance measures also are used in surgical pathology and cytopathology laboratories. For new procedures or equipment, only some test characteristics are put forward by the manufacturer or by the clinician, and these are usually the ones that portray these procedures and equipment in the best light. It is helpful if we know how to work through the math. For additional reading on this topic, see the references below.

S. Raab, M.D.

References

1. Jones RH, McClatchey MW: Beyond sensitivity, specificity, and statistical independence. *Statistical Med* 7:1289–1295, 1988.
2. Galen RS, Gambino SR: *Beyond Normality: The Predictive Value and Efficiency of Medical Diagnoses.* New York, John Wiley & Sons, 1975, pp 49–51.

Tetrault G: Sensitivity and specificity of clinical tests. Am J Clin Pathol 96:556, 1991.

Suggested Reading

Goldman DA, Simpson DM: Survey of El Paso physician's breast and cervical screening attitudes and practices. *J Comm Health* 19:75–85, 1994.

Janerich DT, Hadjimichael O, Schwartz PE, et al: The screening histories of women with invasive cervical cancer, Connecticut. *Am J Public Health* 85:791–794, 1995.

Morrell D, Curtis P, Mintzer M, et al: Perceptions and opinions on the performance of Pap smears: A survey of clinicians using a commercial laboratory. *Am J Prev Med* 12:271–276, 1996.

▶ Of all malpractice suits that pathologists must face, suits involving Pap smears are one of the most frequent. Malpractice suits involving Pap smears also may involve clinicians, and since clinicians serve as the gateway for our receiving Pap smears, it is important to know their perceptions and opinions. Morrell, et al. surveyed 149 North Carolina clinicians who came from a variety of practice settings, ranging from obstetricians/gynecologists to nurse practitioners/physician assistants. As probably should be expected, some of the data show that clinicians have some misunderstandings involving Pap smear interpretation. For example, 19% of respondents felt that squamous cells were not necessary for an adequate smear, and 17.7% felt that mucous was necessary for an adequate smear. Over 4% thought that semen interfered with diagnostic interpretation. These data do not mean that we have to be better educators (although this would be nice) but that we should be aware that what we may think is obvious is not known by all the clinicians. Interestingly, 26.4% of clinicians responded that the most frequent problem in the overall screening process was diagnostic interpretation. The actual false-negative rate due to laboratory error reportedly has ranged from 30% to 50%. Another 9.5% of respondents felt that returning lab reports to clinicians was often a source of error. I wonder what this actually means. Are we really so poor at returning results to clinicians?

S. Raab, M.D.

Schwartz JS, Lewis CE, Clancy C, et al: Internists' practices in health promotion and disease prevention: A survey. *Ann Intern Med* 114:46–53, 1991.

17 Pathology Techniques

Immunohistochemical Identification of Tumor Markers In Metastatic Adenocarcinoma: A Diagnostic Adjunct In the Determination of Primary Site
Brown RW, Campagna LB, Dunn JK, et al (Baylor College of Medicine, Houston)
Am J Clin Pathol 107:12–19, 1997   17–1

Introduction.—Sixty percent of metastatic cancers are composed of metastatic adenocarcinoma of unknown primary site. For many types of cancer, unequivocal identification of the primary site is essential, but using extensive radiographs and endoscopic examinations are time consuming, expensive, inconvenient, and oftentimes unsuccessful. Single tumor markers have been used in a number of previous immunohistochemical studies. A single marker is not available that is site specific for common adenocarcinomas, but the alternative approach of using a panel of markers has shown success. A retrospective study was conducted to determine whether a panel of markers could accurately predict the site of origin of common metastatic adenocarcinomas.

Methods.—Using paraffin section immunohistochemistry, 128 metastatic adenocarcinomas from 5 primary sites (colon, breast, ovary, lung, and upper gastrointestinal-pancreaticobiliary tract) were examined. Eight tumor markers were selected for simultaneous immunohistochemical examination of 128 metastatic tumors. Statistical analysis was used to select the most efficient, cost-effective immunohistochemical panel for routine diagnostic use. Staining results were also compared with results of previous studies (Table 3).

Results.—Carcinoembryonic antigen (CEA, CA19-9, CA125, and breast cancer antigen 225 BCA225) were the most informative markers (Table 4). For colon tumors, the most predictive multiple-marker phenotypes—as determined by a combination of area under the receiver operating characteristic curve, specificity, and percent correct predictions—were CEA$^+$, BCA226$^-$, and CA125$^-$. For breast tumors, they were BCA225$^+$, CEA$^-$, and CA125. For lung tumors, they were BCA225$^+$, CEA$^+$, and CA19-9$^-$. For ovarian tumors, they were CA125$^+$ and CEA$^-$. For upper gastrointestinal tract tumors, they were CEA$^+$, CA19-9$^+$, and CA125$^+$. In 66% of cases, these phenotypes correctly predicted the known primary site.

TABLE 3.—Immunoperoxidase Staining Results of Current Study Compared With Those of Previous Studies Using Paraffin Sections

	Colon	Breast	Lung	Ovary	Upper GI Tract
GCDFP-15					
Current	0	52	0	0	0
Previous[11–13]	0	74	0	4	0
BCA225					
Current	4	96	78	67	28
Previous[5–11]	13	99	77	68	47
B72.3					
Current	68	36	70	67	76
Previous[6,7,10]	69	52	85	69	76
CEA					
Current	96	8	65	7	72
Previous[10,14,15]	99	30	84	4	76
CA19-9					
Current	79	24	13	30	72
Previous[16–18]	71	11	30	48	79
DF3					
Current	61	100	87	100	88
Previous[18]	81	100	94	100	93
CA125					
Current	4	24	35	96	40
Previous[16,20]	9	13	20	91	38
Estrogen receptor					
Current	0	32	0	4	0
Previous[30]	NA	73	NA	NA	NA

Note: All values represent percentages. Reference numbers refer to references within original article.

Abbreviations: BCA225, breast cancer antigen 225; *CEA,* carcinoembryonic antigen; *NA,* insufficient immunohistochemical data available for site.

(Courtesy of Brown RW, Campagna LB, Dunn JK, et al: Immunohistochemical identification of tumor markers in metastatic adenocarcinoma: A diagnostic adjunct in the determination of primary site. *Am J Clin Pathol* 107:12–19, 1997.)

TABLE 4.—Multiple-Marker Phenotypes Most Predictive of Primary Site

	Colon	Breast	Lung	Ovary	Upper GI Tract
Two-marker phenotype	CEA⁺, BCA225⁻	BCA225⁺, CEA⁻	CEA⁺, CA19-9⁻	CA125⁺, CEA⁻	CEA⁺, CA19-9⁺
Three-marker phenotype	CEA⁺, BCA225⁻, CA125⁻	BCA225⁺, CEA⁻, CA125⁻	BCA225⁺, CEA⁺, CA19-9⁻	CA125⁺, CEA⁻, CA19-9⁻	CEA⁺, CA19-9⁺, CA125⁺
Four-marker phenotype	CEA⁺, BCA225⁻, CA125⁻, CA19-9⁺	BCA225⁺, CEA⁻, CA125⁻, CA19-9⁺	BCA225⁺, CEA⁺, CA19-9⁻, CA125⁺	CA125⁺, CEA⁻, CA19-9⁻, BCA225⁺	CEA⁺, CA19-9⁺, CA125⁺, BCA225⁻

Note: Panel included breast cancer antigen 225 *(BCA225),* carcinoembryonic antigen *(CEA),* CA19-9, and CA125. Most predictive phenotype is defined as that which produces highest area under receiver operating characteristic curve, specificity, and correct predictions. Plus and minus signs indicate whether a positive or negative result is predictive of that primary site.

Abbreviation: GI, gastrointestinal.

(Courtesy of Brown RW, Campagna LB, Dunn JK, et al: Immunohistochemical identification of tumor markers in metastatic adenocarcinoma: A diagnostic adjunct in the determination of primary site. *Am J Clin Pathol* 107:12–19, 1997.)

Conclusion.—A panel of selected immunohistochemical markers is the best means for suggesting or excluding the origin of metastatic adenocarcinoma until single highly sensitive and specific markers are developed.

► There is an ongoing attempt to find the best set of phenotypic markers to identify metastatic adenocarcinomas, especially those involving the pleura. This paper, however, goes beyond the usual attempt. First, it is not limited to differentiating mesothelioma from adenocarcinoma; second, it makes good use of previously published studies; and, third, it uses statistical tools beyond sensitivity and specificity, i.e., receiver operating characteristic curves, to analyze the data. The data are best summarized in the 2 included tables. Despite all of this, the phenotypic profile correctly identified the primary in only two thirds of cases. Although this paper clearly adds to the existing literature, it is also clear that more, better studies are needed.

M.B. Cohen, M.D.

Comparison of p53 Immunoreactivity in Fresh-cut versus Stored Slides With and Without Microwave Heating

Shin HJC, Kalapurakal SK, Lee JJ, et al (Univ of Texas, Houston)
Mod Pathol 10:224–230, 1997   17–2

Background.—A *p53* gene alteration may be the most common genetic abnormality in human carcinomas. Expression of p53 in tumor cells may be predictive of outcome in patients with various types of cancer. Technical problems in immunohistochemical staining methods can cause antigens to be masked or lost. To avoid such problems, enzymatic tissue digestion and microwave heating have been used to retrieve masked epitopes of p53 and other antigens. Decreased immunoreactivity of p53 in tissue samples kept at room temperature was investigated.

Methods.—In 13 head and neck squamous cell carcinomas and 13 non–small-cell lung carcinomas, p53 immunohistochemical staining was done. Results of p53 immunostaining in fresh-cut and stored slides with and without microwave heating were compared. Stored slides were between 4 and 25 years old and stored at room temperature for 6–48 months.

Results.—Positivity for p53 was seen in 12 head and neck squamous cell carcinomas and 6 lung carcinomas. For cases showing p53 positivity, each case consistently showed p53 positivity regardless of age of block, length of storage, or microwave heating. Substantially less staining intensity was seen in stored slides than in fresh-cut slides. This difference was statistically significant, but the mean difference was only 3.6%, which may not be meaningful. Microwave heating significantly improved staining intensity and the percentage of positivity for stored and fresh-cut slides. With microwave heating, there was no significant difference in staining intensity between the 2 types of slides, but the difference in percentage of positivity was significant.

Discussion.—Significantly less p53 immunoreactivity was seen in stored slides. Microwave heating enabled the p53 antigen to be retrieved without changing p53 status. Results of p53 immunostaining in fresh-cut slides and stored slides using a microwave heating retrieval method in a metal-containing solution should be comparable providing that staining intensity is not the only outcome measure.

▶ Recent concerns have emerged about the feasibility of performing immunohistochemical staining on sections that have been previously cut and subsequently stored. Antigenic loss for unknown reasons is the major concern, resulting in false negative staining. In this study, using p53 as a model, the authors show that this can be overcome with antigen retrieval; this protocol utilized a metal-containing (Zn) procedure. Their results indicate that using the antibody DO-7, staining could be identified. I would add that the 1801 antibody is also a good antibody that gives similar but not fully overlapping results. It may be useful to use both of these antibodies for p53 analysis.

M.B. Cohen, M.D.

Suggested Reading

Thomas MD, McIntosh GG, Anderson JJ, et al: A novel quantitative immunoassay system for p53 using antibodies selected for optimum designation of p53 status. *J Clin Pathol* 50:143–147, 1997.

Development of an Optimal Protocol for Antigen Retrieval: A 'Test Battery' Approach Exemplified With Reference to the Staining of Retinoblastoma Protein (pRB) in Formalin-fixed Paraffin Sections
Shi S-R, Cote RJ, Yang C, et al (Univ of Southern California, Los Angeles; Baylor College of Medicine, Woodlands, Tex)
J Pathol 179:347–352, 1996   17–3

Background.—The retinoblastoma (RB) gene encodes the nuclear RB protein (pRB) and may have a role in cell cycle control and cell differentiation. Studies have shown that loss of RB function may be involved in the formation of tumors and the progression of bladder, lung, breast, prostate, and other human cancers. It may be valuable and economical to combine immunohistochemical detection of pRB expression in formalin-paraffin sections of cancer with routine surgical pathology practice. There have been inconsistent results using pRB antibodies on routinely processed, paraffin-embedded tissue. The antigen retrieval method was used for immunohistochemical detection of pRB expression in paraffin-embedded tissue, and a test battery approach was used to develop the best antigen retrieval protocol.

Methods.—The test battery approach uses buffered solutions at pH 1, 6, and 10, and microwave heating at 120°C, 100°C, and 90°C. Data were presented for the antibody RB-WL-1, for which the low pH solution and heating at 100°C were most effective. To compare pRB immunostaining, fresh and routinely processed formalin-paraffin tissues of normal and bladder carcinoma were used. To evaluate the antigen retrieval method, a comparison was made of immunohistochemical staining results on routinely processed formalin-paraffin sections with frozen sections of the same tumor.

Results.—A consistent intensity of immunohistochemical staining for pRB was seen with the antigen retrieval protocol identified as optimal on formalin-paraffin sections. All slides showed positivity for pRB in normal mesenchymal and epithelial tissues, with similar patterns of pRB localization and staining intensity to that seen in frozen sections, although the intensity in paraffin sections was somewhat stronger than in frozen sections. Consistent pRB immunostaining results were seen in tests of the identified protocol in routinely processed paraffin tissue sections of 245 cases of bladder cancer.

Discussion.—An optimal antigen retrieval protocol for immunohistochemical detection of pRB expression in paraffin-embedded tissue is easy to perform and gives reproducible results. The study used the test battery approach, which can be used with any new antibody being evaluated. The test battery approach may contribute to the standardization of antigen retrieval immunostaining because it allows rapid identification of the protocol that offers maximal retrieval.

▶ The identification of antigenic epitopes by immunohistochemistry is now well established in anatomical pathology. Historically, there was difficulty in identifying the majority of these epitopes with polyclonal and monoclonal antibodies. This was a result of masking because of formalin fixation. With the advent of antigen retrieval, many of these antibodies can now be successfully applied to tissues prepared in this manner. As pointed out by the authors, each antibody must be worked up individually to determine the best staining protocol. This paper has identified a useful test battery based on different pHs (1, 6, and 10) and heating times (autoclave or microwave; 90°C to 120°C; all for 10 minutes) to determine that best protocol. Although applied to Rb staining, this approach will, hopefully, be useful in the case of other antibodies that are being introduced into the laboratory.

M.B. Cohen, M.D.

Lack of Correlation Between Flow Cytometric and Immunohistologic Proliferation Measurements of Tumors

Linden MD, El-Naggar AK, Nathanson SD, et al (Henry Ford Hosp, Detroit; M.D. Anderson Cancer Ctr, Houston)
Mod Pathol 9:682–689, 1996   17–4

Background.—Patients with transmurally invasive, lymph node negative, colorectal adenocarcinoma have a reported 5-year disease-free survival rate of 54% to 85%. In colon carcinoma, histologic grade, lymphocytic infiltrate, and angiolymphatic invasion are correlated with prognosis.

The subjective evaluation of these factors does not provide useful prognostic information. An additional problem is the subset of patients with colorectal carcinoma without lymph node involvement or distant metastases. These patients may benefit from an objective means of tumor evaluation.

Methods.—A comparison was made of flow cytometric and immunohistologic analyses of tumor proliferative activity. Immunohistologic analysis was made of formalin-fixed, paraffin-embedded tissue. Evaluations were made of 84 cases of Dukes' stage B colorectal adenocarcinoma to identify patients who might benefit from adjunctive therapy. The specimens were from 40 men and 44 women between the ages of 20 and 104 years. Flow cytometric analysis involved a modified Hedley method with a combined S+G2/M phase proliferative fraction calculated using a rectangular model after debris subtraction. Immunohistologic analysis of tumor proliferation involved serial step sections from the same blocks used for flow cytometric analysis with antibodies to proliferating cell nuclear antigen (PCNA) and Ki-67 (MIB-1).

Results.—For flow cytometric analysis, the proliferative fraction ranged from 5% to 27%, with a mean of 14.8%. The PCNA tumor proliferation indices ranged from 4% to 90%, with a mean of 43.2%. The MIB-1 tumor proliferation indices ranged from 2% to 47%, with a mean of 16.2%. There was no correlation between the flow cytometric proliferative fraction and immunohistologic tumor proliferation, or between PCNA and MIB-1 indices.

Discussion.—The lack of correlation between flow cytometric and immunohistologic findings may have resulted from using formalin-fixed, paraffin-embedded tissue for flow cytometric evaluation, with greater debris and lower accuracy of cell cycle measurements. The lack of correlation between PCNA and MIB-1 indices may have resulted from inherent problems with anti-PCNA antibody staining of formalin-fixed tissue. It may be useful for future prospective studies to use fresh tissue with 2-color multiparameter flow cytometric analysis. Histogram-dependent background fitting may also be useful in defining the relationship between flow cytometric and immunohistologic findings of tumor proliferative activity.

▶ In this study, proliferation was assessed in a series of colon adenocarcinomas by either flow cytometric analysis (looking for the S+G2/M fraction) or immunohistochemically using 1 of 2 anitbodies (PC-10, which recognizes PCNA, and MIB-1, which recognizes the Ki-67 antigen). Because all these methods measure slightly different aspects of "proliferation," it should not be surprising that no correlation was identified between the various markers. It would have been useful if the authors had examined some other parameters of outcome to see if some predictive value could be associated with one or more of the markers, e.g., 5-year survival. The results noted here reflect the considerable variability in applying "prognostic markers." Further, they also highlight the difficulty of interpreting results between various laboratories. In a related article about flow cytometry,[1] it is clear that ploidy analysis is only variably used, especially in non-breast cancers.

M.B. Cohen, M.D.

Reference

1. McCoy JP Jr, Overton WR: A survey of current practices in clinical flow cytometry. *Am J Clin Pathol* 106:82–86, 1996.

Molecular and Immunological Detection of Circulating Tumor Cells and Micrometastases From Solid Tumors
Pelkey TJ, Frierson HF Jr, Bruns DE (Univ of Virginia, Charlottesville, VA)
Clin Chem 42:1369–1381, 1996   17–5

Introduction.—Histologic, immunologic, and molecular techniques are used in the detection of micrometastases from nonhematopoietic malignancies. Reverse transcriptase-polymerase chain reaction is the newest method and has been used for detecting micrometastases of the esophagus, stomach, liver, colorectum, pancreas, lung, breast, and prostate. It has also been used in melanoma, neuroblastoma, and hematopoietic malignancies. Because long-term follow-up information is not yet available, the role of reverse transcriptase-polymerase chain reaction for detecting micrometastases in cancer staging is unknown. Data from the literature on micrometastasis detection using immunologic and molecular methods were reviewed.

Immunologic Methods.—Most of the studies on the prognostic value of immunologic detection of bone marrow micrometastases have focused on patients with breast cancer. These studies have reported that recurrent disease can be predicted by detection of bone marrow micrometastases using immunologic methods. For lung, gastric, and colorectal carcinomas, detection of bone marrow micrometastases can be predictive of recurrent disease and findings have correlated with clinicopathologic staging. Although the detection of bone marrow micrometastases can have prognostic value, this protocol is not used extensively in cancer staging protocols, and standardization of techniques has been recommended.

Reverse Transcriptase-Polymerase Chain Reaction.—This is the most common molecular method for detecting micrometastases. It has been used for detecting micrometastases of prostate cancers, but its clinical value is doubted by some authors because negative results have occurred in some untreated patients with prostate cancer and known metastatic disease. Its value as a staging tool in guiding adjunctive therapy or as a predictor of recurrent disease has not been demonstrated. In the future, reverse transcriptase-polymerase chain reaction must show superiority over current staging techniques and the new ultrasensitive prostate-specific antigen assays before it gains acceptance in the detection and staging of prostate cancer and detection of recurrent disease.

Discussion.—It has been 100 years since circulating tumor cells were first detected. Our understanding of cancer and micrometastasis has increased with the development of immunologic and molecular techniques. The clinical value of current methods of detecting circulating tumor cells and the role of micrometastasis detection in the staging of solid tumors are not yet clear. Many studies on these topics are discussed in this extensive article, as well as the use of immunologic techniques in detecting lymph node micrometastases, reverse transcriptase-polymerase chain reaction in nonprostatic micrometastases, reverse transcriptase-polymerase chain reaction vs. immunologic methods, and false positive diagnostic results.

▶ This review article, based on published literature between January 1976 and December 1995, includes 163 references. The article is comprehensive and focuses on immunologic methods and reverse transcriptase-polymrase chain reaction. The latter has received a lot of recent attention, particularly as it applies to the detection of circulating prostate cancer cells by using prostate-specific antigen mRNA as the basis of the assay. Although few, if any, of the methods are imminently being introduced into patient care, I do think that this will be part of the future management of patients with various malignancies.

M.B. Cohen, M.D.

Feasibility of Using Decades-old Archival Tissues In Molecular Oncology/Epidemiology
Iwamoto KS, Mizuno T, Ito T, et al (Hiroshima Univ, Japan)
Am J Pathol 149:399–406, 1996   17–6

Introduction.—Molecular biology has been revolutionized by polymerase chain reaction. A plethora of genes can be studied with nanogram quantities of tissue DNA. Reliance on archival tissues is essential in fields such as molecular oncology/epidemiology. It has never been shown that a large number of decades-old samples (20 or more years) could be used for analysis by polymerase chain reaction. Such archival tissues are found in the tumor and tissue registries of atomic bomb survivors. Using archival materials collected from atomic bomb survivors in comparison with recently procured samples, the feasibility and limitations of an expansive molecular epidemiology study were tested.

Methods.—The study included 275 hepatocellular carcinoma cases and 41 skin cancer cases from the tumor registry of atomic bomb survivors. These were compared with 23 cases of thyroid papillary carcinoma involving people who lived near the Chernobyl nuclear reactor accident. After DNA extraction and polymerase chain reaction amplification, radioactive labeling was performed.

Results.—In autopsy hepatocellular carcinoma samples, degradation of DNA is severe, but can be compensated for by deceasing the polymerase chain reaction product size. The amplification efficiency was improved from 60% to 80% by increasing the amount of DNA used by a factor of 8. By comparison, polymerase chain reaction amplification of skin and thyroid tumors was efficient. When liver cases that were less than 10 years old were compared with the controls, it was found that the former had a substantial degree of degradation. The source of procurement was a greater problem than the age of the sample.

Conclusion.—All types of assays that require polymerase chain reaction amplification can take advantage of extracted DNA. Assays include restriction fragment length polymorphism, single-strand conformation polymorphism, and direct sequencing.

▶ The field of molecular epidemiology is one of the hot areas at the moment. Because retrospective studies require the use of archival specimens, typically formalin-fixed and paraffin-embedded, the isolation of usable genetic material is key to the success of any study. Most of these studies use one or more polymerase chain reaction–based approaches to identify abnormalities at the DNA level, including the identification of point mutations; gene rearrangements; gene amplification; and, rarely, restriction fragment length polymorphism. This study, using 2 sets of tissues (from Japanese atomic bomb survivors and survivors of the Chernobyl accident), shows that this approach is feasible. Success, although limited, was also feasible with autopsy tissues.

One of the key elements in success is to design appropriate primers so that the resultant product is of a size that can be reliably amplified. Those interested in this area may also want to look at an article by Farkas et al.[1] which may be of use for prospectively storing specimens. Another interesting and related article[2]; describes the use of microdissection and identification of point mutations by polymerase chain reaction analysis of isolated DNA.

M.B. Cohen, M.D.

References

1. Farkas DH, Kaul KL, Wiedbrauk DL, et al: Specimen collection and storage for diagnostic molecular pathology investigation. *Arch Pathol Lab Med* 120:591, 1996.
2. Moskaluk CA, Kern SE: Microdissection and polymerase chain reaction amplification of genomic DNA from histological tissue sections. *Am J Pathol* 150:1547–1552, 1997.

Critical Evaluation of Prognostic Factors
Dhingra K, Hortobagyi GN (MD Anderson Cancer Ctr, Houston)
Semin Oncol 23:436–445, 1996   17–7

Introduction.—Treatment strategy for breast cancer can be difficult because the disease is so variable and survival varies. Biological markers can help predict the natural history of this disease, help doctors decide

---

TABLE 3.—Challenges in Developing Definitive Prognostic Markers in
Breast Cancer

Heterogeneity of disease
Heterogeneity of intervention, especially systemic adjuvant
 therapy
Redundancy of growth stimulatory pathways in tumors
Temporal/spatial heterogeneity of expression of relevant bio-
 logical changes
Consistency/reproducibility of technical assays
Failure to duplicate optimized cutoff points identified in initial
 studies

(Courtesy of Dhingra K, Hortobagyi GN: Critical evaluation of prognostic factors. *Semin Oncol*
23:436–445, 1996.)

---

which treatment to pursue, and help predict the outcome. To determine the risk of systemic relapse, tumor size, lymph node metastases, and histopathologic features have been used in the past. The discovery of a number of specific genetic and biochemical markers has led to the molecular era of prognostic factors. There have been changes in predicting the presence of micrometastases, in the sensitivity of micrometastases to planned therapy, and in site of and time to manifestation of metastases.

Conventional predictors.—The best predictor of systemic micrometastases has been the presence of tumor cells in axillary lymph nodes; however, some individuals in this group have been cured by local therapy alone. A poor response to chemotherapy has been found in those individuals who exhibit multidrug resistance-associated protein or P-glycoprotein. Predictors of organ-specific metastases are PTHrP-expression, vimentin, bone marrow micrometastases, and L-*myc* polymorphisms. Predictors of the efficacy of systemic adjuvant therapy are hormone receptors ER and PR, *neu* amplification, and *p53* mutations.

Molecular predictors.—Molecular changes such as dysregulated proliferation, invasion, and metastases can determine malignancy. The risk of relapse may be better determined with molecular predictors than by conventional methods. Amplification/overexpression of the HER-2/*neu* oncogene is a marker of increased risk of relapse after locoregional therapy of breast cancer. Sensitivity to chemotherapeutic drugs may also be ascertained with this oncogene.

Conclusion.—Some of the potential complexities involved in predicting the biological behavior of breast cancers with prognostic markers are heterogeneity of disease, heterogeneity of intervention, and redundancy of growth (Table 3). Conventional histopathologic and clinical prognostic assessment must be integrated with the large body of data generated for potential use in regard to the newer molecular prognostic factors.

▶ This review article focuses on predicting the biology of human breast cancer. It is a balanced overview that concludes, and I think appropriately,: "...the large body of data generated regarding the potential utility of newer, molecular prognostic factors is yet to be fully integrated with conventional histopathological and clinical prognostic assessment." Those of us who still push chemotoxylin-eosin–stained glass still have a job, but this is a rapidly evolving field—so stay tuned.

M.B. Cohen, M.D.

Lessons From Hereditary Colorectal Cancer
Kinzler KW, Vogelstein B (Johns Hopkins Oncology Ctr, Baltimore, Md; Howard Hughes Med Inst, Baltimore, Md)
Cell 87:159–170, 1996   17–8

Introduction.—There is much evidence that accumulated genetic changes precede the development of neoplasia. This process is seen in colorectal cancers that develop over decades and seem to require 7 genetic events or more for completion. The inheritance of a single altered gene can increase the risk of colorectal cancer in familial adenomatous polyposis and hereditary nonpolyposis colorectal cancer. In familial adenomatous polyposis, the genetic defect seems to affect the rate of tumor initiation by targeting the gatekeeper function of the *APC* gene, but in hereditary nonpolyposis colorectal cancer, the defect seems to affect tumor progression by targeting the genome guardian function of DNA mismatch repair.

Familial Adenomatous Polyposis.—This is an autosomal, dominantly inherited disease with an incidence of about 1 in 7,000 individuals. Hundreds to thousands of benign colorectal tumors develop when patients are in their 20s and 30s. Although these tumors are not life threatening, their large numbers assure that some will progress to invasive lesions. Patients with this disease often have retinal lesions, osteomas, desmoids of the skin, brain tumors, and other extracolonic manifestations.

Genetic Instability in Cancer.—Studies of colorectal cancer have shown that multiple mutations are necessary for malignancy to develop (Fig 7). As both alleles of the tumor suppressor genes are inactivated, at least 7 independent genetic events seem to be required. Previously, it was unclear whether normal rates of mutation were high enough to account for the accumulated mutations, or whether tumor cells had higher mutation rates. Studies of hereditary nonpolyposis colorectal cancer have shown that, in some cancers, mutation rates in tumor cells with *MMR* deficiency are 2 to 3 orders of magnitude higher than in normal cells.

Discussion.—Knowledge of the hereditary bases of familial colorectal cancer is valuable to patients because genetic testing can improve diagnosis. Individuals who test negative for specific *APC* or *MMR* gene mutations will not have to have repeated medical and endoscopic examinations. Those who have inherited a mutant gene can be more closely monitored. Development of practical methods for detecting germline alterations will be complex. Other topics discussed in this extensive article include rate-limiting events in tumorigenesis; phenotype vs. genotype; hereditary vs.

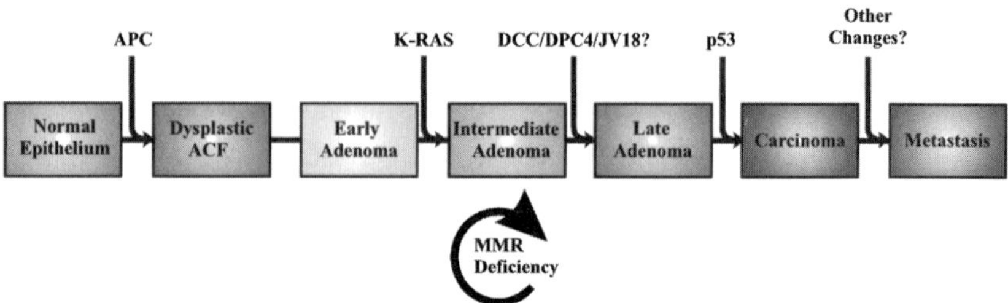

FIGURE 7.—Genetic changes associated with colorectal tumorigenesis. *APC* mutations initiate the neoplastic process, and tumor progression results from mutations in the other genes indicated. Patients with familial adenomatous polyposis inherit *APC* mutations and numerous dysplastic aberrant crypt foci develop, some of which progress as they acquire the other mutations indicated in the figure. The tumors from patients with hereditary nonpolyposis colorectal cancer go through a similar, though not identical, series of mutations; MMR deficiency speeds up this process. *K-RAS* is an oncogene that requires only 1 genetic event for its activation. The other specific genes indicated are tumor suppressor genes that require 2 genetic events (1 in each allele) for their inactivation. Chromosome 18q21 may contain several different tumor suppressor genes involved in colorectal neoplasia, with *DCC*, *DPC4*, and *JV18–1* genes proposed as candidates. A variety of other genetic alterations have each been described in a small fraction of advanced colorectal cancers. These may be responsible for the heterogeneity of biologic and clinical properties observed among different cases. (Courtesy of Kinzler KW, Vogelstein B: Lessons from hereditary colorectal cancer. *Cell* 87:159–170. Copyright 1996 by Cell Press.)

environment; rare syndromes, common cancers, and gatekeepers; and mutagens and cancer.

▶ This review, although not truly a techniques article, is of interest to pathologists, and others. Much of our current understanding of neoplastic development and progression in colorectal cancer has come from the Vogelstein laboratory. An earlier review by Fearon and Vogelstein was widely read.[1] The molecular genetic alterations that underlie progression in colon cancer have been in large part based on the contributions of this laboratory. Further, colorectal adenocarcinoma has been used as a paradigm to investigate other carcinomas. Consequently, this may be 1 article that you would want to read in its entirety.

M.B. Cohen, M.D.

Reference

1. Fearon ER, Vogelstein B: A genetic model for colorectal tumorigenesis. *Cell* 61:759–767, 1990.

PART II

LABORATORY MEDICINE

———

18 Transfusion Medicine and Hemostasis

Evaluation of Original and Modified APC-resistance Tests in Unselected Outpatients With Clinically Suspected Thrombosis and in Healthy Controls
Svensson PJ, Zöller B, Dahlbäck B (Univ of Lund, Sweden; Univ Hosp, Malmö, Sweden)
Thromb Haemost 77:332–335, 1997   18–1

Background.—Most functional tests currently used for activated protein C (APC) resistance are only 85% to 90% sensitive and specific for the factor V gene (FVR506Q) mutation. Several factors influence the original APC-resistance test. A modified test, including predilution of patient plasma in factor V–depleted plasma, has increased the sensitivity and specificity for the factor V mutation. To date, however, neither the original nor the modified APC-resistance test has been assessed in patients with acute thrombotic events.

Methods.—A total of 220 patients with clinically suspected acute deep venous thrombosis (DVT) and 278 control subjects were recruited from an emergency department between March 1994 and January 1996. Patients were classified as *DVT-negative* or *DVT-positive*, depending on contrast phlebography findings.

Findings.—The DVT-positive patients with a normal factor V genotype had significantly lower APC ratios than the corresponding group of DVT-negative patients (Fig 1). Because of the reduced APC ratios in DVT-positive patients with normal factor V genotype, compared with the control subjects, the specificity of the APC-resistance test for the mutation among DVT-positive patients was only 28% at a cutoff value ensuring a 100% sensitivity for the mutation test. The modified APC-resistance test had a 98.8% specificity at an APC ratio cutoff value of 2.1, ensuring a 100% sensitivity for the FVR506Q mutation.

Conclusions.—The modified APC-resistance test using factor V–depleted plasma is a useful, easy-to-perform screening test for the FVR506Q allele. This test can be used in clinical practice for patients with acute

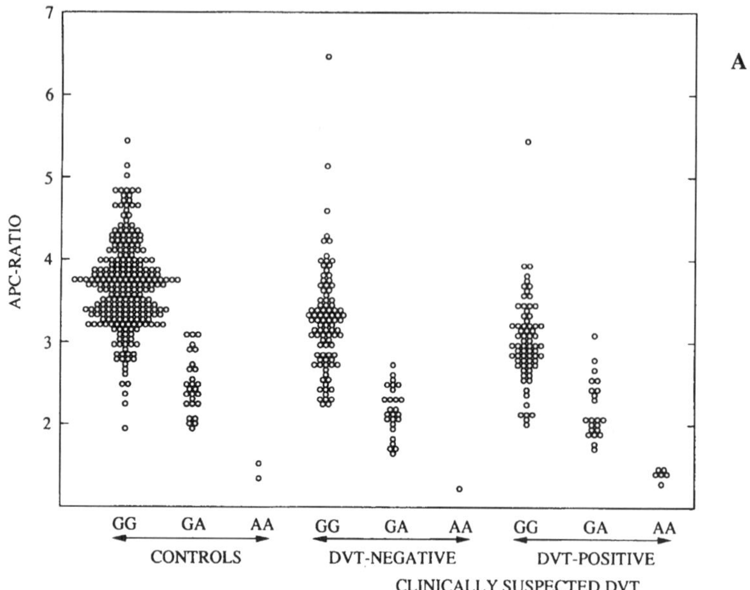

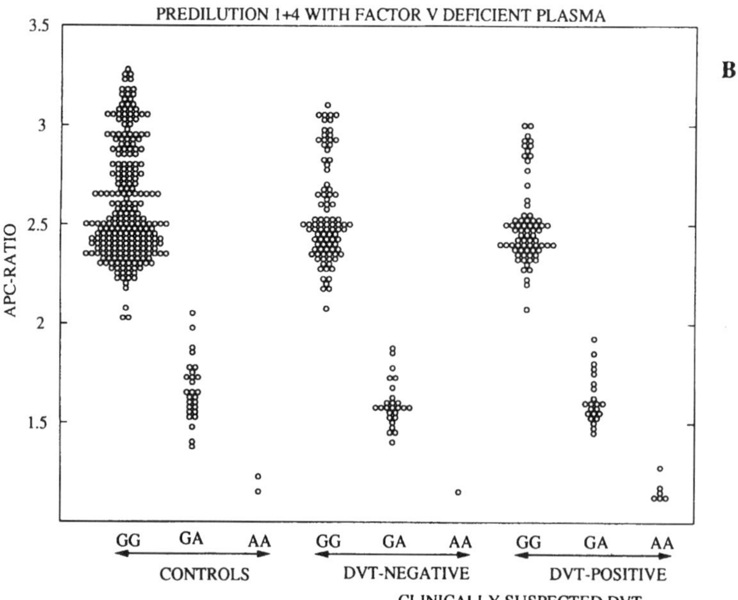

FIGURE 1.—Original (A) and modified (B) APC-resistance test in patients with clinically suspected acute DVT and in controls. A, The original APC-resistance test was performed in controls and in patients with clinically suspected DVT, and the individuals were grouped according to factor V genotype and whether they had thrombosis according to phlebography. APC ratios are plotted, and each circle represents one individual. B, The same analysis as in A but with the modified APC-resistance test. (Courtesy of Svensson PJ, Zoller B, Dahlback B: Evaluation of original and modified APC-resistance tests in unselected outpatients with clinically suspected thrombosis and in healthy controls. *Thromb Haemost* 77:332–335, 1997.)

thrombosis without being influenced by sex or acute venous thrombotic events.

▶ APC-resistance caused by a single point mutation in the factor V gene (FVR506Q) is the most common inherited disorder predisposing an individual to venous thromboembolism. It can be definitively identified by molecular diagnostic techniques, but these are generally not practial to use as screening tests. A coagulation-based, functional test for APC-resistance has been used for screening. However, this test is influenced by numerous factors including oral anticoagulants and heparin. A modified functional test, in which the patient's plasma is diluted 1:5 in factor V–deficient plasma, was developed to screen patients being treated with warfarin or heparin. Neither of these tests had been previously evaluated in patients who were being treated for active DVT. This paper demonstrates that the modified, but not the original, functional test for APC-resistance is highly specific in detecting patients with the FVR506Q mutation. Use of the modified test should allow rapid evaluation of patients with active DVT at the time of presentation, allowing informed decisions to be made regarding long-term anticoagulation.

A.J. Schlueter, M.D., Ph.D.

Association Between High Values of D-dimer and Tissue-plasminogen Activator Activity and First Gastrointestinal Bleeding in Cirrhotic Patients
Violi F, and the CALC Group (Università "La Sapienza," Rome)
Thromb Haemost 76:177–183, 1996   18–2

Introduction.—After gastrointestinal bleeding, the prognosis of patients with liver cirrhosis is poor. For the future treatment of patients with cirrhosis, the identification of risk factors of first bleeding may be of potential clincial relevance. In patients with cirrhosis with a clinical history of bleeding, it has not been investigated whether hyperfibrinolysis increases the risk of gastrointestinal bleeding. These patients may have high values of tissue plasminogen activator activity and D-dimer, markers of thrombin and plasmin activation, suggesting that the clinical course of cirrhosis is complicated by hyperfibrinolysis. In an unselected cohort of patients with cirrhosis with mild to severe liver failure, it was analyzed whether hyperfibrinolysis increases the risk of bleeding. The association of hyperfibrinolysis and clinical variables was examined.

Methods.—One hundred twelve patients with cirrhosis with esophageal varices but no previous upper-gastrointestinal bleeding were followed up for 3 years every 2–4 months. Their plasma values of D-dimer and tissue plasminogen activator activity wcrc measured, and if both showed high values, the patients were considered to have hyperfibrinolysis. Follow-up included a study of coagulation and fibrinolytic system.

Results.—Thirty-four patients (30%) bled during the follow-up. Compared with patients who did not bleed, the patients who bled had more severe liver failure and variceal size, higher prevalence of ascites, varices with red signs, and hyperfibrinolysis. The bleeders also had higher serum values of bilirubin and lower blood values of albumin, fibrinogen, and prothrombin activity. Hyperfibrinolysis was found to be the only marker predictive of bleeding. All patients with hyperfibrinolysis had ascites; however, 47% of patients with ascites did not have hyperfibrinolysis.

Conclusion.—To identify patients at risk for bleeding, screening for hyperfibrinolysis may be useful.

▶ Gastrointestinal hemorrhage is a major source of morbidity and mortality in patients with cirrhosis. Identification of a reliable predictor of bleeding would potentially be very useful in treating these patients. Hyperfibrinolysis has been associated with severe liver disease and gastrointestinal bleeding in previous studies.[1-3]

These authors extend the findings of the previous investigations to a larger group of patients who were approximately equally distributed between Child's class A, B, and C. They prospectively studied a group of 112 patients with cirrhosis who had not yet experienced an incident of gastrointestinal bleeding. Their study group was composed of a large proportion of patients with cirrhosis resulting from hepatitis B and C (73%) and a relatively few patients with alcoholic liver disease (8%). They report that 2 measures of hyperfibrinolysis, elevations in D-dimer (as measured by enzyme-linked immunosorbent assay) and tissue plasminogen activity, are predictive of future gastrointestinal bleeding, even when the population was controlled for other parameters associated with liver disease such as albumin, fibrinogen, bilirubin, prothrombin time, and size of varices. The authors do not report the predictive value of these 2 variables when used independently, and they did not assess the utility of fibrin degradation product measurement in identifying patients at risk for gastrointestinal bleeding.

A.J. Schlueter, M.D., Ph.D.

References

1. Francis RB, Feinstein DL: Clinical significance of accelerated fibrinolysis in liver disease. *Hemostasis* 1434:460–465, 1984.
2. Boks AL, Brommer EJP, Schalm SW, et al: Hemostasis and fibrinolysis in severe liver failure and their relation to hemorrhage. *Hepatology* 6:79–86, 1986.
3. Violi F, Ferro D, Basili S, et al: Hyperfibrinolysis increases the risk of gastrointestinal hemorrhage in patients with advanced cirrhosis. *Hepatology* 15:672–676, 1992.

HLA Class I-eluted Platelets as an Alternative to HLA-matched Platelets
Novotny VMJ, Huizinga TWJ, van Doorn R, et al (Red Cross Blood Bank, Leidsenhage, The Netherlands; Univ Hosp Leiden, The Netherlands)
Transfusion 36:438–444, 1996   18–3

Introduction.—Formation of HLA antibodies occurs in up to 50% of patients with a history of nonleuko–reduced transfusions or pregnancies.

For some patients, there are few if any HLA-compatible or crossmatch-negative donors because the HLA system is very polymorphic. In patients with alloantibodies, high-dose IV immunoglobulin to inhibit Fc-receptor-dependent destruction of platelets appears not to be effective. The surface class I major histocompatibility complex molecules could be removed from viable mononuclear cells and platelets with brief exposure to an acid-buffered solution at pH 3.0, while the platelets retained their specific antigens. In 2 refractory, alloimmunized patients with thrombocytopenia, the transfusion results obtained with HLA-eluted platelets were described.

Methods.—Citric acid was incubated with random-donor platelet concentrates, which were washed and transfused to 2 patients.

Results.—No effect was seen on platelet-specific glycoproteins, whereas HLA expression decreased below 25% of the initial expression. Because of a rare HLA type, 1 alloimmunized patient had no compatible donors and had repeated transfusions with acid-treated platelets. With acid-treated platelets, posttransfusion increments up to 47×10^{-9} per L were obtained, in contrast to the results with random-donor platelet transfusions. Profuse gastrointestinal bleeding stopped after three acid-treated platelet transfusions (30 donor units) and there was resolution of multiple skin hemorrhages. There were no observed side effects. After 1 transfusion with acid-treated platelets expressing 30% of the original HLA antigens, the other patient had a severe transfusion reaction with platelet increment, and more transfusions were not given.

Conclusions.—It is necessary to standardize the acid elution technique and validate the technique in patients. A place in platelet transfusion therapy may be reserved for HLA-eluted platelets prepared under specific conditions.

▶ The alloimmunized, platelet refractory patient with thrombocytopenia who is bleeding presents a frustrating and often desperate clinical dilemma. The usual therapeutic options in such patients include administration of high-dose IV immunoglobulin, antifibrinolytic agents such as aprotinin or Amicar, HLA-matched platelets, crossmatch-compatible platelets, or platelets from sibling donors.

This article and 1 other[1] offer preliminary data suggesting that another relatively simple option might be available to treat such patients. By eluting greater than 80% of the HLA antigens from the surface of platelets, platelet survival in some patients who are platelet refractory is increased. Because the procedure requires treatment with acidic solutions and several centrifugation steps, concern about platelet function is an issue. In vitro studies have provided evidence for retention of platelet function after HLA antigen elution; this article provides the first evidence of clinical improvement after infusion of several units of platelets treated in this fashion.

A.J. Schlueter, M.D., Ph.D.

Reference

1. Shanwell A, Sallander S, Olsson I, et al: An alloimmunized, thrombocytopenic patient successfully transfused with acid-treated, random-donor platelets. *Br J Haematol* 79:462–465, 1991.

Placental Blood as a Source of Hematopoietic Stem Cells for Transplantation Into Unrelated Recipients

Kurtzberg J, Laughlin M, Graham ML, et al (Duke Univ, Durham, NC; New York Blood Ctr)

N Engl J Med 335:157–166, 1996   18–4

Background.—The lack of human leukocyte antigen (HLA)-matched donors and the risk of graft-vs.-host disease (GVHD) limit bone marrow transplantation (BMT) from unrelated donors. Hematopoiesis can be reconstituted with placental blood from sibling donors. The preliminary findings of transplantation using partially HLA-mismatched placental blood from unrelated donors were reported.

Methods.—Twenty-five consecutive patients with a variety of malignant and nonmalignant conditions were given placental blood from unrelated donors and examined for hematologic and immunologic reconstitution and GVHD. Most patients were children. Before transplantation, HLA matching was performed by serologic typing for class I HLA antigens and low-resolution molecular typing for class II HLA alleles. High-resolution class II HLA typing was performed retrospectively in donor–recipient pairs differing by no more than 1 HLA antigen or allele. For donor–recipient pairs mismatched for 2 HLA antigens or alleles, high-resolution typing was done prospectively to determine the best match for HLA-DRB1.

Findings.—Twenty-four donor–recipient pairs were discordant for 1–3 antigens. The infused hematopoietic stem cells engrafted in 23 recipients. Acute grade III GVHD occurred in 2 of 21 assessable patients. Two patients had chronic GVHD. Sixty days after transplantation, in vitro proliferative responses of T and B cells to plant mitogens were found. With a median 12.5-month follow-up, the overall 100-day survival rate was 64%. Overall event-free survival was 48%.

Conclusions.—Partially mismatched placental blood from unrelated donors can provide an alternative source of stem cells for hematopoietic reconstitution. With placental blood differing by 1–3 alleles, donor chimerism was 100%, and immune reconstitution was achieved. Cases of GVHD were generally treatable.

▶ Placental blood has been used successfully as a source of hematopoietic stem cells for pediatric HLA-matched allogeneic transplants, primarily between siblings, since 1989. When compared with bone marrow as a source for stem cells, placental blood transplants are associated with a lower than expected incidence of GVHD. Based on this observation, these authors report their experience using placental blood from unrelated, HLA-mismatched donors as a source of stem cells for 25 consecutive children requiring transplants. Their observation of low rates of severe GVHD as well as successful trilineage engraftment in the majority of their patients provides evidence that unrelated, mismatched placental blood transplants may be a viable option for children who do not have an HLA-matched, related donor. A major advantage to this method of transplantation is the relatively short time to donor identification and transplant compared with unrelated bone marrow donor searches. Long-term follow-up of these patients will determine whether an increased risk of disease relapse because of lack of "graft-vs.-leukemia effect" is associated with the observed low incidence of GVHD.

A.J. Schlueter, M.D., Ph.D.

Effect of 3.2% vs. 3.8% Sodium Citrate Concentration on Routine Coagulation Testing
Adcock DM, Kressin DC, Marlar RA (Univ of Colorado, Denver; Denver VA Med Ctr)
Am J Clin Pathol 107:105–110, 1997   18–5

Background.—Routine coagulation assays can be affected by many preanalytic variables. These variables can be classified into 3 main categories: specimen collection, transportation and storage, and processing. In the United States, most laboratories use an evacuated tube collection system for routine blood collection. Differences in these tubes include a citrate concentration of 3.2% or 3.8%, stopper type, tube composition, lubrication, and siliconization. The effect of these differences in evacuated tube systems on routine coagulation assays is unknown in most laboratories. The effect of 2 common sodium citrate concentrations on routine coagulation assays was analyzed.

Methods.—The variability of 3.2% and 3.8% citrate concentrations was tested in 5 populations: healthy volunteers, inpatients not receiving anticoagulant therapy, inpatients receiving IV heparin therapy, inpatients receiving both IV heparin and oral anticoagulant therapy, and outpatients receiving oral anticoagulant therapy. To determine the effect of reagent sensitivity, 2 prothrombin times and activated partial thromboplastin times were used, one responsive and the other relatively nonresponsive.

Results.—With the use of nonresponsive prothrombin time and activated partial thromboplastin time reagents, there was little effect of the citrate concentration on assay results, except in patients receiving IV heparin therapy. When responsive prothrombin time and activated partial thromboplastin time reagents were used, citrate concentrations had a significant effect on assay results. A change of less than 0.7 International Normalized Ratio units between citrate concentrations was seen in 18% of samples from patients receiving oral anticoagulant therapy. A greater than 7-second difference was seen in 19% of patients receiving IV heparin therapy when comparing results of activated partial thromboplastin times.

Discussion.—Citrate concentration can affect clotting time because the amount of citrate directly affects calcium concentration. Prothrombin time and activated partial thromboplastin time are typically longer in tubes with 3.8% sodium citrate. In the United States, of 942 laboratories polled, 21% used 3.2% sodium citrate and 79% used 3.8% sodium citrate. In Europe, the majority of laboratories used 3.2% citrate. The citrate concentration is not recorded on collection tubes. Until a standard citrate concentration is adopted, laboratory staff should be aware of this difference and take steps to ensure that the same citrate concentrations are used. The 3.2% citrate is recommended for all coagulation tests.

▶ Most specimens submitted for routine coagulation testing are drawn into tubes containing sodium citrate anticoagulant. The effect of citrate concentration on prothrombin in time and activated partial thromboplastin time test results has been underappreciated. This paper demonstrates that prothrombin time values obtained with sensitive reagents can be affected by the citrate concentration to a degree that would influence patient management. Activated partial thromboplastin time values are also affected but to a degree that would not be clinically significant in the majority of cases. Additionally, differences in citrate concentrations between the reagent International Sensitivity Index and the specimen may affect the International Normalized Ratio calculation. The authors make several recommendations to address these issues that should be fairly easy to implement. These include ensuring that all the specimens tested in the laboratory are drawn into the same concentration of anticoagulant (including specimens received from remote sites) and establishing normal ranges based on that same citrate concentration. These considerations are likely to apply to many special coagulation tests performed in reference laboratories as well. Although still under consideration, it is likely that recommendations to use only 3.2% sodium citrate will be forthcoming.

A.J. Schlueter, M.D., Ph.D.

The Risk of Transfusion-transmitted Viral Infections
Schreiber GB, for the Retrovirus Epidemiology Donor Study (Westat Inc, Rockville, Md; et al)
N Engl J Med 334:1685–1690, 1996   18–6

Background.—The greatest threat to the safety of the blood supply is donations from individuals during the infectious window period when seronegative donors are undergoing seroconversion. The residual risks of transmitting disease can be determined by combining rates of seroconversion with estimates of probability that blood was donated during a donor's window period. The incidence rates of seroconversion in blood donors for HIV, human T-cell lymphotropic virus, hepatitis C virus, and hepatitis B virus from 1991 through 1993 were determined.

TABLE 2.—Residual Risks to the Blood Supply Associated With Window-period Donations by Seroconverting Donors

Virus*	Length of Window Period (days)		Residual Risk (per million donations)	
	Estimate	Range	Estimate†	Range‡
HIV	22§	6–38	2.03	0.36–4.95
HTLV	51¶	36–72	1.56	0.50–3.90
HCV	82‖	54–192	9.70	3.47–36.11
HBV				
HBsAg	59**	37–87	6.65	2.87–13.43
Total HBV††	—	—	15.83	6.82–31.97

*Markers for each virus were assayed as described in the Methods section.
†Calculated by multiplying the adjusted incidence rate of seroconversion by the length of the window period.
‡The lower and upper bounds of the range were calculated by multiplying the lower and upper limits of the window-period range by the lower and upper limits of the 95% confidence interval for the adjusted incidence rate, respectively.
§Data were obtained from Busch et al.
¶Data were obtained from Manns et al.
‖Data were obtained from Busch et al, and Lelie et al.
**Data were obtained from Mimms et al.
††Data were adjusted for transient antigenemia by multiplying the estimated residual risk of HBsAg seroconversion and the range by 2.38 on the assumption that 42% of hepatitis B virus infections are detected by the assay for HBsAg.
Abbreviations: HTLV, human T-cell lymphotropic virus; *HCV*, hepatitis C virus; *HBV*, hepatitis B virus; *HBsAg*, hepatitis B surface antigen.
(Reprinted by permission of *The New England Journal of Medicine*, from Schreiber GB, for the Retrovirus Epidemiology Donor Study: The risk of transfusion-transmitted viral infections. *N Engl J Med* 334:1685–1690, 1996. Copyright 1996, Massachusetts Medical Society. All rights reserved.)

Methods.—Data from 586,507 individuals who donated blood more than once during the study period and whose blood units passed all screening tests were used. For each virus, crude incidence rates were determined by dividing the number of donors undergoing seroconversion by the total number of person-years at risk. The total number of person-years was determined by totaling the intervals between donations for all donors.

Results.—Data from more than 2,300,000 allogeneic donations were used. Among these donors, the risks of donating blood during an infectious window period were 1 in 493,000 for HIV, 1 in 641,000 for human T-cell lymphotropic virus, 1 in 103,000 for hepatitis C virus, and 1 in 63,000 for hepatitis B virus (Table 2). The aggregate risk was 1 in 34,000, and hepatitis B virus and hepatitis C virus accounted for 88% of this risk. These risks could be reduced by 27% to 72% by the new screening tests that shorten the window period.

Discussion.—The estimates of residual risk are the probability that a unit is infectious, but was donated in the window period before seroconversion. The incidence of seroconversion in one-time donors could not be calculated, but these donors accounted for only 20% of the donations in this study. A previous study estimated that up to 22% of donors infected with human T-cell lymphotropic virus-II are missed by current screening tests. A 1992 investigation by The Centers for Disease Control and Prevention suggested that up to 10% of individuals with hepatitis C virus infection are missed by current screening tests. The current findings may not reflect national averages. The blood centers in this study account for about 9% of blood donations in the United States.

▶ This paper provides the most recent data on the risk of transfusion-transmitted viral infections from individuals giving multiple donations (more than 80% of the U.S. blood supply). Figures are based on more than 2 million donations, corresponding to about 9% of the annual collections in the United States. They are based on the most recent antibody tests available for human T-cell lymphotropic virus, HIV, hepatitis B virus, and hepatitis C virus, but do not include data on p24 antigen testing for HIV. Because units that test positive for one of the above infectious disease markers are discarded, the risk of transfusion-associated infection was based on the seroconversion rate and the estimated antibody negative "window period" following infection. This approach necessitated exclusion of first-time donors from the calculations; however, these individuals constitute less than 20% of the donor population and the authors chose not to adjust their calculations for this factor. The risk of viral transfusion-transmitted infection remains quite low, and continues to decrease from earlier estimates.

A.J. Schlueter, M.D., Ph.D.

Crossmatch-Compatible Platelets Improve Corrected Count Increments in Patients Who Are Refractory to Randomly Selected Platelets
Gelb AB, Leavitt AD (Univ of California, San Francisco)
Transfusion 37:624–630, 1997   18–7

Background.—Thrombocytopenic patients refractory to randomly selected platelets are often supported with HLA-matched and crossmatch-compatible platelets. Studies showing the efficacy of crossmatch-compatible platelets have been primarily limited to refractory patients previously shown to be alloimmunized. The effectiveness of crossmatch-compatible platelets in unselected refractory patients was investigated.

Methods.—The records of all patients receiving crossmatch-compatible platelets between January 1991 and May 1994 were reviewed. Sixty-six patients refractory to random-donor platelets, having 2 consecutive corrected count increments (CCIs) of less than 10,000, were evaluable.

Findings.—A total of 475 crossmatch-compatible platelet components were administered. Compared with randomly selected platelets, crossmatch-compatible platelets had a significantly improved mean CCI, increased by 8,000. The mean CCI improved to at least 7,500 in 59% of the patients and to at least 10,000 in 41%. When the 10 patients for whom crossmatch-compatible platelets could not be identified were included in the analysis, the mean CCI improved to at least 7,500 in 51% and to at least 10,000 in 36%. Continued use did not reduce the efficacy of crossmatch-compatible platelets.

Discussion.—Many factors reportedly contribute to the development of refractoriness to platelet transfusion. These include fever, infection, sepsis, disseminated intravascular coagulation, bleeding, hypersplenism, and alloimmunization to HLA-, ABO-, or platelet-specific antigens. Immune-mediated processes are estimated to account for 25% to 55% of all refractoriness. This study shows that crossmatch-compatible platelet components significantly improve the mean CCI for about one half of refractory patients, even when patients are not preselected on the basis of alloimmunization.

▶ Patients may become refractory to random-donor platelets by immune or nonimmune (sepsis, splenomegaly, disseminated intravascular coagulation, etc.) mechanisms. In many institutions, patients who fail to show adequate increments to random donors must demonstrate alloantibodies to platelet, HLA, or ABO antigens before they become eligible to receive crossmatched platelets. These authors report their success rate using crossmatch-compatible platelets in an unselected group of platelet refractory patients. Their success rate of 36% to 59% (depending on the definition of adequate platelet increment) suggests this approach to finding compatible units n v be useful.

The authors also demonstrate that the patients who responded to several crossmatch-compatible units were unable to respond to intermittent random-donor platelet transfusions and argue that loss of refractoriness was not the reason for continued response to crossmatched units. No data are provided on the clinical condition of the patients in the study for determination of whether clinical factors might help predict the response to crossmatched platelets. Intuitively, the relatively high response rate of unselected patients to crossmatched units suggests cost effectiveness, but these authors did not perform cost analysis to formally demonstrate this point.

A.J. Schlueter, M.D., Ph.D.

Loss of Volunteer Blood Donors Because of Unconfirmed Enzyme Immunoassay Screening Results
Ownby HE, and the Retrovirus Epidemiology (Donor Study, American Red Cross Blood Services, Detroit)
Transfusion 37:199–205, 1997   18–8

Background.—A major problem for blood banks today is the loss of donors who repeatedly test reactive on enzyme immunoassay (EIA) but who are not confirmed to test positive on further assessment. Although 4% of units are discarded because of EIA reactivity, less than 1 in 10 of these potential donors test positive in subsequent testing. Few data are reported on the demographic features of false positive donors.

Methods and Findings.—Data were obtained from the Retrovirus Epidemiologic Donor Study database, which included more than 2 million allogeneic whole-blood donations collected from 1991 through 1993. The prevalences of both false positive and indeterminate donations were significantly greater among donations from females compared with males and among units from first-time donors. The prevalence of false positive donations from blacks was higher compared with other racial groups, as well as in directed donations compared with community donations. For HIV testing, there was also a trend toward a declining prevalence with increasing age.

Discussions.—A large body of evidence indicates that most blood donors with stable, unconfirmed reactions are not infected. The most plausible explanation for the hepatitis C virus (HCV) findings—with more than two thirds of EIA–repeatably reactive but unconfirmed donations testing indeterminate—is cross-reactivity to similar HCV antigens, as HCV screening and confirmatory assays contain similar and sometimes identical HCV recombinant proteins. Twenty-eight percent of HIV EIA–repeatably reactive but unconfirmed donations were indeterminate. In such cases, cross-reactivity may be occurring to different antigen specificities in the 2 assays. It is unclear which hypothesis best explains why two thirds of human T-lymphotropic virus–repeatably reactive unconfirmed donations were indeterminate.

▶ Presently, testing for 7 infectious disease markers is required by the Food and Drug Administration on each unit of blood product transfused in the United States. To maximize safety of the blood supply, units that are repeatably reactive on the screening assays are discarded and the donors are deferred, despite the fact that these results are almost invariably false positives. This loss accounts for approximately 4% of the blood products collected, in addition to the loss of future donations from the deferred donors. The Retrovirus Epidemiology Donor Study database, established in 1989, contains information on all donations from 5 major, geographically distributed United States blood collection facilities.

In this paper, the study group analyzed the demographics of the donors of units that tested positive on screening assays but were negative by confirmatory testing. Their results identified groups of donors that are more likely than the general donor population to test falsely positive by current testing methods. These data should provide the basis for focused investigations into the reasons for false positivity on infectious disease screening tests and, ultimately, the design of screening tests with equivalent sensitivity but higher specificity. This, in turn, should decrease unnecessary loss of uninfected units from the blood supply.

A.J. Schlueter, M.D., Ph.D.

A Common Genetic Variation in the 3′-Untranslated Region of the Prothrombin Gene Is Associated With Elevated Plasma Prothrombin Levels and an Increase in Venous Thrombosis

Poort SR, Rosendaal FR, Reitsma PH, et al (Leiden Univ, The Netherlands)
Blood 88:3698–3703, 1996   18–9

Introduction.—Genetic risk factors for thrombotic disease have been verified in selected families. An analysis of the prothrombin genes of selected research subjects with a history of venous thrombophilia was performed using polymerase chain reaction (PCR) and direct sequencing of the coding regions and their flanking splice junctions and the 5′- and 3′-untranslated (UT) regions.

Methods.—Families of 28 of 113 probands with a personal and family history of venous thrombophilia were randomly selected for PCR and sequencing analysis. Patients with a first episode of deep-vein thrombosis acted as controls. The mean patient and control age was 47 years. Blood was collected from both patient groups and underwent PCR and sequencing analysis.

Results.—There were no deviations in the coding regions or the 5′-UT region, except for known polymorphic sites. In the sequence of the 3′-UT region, 1 nucleotide change of a G to an A transition was detected at position 20210. The 20210 AG genotype was detected in 18% and 1% of the patient and control groups, respectively. This sequence was confirmed by restriction enzyme analysis using 1 mutagenic primer. The relevance of the 20210 A allele in the general population was analyzed via a population-based, patient-control study (Leiden Thrombophilia Study [LETS]).

The prevalence of the 20210 A allele was 1.2% in healthy controls. The prevalence of the 20210 AG genotype was 6.2% in patients and 2.3% in healthy controls. There was a relative risk of 2.8 for thrombosis associated with the 20210 A allele. Its presence was associated with increased risk of venous thrombosis in all age groups. There was a correlation between the presence of the 20210 A allele and elevated prothrombin time; 87% of patients with the 20210 A allele were in the highest quartile of plasma prothrombin levels. Elevated prothrombin was a risk factor for venous thrombosis. Patients with a prothrombin level greater than 1.15 U/mL had a 2.1–fold increased risk for venous thrombosis.

Conclusion.—The presence of the 20210 A allele is a moderate risk factor for venous thrombosis. Carriers of the allele have significantly higher prothrombin levels than noncarriers. The elevated prothrombin level itself is a risk factor for venous thrombosis, suggesting that the 20210 A allele may act through the elevated prothrombin levels. The LETS detected an incidence of the 20210 A allele in 6.3% of unselected patients with a first episode of deep vein thrombosis, suggesting that the allele is a relatively common risk factor for venous thrombosis.

▶ A large proportion of patients with venous thromboembolism have no currently identifiable hereditary or acquired risk factors for this condition. Patients in whom hereditary risk factors can be identified are considered more strongly for long-term anticoagulation to prevent recurrent disease than those without identifiable risks. Thus, there is continuing interest in identification of genetic defects associated with venous thrombosis.

This paper describes a genetic variation in the 3'-UT region of the prothrombin gene which was found to be more common in patients with venous thrombosis than in case controls. The study populations were the same as those used for 2 previous studies attempting to identify risk factors for venous thrombosis, including the study that identified activated protein C resistance as a risk factor.[1, 2] The individuals with the prothrombin gene mutation also had elevated plasma prothrombin activity (although not all individuals with elevated prothrombin activity had the described mutation). The authors hypothesize that the mutation causes elevated prothrombin activity and that this is responsible for increased risk of venous thrombosis, but these links have not yet been formally demonstrated.

In addition to its importance in providing evidence for another, potentially common hereditary risk factor for venous thrombosis, this paper demonstrates a powerful approach for identifying other risk factors for thrombophilia. By maintaining a bank of DNA from patients with thrombosis and case controls, the risk associated with any potential mutation that might influence thrombus formation can be quickly assessed. This approach should lead to rapid identification of other mutations associated with thrombophilia.

A.J. Schlueter, M.D., Ph.D.

References

1. Kierkegaard A: Incidence of acute deep vein thrombosis in two districts: A phlebographic study. *Acta Chir Scand* 146:267–269, 1980.
2. Engesser L, Brommer EJ, Kluft C, et al: Elevated plasminogen activation inhibitor (PAI), a cause of thrombophilia? A study in 203 patients with familial or sporadic venous thrombophilia. *Thromb Haemost* 62:673–680, 1989.

Potentially Clinically Important Inaccuracies in Testing for the Lupus Anticoagulant: An Analysis of Results From Three Surveys of the UK National External Quality Assessment Scheme (NEQAS) for Blood Coagulation

Jennings I, for the UK Natl External Quality Assessment Scheme for Blood Coagulation (Royal Hallamshire Hosp, Sheffield, England)
Thromb Haemost 77:934–937, 1997

18–10

Background.—The most widely used and sensitive tests for confirming the presence of lupus anticoagulant (LA) have a low concentration of phospholipid, such as the kaolin clotting time (KCT), dilute Russell's viper venom time (DRVVT), and thromboplastin dilution test. Preanalytic variables influence the test results in LA assays, especially those affecting the phospholipid concentration of the test plasma because of platelet contamination and activation. These features have resulted in inaccuracies in LA testing results.

Methods.—Lyophilized plasma samples from 3 subjects with strong, weak, and absent LA were tested in 220 centers. The tests most commonly used were activated partial thromboplastin time (APTT), DRVVT, and KCT.

Findings.—For the strong, weak, and absent LA samples, median DRVVT ratios were 1.75, 1.17, and 1.10, respectively. Four percent of the laboratories did not detect the presence of a strong LA. Ninety-four percent of DRVVT users and 85% of KCT users made an accurate diagnosis from the speciman containing a strong LA. More than half the centers did not detect a weak LA. With this sample, correction of APTT, DRVVT, or KCT was frequently observed on addition of plasma and also in platelet neutralization. Thirty-seven percent of DRVVT users and 27% of KCT users made corrected diagnoses. About one fourth of the laboratories falsely detected LA in a factor IX–deficient plasma. The absence of LA was reported correctly by 73% of DRVVT users and 69% of KCT users.

Conclusion.—The suboptimal accuracy of LA testing is likely to have important clinical consequences. Greater conformity is needed in the selection and performance of LA tests. Using standard plasma for internal quality assessment in individual laboratories may be helpful.

▶ The identification of antiphospholipid antibodies in patients with recurrent thrombosis, particularly those without coexisting autoimmune disease, has important implications for institution of long-term anticoagulation. Numerous tests are in use to identify this heterogeneous antibody population. This report summarizes the results of 3 challenges for the detection of LA distributed to approximately 220 laboratories in the United Kingdom. Based on reference laboratory testing, 1 sample was strongly positive for LA, 1 was weakly positive for LA, and the third contained no detectable LA activity but was from a factor IX–deficient patient. The laboratories could perform any tests they wished to identify LA activity, and they reported results of the individual tests as well as a global interpretation of the test results (i.e., presence or absence of LA in the specimen).

The poor performance of the participating laboratories on the latter 2 samples (44% correct on the specimen with weak LA activity and 74% correct on the sample with no LA activity) re-emphasizes the suboptimal performance of certain test methods for LA and the need for standardization of these procedures between laboratories. In addition, the role of preanalytic variation in these specimens is discussed, particularly the degree of plasma contamination with platelet phospholipid.

A.J. Schlueter, M.D., Ph.D.

Removing IgG Antibodies From Intact Red Cells: Comparison of Acid and EDTA, Heat, and Chloroquine Elution Methods

des Roziers NB, Squalli S (Établissement de Transfusion Sanguine de Languedoc-Roussillon, Nîmes, France)

Transfusion 37:497–501, 1997   18–11

Background.—Typing red blood cell (RBC) antigens in patients with warm autoimmune hemolytic anemia and a strongly positive direct antiglobulin test (DAT) is difficult. Phenotyping these RBCs by indirect antiglobulin methods requires an effective technique for dissociating IgG molecules from human RBCs without changing blood group antigen expression. The current study determined the relative abilities of chloroquine diphosphate dissociation, acid/ethylenediamine tetraacetic acid (EDTA) elution, and heating at 56°C for 10 minutes to produce intact antibody-free RBCs from 50 DAT-positive RBCs coated in vitro or in vivo. The integrity of common blood group antigens was also assessed, and the activities of the antibodies eluted by the acid/EDTA method or with heat were compared.

Methods and Findings.—Warm-reactive autoantibodies (red cells sensitized in vivo) from 8 patients and alloantibodies (sensitized in vitro) from 42 patients were studied. Acid/EDTA and heat reduced the conventional tube DAT positivity more strongly than did chloroquine. Compared with heat, the acid/EDTA technique eluted significantly more agglutinating Rh system alloantibodies, Kell system alloantibodies, and warm autoantibodies. Agglutination scores of acid/ECTA eluates were greater than heat elution scores in 43 of 50 instances and were similar in 3. Neither acid/EDTA nor chloroquine treatment affected antigens in the Rh, Kidd and Duffy systems, or S and s. However, acid/EDTA rendered K, k, and Kp^b completely nonreactive. All blood group antigens assessed were expressed more weakly after heat elution. End-point titrations demonstrated that accurate typing of RBCs after heat elution was possible for all specificities by using fourfold greater concentrations of typing sera in the gel low–ionic-strength saline indirect antiglobulin test or tube tests, except for K typing, for which a tenfold higher concentration of anti-K was needed.

Conclusion.—Obtaining large amounts of RBCs from patients with positive DATs is often difficult. An elution procedure for these patients should provide undamaged, antibody-free RBCs for antigen phenotyping and adsorption methods, while yielding potent eluates that can be used for serologic investigations. The acid/EDTA elution technique meets all these criteria and seems optimal for routine typing of RBCs coated with warm-reactive IgG alloantibodies or autoantibodies.

▶ It is occasionally desirable to phenotype the RBCs of patients who have a positive DAT, particularly those who have a broadly reacting antibody in their eluate with a specificity which is difficult to determine. Because of sample size and time limitations, it would also be useful if the technique used to generate the eluate could provide RBCs with intact antigens for phenotyping. These authors compared chloroquine, heat, and acid/EDTA elution methods for their ability to provide a high titer eluate and antigen-intact RBCs. In vitro sensitization of RBCs with representative high titer antisera for virtually all of the clinically relevant antigens (in addition to evaluation of 8 specimens containing a warm autoantibody) ensured that the study results would be broadly applicable.

The acid/EDTA method proved, in general, to be the most useful for both eluate and RBC preparation, but suffered from the significant flaw of completely destroying K, k, and Kp^b antigen reactivity on the RBCs. The authors do not suggest a solution to this problem; however, the heat elution method was successful in retaining reactivity to these antigens and might be used in addition to acid/EDTA elution when phenotyping for these antigens is relevant.

A.J. Schlueter, M.D., Ph.D.

Reliability of Five Rapid D-Dimer Assays Compared to ELISA in the Exclusion of Deep Venous Thrombosis
Janssen MCH, Heebels AE, de Metz M, et al (Univ Hosp, Nijmegen, The Netherlands; Canisius Wilhelmina Hosp, Nijmegen, The Netherlands)
Thromb Haemost 77:262–266, 1997   18–12

Background.—More than half the patients with symptoms suggesting deep venous thrombosis (DVT) do not have thrombosis. Ascending venography is still the definitive test for diagnosing DVT. A simple, reliable blood test to exclude DVT would have practical and cost-efficient advantages. The efficacies of 5 novel, rapid D-dimer (DD) assays for excluding DVT in outpatients with suspected DVT were assessed and compared with that of enzyme-linked immunosorbent assays (ELISA).

Methods.—One hundred thirty-two patients suspected of having DVT were included in the study. The tests compared included a rapid ELISA (VIDAS), a classical ELISA DD assay (Organon Mab Y18), and 4 novel latex DD tests (Tinaquant, Minutex, Ortho, and SimpliRed).

Findings.—The overall prevalence of DVT was 67%. Proximal DVT was found in 59% and distal DVT in 8%. At a cut-off level of 500 ng/ml, the overall sensitivity was 98% for ELISA, 100% for VIDAS, and 99% for Tinaquant. The negative predictive values of these 3 assays were 88%, 100%, and 93%, respectively. The other latex tests had considerably lower sensitivities: 61% for SimpliRed, 77% for Minutex, and 51% for Ortho.

Conclusions.—VIDAS and Tinaquant may be used instead of ELISA DD to exclude DVT. Both assays, which require 20 minutes and 35 minutes to perform, respectively, may be used in routine screening. Large clinical management studies are now needed to confirm these findings.

▶ Clinical criteria for the diagnosis of DVT are notoriously poor, and the use of radiologic procedures has become the gold standard for making this diagnosis. These tests are often difficult to obtain rapidly, and a simple laboratory test to exclude the diagnosis of DVT would be a useful advance in patient care. Elevated plasma D-dimer levels have been proposed as one such test. Most studies demonstrating the usefulness of D-dimer levels in this setting have utilized an ELISA test with a relatively long turnaround time. This study compares a rapid ELISA technique and four latex agglutination tests for D-dimer against a gold standard of compression ultrasound for making the diagnosis of DVT. The high sensitivity of the ELISA test (VIDAS) and one of the latex agglutination tests (Tinaquant) suggests they may be useful in excluding the diagnosis of DVT in patients with a negative test result. As expected, DVT could not be ruled in by any of these test methods as there are numerous reasons for elevated D-dimer levels besides DVT. Unfortunately, the utility of these tests in a point of care setting was not clearly addressed, as the authors chose to separate the plasma from the erythrocytes and freeze the plasma until the time of testing, and then reconstitute the specimens with erythrocytes prior to performing the tests. This adds an extra preanalytic variable that would not normally exist were this test performed in an emergency room, for example. The prevalence of DVT was relatively high in this study (67%), but this should not adversely affect the reported negative predictive value of the tests. The results indicate that D-dimer testing in a point of care setting may be useful for ruling out DVT, but the value of the test result may vary significantly with the choice of test kit.

A.J. Schlueter, M.D., Ph.D.

Cytokine Induction of Platelet Activation

Lumadue JA, Lanzkron SM, Kennedy SD, et al (Johns Hopkins Hosp, Baltimore, Md)
Am J Clin Pathol 106:795–798, 1996   18–13

Background.—Significant levels of cytokines accumulate in the plasma of stored platelet concentrates with white blood cell contamination over time. The current study assessed the level of cytokines that accumulate during platelet storage; these cytokines can cause platelet activation in vitro.

Methods.—Interleukin-6 and -8 (IL-6, IL-8) levels were assessed for random donor platelet concentrates on days 1–4 of storage. Activation was assayed by measuring the expression of p-Selectin (CD62) on the platelet surfaces. Fresh platelets were then incubated with these concentrations of exogenous cytokines. Activation was measured by flow cytometry using a monoclonal antibody directed against p-Selectin.

Findings.—Cytokine concentrations usually present on days 3 and 4 of shelf life were associated with significant platelet activation. There were no increases in activation using cytokine concentrations present on days 1 and 2 of storage.

Conclusions.—IL-6 and -8 concentrations found routinely in 3- and 4-day-old nonleukoreduced platelet products consistently result in increased platelet activation when platelets are exposed to these cytokine levels for 1 hour. The levels of platelet activation in these products may be decreased by prestorage leukoreduction or by adding chemical inhibitors of cytokine generation.

▶ The accumulation of cytokines (particularly IL-1 β, IL-6, and tumor necrosis factor α) in platelet units as a result of deterioration of contaminating leukocytes has been described[1] . These cytokines are thought to be responsible for an increased incidence of febrile transfusion reactions in recipients of these products. The effect of cytokines on platelet function has not previously been reported. These authors studied the effect of IL-6 and IL-8 on platelet activation, specifically the expression of the cell surface antigen CD62. Both of these cytokines were capable of inducing platelet activation at concentrations routinely found in 3- to 4-day-old platelet concentrates. These results suggest that leukoreduction, in addition to decreasing the risk of cytomegalovirus transmission and rates of febrile transfusion reactions and alloimmunization to human leukocyte antigens, may actually provide a platelet product with improved function. Direct studies of platelet function following exposure to these cytokines have yet to be performed.

A.J. Schlueter, M.D., Ph.D.

Reference

1. Muylle L, Joos M, Wouters E, et al: Increased tumor necrosis factor α (TNFα), interleukin 1 and interleukin 6 (IL-6) levels in the plasma of stored platelet concentrates: Relationship between TNFα and IL-6 levels and febrile transfusion reactions. *Transfusion* 33:195–199, 1993.

19 Microbiology

Blood Culture Quality Improvement: A College of American Pathologists Q-Probes Study Involving 909 Institutions and 289,572 Blood Culture Sets
Schifman RB, Bachner P, Howanitz PJ (Univ of Arizona, Tucson; Univ of Kentucky, Lexington; Univ of California, Los Angeles)
Arch Pathol Lab Med 120:999–1002, 1996   19–1

Background.—In patients with sepsis, the occurrence of bacteremia cannot be predicted reliably by clinical parameters. Analysis of blood cultures is needed to establish the diagnosis and guide treatment. Solitary blood culture (SBC) collection may be less sensitive than multiple specimen collections, thereby compromising patient management. The usefulness of SBC collections as a preanalytic quality indicator of blood culture practice was determined.

Methods.—Two College of American Pathologists Q-Probes laboratory quality improvement studies were performed. The proportion of and reasons for SBC collections in 909 centers were assessed prospectively. Data on 289,572 blood culture sets were analyzed.

Findings.—In the first and second studies, the median proportion of SBCs per center was 10.1% and 12.1%, respectively, in adult inpatients; 25.4% and 33.3% among adult outpatients; and 89% and 100% among children. The most common reasons for not obtaining a second culture in adults were that the test was not indicated and that the physician believed that 1 was sufficient. A significantly greater proportion of outpatient SBCs than inpatient cultures were classified as *not indicated*. Institutions that continued to monitor SBCs had a significant decrease in SBC rates.

Conclusions.—Q-Probe findings help set performance benchmarks for an important preanalytic component of the blood culture procedure. The current data also indicate that interinstitutional quality assessment and continuous monitoring are associated with improved performance.

▶ The Q-Probes program is a voluntary subscription program of the College of American Pathologists that conducts periodic multi-institutional studies dealing with quality assessment, improvement, and benchmarking in pathology and laboratory medicine. This report describes the results of Q-Probes studies conducted to evaluate current practices for assessing and improving blood culture practices. Specifically, the studies were designed to examine the frequency of SBC collections and to understand the reasons for which SBCs are collected. The rationale behind the focus on SBCs was that they may compromise patient care by being less sensitive and less reliable diagnostically than multiple specimen collections. Data from this study indicate that the median SBC rate among adult inpatients is 10% to 12%, with substantial interinstitutional variation. Not surprisingly, the SBC rate was highest among adult outpatients (25% to 33%) and infant and pediatric patients (89% to 100%). The following are the most common reasons cited for not performing more than 1 culture: (1) the physician thought that 1 was sufficient; (2) the test was not clinically indicated; (3) miscommunication or improper test ordering. Among 198 laboratories that participated in each of 2 different study years and that provided complete information, continued monitoring of SBC submissions was associated with a declining SBC rate. This study suggests the following: (1) many blood cultures may not be indicated; (2) education regarding proper use of blood cultures should be performed; (3) quality assessment and continuous monitoring of test-ordering practices are associated with performance improvement.

M.A. Pfaller, M.D.

Clinical Prediction Rules to Optimize Cytotoxin Testing for *Clostridium difficile* in Hospitalized Patients With Diarrhea
Katz DA, Lynch ME, Littenberg B (White River Junction [VT] VA Med Ctr; Dartmouth-Hitchcock Med Ctr, Lebanon, NH)
Am J Med 100:487–495, 1996   19–2

Background.—Routine testing of hospitalized patients with diarrhea for *Clostridium difficile* cytotoxin has been advocated as a high-yield procedure. However, some authorities have questioned the rationale for this. The current study derived a clinical decision rule for predicting the results of the *C. difficile* cytotoxin assay in hospitalized adults with diarrhea in an attempt to target a low-yield subgroup for whom routine testing could be deferred.

Methods.—Antibiotic use within 30 days before testing and a history of significant diarrhea were hypothesized to strongly predict cytotoxin results. Data were obtained on 480 consecutive patients undergoing diagnostic testing for *C. difficile.* To develop a more detailed model, additional data were obtained on 68 test-positive (case) patients and 265 randomly selected test-negative (control) patients in the cohort.

Findings.—Overall, the prevalence of positive cytotoxin assays was 14%. Factors independently predicting cytotoxin assay results were previous antibiotic treatment, significant diarrhea, and abdominal pain. The model was able to discriminate between patients with positive and negative assays with a receiver operating characteristic (ROC) area of 0.68. The observed and predicted probabilities of a positive cytotoxin assay were correlated well over the range of observed probabilities. A decision rule, defined as *positive* if previous antibiotic use and either significant diarrhea or abdominal pain are present, had an 86% sensitivity and a 45% specificity. A simplified a priori rule, defined as *positive* if both previous antibiotic use and history of significant diarrhea are present, had a sensitivity of 80%, a specificity of 45%, a positive predictive value of 18%, and a negative predictive value of 94% when applied to the entire data set. Of the cytotoxin assays done in this cohort, 39% could have been avoided had this rule been applied.

Conclusions.—Patients without previous antibiotic use and either significant diarrhea or abdominal pain are unlikely to have positive *C. difficile* cytotoxin assay results. Thus, routine cytotoxin testing may not be indicated in such patients.

▶ *Clostridium difficile*–associated diarrhea remains a major challenge for infection control personnel and is an important source of morbidity in hospitalized patients. The use of laboratory tests to detect *C. difficile* cytotoxin in stool has been advocated as a high-yield diagnostic procedure. However, indiscriminate testing is common, and it has been estimated that approximately 40% of cytotoxin assays for *C. difficile* could be eliminated by using selective criteria. This study used a case-control format to develop a model to discriminate patients likely to have positive and negative *C. difficile* toxin tests. Among a population of 480 consecutive patients who underwent *C. difficile* testing, the prevalence of a positive cytotoxin assay was 14%. Independent predictors of a positive toxin test were prior antibiotic therapy, significant diarrhea, and abdominal pain. A simplified a priori rule, defined as positive if both prior antibiotic use and history of significant diarrhea are present, demonstrated a sensitivity, specificity, positive and negative predictive value of 80%, 45%, 18%, and 94%, respectively. Only 6% of those predicted to be toxin-negative actually tested positive. Use of the rule would have eliminated 39% of the cytotoxin assays performed in the study population.

This study provides a rational approach to the use of laboratory resources. Patients without prior antibiotic exposure and either significant diarrhea or abdominal pain are unlikely to have positive *C. difficile* toxin assay results and may not require routine toxin testing. Patients at low risk for *C. difficile* associated diarrhea should be tested only if their condition worsens or if acute diarrhea persists despite supportive measures.

M.A. Pfaller, M.D.

Cryptosporidiosis in Washington State: An Outbreak Associated With Well Water

Dworkin MS, Goldman DP, Wells TG, et al (Ctrs for Disease Control and Prevention, Altanta, Ga; Washington State Dept of Health, Spokane; Madigan Army Med Ctr, Tacoma, Wa)
J Infect Dis 174:1372–1376, 1996   19–3

Background.—In August 1994, routine testing of a rural water system in Walla Walla County, Washington, revealed total coliforms in 2 wells. Although chlorination treatments were performed twice, total and fecal coliforms were identified again 3 weeks later, prompting a boil-water order. Thereafter, many residents called the local health department to report GI illness. An epidemiologic and environmental study was conducted to investigate this apparent outbreak.

Methods and Findings.—Stool specimens from confirmed case patients were found to contain *Cryptosporidium parvum* oocysts. Probable case patients had diarrhea persisting for 5 days or longer. A survey was sent to the 91 households served by the 2 affected wells. Sixty-two responded, for a rate of 68.1%. Fifteen confirmed and 71 probable case patients were identified. Drinking unboiled well water was associated with being a case patient, with a relative risk of 1.84. There was a significant dose–response relationship between water consumption and illness. Water thought to be treated wastewater from a piped irrigation system was found dripping along the outer casing of one well. This casing was rusted extensively. Presumptive *Cryptosporidium* oocysts were identified in the well water and in the treated wastewater.

Conclusions.—This community outbreak was caused by well water contaminated with *C. parvum*. These and previous data demonstrate that both deep and shallow wells may be at risk for contamination because of suboptimal construction or maintenance. Well-water systems should be inspected periodically for structural defects and vulnerability to contamination.

▶ Waterborne disease outbreaks caused by contamination of water supplies with gastrointestinal pathogens such as C. *parvum* are becoming increasingly common. The ability of these coccidian parasites to resist many water-treatment efforts and to contaminate local wells and even municipal water supplies, resulting in symptomatic diarrheal disease, is now well known. This report provides yet another example of how contamination of a water supply with C. *parvum* can result in a community-wide outbreak. In this case, 2 deep, unchlorinated wells became contaminated, presumably from treated wastewater. The attack rate among individuals drinking unboiled water was 50%. Water-quality issues will likely continue to be important as we approach the millennium. The diagnostic laboratory can play an important role in early detection of such outbreaks by performing appropriate diagnostic testing and by promptly reporting clusters of cases to public health officials.

M.A. Pfaller, M.D.

Detection of Extended-Spectrum β-Lactamase (ESBL)-Producing Strains by the Etest ESBL Screen

Cormican MG, Marshall SA, Jones RN (Univ of Iowa, Iowa City)
J Clin Microbiol 34:1880–1884, 1996   19–4

Background.—Recently, emerging resistance to antimicrobial agents has been difficult to recognize in the laboratory, especially by rapid susceptibility test methods. One phenomenon that is difficult to recognize is resistance to plasmid-encoded extended-spectrum β-lactamase (ESBL) enzymes. The detection of ESBL-producing strains by the Etest ESBL screen was reported.

Methods and Findings.—The Etest ESBL screen uses stable gradient technology to assess the MIC of ceftazidime alone, compared with that of ceftazidime with clavulanic acid, to facilitate recognition of strains expressing inhibitable enzymes. Seventeen *Escherichia coli* transconjugants, ESBL-producing strains, were used to identify interpretive criteria. The criteria of ceftazidime MIC reduction by more than 2 $\log_2$ dilution steps in the presence of clavulanic acid defined 92 probable ESBL-positive organisms among the 225 tested strains of *Klebsiella* sp. and *E. coli* with suspicious antibiogram phenotypes. In a subset of 82 clinical strains, the Etest ESBL screen proved more sensitive than the disk approximation test, those values being 100% and 87%, respectively. Also, the Etest ESBL screen was more convenient. The MICs of ciprofloxacin, gentamicin, and tobramycin, at which 50% of isolates are inhibited, were 16- to 128-fold greater for the ESBL screen-positive group of strains than they were for the negative strains. Some strains with increased cephalosporin MICs, which were Etest ESBL screen-negative were also cefoxitin resistant, consistent with a chromosomally mediated AmpC resistance phenotype.

Conclusions.—The Etest ESBL screen test with the ceftazidime substrate appears useful for detecting or validating the presence of enteric bacilli potentially producing this type of β-lactamase. The use of this test may assist in the wider recognition and careful monitoring of this emerging resistance problem among *E. coli* and *Klebsiella* spp.

▶ Antibiotic resistance among bacteria is a problem of worldwide importance. Notably, resistance to contemporary, broad-spectrum β-lactam antibiotics among gram-negative bacilli is increasing and is often mediated by ESBL enzymes. Detection of ESBL-mediated resistance in the clinical laboratory may be quite difficult, and errors in detection may lead to poor clinical outcomes and further spread of resistant organisms within the hospital environment. The development of simple and accurate methods for characterization of ESBL-producing strains is essential. The newly developed Etest

ESBL screen (AB BIODISK, Solna, Sweden) uses stable gradient technology to determine the MIC of ceftazidime alone, compared with the MIC of ceftazidime with clavulanic acid (2 µg/mL) to facilitate recognition of strains expressing ESBL type inhibitable enzymes. This study demonstrates that the Etest ESBL screen was actually more sensitive (100%) than the more cumbersome disk approximation reference test (87%) and more convenient. The availability of this more convenient and sensitive ESBL detection method may contribute to a wider recognition and more careful monitoring of the emerging ESBL-mediated resistance problem among some Entero-bacteriaceae (*E. coli* and *Klebsiella* spp.).

M.A. Pfaller, M.D.

Diagnosis of Vascular Catheter-related Bloodstream Infection: A Meta-analysis

Siegman-Igra Y, Anglim AM, Shapiro DE, et al (Tel-Aviv Univ, Israel; Harvard School of Public Health, Boston; Univ of Virginia, Charlottesville)
J Clin Microbiol 35:928–936, 1997
19–5

Introduction.—During the 1980s, the incidence of primary nosocomial bloodstream infection increased threefold, mostly because of catheter infection. A recent study indicated that the excess hospital cost associated with this was $40,000 per patient. Central venous catheters were associated with more than 90% of catheter-related bloodstream infections, but diagnosing these infections was difficult. To diagnose these infections, 16 methods and 17 variations have been proposed, but it is still unclear which is the most cost-effective and accurate. To determine which method is accurate, a meta-analysis of published studies was conducted.

Methods.—The meta-analysis had 22 studies that evaluated 6 test methods that met the criteria. Pooled sensitivity and specificity and summary receiver-operating characteristic curve analysis were determined. Methods published by the College of American Pathologists were used to estimate the cost for each test. In the cost-per-accurate-test result, costs of catheter replacement and antibiotic therapy for false positive results were included. The 6 methods were qualitative, semiquantitative, and quantitative catheter segment culture; and unpaired qualitative, unpaired quantitative, and paired quantitative blood culture from catheter.

Results.—Largely because of an increase in specificity, the accuracy increased in receiver-operating characteristic analysis for catheter segment cultures with increasing quantitation. The quantitative catheter segment culture resulted in the highest Youden index, with a mean of 0.85. This was the only method that had a pooled specificity and sensitivity above 90%. There was no statistically significant trend toward increased accuracy in the blood culture methods. The lowest cost-per-accurate-test result was the unpaired quantitative catheter blood culture, but it had only a 78% sensitivity.

Conclusions.—For catheter segment culture, quantitative culture was the most accurate method, and may be the most optimal test, for catheters in place less than 2 weeks. The single most cost-effective test was the unpaired quantitative catheter blood culture, particularly for long-term catheters.

▶ Catheter-related bloodstream infections are important causes of morbidity, mortality, and excess hospital costs. Numerous approaches to the laboratory diagnosis of catheter-related bloodstream infections have been published, but there has been no consensus on the optimal method in sensitivity, specificity, and cost-effectiveness.

Siegman-Igra and colleagues have attempted to address this issue by performing a meta-analysis of published studies on the accuracy of methods for diagnosing catheter-related bloodstream infections. Twenty-two studies evaluating 6 test methods met inclusion criteria for the meta-analysis. The results of the meta-analysis confirmed the superiority of quantitative techniques for catheter segment culture. Quantitative catheter segment culture was the most accurate method, being the only one with pooled sensitivity and specificity above 90%.

The quantitative catheter segment culture may be the optimal test for epidemiologic studies involving catheters in place for less than 2 weeks. Unfortunately, this test requires removal of the catheter and thus is of no use in deciding prospectively whether the catheter can remain in place or must be removed from a potentially infected patient. The quantitative blood culture aspirated from the catheter provides prospective information and was the most cost-effective test ($198.18 per accurate result); however, the sensitivity of quantitative blood cultures from catheters was low (78%), especially for short-term catheters.

M.A. Pfaller, M.D.

Evaluation of Automated COBAS AMPLICOR PCR System for Detection of Several Infectious Agents and Its Impact on Laboratory Management
Jungkind D, DiRenzo S, Beavis KG, et al (Thomas Jefferson Univ, Philadelphia)
J Clin Microbiol 34:2778–2783, 1996   19–6

Introduction.—In much the same way that labor-intensive sections of the clinical chemistry laboratory were automated during the past 3 decades, polymerase chain reaction (PCR) holds the potential for allowing automation of parts of the clinical microbiology laboratory. The first-generation microwell plate assays were compared with an automated COBAS AMPLICOR (CA) PCR system (Roche Diagnostic Systems, Branchburg, NJ). Amplifying target DNA, the CA system captures the biotinylated amplification products with magnetic particles coated with specific oligonucleotide probes and detects the bound products colorimetrically. With emphasis on determining the degree of concordance between the microwell plate assay and the CA assay systems when tested with separate aliquots from clinical samples, the study was designed as a preclinical trial.

Methods.—The reference method was the Roche AMPLICOR microwell plate PCR. In comparing *Mycobacterium tuberculosis*, there were 230 samples, including 20 culture-positive samples. The comparison of hepatitis C virus involved 214 samples, including 60 positive samples. For *Chlamydia trachomatis* and *Neisseria gonorrhoeae*, there were 199 cervical specimens, including 10 *C. trachomatis* and 3 *N. gonorrhoeae* culture-positive samples. The College of American Pathologists workload recording method was used to determine the total hands-on time.

Results.—The correlation of the results of CA tests with those of microwell plate tests was 100% for *Mycobacterium tuberculosis*, 100% for hepatitis C virus, and 100% for *C. trachomatis*, *N. gonorrhoeae*, and the internal control. Overall, the agreement was 100% for all 832 comparisons with the PCR methods. There was no carryover cross-contamination of negative samples after spiking alternating amplification tubes in the CA system with 10 to 14 copies of the *Chlamydia* amplicon per milliliter. For *Mycobacterium tuberculosis*, the total hands-on time to produce CA PCR results was 4.4 minutes; for hepatitis C virus, it was 7.9 minutes; and for *Chlamydia* plus gonorrhea and an internal control, it was 3.3 minutes.

Conclusions.—True PCR automation can be brought to laboratories with the CA system. The CA system supports both MultiPlex amplification and sequential algorithm detection of analytes, provides labor savings, and provides accuracy of automated results.

▶ A number of commercially available PCR-based methods are now commonly used in the clinical laboratory for the detection of infectious agents. The PCR kits developed by Roche Diagnostic Systems include tests for detection of *M. tuberculosis*, *C. trachomatis*, *N. gonorrhoeae*, and hepatitis C virus. Although kits for each of these infectious agents have been useful as manual stand-alone assays, there clearly is a role for automation of such assays, particularly in high-volume laboratories.

The investigators in this article describe the first evaluation of an automated COBAS AMPLICOR (CA) PCR System that will provide complete automation of the amplification and detection steps required to detect the 4 infectious agents noted above. The authors compared the CA system to the more manual microwell plate assays available for each agent. They found essentially complete concordance between the manual microwell plate assay and the CA system for all infectious agents tested. Furthermore, they found that the automated CA system offered standardized testing in a highly efficient manner. The CA system provides accurate automated results, labor savings, and containment of the amplification and detection components of PCR, and it supports both Multiplex amplification (more than 1 agent detected simultaneously in a single specimen) and sequential algorithm detection of analytes. Further development of this prototype automated PCR system will be of great value to clinical laboratories.

M.A. Pfaller, M.D.

Fluconazole and Amphotericin B Antifungal Susceptibility Testing by National Commitee for Clinical Laboratory Standards Broth Macrodilution Method Compared With E-test and Semiautomated Broth Microdilution Test

Eldere JV, Joosten L, Verhaeghe A, et al (Katholieke Universiteit Leuven, Belgium)
J Clin Microbiol 34:842–847, 1996   19–7

Introduction.—The frequency and clinical importance of invasive fungal infections are increasing, particularly to the growing group of immunocompromised patients. To guide antifungal therapy and monitor local resistance patterns, there is a need for a precise, clinically relevant easy-to-perform in vitro susceptibility testing method. For the determination of MIC end points for amphotericin B and fluconazole against *Candida* species, a comparison was made between the National Committee for Clinical Laboratory Standards (NCCLS) macrodilution method, which is labor-intensive and time-consuming, with the E-test and with the new broth microdilution method, which uses a computer-controlled dispenser-shaker-incubator-turbidometric reader to reduce preparation time and culture medium volume needed. The broth microdilution and E-test methods were evaluated as possible alternatives for routine fungal susceptibility testing.

Methods.—The 3 test methods were used with 68 clinical *Candida* species isolates to compare fluconazole and amphotericin B susceptibility testing. The E-test is an agar diffusion method. The NCCLS method is a broth macrodilution method. The newer method is an in-house prepared semi-automated broth microdilution method based on the Bioscreen turbidometer. Precise and objective determination of end points was permitted with continuous measurement of the growth of the yeasts by the Bioscreen automatic turbidometer in the microdilution method. For the microdilution method and the E-test, MIC end points were read after 24 hours.

Results.—In 89% of the tests, amphotericin B susceptibility testing had comparable results with the NCCLS method and the E-test. In these 2 methods, the end points were identical or differed by no more than 2 twofold dilutions. There was a score of 97% in comparable results with the broth microdilution test and the NCCLS tests. There were 90% comparable results with the E-test and broth microdilution tests. With the NCCLS and the E-tests, there was a 96% score in comparable results with fluconazole susceptibility testing, 98.5% comparable results with the E-test and microdilution method, and 100% comparable results with the microdilution methods and the NCCLS method.

Conclusions.—For routine susceptibility testing of *Candida* species with fluconazole and amphotericin B, valuable alternatives to the more time-consuming NCCLS method are the E-test and the Bioscreen microdilution method.

▶ The development of a standardized reference broth dilution susceptibility testing method for in vitro testing of yeast isolates has provided a touchstone for the development of alternative testing methods. There is a need for a precise, clinically relevant, and convenient antifungal susceptibility testing method for use in the clinical laboratory. Since the publication of the NCCLS reference method, a number of alternative testing methods have been described. In the study of van Eldere et al., the authors provided comparative data with the NCCLS reference method, the agar-based E-test, and a microdilution modification of the reference method. In vitro testing of amphotericin B and fluconazole produced comparable MIC values with all 3 test methods. This study provides further confirmation that broth microdilution and E-test methods are valuable alternatives to the NCCLS reference method for susceptibility testing of *Candida* species against fluconazole and amphotericin B.

M.A. Pfaller, M.D.

Misdiagnosis of Multidrug-resistant Tuberculosis Possibly Due to Laboratory-related Errors

Nitta AT, Davidson PT, de Koning ML; et al (Tuberculosis Control, Los Angeles; Univ of California, Los Angeles; Univ of Southern California, Los Angeles)
JAMA 276:1980–1983, 1996   19–8

Background.—Although the need for rapid identification and susceptibility testing of *Mycobacterium tuberculosis* complex organisms is well recognized, definitions, methods and reporting procedures have not been standardized. Because of the serious clinical and public health consequences of the diagnosis of multidrug-resistant tuberculosis (MDRTB), this diagnosis was examined in a series of 70 consecutive patients identified by Tuberculosis Control in Los Angeles.

Methods.—Between August 1993 and August 1994, detailed clinical consultation was performed for 70 patients found to have MDRTB, defined as culture-confirmed tuberculosis with in vitro resistance to isoniazid and rifampicin. The MDRTB unit within Tuberculosis Control reviewed medical records and all available culture and susceptibility reports for these patients. Cases were reviewed monthly and presented to a group of tuberculosis experts when any discrepancies were detected.

Results.—Among the 70 patients in this series, pulmonary MDRTB was misdiagnosed in 9. The reasons for the incorrect diagnosis were as follows: growth of MDRTB from an old tuberculosis lesion in 1 patient, documented contamination with *Mycobacterium avium* complex in 1 patient, suspected cross-contamination in 1 patient, suspected mislabeling in 1 patient, successful treatment after report of resistance in 4 patients, discrepant susceptibility results in further samples in 2 patients, and no clinical evidence of tuberculosis in 3 patients.

Conclusions.—Because the diagnosis of MDRTB has important clinical and public health consequences, standardization and quality control of mycobacterial methods are essential. Susceptibility results without clinical correlation should not be considered sufficient to diagnose MDRTB.

▶ Recent outbreaks of MDRTB have emphasized the need for rapid detection, identification, and susceptibility testing of *M. tuberculosis* complex organisms. Unfortunately, the methods of identification, concentrations of drugs used in susceptibility testing, culture media used in culture and susceptibility testing work, and reporting formats for transmitting results from laboratory to clinician are not standardized. Lack of standardization of test procedures in the laboratory may lead to errors of omission or commission, with resultant misdiagnosis of infectious disease processes. In this study, misdiagnosis of MDRTB occurred in 9 of 70 cases (13%) possibly as a result of laboratory-related errors. These errors included possible cross-contamination of specimens (4 patients), erroneous or nonreproducible susceptibility test results (4 patients), and specimen mislabeling (1 patient).

Factors that may contribute to such errors include inattention to accurate labeling of specimens, use of common dispensers of reagents (increasing risk of cross-contamination), failure to ensure pure cultures (susceptible *M. tuberculosis* complex may be mixed with resistant nontuberculosis mycobacteria), staff shortages relative to the workloads, lack of experience, and, importantly, failure of the clinician to discuss incongruent results with laboratory staff. Although improved standardization and quality control of laboratory methods will go a long way toward minimizing such errors, careful clinical correlation of laboratory data cannot be overemphasized. The diagnosis of MDRTB should be questioned if the patient has no risk factors and the clinical course is not compatible with the diagnosis.

M.A. Pfaller, M.D.

Use of Gen-Probe AccuProbe Group B Streptococcus Test to Detect Group B Streptococci in Broth Cultures of Vaginal-Anorectal Specimens From Pregnant Women: Comparison With Traditional Culture Method
Bourbeau PP, Heiter BJ, Figdore M (Geisinger Med Ctr, Danville, Pa)
J Clin Microbiol 35:144–147, 1997   19–9

Background.—Group B streptococci (GBS) are the major cause of infectious morbidity and mortality in American neonates. Early-onset GBS disease is caused by GBS transmission from the maternal anogenital region to the neonate. The standard method of detecting maternal GBS colonization is labor-intensive and involves primary incubation in selective broth followed by subculture to plated media with identification of GBS. In this study, this rigorous culture method was compared with a more rapid commercially produced GBS genetic probe, the AccuProbe GBS Culture Identification Test (GPGB).

Methods.—Anogenital specimens were obtained from women receiving prenatal care at Geisinger primary care sites. One swab was used to inoculate 1 trypticase soy agar plate containing 5% sheep blood and 1 Columbia agar plate containing sheep blood, nalidixic acid, and colistin. This swab was also immersed in a tube of Todd-Hewitt broth with nalidixic acid and colistin. After overnight incubation, the plates were examined. If results were negative, the broth was subcultured. The second test swab was refrigerated and batch tested within 72 hours with the GPGB after culture in Todd-Hewitt broth with nalidixic acid and colistin broth.

Results.—There were 502 samples tested in this study. Both the standard culture method and GPGB detected 90 or 95 GBS-positive specimens. There were 2 false-positive GPGB results. Estimated costs were $3.68 for a standard negative culture and $5.41 for a standard positive culture. Cost for the GPGB was $5.16 per test.

Conclusions.—In a large series of tests for GBS, the GPGB performed as well as the standard culture method for the identification of GBS. The time to completion of this test could be as much as 48 hours shorter than that of the culture method. Overall costs are slightly higher for the GPGB, but its advantages include lower labor costs, incremental savings at high test volumes, and the ability to interface with laboratory computer systems.

▶ Group B streptococcal disease in neonates is an important and potentially preventable cause of morbidity and mortality. Recommended strategies for prevention of GBS disease have been outlined in a recent consensus statement and include efforts to detect maternal vaginal and anorectal colonization by culturing all pregnant women at 35 to 37 weeks of gestation. Recommended culture methods include the use of a selective enrichment broth followed by subculture to plated media with subsequent identification of GBS from the subculture-plated media. An alternative approach to subculture would be the use of a specific nucleic acid probe to identify GBS directly in the broth media. This approach would provide specific results as much as 48 hours sooner than the more labor-intensive subculture method. In a comparative study of 502 specimens, broth cultures were performed and GBS were identified either by the traditional subculture approach or by testing the broth directly with the GPGB. The method incorporating the GPGB was equivalent in sensitivity to the standard culture method. Depending on the frequency with which the GPGB was performed in the laboratory (batch testing is preferred), the time for test completion for the GPGB could be as much as 48 hours shorter than that of culture. Although the overall costs for the GPGB method are slightly higher, the GPGB has lower labor costs, offers the potential for automated test reading, and offers incremental savings at higher test volumes.

M.A. Pfaller, M.D.

Reliability of Nucleic Acid Amplification for Detection of *Myobacterium tuberculosis*: An International Collaborative Quality Control Study Among 30 Laboratories

Noordhoek GT, van Embden JDA, Kolk AH (Public Health Laboratory, Leeuwarden, The Netherlands; Natl Inst for Public Health and Environmental Protection, Bilthoven, The Netherlands; Royal Tropical Inst, Amsterdam)
J Clin Microbiol 34:2522–2525, 1996   19–10

Background.—Polymerase chain reaction and other nucleic acid amplification techniques for detection of *Mycobacterium tuberculosis* are becoming common laboratory tools. The sensitivity and specificity of these tests have been questioned, and there are no standardized reagents for quality control procedures.

Methods.—An interlaboratory study was conducted of 30 laboratories in 18 countries. Blinded panels of 20 sputum samples were prepared. The samples contained 0, 100, or 1,000 mycobacterial cells. Each laboratory was to detect *M. tuberculosis* by their routine method of nucleic acid amplification.

Results.—The presence or absence of mycobacterial DNA in all 20 specimens was detected by only 5 laboratories. Seven laboratories correctly detected DNA in all positive samples and 13 laboratories correctly detected DNA in all negative samples. Lack of specificity was a greater problem than lack of sensitivity. Reliability was not associated with any particular method of nucleic acid amplification.

Discussion.—Nucleic acid amplification assays for detecting *M. tuberculosis* in clinical samples are unreliable and many laboratories do not have adequate quality controls. There is a need for standardized laboratory procedures and reference reagents to monitor the whole assay, including pretreatment of samples. Further steps to ensure quality control of nucleic acid amplification techniques for detecting *M. tuberculosis* were described in the paper.

▶ Rapid detection of *M. tuberculosis* in clinical specimens has been greatly facilitated by the development of nucleic acid amplification techniques. The commercial availability of at least 2 amplification-based methods has resulted in the use of these approaches in the clinical diagnostic laboratory. However, the sensitivity and specificity of these tests may be questioned, and no standardized reagents for quality control assessment are available.

In this study, the authors conducted a proficiency survey of 30 laboratories in 18 countries to assess the performance of amplification tests for routine diagnosis of tuberculosis. Blinded panels of 20 sputum samples containing varying numbers of mycobacterial cells were sent to each laboratory. Each laboratory was asked to detect *M. tuberculosis* by their routine method of nucleic acid amplification.

Only 5 laboratories (17%) correctly detected the presence or absence of mycobacterial DNA in all 20 samples. In the remaining laboratories, both false positive and false negative results were reported. Errors were observed in laboratories using commercial kits as well as "home brew" amplification methods. The results show that nucleic acid amplification methods for the detection of *M. tuberculosis* may be unreliable. The outcome of the study underscores the need for reference reagents and standardized operating procedures that would enable experienced personnel to perform reliable quality control assessment of nucleic acid amplification methods.

M.A. Pfaller, M.D.

Multiplex PCR for Diagnosis of AIDS-related Central Nervous System Lymphoma and Toxoplasmosis

Roberts TC, Storch GA (Washington Univ, St Louis)
J Clin Microbiol 35:268–269, 1997   19–11

Introduction.—The leading causes of focal brain disease in patients with advanced AIDS are *Toxoplasma* encephalitis and Epstein-Barr virus (EBV)–associated primary central nervous system lymphoma (P-CNSL). It is difficult to distinguish between these 2 entities. Reported is a novel multiplex polymerase chain reaction (PCR) assay capable of detecting EBV and *T. gondii* DNA simultaneously.

Methods.—Cerebrospinal fluid (CSF) samples from 52 patients with advanced AIDS were tested. All CSF samples were analyzed with 3 different PCR assays: 1 for *T. gondii* DNA alone, 1 for EBV DNA alone, and the multiplex for *T. gondii* and EBV together.

Results.—The multiplex assay for *T. gondii* matched those of the separate *T. gondii* assay in all except 1 sample in a patient with presumed toxoplasmosis who was positive by the multiplex assay and negative for the *T. gondii* assay. The multiplex assay for EBV matched except for 3 specimens from patients with confirmed P-CNSL. These were negative by the multiplex assay, but positive by the separate EBV assay.

Conclusion.—The multiplex PCR assay may be helpful in making a specific diagnosis in AIDS patients with intracranial mass lesions.

▶ Among patients with advanced AIDS, *Toxoplasma* encephalitis and Epstein-Barr virus (EBV)-associated primary central nervous system lymphoma (P-CNSL) are the leading causes of focal brain disease. Distinguishing between these two entities is important for therapy and may not be possible using non-invasive clinical and radiographic approaches. In the present study, the authors describe a novel multiplex PCR method that allows simultaneous detection of both *T. gondii* and EBV DNA in cerebrospinal fluid (CSF). CSF samples from 52 AIDS patients (8 with *Toxoplasma* encephalitis and 14 with P-CNSL) were analyzed. The nested multiplex PCR assay detected *T. gondii* DNA in 8 of 8 patients with *Toxoplasma* encephalitis and EBV DNA in 9 of 14 patients with P-CNSL. The availability of assays capable of detecting multiple infectious agents that may cause similar or identical clinical syndromes is highly desirable. This study demonstrates the feasibility of such an approach and suggests that it should be useful in conjunction with other clinical data in selecting effective therapy.

M.A. Pfaller, M.D.

Pilot Studies for Proficiency Testing Using Fluorescence In Situ Hybridization With Chromosome-specific DNA Probes: A College of American Pathologists/American College of Medical Genetics Program
Dewald GW, Brothman AR, Butler MG, et al (Mayo Clinic, Rochester, Minn; Univ of Utah, Salt Lake City; Vanderbilt Univ, Nashville, Tenn; et al)
Arch Pathol Lab Med 121:359–367, 1997   19–12

Introduction.—Fluorescence in situ hybridization (FISH) with chromosome-specific probes is being used with increasing frequency for certain congenital and neoplastic disorders. Three pilot studies were designed to determine if proficiency testing is possible for FISH. Nineteen representative laboratory directors were invited to participate in each pilot study. Reported is data from these proficiency tests.

Findings.—Fixed cells or microscope slides with fixed cells were prepared using standard cytogenetic methods. The first pilot used probes for X and Y chromosomes to evaluate metaphase spreads and interphase nuclei. The second pilot used probes for *bcr* and *abl* to detect *bcr/abl* fusion in interphase nuclei in chronic myelogenous leukemia. The third pilot used a D22S75 probe to detect microdeletions in metaphase spreads in a patient with velocardiofacial syndrome. Nine of 19 cytogenetic laboratories participated in all 3 pilot studies. Proficiency testing for FISH was possible in the 3 pilot studies using either metaphase or interphase preparations. Both microscope slides and fixed cell pellets were acceptable.

Conclusion.—Proficiency testing for FISH with chromosome-specific DNA probes is feasible and can be accomplished at a relatively low cost. It can produce objective data with high concordance among laboratories.

▶ Fluorescence in situ hybridization (FISH) using chromosome-specific DNA probes is an important adjunct to standard cytogenetics and is useful for classifying certain congenital and cytogenetic disorders. As newer testing methods become part of routine clinical practice, the need for proficiency testing becomes acute. The development of useful proficiency surveys is not a simple matter and as such requires considerable planning and effort. The paper by Dewald et al. describes initial efforts and pilot studies for proficiency testing using FISH. The results of these studies indicate that such proficiency testing is feasible and necessary. The authors describe a system that can be expanded to larger numbers of laboratories and present data suggesting that there is clearly a need for such a program to aid in the development of testing standards and guidelines. Although most of the laboratories participating in these pilot studies were quite experienced in the use of FISH, there were notable differences in the application and interpretation of the results of this technique. Thus proficiency testing for FISH with chromosome-specific DNA probes is attainable and can be done at relatively low cost. The development of such a proficiency testing program is important for the incorporation of FISH into clinical practice.

M.A. Pfaller, M.D.

Rapid Prediction of Rifampin Susceptibility of *Mycobacterium Tuberculosis*

Ohno H, Koga H, Kuroita T, et al (Nagasaki Univ, Japan; Toyobo Gene Analysis Co Ltd, Tsuruga, Japan)
Am J Respir Crit Care Med 155:2057–2063, 1997   19–13

Background.—Although rifampin is considered effective in the treatment of tuberculosis, the incidence of infection with drug-resistant *Micobacterium tuberculosis* in patients with AIDS is increasing. Moreover, *M. tuberculosis* strains resistant to rifampin only have been reported. The relationship between rifampin susceptibility and amino acid substitution in the *rpoB* gene of *M. tuberculosis* and the value of *rpoB* gene sequencing in the rapid prediction of rifampin susceptibility of *M. tuberculosis* in clinical specimens were studied.

Methods and Findings.—Rifampin-resistant *M. tuberculosis* strains were collected from geographically different regions of Japan. Seventy-six genetic alterations in the 69-bp core region of *rpoB* gene were identified in 74 of 130 *M. tuberculosis* strains. The correlation between the minimum inhibitory concentrations (MICs) of rifampin and amino acid substitutions in the 69-bp core region of *rpoB* gene was determined. All 43 strains containing amino acid substitution with Leu or Trp in codon 531 showed rifampin-resistant phenotypes, with MICs of 64 µg/mL or greater. By contrast, the level of rifampin susceptibility varied among strains containing amino acid substitutions in codon 516 or 526. In a clinical study, 26 sputum samples, 2 gastric lavages, and 1 synovial fluid sample were obtained from patients with tuberculosis. The rifampin susceptibility predicted by direct *rpoB* sequencing was compatible with the findings of the rifampin-susceptibility test and the MICs of rifampin against isolated organisms.

Conclusion.—Alterations in the 69-bp region of *rpoB* gene were detected in 95% of these rifampin-resistant *M. tuberculosis* strains. Screening for such alterations may provide an accurate, rapid prediction of rifampin-resistant *M. tuberculosis*.

▶ The application of molecular methods to the detection and characterization of microorganisms promises to revolutionize clinical microbiology. Although rapid and sensitive amplification-based methods have been shown to be extremely useful in detecting the presence of pathogenic organisms in clinical specimens, the need to determine the susceptibility of the infecting organism to antimicrobial agents is considered necessary for optimal therapy. Recent advances in molecular biology have revealed some of the genetic mechanisms of drug resistance of organisms such as *M. tuberculosis*. Detection of point mutations in the core region of the *rpoB* gene, which encodes the β subunit of RNA polymerase, has been shown to predict resistance of *M. tuberculosis* to rifampin.

In this paper, the authors have developed a polymerase chain reaction (PCR)-based approach that allows both detection of *M. tuberculosis* and prediction of rifampin susceptibility directly in clinical specimens. The technique uses PCR amplification of the *rpoB* gene followed by direct sequencing to detect point mutations within the 69-bp core region. The rifampin susceptibility predicted by direct *rpoB* sequencing was satisfactorily compatible with the results of in vitro susceptibility testing and could be completed within 3 to 5 days, as opposed to 30 to 90 days for the phenotypic test. The association of rifampin resistance with multidrug resistance in *M. tuberculosis* makes this direct approach even more attractive. These results provide an example of the use of molecular biology to both diagnose and predict response to therapy and are a model for future applications of molecular biology to infectious diseases.

M.A. Pfaller, M.D.

Viral Load and Disease Progression in Infants Infected With Human Immunodeficiency Virus Type 1

Shearer WT, for the Women and Infants Transmission Study Group (Baylor College of Medicine, Houston; et al)
N Engl J Med 336:1337–1342, 1997   19–14

Introduction.—Measurement of the viral load may be important in understanding the pathogenesis of perinatally acquired HIV type I (HIV-1) infection and in managing the infection. Prospective data from the Women and Infants Transmission Study were used to evaluate the relationship between viral load and clinical outcome in infants and children with HIV-1 infection.

Methods.—Plasma samples were collected from 106 infants with HIV infection at birth; at 1, 2, 6, 9, 12, 15, and 18 months; then every 6 months. Reverse-transcription polymerase chain reaction was used to assay HIV-1 RNA. Only 21% of the mothers of these infants received treatment with zidovudine while pregnant.

Results.—The median RNA load was under the cutoff level at birth (greater than 400), then rose to 318,000 and 256,000 copies per mL at 1 and 2 months, respectively. There was a gradual decline to a median of 34,000 copies per mL at 24 months. Infants with early HIV-1 infection (in utero transmission) had significantly higher median HIV-1 RNA values in the early months of life, compared with infants with late infection (peripartum transmission). Infants who had a first positive HIV-1 culture within 48 months of birth had significantly higher HIV-1 RNA levels during the first 2 months of life, compared with those with a first positive culture 7 or more days after birth. Infants with rapidly progressing disease had significantly higher peak HIV-1 RNA levels during the first 2 months of life and a significantly higher geometric mean value during the first year of life, compared with infants without rapid disease progression.

Conclusion.—Infants infected perinatally had high HIV-1 RNA levels that gradually declined in the first 2 years of life. Infants with high viral loads in the first months of life were at increased risk of rapidly progressing disease. Such infants may need early treatment with antiretroviral agents.

▶ Relatively little is known of the progression of HIV-1 infection in perinatally infected infants. The availability of viral load determinations using quantitative polymerase chain reaction (PCR) provides a unique opportunity to conduct studies designed to understand the dynamics of HIV-1 infection and its relationship to disease progression.

In this study, serial plasma samples were obtained from 106 HIV-infected infants and analyzed for HIV viral load by PCR. Plasma HIV-1 RNA levels peaked at 1–2 months of age and then slowly fell over the first 24 months of life. Infants with early infection (positive culture within the first 48 hours of life) had higher peak RNA levels than those with late infection (positive culture at 7 days or more after birth). Infants with progressive disease had both higher peak levels of RNA and higher mean levels during the first year of life. Infants with very high viral loads during the first months of life are at increased risk of rapid progression of disease, which suggests that early treatment with antiretroviral agents may be indicated.

M.A. Pfaller, M.D.

20 Molecular Pathology

Association of Plasma Human Immunodeficiency Virus Type 1 RNA Level With Risk of Clinical Progression in Patients With Advanced Infection
Coombs RW, for the AIDS Clinical Trials Group (ACTG) 116B/117 Study Team and the ACTG Virology Committee Resistance and HIV-1 RNA Working Groups (Univ of Washington, Seattle; et al)
J Infect Dis 174:704–712, 1996   20–1

Background.—Laboratory markers of HIV-1 replication are needed urgently to assess the efficacy of antiretroviral drug treatments. The value of plasma HIV-1 RNA levels as a surrogate marker for disease progression was determined in a clinical trial of advanced HIV-1 infection.

Methods.—A subset of 913 subjects were studied. They had been previously receiving at least 16 weeks of zidovudine treatment in AIDS Clinical Trials Group protocol 116B/117, and their status was followed for a mean of 48 weeks. In that protocol, disease progression was defined as a new AIDS event or death. At baseline, 100 of these patients had plasma available for HIV-1 RNA analysis. At week 4, 71 patients had plasma available for analysis, and at week 24, 49 patients had plasma available for analysis.

Findings.—Baseline HIV-1 RNA levels independently predicted disease progression, with a relative hazard of 1.26 for each doubling of HIV-1 RNA level after adjustment for the following: week 4 changes in HIV-1 RNA levels, baseline CD4 cell counts, syncytium-inducing phenotype, clinical status at study entry, and treatment randomization. During the study, a 50% decrease in HIV-1 RNA level was correlated with a 27% reduction in the adjusted risk of disease progression.

Conclusions.—Baseline levels of HIV-1 replication, determined by the plasma-associated HIV-1 RNA level, are independently associated with the risk of disease progression in HIV-infected patients. It may be possible to use HIV-1 RNA as a predictor for end points in clinical trials and practice.

▶ The use of quantitative nucleic acid amplification assays to estimate viral load in the blood of HIV-infected patients is becoming a standard means of assessing disease progression and response to antiviral therapy. In this study, the authors evaluated the HIV RNA level in plasma as a surrogate marker for disease progression in a clinical trial of advanced HIV infection. Baseline HIV RNA level was an independent predictor of disease progression. The change in plasma HIV RNA observed in association with antiretroviral therapy approached statistical significance as an independent predictor for the risk of disease progression. Thus, the quantitative assessment of plasma HIV RNA using polymerase chain reaction or other amplification-based nucleic acid detection methods promises to be useful in both clinical trials and practice.

M.A. Pfaller, M.D.

Antenatal Screening for Cystic Fibrosis
Cuckle H, Quirke P, Sehmi I, et al (Univ of Leeds, England; Leeds Gen Infirmary, England)
Br J Obstet Gynaecol 103:795–799, 1996   20–2

Background.—Cystic fibrosis (CF) is the most common autosomal recessive disorder in the United Kingdom. Antenatal screening appears to be the best way to identify carrier couples. The practicality of implementing such screening in Yorkshire was investigated.

Methods.—Antenatal screening at 2 hospitals and 8 general practices was offered to all pregnant Yorkshire residents. Testing for the ΔF508 mutation, which accounts for about 85% of the carriers in Yorkshire, was performed. The reproductive partners of women found to be cystic fibrosis carriers were then tested.

Findings.—A total of 3,773 women (62% of the eligible population) participated in the screening. The uptake rates for the 2 hospitals were 78% and 60%, respectively, and for the general practices, 67%. A total of 130 (3.4%) women were found to be carriers. Further analysis identified 3 carrier couples. Median time to laboratory results was 5 days. The mean cost was £16.

Conclusions.—Antenatal screening for cystic fibrosis poses no practical difficulties. Introducing it as a routine practice in Yorkshire is feasible.

▶ Antenatal screening for genetic diseases appears to be an efficient way of identifying carrier couples who can then be offered invasive diagnostic procedures and, where appropriate, selective termination of pregnancy. In screening for CF carriers, testing for the ΔF508 mutation and the next 3 most common mutations will identify 80% to 90% of carriers. This article describes a prospective study in which all pregnant women were offered testing for the ΔF508 mutation, which accounts for about 85% of carriers in Yorkshire. In screening 3,773 women, investigators found 130 (3.4%) carriers and identified 3 carrier couples. The median time interval for the laboratory to produce a result was 5 days. The cost of performing CF screening was estimated to be higher than that of established antenatal screening services such as Down's syndrome screening. It appears that antenatal screening for CF would be feasible to introduce into routine practice.

M.A. Pfaller, M.D.

Genetic Testing Is Important in Families With a History Suggestive of Hereditary Non-polyposis Colorectal Cancer Even if the Amsterdam Criteria Are Not Fulfilled
Beck NE, Tomlinson IPM, Homfray T, et al (John Radcliffe Hosp, Oxford, England; St Mark's and Northwick Park Hosps Trust, Harrow, England)
Br J Surg 84:233–237, 1997
20–3

Introduction.—The most common form of inherited colorectal cancer is hereditary nonpolyposis colorectal cancer (HNPCC), an autosomal dominant disorder. Characterized by a familial aggregation of early-onset colorectal and uterine cancer and an increased incidence of gastric, pancreatic, ovarian, and upper urinary tract malignancies, it accounts for up to 6% of all cases of colorectal cancer. Up to 90% of gene mutations in these families are found in *hMSH2* and *hMLH1*; however, screening for these genes is time-consuming and expensive. At the second meeting of the International Collaborative Group on HNPCC in Amsterdam in 1990, minimum criteria were agreed on, but they have been criticized because they do not take into account family members with extracolonic cancers, which may lead to an underdiagnosis of this disease.

Methods.—In 10 families who had pedigrees with features suggestive of HNPCC in which the Amsterdam criteria were not satisfied, germline mutations were sought in the *hMSH2* and *hMLH1* genes. The Amsterdam criteria are: there should be at least 3 family members with colorectal cancer with 1 a first-degree relative of the other 2; at least 2 generations should be affected; and at least 1 individual is younger than 50 years at time of diagnosis. Germline mutations in the 2 genes were sought using the technique of single-strand conformational polymorphism analysis.

Results.—In 6 families, mutations were identified and all were present as a heterozygote with the wild-type allele. There were 3 mutations in each gene: 3 missense, 1 nonsense, 1 frameshift, and 1 putative splice-site mutation.

Conclusions.—Even if the Amsterdam criteria are not fulfilled, all families with a pedigree suggestive of HNPCC should be referred to a geneticist. Targeted surveillance and early surgical intervention that could be curative are possible with a knowledge of the gene carrier status.

► Hereditary nonpolyposis colorectal cancer is an autosomal dominant disorder characterized by a familial aggregation of early-onset colorectal and uterine cancer and an increased incidence of gastric, pancreatic, ovarian, and upper urinary tract malignancies. Germline mutation of 1 of the genes responsible for repairing base-pair mismatches in newly synthesized DNA has been identified as the genetic basis for this disease. The Amsterdam criteria were established to facilitate the collection of uniform data about HNPCC. It is now clear that families that do not fulfill the Amsterdam criteria but with a pedigree suggestive of HNPCC may have germline mutations indicating a predisposition toward malignancies.

In this study, the authors used polymerase chain reaction followed by single-strand conformational polymorphism analysis to detect germline mutations in the known mismatch repair genes *hMSH2* and *hMLH1*. Defects in these genes have been shown to account for more than 90% of mutations found in families with HNPCC. Germline mutations were detected in the mismatch repair genes in 6 of 10 HNPCC families studied. None of these families fulfilled the Amsterdam criteria. This study shows that families with a pedigree suggestive of HNPCC should be referred to a geneticist even if the Amsterdam criteria are not fulfilled. A full family history can then be taken and, if appropriate, genetic testing can be offered. A knowledge of the gene carrier status will enable targeted surveillance and the possibility of early surgical intervention that may be curative.

M.A. Pfaller, M.D.

Prenatal Diagnosis of Cystic Fibrosis in a Highly Heterogeneous Population

Casals T, Gimenez J, Ramos MD, et al (Hosp Duran i Reynals, Barcelona)
Prenat Diagn 16:215–222, 1996   20–4

Background.—Cystic fibrosis (CF) is the most common autosomal recessive disease among whites. The CF gene, the CF transmembrane conductance regulator (CFTR), was cloned in 1989 and the most common mutation, ΔF5087, has been identified. More than 500 other CF mutations have been identified. The Spanish CF population is extremely heterogeneous, with more than 73 identified CF mutations. Molecular diagnosis of CF by mutational detection is difficult in the Spanish population. This report describes the method used to perform prenatal diagnoses for Spanish families with CF.

Methods.—Beginning in 1990, 81 prenatal CF diagnoses were performed for 74 couples. The gestational age ranged from 10 to 20 weeks. To perform the diagnosis, a flexible scheme was adopted. It was based on the couple's risk, the availability of a previous genetic study, the information from mutations and polymorphisms, the gestational age, and the availability of genetic material from a family member with CF.

Results.—Among the 81 cases, direct genetic analysis was possible in 36. Polymorphic markers were also employed in 24 cases, microvillar enzymatic analysis was also used in 5 cases, and in 16 cases only indirect analysis was possible. Nine different mutations, including the most common CF mutation, were detected in families in this series, and 10 more were detected after prenatal diagnosis.

Conclusions.—The Spanish population is extremely heterogeneous for CF mutations, which makes direct genetic analysis for prenatal diagnosis difficult. The strategy used in this report involves both direct and indirect methods. The first step is to analyze directly for the 2 most common mutations and to analyze indirectly for the intragenic markers IVS8CA, IVS17BTA, and IVS17BCA. If necessary, the patient is screened for mutations associated with the CFTR microsatellite haplotypes. The final step, if the first 2 steps are insufficient, is a specific search for unknown mutations. This diagnostic strategy permits rapid, accurate, and reliable prenatal CF diagnosis for most Spanish couples. A similar strategy might also be effective for other genetic disorders in which heterogeneity is common.

▶ Cystic fibrosis is the most common autosomal recessive disease in white populations. The Spanish CF population is highly heterogeneous, with more than 70 different mutations causing CF. Prenatal diagnosis of CF by direct analysis of the molecular defect of the CFTR gene is only possible in those families in which the specific mutations responsible for the disease have been identified. In geographic regions where the frequency of the ΔF508 mutation is about 50% and there is high mutation heterogeneity, direct analysis of the CF defect is only feasible for about two thirds of cases, after a comprehensive mutation search. A 3-step strategy for molecular diagnosis of CF in the heterogeneous Spanish population is described. The first step is direct analysis for the two most frequent mutations (ΔF508 and G542X) and indirect analysis with the intragenic markers IVS8CA, IVS17BTA, and IVS17BCA. The second step consists of screening for the mutations already associated with the CFTR microsatellite haplotypes, and the third step is a specific search for unknown mutations. This diagnostic strategy, although not ideal, provides rapid, accurate, and reliable prenatal diagnosis for most couples. This type of approach can be generalized to other genetic disorders for which high heterogeneity has been described.

M.A. Pfaller, M.D.

Reverse Transcription/Polymerase Chain Reaction (RT/PCR) Amplification of Very Small Numbers of Transcripts: The Risk in Misinterpreting Negative Results

Melo JV, Yan X-H, Diamond J, et al (Hammersmith Hosp, London)
Leukemia 10:1217–1221, 1996   20–5

Background.—Technical changes to the reverse transcription–polymerase chain reaction (RT/PCR amplification method now allow detection of amplified products from even 1 abnormal cell, either isolated or mixed with normal cells. The reproducibility of such results was examined using low numbers of cells from patients with chronic myeloid leukemia, and chronic myeloid leukemia cell lines in quintuplicate 2-step RT/PCR that amplifies BCR-ABL sequences.

Results.—An amplification product was obtained in each test when one K562 or KYO1 cell was diluted in 10^3 nonchronic myeloid leukemia HL60 cells. BCR-ABL transcripts were detected erratically at greater dilutions.

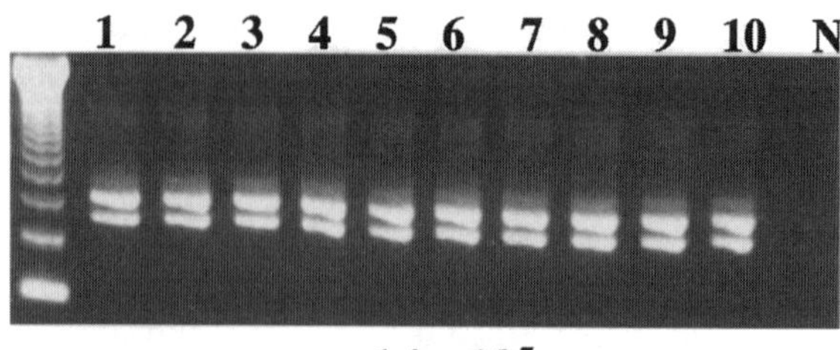

1 in 10⁵

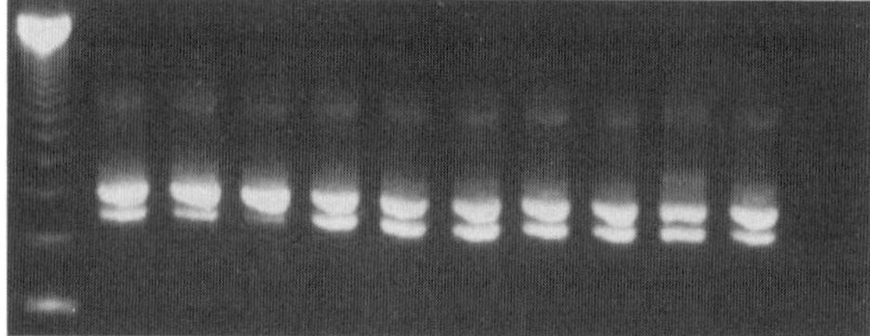

1 in 10⁶

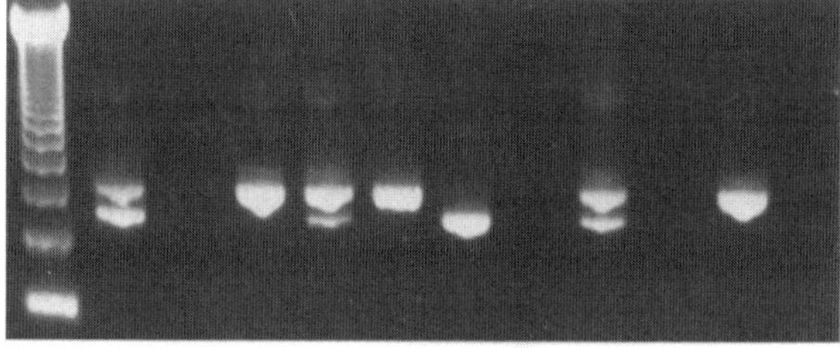

1 in 10⁷

FIGURE 4.—The sampling effect. Ten replicate polymerase chain reaction tests on 3 different dilutions of complementary DNA (cDNA) from cells expressing both b3a2 and b2a2 BCR-ABL transcripts in 1 patient. *Abbreviation:* N, no cDNA, negative control reaction. (Courtesy of Melo JV, Yan X-H, Diamond J, et al: Reverse transcription/polymerase chain reaction amplification of very small numbers of transcripts: The risk in misinterpreting negative results. *Leukemia* 10:1217–1221, 1996.)

Titration of complementary DNA (cDNA) synthesized from 5×10^7 cells from 4 patients with chronic myeloid leukemia showed amplification of positive BCR-ABL sequences in some tests with a 1 in 10^7 dilution of cDNA template, but the dilution threshold for reproducible amplification was shown to be about 1 to 5 in 10^5. Quantitative PCR analysis showed that reactions from 1 in 10^7 diluted cDNA had fewer than 10 BCR-ABL transcripts as the starting template. The stochastic nature of amplification from small numbers of transcripts was seen in results of 10 replicate PCR tests on cDNA from a patient expressing b3a2 and b2a2 transcripts: dilutions of cDNA up to 1 in 10^5 showed dual amplification in the 10 tests, but the 1 in 10^7 cDNA dilution showed b3a2 and b2a2 in 3 tests, b3a2 alone in 3 tests, b2a2 alone in 1 test, and no amplification in 3 tests (Fig 4).

Discussion.—These findings suggest that this sampling effect may give false negative results and allow misinterpretation of data on gene expression when only a small amount of target material is available.

▶ The PCR has proven extremely useful in detecting small numbers of abnormal cells within a larger population of "normal" cells in a clinical specimen. An example of this approach is the detection of as few as 1 cell containing BCR-ABL sequences in the blood of a patient with chronic myeloid leukemia. The authors have shown that there is a threshold of sensitivity in a PCR assay and that at this threshold, there is an even chance of a target sequence being present or absent in the reaction mixture. Thus, even though it is possible to observe a positive PCR amplification, the outcome of the process at this level is unreliable.

When working at the limits of sensitivity of an assay, sampling becomes a major variable and sensitivity is further impacted when the assay requires co-amplification of targets competing for the same primers and other reagents. The limitations of sampling when trying to detect very small numbers of transcripts in clinical specimens are such that a random and unpredictable amplification occurs. This variability casts doubt on the reliability of a single negative PCR test when one is attempting to detect the presence of a very small number of cells.

M.A. Pfaller, M.D.

Quantitative Polymerase Chain Reaction-based Homogeneous Assay With Fluorogenic Probes to Measure *c-erb*B-2 Oncogene Amplification

Gelmini S, Orlando C, Sestini R, et al (Univ of Florence, Italy; Perkin-Elmer Italy, Milan)
Clin Chem 43:752–758, 1997

20–6

Background.—The use of fluorogenic probes to detect specific polymerase chain reaction (PCR) products has recently been proposed. An assay for measuring *c-erb*B-2 amplification in DNA from human breast tumors has been developed to verify the applicability of this approach to quantitative PCR. The PCR-based assay, using the TaqMan™ system, was described.

Methods and Findings.—Two fluorogenic probes anneal to the target between primers for *c-erb*B-2 and β-globin genes. They contain both a reporter dye and a quencher dye. During the extension phase of the PCR cycle, the $5'{\rightarrow}3'$ exonuclease activity of *Taq* polymerase cleaves the hybridized fluorogenic probe. This results in increased fluorescence emission of the reporter dye that is quantitative for the amount of PCR product and, under appropriate conditions, for the amount of template. The assay was found to have adequate precision, a lower detection limit, and a good correlation with the findings of a competitive PCR assay.

Conclusion.—The homogeneous assay described appears to be suitable for determininig *c-erb*B-2 oncogene amplification in tumor specimens. The assay is time-saving and avoids the usually cumbersome postamplication procedures that can be additional sources of inaccuracy and contamination.

▶ Quantitative PCR has provided unique insights into various disease processes and, in some instances, has been useful as both a diagnostic and a prognostic marker. In the field of oncology, detection of oncogene amplification can serve as a marker for prognosis. In particular, several authors have reported a direct correlation between *c-erb*B-2 amplification in breast carcinoma and clinical outcome. In this study, the authors have used the instrumentation and the fluorogenic probes of the Perkin-Elmer Cetus TaqMan System to develop a PCR-based assay for determining *c-erb*B-2 oncogene amplifications in breast cancer.

In this assay, 2 fluorogenic probes anneal to the target between primers for *c-erb*B-2 and β-globin genes and contain both a reporter dye and a quencher dye. During the extension phase of the PCR cycle, the 5′→3′ exonuclease activity of Taq polymerase cleaves the hybridized fluorogenic probe, resulting in an increase of fluorescence emission of the reporter dye that is quantitative for the amount of PCR product and, under appropriate conditions, the amount of template.

The assay is simple, homogeneous, and has adequate precision and sensitivity. It provides simultaneously both quantitative and qualitative information. The authors demonstrate good agreement between the TaqMan assay and competitive PCR for determining the extent of *c-erb*B-2 amplification. Further methodologic studies will be necessary to confirm that the TaqMan methodology can be considered an accurate and sensitive quantitative PCR method.

M.A. Pfaller, M.D.

21 Hematopathology and Immunopathology

Hemoglobin A₂ Levels in Healthy Persons, Sickle Cell Disease, Sickle Cell Trait, and β-Thalassemia by Capillary Isoelectric Focusing
Craver RD, Abermanis JG, Warrier RP, et al (Louisiana State Univ, New Orleans; Children's Hosp, New Orleans, La)
Am J Clin Pathol 107:88–91, 1997   21–1

Introduction.—Normal reference intervals for hemoglobin (Hb)A₂ have not been determined for capillary isoelectric focusing (cIEF). If this information were available, it might help determine the concentration of HbA₂ in sickle cell anemia, sickle cell trait, and β-thalassemia. Mean values and reference intervals of HbA₂ were established using 862 quantitative cIEF Hb typings.

Methods.—Over a 2-year period, 862 quantitative cIEF Hb typings were performed in research subjects with an age range of 1 day to adulthood. Seven hundred twenty-four subjects were 1 year of age or older. Of the 862 research subjects, 318 had normal Hb, 98 had sickle cell trait, 48 had sickle cell anemia, 32 had β-thalassemia, and 228 had other findings. Subjects with normal Hb were grouped, according to age, as 5 months or younger, 6 months to 1 year, and 1 year or older. Mean values of research subjects with sickle cell trait, sickle cell anemia, and β-thalassemia were compared with age-matched values of subjects with normal Hb.

Results.—Research subjects 1 year of age or older with sickle cell trait, sickle cell anemia, or β-thalassemia were significantly different from subjects with normal values. Mean values for sickle cell anemia and sickle cell trait were not significantly different from one another but were different from those for β-thalassemia.

Conclusion.—There is a distinct difference between HbA₂ levels in healthy persons and in patients with sickle cell anemia, sickle cell trait, and β-thalassemia. With cIEF, reference HbA₂ levels are comparable with other methods.

▶ Determination of HbA₂ has presented a problem in clinical laboratories for some time. The usual ion exchange methodologies are often obfuscated by the co-binding and elution of other variant Hb, precluding accurate A₂ measurements. These authors have evaluated a cIEF method that could be of considerable practical value in the routine clinical laboratory. They have shown the method to be effective in determining the concentration of HbA$_2$ in normal individuals and in those with sickle cell disease, sickle trait, and β-thalassemia. In addition, they generated reference ranges in the population by age.

Their data are compared with other, more commonly used methodologies and demonstrate the vital importance of each laboratory determining the prevalent range in their population of healthy individuals when using their own test method. This is an example of testing in which extrapolating data from the literature or from other methods could be very dangerous. Of interest, this cIEF method should also be effective in identifying abnormal Hb.

Information lacking in this manuscript that is of critical importance for laboratories desiring to use this method is comparison of cost. In general, isoelectric focusing gels—particularly the ampholines needed—are expensive. It is certainly possible that at the capillary level, these methods would be cost effective.

J.D. Olson, M.D., Ph.D.

Automation of Human Sperm Cell Analysis by Flow Cytometry
Ferrara F, Daverio R, Mazzini G, et al (Scientific Inst HS Raffaele, Milan, Italy; Natl Research Council, Pavia, Italy)
Clin Chem 43:801–807, 1997   21–2

Introduction.—Sperm analysis is usually performed via manual techniques and microscopic evaluation, methods that are tedious, expensive, and unstandardized. The clinical validity is questionable as the analysis is subject to wide imprecision. Sperm viability was assessed using flow cytometry to do cell counts and typing via a new membrane-permeant nucleic acid stain.

Methods.—The comparison of manual and automated methods for sperm counts was conducted by means of the Bland and Altman method of statistical analysis.

Results.—The mean difference, according to the Bland and Altman method, was 0.243 × 10^6 sperms/mL. Using the whole sperm, the precision of the flow cytometry analysis was 7.5% for the between-run CV and 2.5% for the within-run coefficient of variation.

Conclusion.—The precision of the flow cytometry analysis was acceptable, with observed CVs significantly better than those observed for the manual method. The high precision, accuracy, and low cost of flow cytometry make it a viable option for routine clinical use.

▶ Semen analysis is frequently performed in point-of-care laboratories supporting fertility clinics within urology, obstetrics, or combined practices. Occasionally, the laboratory support for these fertility workups will be performed in central hospital laboratories. Those who have been involved with such analyses know that the manual counting of spermatozoa, with normal counts of 70–80 $\times 10^6$ sperm per mL, is very imprecise, with sperm counts being overestimated in as many as 30% of cases.

No single laboratory performs high-volume semen analyses, making the application of flow cytometric techniques impractical because of the high costs of instrumentation. However, many laboratories have flow cytometers used for a variety of other cell-surface–marker studies. In that setting, the application of the flow cytometer to sperm counts has been demonstrated by these investigators to be low in direct costs (assuming the fixed cost of the instrument is already covered), easy to perform, and of very high precision.

Similar high-precision measurements were shown to be useful in determining sperm viability. In addition, once methodologies for analyzing spermatozoa by flow cytometric methods are developed within the laboratory, further investigation of other potentially important antigenic structures on the surface of the sperm may become feasible, opening new areas for investigation into problems of infertility. The methods described here are clearly applicable at the present time for laboratories that have flow cytometry technology.

J.D. Olson, M.D., Ph.D.

Flow Cytometry of Neonatal Platelet RNA

Joseph MA, Adams D, Maragos J, et al (Univ of Illinois, Peoria)
J Pediatr Hematol Oncol 18:277–281, 1996   21–3

Introduction.—A rapid, noninvasive test to help determine the mechanism of neonatal thrombocytopenia would be helpful, as appropriate treatment depends upon whether low platelet count is caused by decreased platelet production or increased platelet destruction. Flow cytometry analysis was performed on term and preterm infant cord blood and adult blood samples to determine platelet differences in these populations.

Methods.—Blood samples of 18 normal adults, 42 healthy term infants, and 27 preterm infants were evaluated. Infants were classified according to vaginal or cesarean section delivery. The platelet-rich plasma from adult whole blood and infant cord blood samples was partitioned into aliquots containing 5×10^6 platelets. These samples were fixed with 1% paraformaldehyde and stained with thiazole orange for analysis of RNA content. Flow cytometry was used to assess the percentage of RNA-positive reticulated platelets in each aliquot.

Results.—Reticulated platelets were higher in adults than in preterm or term infants. Preterm infant values for reticulated platelets were not significantly higher than term infant values. There were no differences in percentage of reticulated platelets based on delivery type within 1 gestational group. Infants delivered by cesarean section had a more homogeneous size and density distribution on the contour plot, compared with infants of vaginal deliveries.

Conclusion.—This is the first known trial comparing term and preterm infant RNA content using flow cytometry. It validates flow cytometry as feasible and reproducible in this vulnerable patient population.

▶ Since the early 1990s, there has been a growing interest in the counting of young (reticulated) platelets as an index of the rate of platelet production in the bone marrow. Studies have been reported that demonstrate that platelets with elevated RNA content (measured by flow cytometry) are actually less than 24 hours old and that they are increased in patients with rapid platelet turnover.

This study is the first to examine the utilization of the reticulated platelet in the neonate. The evaluation of neonatal thrombocytopenia is of importance, and this first look at reticulated platelets in preterm and full-term neonates, in comparison with adults, is a helpful first step in evaluating platelet production in this clinical setting. The authors' finding that the proportion of platelets with increased RNA in the adult is significantly greater than that seen in the neonate, regardless of the neonatal age, is somewhat surprising.

Because of its high cellularity in the normal state, the neonatal bone marrow has a limited capacity to respond to the stress of rapid peripheral destruction, as seen in hemolysis and immune thrombocytopenia. It will be interesting to see future studies that will examine the relationship of the reticulated platelet count in neonates with clinical thrombocytopenia.

J.D. Olson , M.D., Ph.D.

Platelet Distribution Width for Differential Diagnosis of Thrombocytosis
Osselaer J-C, Jamart J, Scheiff J-M (Mont-Godinne UCL Univ Hosp, Belgium; St-Luc–UCL Univ Hosp, Belgium)
Clin Chem 43:1072–1076, 1997   21–4

Introduction.—Because of the various causes of thrombocytosis, differential diagnosis is not always obvious. The use of routine clinical chemistry has limited use in distinguishing reactive thrombocytosis (RT) and autonomous thrombocytosis. Platelet parameters, such as mean platelet volume (MPV) and the platelet distribution width (PDW), are available, but their clinical usefulness is unclear. The clinical use of PDW was evaluated in a population of patients with high platelet count (PLT) to determine whether PDW is dependent on both MPV and PLT. The combined interpretation of these 3 parameters was examined to determine whether it could improve discrimination between patients with RT and autonomous thrombocytosis.

Methods.—During a 3-month period, 250 patients with platelet counts above $500 \times (10^9/L)$ were evaluated. Of these patients, 174 had RT, 42 had a diagnosis of myeloproliferative disease (MPD), and 34 were excluded because of hemopathy different from MPD. Values for PLT, MPV, PDW, and $PDW_{residual}$ ($PDW_{residual} = PDW_{observed} - PDW_{expected}$) were compared for RT and MPD.

Results.—In the RT group, there was a correlation between PLT, MPV, and PDW. When the discrimination between reactive and autonomous thrombocytosis calculated with $PDW_{residual}$ was compared with that calculated with either PDW, MPV, or PLT, the $PDW_{residual}$ was more powerful than each of the other parameters used separately; 76% of patients with MPD had a $PDW_{residual}$ above the 95th percentile value of the RT population, and none of the patients with MPD had a $PDW_{residual}$ below the 50th percentile.

Conclusion.—The combined interpretation of PLT, MPV, and PDW through the use of $PDW_{residual}$ seems to be of value in the differential diagnosis of thrombocytosis. This approach is free of cost and effortless, requiring only the creation of a laboratory database and use of a simple linear multiple regression model.

▶ The differential diagnosis of patients seen with thrombocytosis can, on occasion, be difficult. Distinguishing reactive from myeloproliferative processes manifesting in this way is, of course, important in the subsequent follow-up and care of the patient. Clinicians occasionally resort to examining the platelet function in an effort to make this distinction, a methodology which provides very poor discrimination.

These authors have observed that the PDW in RT can be predicted by the PLT and the MPV. In addition, this predicted PDW deviates significantly from the measured PDW in patients with myeloproliferative disorders. Therefore, by simply determining the deviation of the observed from the expected PDW, it is possible to discriminate the reactive from the myeloproliferative disorders. Values for the MPV and the PDW reported by new analyzers have appeared to be analyses seeking diagnostic usefulness. In this paper, the authors have demonstrated value of the PDW (residual) in the diagnosis of patients with thrombocytosis.

J.D. Olson, M.D., Ph.D.

Laboratory Diagnosis of Anemia and Related Diseases Using Multivariate Analysis
Shiga S, Furukawa T, Koyanagi I, et al (Kyoto Univ, Japan; SRL Inc, Tokyo; Kobe Gen Hosp, Japan; et al)
Am J Hematol 54:108–117, 1997   21–5

Introduction.—With the vast amount of laboratory information received by physicians, it would be useful to have simple diagnostic systems available that used routine laboratory results. A computer program was developed for the differential diagnosis of anemia and related disorders.

Methods.—Data were gathered for computer analysis from 51 healthy control subjects and 48 patients with anemia or related disorders who had not been treated. Eight laboratory tests were transformed to normal distribution, then applied to principal component analysis to evaluate their independence: white blood cell count, red blood cell count, hemoglobin, hematocrit, mean corpuscular volume, mean corpuscular hemoglobin content, mean corpuscular hemoglobin concentration, and platelet count. The final diagnoses for research subjects in the patient group were as follows: 21 aplastic anemia, 14 myelodysplastic syndrome, 3 iron deficiency anemia, 3 polycythemia vera, and 7 idiopathic thrombocytopenic purpura.

Results.—The relationships between Ht and Hb and between MCV and MCH were almost equipollent. Two sets of laboratory results were constructed and used for further analysis: (1) RBC, MCH, Hb, PLT, and WBC and (2) RBC, MCV, Ht, PLT, and WBC. Two canonical components provided good discrimination of the 5 diseases and of normal research subjects. Use of this analysis for disease prediction yielded correct prediction in 37 of 48 patients (77.1%). When 2 disease predictions were allowed, the correct diagnosis was made in all patients. There were overlaps, particularly in AA and MDS, and with normal research subjects. Additional parameters of age and sex were added to provide a 3-dimensional analysis, which resulted in clearer discrimination. This procedure is being developed in research subjects who are not taking medications; thus, application of this analytic procedure should be used only in individuals not taking medications.

Conclusion.—This is a demonstration project that appears to be promising. Further investigation should include more patients and more disorders.

▶ This interesting article is chosen because of its future implications rather than its current practical application. Most clinical settings are now moving toward computer-based patient records with decision support for clinicians. In their infancy, these decision-support systems merely remind clinicians not to duplicate laboratory orders or warn clinicians about potential drug interactions or allergies. This article demonstrates the probability that these expert systems can be advanced to provide useful additional clinical information based on laboratory data and, eventually, other clinical information. At last count, using the automated analyzer in our laboratory, there are more than 20 different variables generated on each blood specimen analyzed. The trained clinician does the task that these authors are trying to teach the computer to do, that is, to analyze all of these pieces of information and make the maximum use of that information in determining a differential diagnosis and design for their testing. These authors have demonstrated that using a relatively simple two-dimensional canonical analysis, it is possible for the computer to sort with very high probability several common hematologic disorders. The potential for the data generated from both automated hematology and automated chemistry instruments to be analyzed in a stepwise regression, multidimensional canonical analysis, or by both methods to provide probabilities of diagnosis for clinicians as a part of the laboratory report, is demonstrated as being on the near horizon. There is, of course, a considerable amount of work to be done in getting physician input and diagnoses with related laboratory variables into such programs; however, practical use of such devices by the millennium is certainly feasible.

J.D. Olson, M.D., Ph.D.

Immunophenotyping of Blood Lymphocytes in Childhood: Reference Values for Lymphocyte Subpopulations

Comans-Bitter WM, de Groot R, van den Beemd R, et al (Univ Hosp Rotterdam, The Netherlands; Erasmus Univ, Rotterdam, The Netherlands)

J Pediatr 130:388–393, 1997   21–6

Introduction.—Immunophenotyping of blood lymphocytes provides valuable information in the diagnosis of immunologic and hematologic disorders. Relative and absolute size of lymphocyte subpopulations vary with age, so it is important to use age-matched reference values. Reference values for immunophenotyping of blood lymphocytes were created by analyzing blood samples from healthy children.

Methods.—Age of research subjects was 16 years or younger. The lysed whole blood method for analysis of lymphocyte subpopulations was used to evaluate blood samples from 20 neonates (blood samples from the umbilical cord immediately after birth), 358 healthy children, and 51 healthy adults. Age groups of children were as follows: 1 week to 2 months (n = 13); 2 to 5 months (n = 46); 5 to 9 months (n = 105); 9 to 15 months (n = 70); 15 to 34 months (n = 33); 2 to 5 years (n = 33); 5 to 10 years (n = 35); 10 to 16 years (n = 23).

Results.—The absolute number of CD19$^+$ B lymphocytes rises immediately after birth, remains stable until 2 years of age, and gradually diminishes 6.5-fold from 2 years to adulthood. The CD3$^+$ T lymphocytes increase 1.5-fold immediately after birth, then decrease 3-fold from 2 years to adulthood. The absolute size of the CD3$^+$/CD4$^+$ T-lymphocyte subpopulation follows the identical pattern as the total CD3$^+$ population. The CD3$^+$/CD8$^+$ T-lymphocytes remain constant from birth to 2 years, then decrease 3-fold toward adult levels. The absolute number of natural killer cells diminishes almost 3-fold in the firth 2 months of life, then remains stable thereafter. Changes in the absolute size of lymphocyte subpopulations were not always consistent with changes in their relative size. This shows that the relative counts of lymphocyte subsets do not reflect their actual size and are of limited value.

Conclusion.—Changes in the absolute size of lymphocytes subpopulations are not always consistent with variations in their relative sizes. Immunophenotyping of blood lymphocytes for the diagnosis of hematologic and immunologic disorders should be based on absolute rather than relative size of subpopulations. The data collected may be used as age-matched reference values for blood lymphocyte immunophenotyping.

▶ Maybe I am pushing the issue of prevalent ranges a bit hard this year. It is critically important, however, to recognize changes in laboratory analyte values as a function of gender ethnicity, age, and other parameters. Obtaining quality reference range information in children is always difficult. There are few hospitals or parents who are comfortable subjecting healthy children to specimen collection required for obtaining values in these normal children. Therefore, anytime raw data can be generated from children of varying ages, it is important to review and pay attention to the information gathered. This does not argue that the same methodology performed in a different laboratory would generate exactly the same reference ranges; however, the relative changes that occur can clearly be valuable in interpreting laboratory data when the laboratory is not able to generate this information. These authors have successfully undertaken the monumental task of collecting specimens from 20 healthy term neonates, 358 healthy children, and 51 adults and performed relative and absolute distribution of several of the most important lymphocyte surface markers. The data provided are valuable when lymphocyte subsets are analyzed in a clinical setting for potential lymphoproliferative, infectious, or immunodeficiency states.

J.D. Olson, M.D., Ph.D.

Laboratory Investigation of Immune Thrombocytopenia
Warner M, Kelton JG (McMaster Univ, Hamilton, Ont; Canadian Red Cross Centre, Hamilton, Ont)
J Clin Pathol 50:5–12, 1997   21–7

Introduction.—Several techniques have been developed for the serologic evaluation of immune thrombocytopenia. Precise measurement of pathologic antibodies on platelets is difficult because of the unique features of the platelet membrane. Three types of assays for measuring platelet antibodies are described.

Assays.—Phase I assays are indirect assays that measure a platelet end point after normal platelets are activated by test serum. These assays have low sensitivity and specificity. Because most alloantibodies and autoantibodies do not stimulate platelets, these assays are not useful, except in the study of heparin-induced thrombocytopenia. Phase II assays measure all immunoglobulin bound to platelets. These are sensitive assays, but lack specificity of immune thrombocytopenia because they measure both pathologic and nonpathologic antibodies associated with platelets (Fig 3). Phase III assays measure the binding of antibody to a specific platelet glycoprotein. The advantage of phase III assays over phase II assays is that they measure platelet-specific antibodies, not nonspecific platelet/antibody interactions.

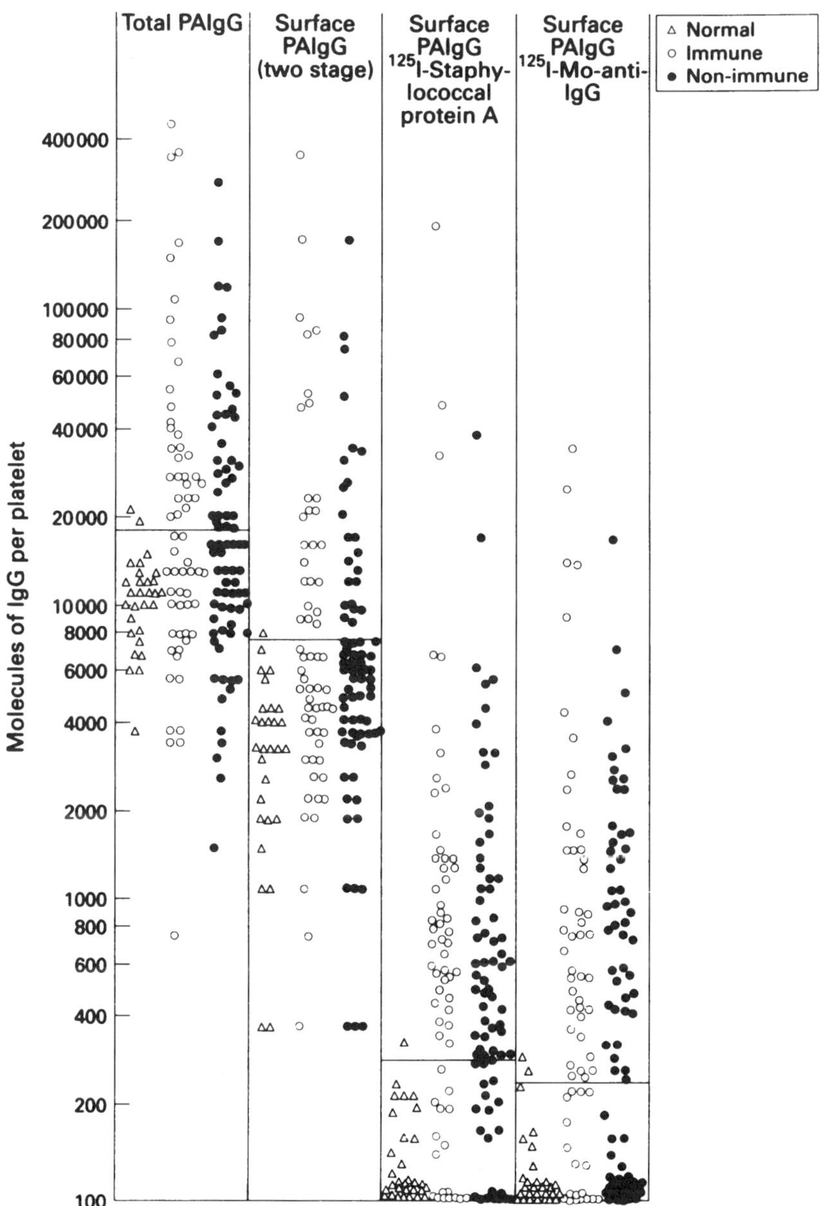

FIGURE 3.—The results of four different assays for PAIgG, representing the different types of PAIgG assays: total PAIgG assays, two stage assays for surface PAIgG, and direct binding assays for surface PAIgG. Normal controls, patients with ITP and nonimmune thrombocytopenia patients are presented in relation to the upper normal ranges, 2 SD above the normal mean values. Reprinted with permission. *Abbreviations*: *PAIgG*, polyclonal anti-IgG; *ITP*, idiopathic thrombocytopenic purpura. (Courtesy of Warner M, Kelton JG: Laboratory investigation of immune thrombocytopenia. *J Clin Pathol* 50:5–12, 1997.)

Conclusion.—The role of phase I, II, and III assays in the diagnosis and classification of immune thrombocytopenia is still unfolding. The ability to classify immune thrombocytopenia according to the interaction between antibody and platelet membrane has been furthered by these technologic advances.

▶ Dr. Kelton has had a long-standing distinguished career focused on the understanding of thrombocytopenia, particularly immune thrombocytopenia. He and Dr. Warner have provided a very nice review of methodologies for the evaluation of immune thrombocytopenia. This concise article nicely explains limitations of assays that are based on the distinction between nonspecific and specific antibodies bound to platelets. One limitation is the lack of good sensitivity specificity data regarding the newer phase III assays for platelet-specific antibody. Despite this, there is considerable useful information on the newer generations of anti-platelet antibody tests and their limitations. These tests have clearly improved the ability of the laboratory to help in supporting the diagnosis of immune thrombocytopenia; however, the overlap seen in the data for normal and affected patients demonstrates the limitations of the laboratory in this disorder.

J.D. Olson, M.D., Ph.D.

Ethnic and Sex Differences in the Total and Differential White Cell Count and Platelet Count
Bain BJ (St Mary's Hosp, London)
J Clin Pathol 49:664–666, 1996
21–8

Introduction.—Ethnic origin and sex influence reference ranges for several hematologic variables. It has been reported that white blood cell (WBC), neutrophil, and platelet counts are lower in persons of African ancestry than Caucasians and that women have higher values of these blood counts than men. Venous blood samples were obtained from male and female Caucasian, African, and Afrocaribbean volunteers to determine reference ranges for WBC and platelet counts for the different ethnic and sex groups.

Methods.—Of 417 volunteers, 201 were women and 216 were men. Ethnic origins were as follows: 200 Caucasian, 115 African, and 102 Afrocaribbean. A geometric mean and 95% range were calculated for total WBC, platelet count, and absolute counts of neutrophils, lymphocytes, monocytes, and eosinophils. Reference ranges were established for each ethnic and sex group.

Results.—Compared with Caucasians, Africans and Afrocaribbeans had lower WBC, neutrophil, and platelet counts, and Africans had lower counts than Afrocaribbeans. Neutrophil and platelet counts were higher in women than men across all 3 ethnic groups.

Conclusion.—These data confirm early findings of lower WBC and neutrophil counts in Africans and Afrocaribbeans than Caucasians and higher counts in women than men. The ethnic differences cannot be explained satisfactorily. The contrasting values between men and women seem to be because of a genuine biologic difference, but the cause for this is unknown. Knowledge of normal ranges of WBC and platelet counts for healthy people of various ethnic and sex groups can help eliminate unnecessary alarm when interpreting hematologic results.

▶ This article is a timely reminder for both laboratories and clinicians concerning the importance of ethnic and gender differences in cell counts and distributions in populations. The article reaffirms information initially alluded to more than 2 decades ago regarding the importance, not only of age, but also of other parameters in determining the prevalent range in the population. These authors have made an extensive comparison of African, African-Caribbean (Afrocaribbean), and Caucasian men and women examining the total white blood cell count, the differential white cell count, and platelet count. They have found statistically significant differences in 47% of these comparisons. It is true from examining the data that, although statistically significant, some of these differences may not be of clinical importance. For example, Caucasian men have a mean monocyte count of 0.34 × 10⁹/L to African at 0.29 × 10⁹/L. This difference is statistically significant; however, I do not believe that it would be of *clinical* importance. In contrast, in thinking about the difficulties of the diagnosis of neutrophilia, the upper limit of the reference range for Caucasian women (7.5 × 10⁹/L) really is a significantly different value than the upper limit of (4.2 × 10⁹/L) seen in African women. To these multiple variables, one must add the difficult variable of the effect of age, particularly in the pediatric population and the geriatric population. This article calls attention to the fact that determining what is "normal or prevalent" in the population is truly multivariate and an overwhelming task to address within a given clinical laboratory. As clinicians and laboratorians approach the problem of cytopenias or cytoses, these differences need to be kept in mind.

J.D. Olson, M.D., Ph.D.

Diurnal Change of Blood Count Analytes in Normal Subjects
Jones AR, Twedt D, Swaim W, et al (Univ of Miami, Fla; VA Med Ctr, Minneapolis; Univ of California, San Francisco)
Am J Clin Pathol 106:723–727, 1996   21–9

Introduction.—In document H26–A, the National Committee for Clinical Laboratory Standards (NCCLS) proposed a goal for automated blood cell analyzers stating, "analytical imprecision should not exceed 25% of the within-person variation of the analyte." This empirical standard for analytic precision using automated blood cell analyzers was reexamined using venous blood samples from 96 healthy volunteers at 3 institutions.

Methods.—Equal numbers of male and female volunteers were instructed not to alter their daily pattern of work, exercise, or relaxation and to avoid fatty foods. Venous blood samples were obtained from each volunteer at about 9 AM on 2 consecutive days. Each specimen was assayed in duplicate at 2 institutions and singly at 1 institution. Duplicate assays were performed to obtain a real-time estimate of analytic imprecision.

Results.—Characteristic changes were observed for each analyte. Negligible changes were seen for properties of erythrocytes, such as mean cell volume and mean cell hemoglobin. Changes in red blood cell count, hematocrit, and hemoglobin were compatible with fluid balance changes. Major changes were observed in total white cell count and some differential count components. These observations raised questions about the confidence limits of clinical decision levels and the validity of commonly used reference intervals. Platelet count changes were characteristically less than analytic imprecision, indicating the need for improvement in this component of analyzer performance.

Conclusion.—Physiologic, short-term diurnal changes in blood count analytes should be considered when interpreting complete blood cell count results. Manufacturers should endeavor to improve the precision and specificity of the platelet count.

▶ Individual variation in blood cell counts is a phenomenon that has been well recognized for several decades. Recently the NCCLS has proposed a precision goal for automated cell analyzers of not more than 25% of the within-person variation of the analyte. The authors of this study have endeavored to examine the diurnal variation of blood cell analytes to determine whether this precision goal is reasonable. In short, the data demonstrate that only the broad variation of the neutrophil count would meet this stringent criteria and that the major cell analyzers used in the study were unable to meet this precision target for any of the other analytes measured. There is a single shortcoming of this study. The investigators made the duplicate sample of the subjects at this same time of the day at 9 AM. For some analytes, this potentially underestimates the variability because of analyte changes that may occur as a function of the time of day. This effect of the time of day is well described among other analytes and is the more commonly used functional definition of diurnal. Nevertheless, the data presented argue strongly that the NCCLS may want to reconsider its precision recommendations for blood cell analyzers.

J.D. Olson, M.D., Ph.D.

Inability of Community-based Laboratories to Identify Pathological Casts in Urine Samples
Rasoulpour M, Banco L, Maut JM, et al (Univ of Connecticut, Farmington; Hartford Hosp, Conn)
Arch Pediatr Adolesc Med 150:1201–1204, 1996   21–10

Introduction.—An important first step in the diagnostic studies of patients with hematuria is to determine whether the cause of bleeding is glomerular disease, tubulointerstitial disease, or disease elsewhere in the genitourinary tract. When this is established, further studies should concentrate on underlying causes so that appropriate treatment and management can be provided. Inaccurate microscopic examination of urine can lead to an incorrect diagnosis. A blinded, prospective evaluation was conducted to determine the ability of 2 large community-based laboratories to identify pathologic casts in the urine of children with glomerulonephritis.

Methods.—Over a period of 4 weeks, 26 fresh morning samples were collected from 7 children with documented glomerulonephritis. Samples were divided into 4 aliquots of at least 10 mL and distributed to 4 different investigation sites within 5 minutes of collection. The investigation sites were 2 community-based laboratories (A and B) and 2 offices of nephrologists (C and D). Participants A, B, and C were blinded to the purpose of the investigation. Participant D was aware of the purpose of the investigation and the diagnosis associated with each specimen.

Results.—Pathologic casts were identified in the 26 specimens as follows: 1 (4%) laboratory A, 2 (8%) laboratory B, 20 (77%) nephrologist C, and 26 (100%) nephrologist D. The investigation sites were significantly different in their reporting of red blood cells, cellular, granular, and mixed cellular/granular casts. Casts were detected more frequently in specimens from patients with severe hematuria by dipstick testing compared with specimens from patients with moderate or mild hematuria.

Conclusion.—The 2 community-based laboratories did not accurately identify pathologic casts in urine specimens from patients with glomerulonephritis. It is not known how well these same results would be observed elsewhere. Primary care providers frequently submit urine specimens of their patients with hematuria to these type of laboratories for examination. These results are cause for concern because misleading reports can lead to improper management and unnecessary evaluations.

▶ This simple study examined 26 urine specimens from 7 children. The specimens were analyzed by experienced observers, nephrologists, and two "community-based" laboratories. Unfortunately, the authors do not adequately define "community-based" laboratories and the quality of the personnel performing the procedures is really unknown. I think it once again represents the difficulty of performing even the simplest of laboratory tests at the point of care with less than the best trained personnel. Quite alarmingly, the identification of both red blood cell and other clinically significant casts (cellular, granular, or mixed casts) differed by more than an order of magnitude. Community laboratories identified casts less than 10% of the time in which they were present.

These findings are both alarming and disappointing. A large proportion of urinalyses are performed in the physician's office by individuals with limited training or experience. The demonstration in this study of the failure to identify casts in such a high percentage is worrisome for the provision of information to assist in the diagnosis, as well as the increased cost of missing useful diagnostic information, leading to misinformation and additional testing to confirm diagnosis. Laboratory procedures should be performed by people with experience who know how to think about the difficulties of the methods.

J.D. Olson, M.D., Ph.D.

The Erythrocyte Cell Hemoglobin Distribution Width Segregates Thalassemia Traits From Other Nonthalassemic Conditions With Microcytosis

Liu T-C, Seong P-S, Lin T-K (Natl Univ Hosp, Singapore; Univ of Singapore)
Am J Clin Pathol 107:601–607, 1997   21–11

Introduction.—Many attempts have been made to distinguish differences between the red blood cells (RBCs) of patients with thalassemia (TH) from those who have other microcytic conditions and between RBCs of patients with β-TH from those with iron deficiency (ID). Three indices of heterogeneity may help distinguish TH traits from ID: red cell distribution width (RDW), cell hemoglobin distribution width (CHDW), and hemoglobin distribution width (HDW). Recursive partitioning methods were used to compare the ability of CHDW, RDW, and HDW to discriminate between TH and nonthalassemic (NT) conditions in 510 patients with microcytosis.

Methods.—A full set of RBC indices (H-3 Hematology analyzer, Baxter) was obtained from routine blood samples collected for hemoglobinopathy screening from 250 patients with TH and 260 patients with NT conditions. The RBC indices included RDW, HDW, and CHDW. These parameters were compared with recursive partitioning methods on a computer program.

Results.—Cell hemoglobin distribution width distinguished patients with iron-replete or iron-deficient NT conditions from patients with TH traits. A CHDW level below 3.05 correctly differentiated 78.4% of patients in a mixed sample of hospitalized patients. With a CHDW/RBC ratio of less than 0.57, sensitivity was 79.2% and specificity was 88.5% for recognizing a TH trait.

Conclusion.—The CHDW was able to separate characteristics of TH from those of NT RBCs. Discrimination of CHDW is enhanced when combined with RBC values. A CHDW ratio of 0.57 correctly identified 79% of patients with TH and 89% of patients with NT microcytosis.

▶ The evaluation of the microcytic blood film presents a significant problem for both clinical laboratories and clinicians. In varying parts of the world the problem of TH is of sufficient prevalence that simple methodologies of separating TH from NT causes of microcytosis would be of value. These authors have evaluated the use of the CHDW, a parameter now generated by some automated analyzers, in distinguishing causes of microcytic disease. They compared this with the more commonly used RCDW and HDW. In addition, they evaluated a number of paired variables (ratios) to try to improve discrimination. They found that the CHDW/RBC ratio provided a discrimination of more than 80%, properly identifying 84% of patients with either TH or NT causes of disease. They used a decision level for TH as a ratio of less than 0.57. It is certainly possible that if the sensitivity for the detection of TH is of importance, that adjustment of this threshold within a given laboratory may improve sensitivity at the cost of some specificity. Utilization of the CHDW/RBC ratio may be of use in planning the further evaluation of the patient with microcytic anemia.

J.D. Olson, M.D., Ph.D.

Hypoplastic Myelodysplastic Syndromes Can Be Distinguished From Acquired Aplastic Anemia by CD34 and PCNA Immunostaining of Bone Marrow Biopsy Specimens
Orazi A, Albitar M, Heerema NA, et al (Indiana Univ, Indianapolis; Univ of Texas, Houston)
Am J Clin Pathol 107:268–274, 1997   21–12

Introduction.—Hypoplastic myelodysplastic syndromes (h-MDSs) are morphologically difficult to discern from acquired aplastic anemia (AA) and many months of follow-up may be needed to establish the correct diagnosis in some patients. Flow cytometric and immunohistochemical trials have indicated that the bone marrow (BM) in AA is typified by a reduced number of CD34+ cells and decreased expression of the proliferating cell nuclear antigen (PCNA). The differences in CD34 and PCNA between h-MDS and acquired AA were evaluated with conventionally processed BM biopsy specimens.

Methods.—Bone marrow biopsy specimens from 23 patients with h-MDS and 27 with acquired AA were retrospectively selected on the basis of paraffin-embedded tissue for immunostaining and complete cytogenetic results. Immunohistochemical staining for CD34 was done using QBEND10, a monoclonal antibody (MoAb) reactive in routinely processed specimens. The PCNA was evaluated by the PC10 MoAb using a microwave oven-based antigen retrieval technique.

Results.—Significantly higher values of PCNA and CD34 were observed in BM specimens of patients with h-MDS compared with BM specimens from patients with acquired AA.

There was an increased incidence of PCNA-positive cells in the marrow of patients with h-MDS with normal cytogenetics compared with the marrow of patients with abnormal kerotypes.

Conclusion.—There was a positive correlation between lower PCNA expression and abnormal cytogenetics in patients with MDS. Other trials have shown that the presence of chromosome abnormalities and decreased proliferative activity in BM cells of patients with MDS are correlated with advanced disease and dismal prognosis. These findings are in agreement with those of decreased proliferative capability and increased apoptotic ratio in patients with MDS and cytogenetically abnormal blasts.

▶ For individuals who interpret BM samples, the distinction between AA and h-MDS can be very difficult on the basis of morphologic findings alone. When this differential is anticipated, the cytogenetic analysis of the marrow has frequently been the most helpful distinguishing characteristic, with cytogenetic abnormalities being common in the myelodysplastic processes and distinctly uncommon among patients with AA. The authors of this article have addressed 2 of the problems that occasionally arise. First, in most clinical settings, the cytogenetic analysis is not performed routinely on every BM specimen, and the distinction between these two similar diagnoses may not have the benefit of a specimen suitable for cytogenetics. Second, there is provided an alternative, immunohistochemical, approach to making this distinction in a retrospective manner using paraffin-embedded tissue. This is particularly helpful in the setting of patients whose diagnosis may be made in the community hospital with subsequent referral for appropriate management, BM transplantation, in an academic center. The preparation of the patient for BM transplantation is different in the two syndromes; therefore distinction is of clinical importance. The authors have demonstrated that in AA, CD34+ cells and the expression of PCNAs are both significantly reduced, features that have not been associated with the myelodysplastic syndrome. Their retrospective approach has successfully distinguished 23 patients with myelodysplastic syndrome from 27 with AA. This is a relatively simple methodology that can be of significant value in this clinical setting.

J.D. Olson, M.D., Ph.D.

Is the Red Cell Morphology Really Useful to Detect the Source of Hematuria?

Favaro S, Bonfante L, D'Angelo A, et al (Univ of Padua, Italy)
Am J Nephrol 17:172–175, 1997   21–13

Introduction.—The validity of morphologic analysis of urinary erythrocytes by phase-contrast microscopy has been supported or questioned by various reports evaluating its ability to detect the source of bleeding within the genitourinary tract. The validity of morphologic analysis of urinary erythrocytes by phase-contrast microscopy was evaluated in 129 patients with persistent microhematuria.

Methods.—Of 129 research subjects with persistent isolated microhematuria, 31 (24.1%) had mild proteinuria (below 1 g/day), and 21 (21.4%) had pathologic albumin levels (above 15 µg/min). Patients were followed up for 6 years. During follow-up, 6 patients (4.6%) had renal biopsy because of recurrent macrohematuria or proteinuria ranging from 2 to 3 g/day. Patients underwent laboratory testing every 6 months and had renal sonograms yearly.

Results.—Morphologic analysis of urinary red blood cells in 129 patients showed erythrocytes were nonglomerular in 109, glomerular in 19, and of mixed type in 1. Erythrocyte dysmorphisms were detected in only a small number of patients. Two of 6 patients with parenchymal nephropathy had histologic findings compatible with renal bleeding. During 6-year follow-up, only 2 patients with dysmorphic red blood cells experienced proteinuria exceeding 1 g/day. None of the patients with nonmomorphic erythrocytes had serious urologic problems.

Conclusion.—These findings are in agreement with others that report that morphologic evaluation of urinary erythrocytes is not a reliable test for identifying the exact origin of hematuria. Morphologic evaluation does not correspond well with actual pathologic findings.

▶ Asymptomatic microscopic hematuria is not an uncommon finding in healthy patients. The difficulty presented to clinicians and laboratorians is identifying or predicting the patient in whom this finding is of clinical significance. Many practitioners believe that the glomerular source of the red cell, and therefore the clinically significant cases, can be identified by the morphology of the red blood cell in the urine. This examination is made by phased-contact microscopy and is still in use in many laboratories. Although the data are not managed in this way in the article, predictive value theory can be applied to the finding of abnormal (glomerular) erythrocytes compared with the presence of evidence of renal disease. The results of such an application yield sensitivity of 16%, specificity of 85%, the predictive value of a positive test result of 25%, and predictive value of a negative test result of 76%. This article makes it clear that evaluation of high urinary red cell morphologic findings in patients with asymptomatic microscopic hematuria may be as frequently misleading as helpful. It should not be a part of the evaluation of such patients.

A second article on the topic of microscopic hematuria[1] evaluated the usefulness of microscopic hematuria in the assessment of patients with urinary tract symptoms and benign prostatic hyperplasia. In this setting the finding of hematuria could not be related to calculi for which patients needed treatment or the presence of tumor within the bladder. Conclusions from this prospective study of more than 750 consecutive patients with benign prostatic hyperplasia were that the finding of microscopic hematuria is extremely common and additional tests to pursue its cause should be performed only in the face of other clinical indications.

J.D. Olson, M.D., Ph.D.

Reference

1. Ezz El Din K, Koch WFRM, de Wildt MJAM, et al: The predictive value of microscopic haematuria in patients with lower urinary tract symptoms and benign prostatic hyperplasia. *Eur Urol* 30:409–413, 1996.

Proficiency Testing of Hemoglobinopathy Techniques in Ontario Laboratories

Lafferty J, Ali MAM, Carstairs K, et al (St Joseph's Hosp, Hamilton, Ont; Toronto Hosp; Laboratory Proficiency Testing Program, Toronto)
Am J Clin Pathol 107:567–575, 1997   21–14

Background.—The Laboratory Proficiency Testing Program (LPTP), a unit of the Ontario Medical Association established 20 years ago, performs proficiency testing in various disciplines of clinical laboratory medicine. The experience of the LPTP with hemoglobinopathy proficiency testing between 1989 and 1994 was reported.

Methods.—Samples distributed for screening, investigation, and identification of hemoglobinopathies were included in the analysis. Six samples for hemoglobin (Hb) S screening were sent to from 37 to 163 laboratories performing screening tests for sickle cell disease, and 10 samples were sent to from 52 to 71 laboratories for Hb electrophoresis.

Findings.—The performance of most laboratories was acceptable. Error rates for sickle cell screening ranged from 2.7% to 19.7%. The lowest performance was noted for Hb SC disease. For Hb electrophoresis, the error rates ranged from 1.4% to 36.8%, with the poorest performance in the assessment of Hb H disease and α-thalassemia trait. Survey performance was noted in the screening for Hb S trait and in the assessment of Hb H disease, illustrating the positive effects of proficiency testing on laboratory services.

Conclusions.—The LPTP has demonstrated acceptable performance by most laboratories licensed to perform the techniques studied, as well as some clinically significant problems. In Ontario, the LPTP has resulted in improved performance through method modification in direct response to the committee's concerns and through educational activities.

▶ This report of the hemoglobinopathy proficiency testing program in Ontario twice a year during a 5-year period demonstrates some important points. First and most importantly, over the course of this study, laboratories improved their performance in identifying hemoglobinopathies and α-thalassemia. Second, laboratories performing only screening for Hb S frequently misinterpreted settings in which Hb S is present as trait or as Hb SC disease. Finally, and most important, is the report of the difficulty experienced by laboratories in identifying Hb H. Twenty-three percent of laboratories made errors in the analysis for interpretation. It is emphasized, as a result of this proficiency testing sample, that: Hb H is difficult to detect with a number of commercially available products; that evaluation of hemoglobinopathy for a microcytic disease in which iron deficiency and α-thalassemia have been excluded, should include examination for Hb H inclusion bodies.

J.D. Olson, M.D., Ph.D.

The Diagnostic Value of the Neutrophil Left Shift in Predicting Inflammatory and Infectious Disease

Seebach JD, Morant R, Rüegg R, et al (Univ Hosp Zürich, Switzerland; Univ of Zürich, Switzerland)
Am J Clin Pathol 107:582–591, 1997   21–15

Background.—Although the association between acute inflammatory or infectious disease (ID) and white blood cell (WBC) count, neutrophil count, increased level of banded neutrophils, and the immature total neutrophil count (I/T) ratio has been known for years, the diagnostic value of the band count as an indicator for ID continues to be debated. The current study further explored the utility of neutrophil left shift parameters in diagnosing inflammatory and ID, using C-reactive protein (CRP) level as the gold standard.

Methods and Findings.—Of 292 patients studied, 79% had a CRP of 1.0 mg/dL or greater. These patients were classified as having inflammation. The remaining 21% had normal levels. In each patient, the neutrophil band count was assessed by microscopic examination of 200 WBCs. The diagnostic value of this count as an ID indicator was determined compared with the WBC count, the neutrophil count, and the left-shift indicators of 2 automated hematologic analyzers. In receiver operating characteristics analysis, the band count was better than the I/T ratio, total WBC count, and neutrophil count. The sensitivity and specificity for identifying ID at designated cutoff points were 53% and 79%, respectively, for band count of 20% or more of the total WBC count; 59% and 63%, respectively, for I/T ratio of 0.25 or greater; 68% and 56%, respectively, for total WBC count of 9.6×10^6 /mL or greater; and 60% and 58%, respectively, for neutrophil count of 8×10^6 /mL or greater. Microscopic assessment to determine the presence of reactive morphologic changes in neutrophils had an 80% sensitivity but a 58% specificity in predicting ID.

Conclusions.—Microscopic and automated neutrophil left shift parameters have a limited diagnostic value as ID indicators. However, morphologic changes have a high specificity or sensitivity in predicting ID. Thus, such changes may be clinically useful.

▶ This study makes yet another attempt to evaluate the left shift. With the evolution of rapidly available CRP measurements from random access analyzers, which have been demonstrated to be superior in detecting inflammatory infectious disease, one would hope that clinicians will eventually stop relying upon the "left shift" as a diagnostic tool. These authors have demonstrated that both the manually and automated generation of neutrophil immaturity have limited value. One small aspect of the study design is important. All of the manual band counts were performed by an individual technologist, a total of 15 technologists participating in data generation. This carries, in one way, some strength in that it is the way that these measurements would be generated in a given laboratory. The difficulty, however, is the tremendous and well-documented variation among different observers in generating manual band counts. Because of this variability, application of the method in individuals is inadvisable even when population data appear useful. The instruments used will generate, very precisely, the same value on the same instrument repeatedly. In contrast, if the same specimen were analyzed manually by all 15 technologists, the degree of variation would be extremely high. In addition, they used 200 manual cell count differentials, a number that exceeds the actual routine cell counting methodologies in most laboratories. In short, this is another paper that demonstrates the limited value of the left shift and the value of encouraging clinicians to evaluate inflammatory and ID possibilities using the CRP.

J.D. Olson, M.D., Ph.D.

22 Clinical Chemistry and Toxicology

Prognostic Implication of Creatine Kinase Elevation Following Elective Coronary Artery Interventions
Kong TQ Jr, Davidson CJ, Meyers SN, et al (Northwestern Univ, Chicago)
JAMA 277:461–466, 1997   22–1

Introduction.—Some patients will have a rise in serum creatine kinase (CK) after elective coronary artery procedures. The prognostic importance of an elevation in CK occurring after percutaneous transluminal angioplasty (PTCA) is unknown. Late cardiac mortality was compared for patients who did and did not have an increase in CK after PTCA.

Methods.—The retrospective study included 373 patients who had undergone elective PTCA. The cases included 253 consecutive patients whose total CK and CK-MB rose after PTCA. The controls were 120 patients who did not have CK elevations. The 2 groups underwent PTCA at about the same time and using the same equipment. They were compared for in-hospital and late cardiac mortality, subsequent myocardial infarction, and a combined end-point of cardiac mortality or myocardial infarction. Both groups were followed up for longer than 3.5 years.

Results.—The 2 groups were comparable in terms of age, sex, extent of coronary artery involvement, left ventricular function, and number of lesions treated. The cases tended to have more complex target lesions, were more likely to have lesions in degenerated saphenous vein grafts, and were more likely to have occluded target vessels. The patients with postprocedural CK elevations showed a significant increase in cardiac mortality. On stratification by peak CK elevation, cardiac mortality was increased for patients with intermediate elevations (1.5 to 3.0 times normal) and high elevations (more than 3 times normal). The main predictors of increased cardiac mortality on multivariate analysis were higher peak CK level and lower ejection fraction. Each 100 U/L increase in CK carried a 1.05 relative risk of cardiac death.

Conclusions.—Elevation of CK after PTCA is an independent prognostic factor for cardiac death. The findings reflect the difficulty of performing percutaneous procedures in patients with previous bypass operations, especially those with lesions in saphenous vein grafts. More study is needed to see if new treatment strategies can alter the long-term prognosis of patients with postprocedural CK elevation.

▶ Percutaneous transluminal coronary angioplasty is performed more than a half million times a year and has become a routine procedure in the treatment of coronary artery disease. It has the advantage of being minimally invasive as opposed to other treatments such as bypass surgery. This paper follows the long-term outcome of 2 groups. The case group experienced elevations in total CK and elevated CK-MB after PTCA, and the matched control group did not have CK elevation.

The case group experienced significantly increased late cardiac death compared with the control group. The average duration of follow-up was 3.5 years. The prediction based on CK levels was independent of clinical variables. When these data are combined with that of other papers that suggest that elevated troponins in patients with unstable angina lead to a poor outcome, it would seem that the destruction of even small amounts of myocardium does not bode well for the patient.

R. Feld, Ph.D.

Evaluating Asymptomatic Patients With Abnormal Liver Function Test Results
Theal RM, Scott K (Kaiser Permanente Med Ctr, Fontana, Calif)
Am Fam Physician 53:2111–2119, 1996   22–2

Introduction.—The family physician occasionally sees an asymptomatic patient with abnormal liver function studies. Management of these cases requires an understanding of the uses and limitations of routine liver function tests. A rational, systematic approach to further evaluation is needed for a cost-effective diagnostic workup.

Abnormal Liver Function Tests in Asymptomatic Patients.—Routine liver function tests screen for cellular integrity, protein synthesis, and excretory function, but they are neither sensitive nor specific for liver disease. When an asymptomatic patient has abnormal results on these tests, the most common findings are fatty liver, alcohol-related liver damage, and chronic viral hepatitis. There are many possible causes of asymptomatic liver disease, including hemachromatosis, Wilson's disease, drug toxicity, chronic autoimmune hepatitis, biliary cirrhosis, primary sclerosing cholangitis, α_1-antitrypsin deficiency, and sarcoidosis. Alternatively, the abnormal results may merely reflect normal variants or laboratory errors.

The evaluation starts with a history and physical examination to seek possible exposure to chemicals, risk factors, and significant liver disease. Screening tests for liver damage can be ordered; the most effective are alanine transaminase, alkaline phosphatase, and bilirubin. If the results are abnormal, the tests shoud be repeated, and confirmatory tests such as creatinine phosphokinase or γ-glutamyltransferase should be ordered. The possibility of biliary obstruction or neoplasm can be assessed by imaging studies. All treatable illnesses should be excluded. The patients may be monitored for 3–6 months to see if progressive symptoms or liver dysfunction develop. This observation period may be followed by further laboratory testing, liver biopsy, or referral to a gastroenterologist.

Discussion.—The problems posed by abnormal liver function test results in an asymptomatic patient are reviewed. The possibilities in these cases range from laboratory error to a serious illness. The article includes an algorithm for patient monitoring, including guidelines for re-evaluation, observation, and referral.

▶ Few things are as frustrating to physicians as abnormal test results for an asymptomatic patient. This is especially so with liver function tests because the diagnostic workup can be involved and expensive. The physician must balance not missing an important, treatable disease with the Ulysses syndrome, for which a long and expensive workup yields no valuable information.

This paper reviews the common liver function tests, and possible causes for abnormal tests and then provides a rational algorithm for approaching the workup of these patients. With estimates of 1% to 2% of the population infected with hepatitis C, homozygous hemochromatosis as common as 3 per 1,000, nonalcoholic steatohepatitis becoming more common as obesity increases, and closet alcoholism common, this paper gives sound guidance to the pathologist and physician faced with the task of developing an approach to the seemingly normal patient with abnormal test results.

R. Feld, Ph.D.

Fasting Total Plasma Homocysteine and Atherosclerotic Peripheral Vascular Disease
Cheng SWK, Ting ACW, Wong J (Univ of Hong Kong)
Ann Vasc Surg 11:217–223, 1997   22–3

Introduction.—In patients with premature atherosclerosis, cerebrovascular diseases, and coronary artery disease, elevated plasma homocysteine levels have been observed. A role may be played by vitamin B_{12}, folate intake, and metabolism. The relation of homocysteine and atherosclerotic peripheral arterial occlusive disease and the association of hyperhomocysteinemia and serum vitamin B_{12} and folate metabolism was investigated in a prospective analysis. In patients with peripheral atherosclerosis, the prevalence and relative risk of mild hyperhomocysteinemia was determined by establishing a normal homocysteine level for the local population.

Methods.—In 100 patients with symptomatic atherosclerotic peripheral vascular disease and 100 age- and sex-matched controls, fasting total plasma homocysteine levels were measured by rapid ion-exchange chromatography. Both groups were measured for demographic data, biochemistry, hematology, and lipid fractions. Recordings were taken of clinical and vascular laboratory disease parameters. Patients with normal homocysteine levels were compared with those with hyperhomocysteinemia, defined as those with fasting homocysteine values exceeding the 90th percentile of the control range. Using objective criteria, homocysteine levels were correlated with disease distribution and severity in the lower limbs.

Results.—In the patient group, total fasting homocysteine concentrations were significantly higher (28.8 ± 14.9 µmol/L) than in the controls (20.3 ± 11.3 µmol/L). Males had higher homocysteine levels than females in both groups. In the healthy controls, homocysteine correlates positively only with age, but not with other risk factors. For peripheral vascular disease, total plasma homocysteine concentration is an independent risk factor, according to multivariate analysis of the biochemical risk factors. Vitamin B_{12} or folate deficiency states are not associated with hyperhomocysteinemia. In the control group, vitamin B_{12} concentration was 591 ± 313 ng/L and it was 682 ± 405 ng/L in the patient group. In the controls, the serum folate concentration was lower (7.2 ± 2.3 µg/L) than in the patients (8.3 ± 2.0 µg/L). In 27% of the patients, mild hyperhomocysteinemia was detected.

Conclusions.—In comparison to patients with a normal homocysteine level, patients with hyperhomocysteinemia had a fourfold increase in risk of peripheral vascular disease. On patient demographics, biochemical risk factors, and disease pattern and severity, there is no significant difference between the 2 groups.

▶ The realization that current known risk factors for atherosclerotic disease such as lipids and fibrinogen do not account for all of the cases observed has encouraged the search for other contributors. Patients with the rare genetic disease homocysteinuria were noted to have premature atherosclerosis. Although the homozygous disease is rare, mutations in the enzymes associated with homocysteine metabolism that lead to reduced activity are common. These enzymes are also dependent on folate, vitamin B_{12}, and vitamin B_6 cofactors, and deficiencies of these micronutrients can lead to elevated homocysteine.

There are many studies showing an association of hyperhomocysteinemia to coronary and cerebral atherosclerosis. This study is concerned with peripheral atherosclerotic disease and does show an independent association of elevated homocysteine with increased risk of peripheral vascular disease.

Measurement of homocysteine is not easy, requiring the use of sophisticated analytical techniques such as high-performance liquid chromatography. An automated method that can be done on a common laboratory instrument is rumored to be available soon. Luckily, the treatment of hyperhomocysteinemia is inexpensive and simple, requiring only supplemental doses of vitamin B_6 and folate with some vitamin B_{12} thrown in to make sure that its deficiency is not masked. Yearly supplementation costs less than $10, which is much less than the cost of a homocysteine assay. Folate supplementation of food is being considered by the Food and Drug Administration as a way to reduce neural tube defects in pregnant women. As the homocysteine level of the population is lowered through treatment and supplementation, perhaps the atherosclerotic component attributable to this compound may decrease.

R. Feld, Ph.D.

A Search for Hepatitis C Virus Polymerase Chain Reaction–Positive but Seronegative Subjects Among Blood Donors With Elevated Alanine Aminotransferase
Prince AM, Scheffel JW, Moore B (Lindsley F Kimball Research Inst of the New York Blood Ctr, New York; Abbott Labs, Abbott Park, Ill)
Transfusion 37:211–214, 1997   22–4

Introduction.—Infections with the hepatitis C virus continue to occur despite the introduction of increasingly sensitive screening tests for this virus. With third-generation screening, it was estimated that 1 in 103,000 donors would be in the seronegative window period of hepatitis C virus infection, and it is know that polymerase chain reaction (PCR) can detect hepatitis C virus RNA before other sensitive assays, including the window-phase hepatitis C virus infections. There were 301 volunteers with elevated alanine aminotransferase levels in which the results of third-generation assays were compared with those of PCR assays.

Methods.—Current and newer versions of assays for anti-hepatitis C virus and PCR assays that were rigidly controlled for specificity and contamination were used to test fresh frozen plasma from 301 donors with alanine aminotransferase levels greater than 100 IU/L. If positive in 2 screening assays and 1 supplemental assay, or if positive in 2 screening assays and 1 PCR, sera were classified as seropositive.

Results.—One hundred percent of seropositive samples were detected with the new versions of screening assays. There was a detection of 87% of seropositive sera with a second-generation immunoblot assay; there was 96% detection with a second-generation recombinant immunoblot assay; and a 98% detection with an enzyme immunoassay for antibody to the envelope protein of hepatitis C virus. Of the 54 seropositive sera, 51 were PCR positive. On PCR, none of the 247 seronegative samples were reproducibly positive.

Conclusions.—In this high-risk donor population, no PCR positive but seronegative donors were found. Using large-scale comparative testing of donor populations, the possible benefit of PCR screening of blood donors can be determined; however, it may be limited to detecting window-phase infections. Unfortunately, routine PCR testing is not feasible presently.

▶ The routine testing of transfused blood for infectious diseases has greatly reduced the posttransfusion infection rate. Those of us who have this responsibility in our laboratories, however, are not excited when the Food and Drug Administration mandates another screening test. It adds greatly to the workload and is 1 more assay that is subject to Food and Drug Administration inspection.

The wisdom of some of these choices is sometimes not evident. It took 10 years to stop alanine aminotransferase-level screening of blood donors. The recent introduction of HIV antigen is estimated to find 5 additional donors a year who are in the window period between infection and the appearance of HIV antibody. The estimated cost of this 1 additional test is $60 million a year, which is probably a gross underestimate.

The introduction of hepatitis C antibody testing in the early 1990s has clearly been a success. Posttransfusion hepatitis already decreased by hepatitis B screening has been further diminished by this testing. Disturbing reports in the last few years have alluded to donors who are hepatitis C antibody negative but in whom hepatitis C RNA can be detected by PCR. Some of these donors are in the window period before antibody development, but others were reported to be beyond this time. If this were true, it would have grave implications for donor testing.

This report describes 301 samples from donors with ALT alanine aminotransferase levels greater than 100 IU/L. Eighteen percent of these donors were hepatitis C antibody positive. Of the 247 with negative hepatitis C antibodies, none were positive by PCR. These results do not confirm a preliminary study by the same authors, who discuss the problem of PCR contamination as a possible explanation. We hope the number of seronegative, PCR positive donors not in the window period is very low.

R. Feld, Ph.D.

Heterophilic Antibodies Produce Spuriously Elevated Concentrations of the MB Isoenzyme of Creatine Kinase in a Selected Patient Population
Sosolik RC, Hitchcock CL, Becker WJ (Ohio State Univ, Columbus)
Am J Clin Pathol 107:506–510, 1997   22–5

Introduction.—A relatively sensitive and specific indicator of ischemic myocardial injury is an increased serum concentration of the MB isoenzyme of creatine kinase. Erroneous results can occur because of the heterophile antibodies, however, such as human antimurine antibodies, which can interfere with assays used to quantitate the MB isoenzyme of creatine kinase. After patients with colorectal carcinoma received an injection of iodine-125–labeled monoclonal antibody directed against a tumor-associated glycoprotein, the serum levels of the MB isoenzyme of creatine kinase were measured. The patients had an increased risk for having human antimurine antibody develop.

Methods.—Approximately 3 weeks after injection, the radiolabeled antibody was used to guide subsequent surgical resection of any metastatic tumor. It was hypothesized that because of human antimurine antibody, these patients had increased concentrations of the MB isoenzyme of creatine kinase and normal creatine kinase activities. To counteract the effect of human antimurine antibody, a heterophile blocking reagent (HBR) was added to their sera. To determine whether the addition of HBR altered pathologically increased serum concentrations of the MB isoenzyme of creatine kinase, the effect of HBR on serum specimens was analyzed from patients who had acute myocardial ischemia.

Results.—A marked increase in the level of the MB isoenzyme of creatine kinase and normal total creatine kinase concentrations was seen in serum specimens from 8 (42%) of the patients. After an HBR was added, the increased concentrations of the MB isoenzyme of creatine kinase, which were attributed to interference by human antimurine antibodies, were substantially reduced in these specimens. In patients who had clinical evidence of acute myocardial ischemia, this reagent did not significantly alter the serum level of the MB isoenzyme of creatine kinase.

Conclusions.—In sandwich-type immunoassays that use murine immunoglobulins, serum specimens from patients who have received monoclonal antibody–based formulations may frequently show heterophilic antibody interference. The implications must be recognized by laboratory personnel. Heterophile blocking reagent may help resolve this problem.

▶ There is an old saying that new solutions lead to new problems. Refrigeration was introduced to prevent food spoilage, but then we learned that chlorofluorocarbons destroy the ozone layer. Monoclonal antibodies have been quickly adopted in many assays used in the clinical laboratory. They can react with very limited epitopes on an analyte, thereby conferring great specificity to an assay. So-called sandwich assays use 1 monoclonal antibody to capture the analyte and a second monoclonal antibody tagged with a reporter molecule to give a signal. Most monoclonal antibodies are made in mouse cells and not only are used in assays but also therapeutically. They can be tagged with a killer molecule that will specifically bind to antigens produced by certain tumors and destroy them.

A problem occurs in sandwich assays because any molecule that links the 2 antibodies will produce a signal like the desired analyte. In patients receiving mouse monoclonals therapeutically, antibodies to the mouse monoclonals can develop, which will link the 2 antibodies and will therefore give a false signal. These human antimurine antibodies also can occur in patients without obvious exposure to mouse monoclonals.

This article describes falsely elevated creatine kinase–MB levels as determined by a sandwich assay in patients receiving an iodine-125–labeled murine monoclonal directed against a tumor-associated glycoprotein. Most assays include mouse serum in their reagents to reduce the effect of human antimurine antibodies. This assay did contain mouse serum, but the effect of human antimurine antibodies could only be overcome by the addition of HBR. Heterophile blocking reagent did not reduce the creatine kinase–MB measured in patients who had myocardial infarctions. Human antimurine antibodies should always be considered when the results of an assay are at odds with the clinical data.

R. Feld, Ph.D.

Disparities in Clinical Laboratory Performance for Blood Lead Analysis

Sargent JD, Johnson L, Roda S (Dartmouth-Hitchcock Med Ctr, Lebanon, NH)

Arch Pediatr Adolesc Med 150:609–614, 1996   22–6

Background.—Direct measurement of blood lead concentrations has recently become a routine part of commercial laboratory profiles. Compared with the current threshold of concern (0.48 µmol/L), acceptable error in such measurement is high. For example, the Centers for Disease Control Blood Lead Proficiency Program would accept any result between 0.29 and 0.68 µmol/L. The validity of blood lead analysis on clinical specimens was investigated.

Methods.—Blood lead samples with known lead concentrations were submitted as clinical specimens to 18 laboratories in a blinded fashion. Each laboratory received 6 specimens with an actual blood lead (ABPb) concentration of 0.43 µmol/L and another 3 specimens with ABPb concentrations of 0.33, 0.89, and 1.59 µmol/L, respectively.

Findings.—Blood lead findings on 157 of the 162 submissions were obtained. One laboratory reported that all specimens had lead levels of less than 0.48 µmol/L. Of 18 (11%) specimens, 2 with ABPb levels of 0.89 µmol/L and 1 of 17 (6%) with a concentration of 1.59 µmol/L were reported as being less than 0.48 µmol/L. Two (11%) of 18 with an ABPb level of 0.33 µmol/L and 44 (42%) of 104 with a level of 0.43 µmol/L were classified as 0.48 µmol/L or higher. The laboratory mean for specimens with an ABPb level of 0.43 µmol/L ranged from 0.23 to 0.52 µmol/L. The coefficient of variation ranged from 3% to 37%. Laboratories using anodic stripping voltammetry were 6.3 times more likely to report findings differing by more than 0.14 µmol/L from the ABPb concentrations than laboratories using atomic absorption techniques.

Conclusions.—The validity of blood lead measures varies widely among clinical laboratories. Some laboratories made large errors, could have resulted in the misclassification of children with significant lead exposure.

▶ Choosing a reference laboratory has never been an easy issue for the physician, and the decision has been made even more difficult with the advent of managed care. Because each managed care organization may have a contract with a different reference laboratory, the physician may have to deal with several laboratories depending on the patient population.

The action level for blood lead measurement in children has been ratcheted down to less than 10 µg/dL over the last 20 years as we have learned more about the deleterious effects of lead on young minds. This paper sent reference samples disguised as patient specimens to laboratories selected from the phone book that offered blood lead testing. All of them were certified under the Clinical Laboratory Improvement Act of 1988. Several labs misclassified samples with known lead levels. Separating good from poor labs was difficult because quality did not depend on the charge or the proficiency testing program used. There was a strong correlation between accuracy and the method of analysis. This paper shows that choosing a reference laboratory is still not easy, and a poor laboratory could have a deleterious effect on patients for this critical analysis.

R. Feld, Ph.D.

Cardiac-specific Troponin I Levels to Predict the Risk of Mortality in Patients With Acute Coronary Syndromes

Antman EM, Tanasijevic MJ, Thompson B, et al (Brigham and Women's Hosp, Boston; Maryland Med Research Inst, Baltimore; Univ of British Columbia, Vancouver)
N Engl J Med 335:1342–1349, 1996   22–7

Objective.—To examine the predictive value of troponin I for myocardial necrosis in patients with unstable angina or non–Q-wave myocardial infarction.

Background.—Unstable angina and non–Q-wave myocardial infarct cannot be distinguished in patients with chest pain at rest with no ST-segment elevation. Although there is a serum marker of myocardial damage, it would be beneficial to have a marker that is more sensitive, reflects the degree of myocardial damage, has predictive value, and is able to be measured quickly. Cardiac troponin I is very specific for cardiac tissue,

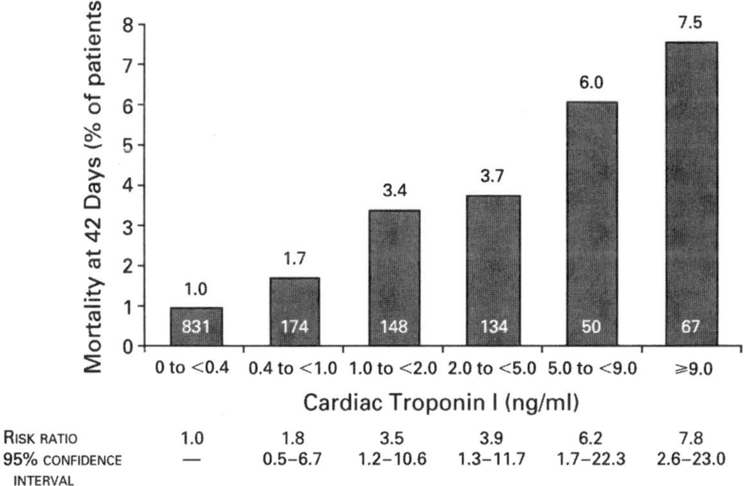

Rɪsᴋ ʀᴀᴛɪᴏ	1.0	1.8	3.5	3.9	6.2	7.8
95% ᴄᴏɴꜰɪᴅᴇɴᴄᴇ ɪɴᴛᴇʀᴠᴀʟ	—	0.5–6.7	1.2–10.6	1.3–11.7	1.7–22.3	2.6–23.0

FIGURE 3.—Mortality rates at 42 days according to the level of cardiac troponin I enrollment. Mortality rates at 42 days (without adjustment for base-line characteristics) are shown for ranges of cardiac troponin I levels measured at base line. The numbers at the bottom of each bar are the numbers of patients with cardiac tropinin I levels in each range, and the numbers above the bars are percentages. P < 0.001 for the increase in the mortality rate (and the risk ratio for mortality) with increasing levels of cardiac troponin I at enrollment. (Reprinted by permission of *The New England Journal of Medicine*, from Antman EM, Tanasijevic MJ, Thompson B, et al: Cardiac-specific troponin I levels to predict the risk of mortality in patients with acute coronary syndromes. *N Engl J Med* 335:1342–1349. Copyright 1996, Massachusetts Medical Society. All rights reserved.)

cannot be detected in healthy individuals, and levels may remain elevated up to 10 days after myocardial necrosis occurs.

Methods.—Blood samples were obtained from 1,404 patients with unstable angina or non–Q-wave myocardial infarction. Patient age was between 21 and 76. Specimens were analyzed for levels of cardiac troponin I, and these levels were correlated to mortality at 42 days.

Results.—At 42 days, mortality was significantly higher in the 573 patients with troponin I levels of 0.4 ng/mL or higher than in the 831 patients with levels lower than this (Fig 3). As levels of troponin I increased, mortality increased. With each increase of 1 ng/mL troponin I, there was a significant increase in the risk ratio for death after adjusting for base-line variables that were found to be independent predictors of death.

Conclusions.—Cardiac troponin I levels have predictive value for increased risk of death in patients with unstable angina or non–Q-wave myocardial infarction. Elevated levels of troponin I appear to be associated with higher mortality even in patients with normal levels of creatine kinase and its MB isoenzyme. The usefulness of this cardiac marker may apply to all patients with acute coronary syndromes.

▶ Troponin I and troponin T have burst upon the scene as the latest and greatest biochemical cardiac markers. This has also led to the troponin wars, which are fought at meetings and in advertising. Troponin I claims better cardiac specificity than T, but T claims better sensitivity in detecting small infarcts.

This paper shows that troponin I may be capable of detecting so-called microinfarcts, just like troponin T. There was a correlation between mortality at 42 days and troponin I levels. This was also true at low I levels where its MB isoenzyme was frequently normal. The journey starting with normal myocardium and ending with infarction travels through an increasing continuum of ischemia. As markers become capable of measuring lower levels of ischemia, physicians will have to decide what this means to their patients. This paper shows that even low levels of ischemia, as demonstrated by increased troponin I levels, may predict the patient's outcome.

R. Feld, Ph.D.

Chemistry Specimen Acceptability: A College of American Pathologists Q-Probes Study of 453 Laboratories
Jones BA, Calam RR, Howanitz PJ (St John Hosp, Detroit; Univ of California, Los Angeles)
Arch Pathol Lab Med 121:19–26, 1997   22–8

Background.—Because specimen adequacy is a critical preanalytic factor in the accuracy and utility of laboratory test results, laboratories have guidelines for assessing the specimens submitted. However, clinicians wish to minimize the amount of blood taken from patients. The frequency and reasons for laboratory rejection of chemistry specimens were studied.

Methods.—A total of 453 laboratories participated in the College of American Pathologists Q-Probes laboratory quality improvement study. Data on rejected chemistry specimens were recorded prospectively.

Findings.—Of 10,709,701 chemistry specimens submitted to these laboratories, 37,208 (0.35%) were rejected before testing. The most common reason cited for rejection was hemolysis. This reason was given 5 times more frequently than the second most commonly cited reason, which was insufficient amount for test performance. A higher proportion of rejected specimens were collected in microcollection tubes than in other containers. Significantly fewer rejected specimens were submitted by laboratory personnel than by other in-hospital staff. Out-of-hospital, nonlaboratory personnel had the best performance. The rejection rates for serum and plasma oxalate and fluoride specimens were significantly lower than they were for other specimen types. Rejection rates were higher for nongel tubes and lower for syringes, compared with gel tubes.

Conclusions.—Laboratory specimen rejection rates should be monitored regularly. Institution-specific factors associated with specimen rejection can be identified and improved.

▶ As part of the College of American Pathologists Q-Probe series, this study examined the rejection rate and cause for over 10 million specimens submitted to the chemistry laboratories of 453 participants. Not surprisingly, hemolysis led the list of reasons for specimen rejection, which averaged 0.35%. Also, not surprisingly, microcollection tubes exhibited a high rate of rejection for hemolysis. Anyone who has ever performed a heelstick or fingerstick on a premature newborn can sympathize with this. Phlebotomists controlled by the laboratory submitted fewer rejected specimens than nurses, medical students, and physicians for whom phlebotomy was not their main function. Education could reduce the rejection rate somewhat, but as long as specimens are obtained by a variety of health care personnel, the problem of rejected specimens will always be with us.

R. Feld, Ph.D.

Screening Children Exposed to Lead: An Assessment of the Capillary Blood Lead Fingerstick Test

Parsons PJ, Reilly AA, Esernio-Jenssen D (Wadsworth Ctr, Albany, NY; State Univ of New York, Albany; North Shore Univ Hosp, Manhasset, NY)
Clin Chem 43:302–311, 1997   22–9

Background.—In 1992 the authors' laboratory initiated a study in which capillary blood collection methods and the extent of contamination from lead occurring during blood collection for lead screening were assessed. The results of a 3–year study of matched pairs of venous and capillary blood specimens taken by fingerstick on the same day during routine visits to a private pediatrician or a public lead screening program were reported.

Methods.—A total of 499 paired venous and capillary blood specimens were analyzed. The rate and proportion of false positive findings were determined at 4 lead levels.

Findings.—The false positive rate at the 100 µg/L threshold for all data was 13%. However, the proportion of false positive results was only 5%. The log ratios of capillary-to-venous lead data showed that, except for 8 outliers, 2 subpopulations that followed a log-normal distribution could be identified. These 2 groups—*core*, consisting of 303, and *shifted*, consisting of 188—generated, on average, a positive bias at 100 µg/L lead of 8.6% and 30.3%, respectively. The log ratios of capillary-to-venous erythrocyte protoporphyrin (EP) data were distributed normally, demonstrating that capillary and venous EP do not differ.

Conclusions.—The relationship of capillary lead to venous lead indicates that the use of the former will result in a 5% to 10% bias in lead determinations at 150 µg/L. The resulting false positive rate will range from 1% to 9%, and the false positive proportion from 0% to 2%, as long as the patient's hands have been washed thoroughly before sampling.

▶ The realization of the detrimental effect of lead on the intellectual development of children sparked a concerted effort to remove lead from the environment, especially from gasoline and paint. The CDC has consistently decreased the acceptable blood lead level in children over the last 30 years to today's standard of less than 100 µg/L. These efforts have been rewarded, and now the geometric mean of blood lead in U.S. children is 28 µg/L.

These changes have led to increased challenges for laboratories. The EP test, which was used for many years as a screening test because it was easy, inexpensive, portable, and not susceptible to contamination, has been abandoned because of its lack of sensitivity to low lead levels. Preanalytical considerations have become increasingly important because only slight contamination could adversely affect the interpretation of results. This study examined paired capillary and fingerstick blood leads in a cohort of children. They carefully examined blood-drawing equipment for lead contamination and outlined the phlebotomy procedure. Under these circumstances, they found excellent correlation between capillary and venous samples. Having been raised at a time when there was much more lead in the environment and the mean blood lead concentration was closer to 300 µg/L (a level which now requires intervention), it is a wonder that any of us in the boomer generation can still add 2 and 2. Maybe I can blame this for my increasing memory lapses.

R. Feld, Ph.D.

Detection of Intrauterine Illicit Drug Exposure by Newborn Drug Testing

Kwong TC, Ryan RM (Univ of Rochester, New York)
Clin Chem 43:235–242, 1997

22–10

Introduction.—Intrauterine drug exposure is a major health concern. Placental abruption and premature labor has been associated with the cocaine use of pregnant women. Increased rates of maternal abruption, prematurity, and decreased growth parameters such as low birth weight have been associated with prenatal amphetamines. In utero opioid exposure can result in prematurity, small fetus size, and striking withdrawal symptoms that require treatment.

Testing.—Physicians can only order a newborn drug test if intrauterine drug exposure is suspected. Identification of intrauterine drug exposure infants could result in programs for improving parenting skills, home assistance, maternal drug treatment, restriction of breast-feeding, and close pediatric follow-up. Early identification of drug-exposed newborns should be the aim of testing. To protect physicians and hospitals involved and to decrease bias, specific guidelines should be written to select newborns for testing. An appropriate second test should confirm all drugs reported as positive.

Methodologies.—The best current options for identifying drug-exposed neonates are urine testing and meconium testing. Because of problems encountered in urine collections and the high thresholds used in current urine assays, urine testing sensitivity is low. Increased labor and time required are the disadvantages to meconium testing. Until technically less demanding assays become available, testing of newborn hair is unlikely. Still in the developmental stages are testing of amniotic fluid or gastric lavage.

Conclusion.—An appropriate modification of current methodologies would be to adopt lower urine assay thresholds for newborn samples, which would also increase sensitivity. Testing can be reserved for infants whose mothers have fewer than 5 prenatal visits, have a history of drug abuse, hepatitis B, AIDS, syphilis, gonorrhea, prostitution, or unexplained placental abruption or premature labor. Testing of infants can also be conducted if the infants have unexplained neurologic complications, evidence of possible drug withdrawal, or unexplained intrauterine growth retardation.

▶ Babies are the innocent victims of maternal drug use, including legal drugs such as tobacco and alcohol. It is well known that illicit drug use by the mother can lead to problems in utero, during delivery, and in development after birth. Because drug use on the part of the mother is difficult to elicit by history and legal issues cloud maternal testing, much of the testing in these situations is performed on the baby. Physicians are protected from legal complications if they perform drug testing on the infant according to certain guidelines and inform the parents that this is being done. These guidelines include both maternal history and physical signs found in the infant.

This paper reviews the limits of different analytic methods in detecting drugs and in the need for confirmatory testing. In addition, the various sample types—such as urine, meconium, and hair—are compared as to their advantages and disadvantages in detecting maternal drug use. There are also guidelines for the laboratory report so that all information is transmitted accurately to the ordering physician and for chain-of-custody documentation in case legal action is contemplated. The consequences of maternal drug use are so important from both a medical and legal standpoint that this testing needs to have a high degree of oversight. In the final analysis, it is the laboratory that answers the question, "Was this infant exposed to harmful and illegal substances during gestation?"

R. Feld, Ph.D.

Quality of Lipid and Lipoprotein Measurements in Community Laboratories
Watson JE, Evans RW, Germanowski J, et al (Univ of Pittsburgh, Pa; West Virginia Univ, Morgantown)
Arch Pathol Lab Med 121:105–109, 1997   22–11

Introduction.—The risk of coronary heart disease is increased by elevated serum cholesterol levels. It is necessary to have precise and accurate laboratory measurements to successfully identify, treat, and monitor patients with elevated blood cholesterol levels. The reliabilities of cholesterol and lipoprotein measurements in local community laboratories were determined to evaluate the level of standardization.

Methods.—Twenty-one laboratories used by physicians participating in the Cholesterol-Lowering Intervention Program measured standardized duplicate serum aliquots at 3 concentrations of low, intermediate, and high of total cholesterol, triglycerides, and high-density lipoprotein (HDL) cholestrol. Values obtained from the Centers for Disease Contol and Prevention (CDC)–standardized Heinz Lipid Laboratories were compared with results obtained from the laboratories and with the means of the entire sample.

Results.—For all 3 levels of total cholesterol, the mean coefficient of variation was 1.3% or less, demonstrating a high degree of precision. All were within the 5% range for the medium and high samples, and more than 80% were within 5% of the Heinz Laboratory low reference value, demonstrating high accuracy. For triglycerides and HDL cholesterol, the mean coefficients of variation were similar to that for total cholesterol; however, for HDL cholesterol in the intermediate concentration, 56% of the values fell outside the Heinz reference range, and for triglycerides in the low concentration, 61% of the values fell outside the range. A higher percentage of laboratories fell outside the CDC range because the Heinz Laboratory has a negative 2.7% bias versus the CDC for total cholesterol and HDL measurements. Sixteen percent of the laboratories were outside the 5% CDC range for medium and high total cholesterol samples, and the value was 58% for the low total cholesterol sample. Sixty-one percent were outside the 5% CDC range for the low samples for HDL cholesterol; values were 56% for the medium samples and 39% for the high samples.

Conclusion.—The reliability of total cholesterol measurements in local laboratories is high, according to the standards set by the National Cholesterol Education Program Laboratory Standardization Panel. For triglycerides and HDL cholesterol measurements, the levels of accuracy are lower.

▶ During the past 2 decades, the role of lipids as a risk factor for heart and circulatory system disease has received much attention. Americans are bombarded with the importance of a healthy low-fat diet, exercise, and having their lipid values measured, so that a new generation of effective lipid-lowering drugs can be used as indicated. Because these important medical decisions of diagnosis and treatment rely exclusively on laboratory values, there has been much emphasis on the accuracy and precision of lipid measurements.

The National Cholesterol Education Program has set goals for laboratories of precision and accuracy of 3%. This study uses frozen serum pools to test community and a few physicians' office laboratories in western Pennsylvania and West Virginia for accuracy and precision of their lipid measurements. In general, precision seems good and meets the National Cholesterol Education tion Program guidelines. Compared with CDC values, however, accuracy is found wanting. Accuracy in cholesterol measurements is not straightforward. The CDC uses a modified Abell-Kendall method for cholesterol because this method was used to establish the cut points for risk. The methods used by the CDC to establish accuracy for HDL cholesterol and triglyceride are also ones not used in practicing laboratories. We have recently switched to the new homogeneous HDL, which does not require precipitation, and find that it agrees well with CDC values. Because of the saving in labor, most laboratories will switch to this method. If accuracy in lipid measurements is defined by the people in Atlanta, then manufacturers must work more closely with the CDC to make sure that their methods meet these goals.

R. Feld, Ph.D.

Noninvasive Blood Glucose Monitoring
Klonoff DC (Univ of California, San Francisco)
Diabetes Care 20:433–437, 1997   22–12

Introduction.—Innovative methods are being developed to monitor blood glucose noninvasively. These methods are based on either radiation or fluid extraction. The most promising technologies employ near-infrared radiation spectroscopy, far-infrared radiation spectroscopy, radio wave impedance, optical rotation of polarized light, fluid extraction from skin, and interstitial fluid harvesting. This article describes the principles of and problems associated with each type of noninvasive monitoring technology.

Near-infrared Spectroscopy.—Glucose absorbs a small amount of light at each wavelength. Spectroscopy is used to detect the amount of near-infrared radiation absorbed by glucose through comparison of a reference with a detection beam. The sum of relative absorptions at selected wavelengths is converted to a blood glucose concentration. The major problem with this technology is the frequent need for calibration. Studies of in vivo glucose measurement with this technology have been disappointing.

Far-infrared Spectroscopy.—Glucose strongly absorbs energy in a band around 9400 nm. The absorption of the thermal energy of the body in the far-infrared glucose band is linearly related to blood glucose concentration. The problems with this technology are the small signal size of human thermal emissions and the need for cryoically cooled infrared detectors.

Radio Wave Impedance.—When a radio wave beam is applied to an aqueous solution, a nonionic solute like glucose can attenuate the amplitude and shift the beam phase, resulting in increased impedance proportional to solute concentration. This can be used to calculate the blood glucose concentration. Impedance is also affected by other factors, which must be accounted for in any calculations. A disposable finger clip is necessary for measurement; this could increase expense and decrease compliance.

Optical Rotation of Polarized Light.—When polarized light passes through a fluid containing glucose, the plane of polarization rotates proportionally to glucose concentration. This method is used to measure the glucose content of the aqueous humor of the eye. The signal size is small. There is also a potential lag between blood and aqueous humor glucose concentrations.

Fluid Extraction From Skin.—This technology could be used to monitor blood glucose levels accurately and continuously without patient effort. A device that used this technology, also called *reverse iontophoresis*, could monitor trends in blood glucose concentrations and could be programed to control an insulin-delivery system. Reverse iontophoresis applies an electric current to the skin, which extracts glucose that can be meaured. Problems include the 20–minute lag time between fluid extraction and final report, accuracy required to measure very small amounts of glucose, weekly recalibration, mild discomfort, interference with results by thick skin or sweat, adverse skin effects, and requirement for technology miniaturization.

Interstitial Fluid Harvesting.—Transcutaneous harvesting of interstitial fluid is not noninvasive, but it is minimally invasive. It involves extraction of fluid from the skin followed by direct measurement of glucose concentration. The problems include lag time and expense of disposable assay systems.

Conclusions.—This review briefly describes 6 promising technologies that are being developed to noninvasively detect and monitor blood glucose levels. A noninvasive blood glucose monitor could significantly improve the lives of many people with diabetes.

▶ The search for the Holy Grail of point-of-care glucose testing may soon come to an end. At least 1 company is submitting data to the Food and Drug Administration on a noninvasive glucose monitor. Millions of persons with diabetes who must obtain blood from their fingers to monitor their glucose levels anxiously await this event. Particularly affected are parents of small children with type I diabetes, who must inflict pain on their children several times a day to monitor the disease.

Currently, 2 main approaches, radiation and fluid extraction, are being tried. Radiation includes near-infrared spectroscopy, far-infrared spectroscopy, radio wave impedance, and polarized light rotation. The principles and major problems of each potential method are discussed. Although significant technical problems remain to be solved, some large companies are devoting significant development capital to this technique. There is no doubt that the first reliable noninvasive glucose instrument will be a great benefit and in great demand. For you *Star Trek* fans, once glucose measurement is possible, can the tricorder be far behind?

R. Feld, Ph.D.

Recommended Prostate-specific Antigen Testing Intervals for the Detection of Curable Prostate Cancer
Carter HB, Epstein JI, Chan DW, et al (Johns Hopkins Univ, Baltimore, Md; Natl Inst on Aging, Baltimore, Md; Merck Research Labs, Blue Bell, Pa)
JAMA 277:1456–1460, 1997   22–13

Background.—The prostate-specific antigen (PSA) test is used to detect prostate cancer, although there is no evidence from clinical trials for the usefulness of early detection and treatment. To avoid unnecessary testing, it would be beneficial to determine which men do not require yearly PSA tests.

Methods.—To examine PSA testing intervals, a historical prospective study of serial PSA measurements at 2– and 4– year intervals was carried out with frozen serum samples from the Baltimore Longitudinal Study of Aging (BLSA). The BLSA is an ongoing, long-term prospective study of aging. As part of this study, serum PSA levels were measured in 681 men at least 55. All male BLSA participants who had at least 1 pair of PSA measurements 1.5 to 2.5 years apart were included in the study. The BLSA study group consisted of 40 patients with cancer and 272 men without evidence of prostate cancer. The probability of detecting curable prostatic cancer at a given serum PSA level was determined from a series of 389 men with nonpalpable prostate cancer who underwent radical prostatectomy between 1989 and 1994.

Results.—When the pretreatment PSA level was no more than 4.0 ng/mL, nonpalpable prostate cancers were extremely likely to be small and curable. When the pretreatment PSA level was between 4.0 and 5.0 ng/mL, cancers were likely to be small and curable. When the pretreatment PSA level was greater than 5.0 ng/mL, 30% of prostate cancers were not curable. PSA levels greater than 5.0 ng/mL did not occur after as long as 4 years when the initial PSA level was less than 2.0 ng/mL, but did occur at higher initial PSA levels.

Conclusions.—The results of this series of older men suggest that it is safer to alter current recommendations for PSA testing. For men between the ages of 50 and 70 without suspicion of prostate cancer on digital rectal examination, a 2–year PSA testing interval is appropriate when baseline PSA is less than 2.0 ng/mL. Above that level, annual PSA testing remains appropriate. This change would avoid unnecessary testing and result in a large health care cost saving.

▶ Cancer is one of the most feared diseases in our society. Like the crab for which it is named, once it grabs hold of you it is difficult to break its grip. A recent controversial article suggested that advances in treatment have been minimal and that more funding should be directed toward prevention and education

There is currently no evidence that PSA screening has been beneficial in prolonging life through early detection. Nevertheless, the use of the test is widespread, and this use leads to many difficult decisions for both the physician who interprets the results and the patient who must choose between watchful waiting and treatment options.

By means of sera collected at intervals in the BLSA, the rate of increase in PSA was determined for those men in whom cancer developed. It is common practice for men 50 to 70 years to obtain yearly PSA values. A value of more than 5.0 ng/mL was chosen as a level at which most cancers were outside the capsule and therefore not curable. The increase to this level from values less than 2.0 ng/mL was not rapid. Because 70% of men between 50 and 70 years have PSA values less than 2.0 ng/mL, for men with negative results of direct rectal examination, a screening schedule of every other year would not increase the risk of missing a curable tumor. This recommendation would decrease unnecessary testing and its cost.

R. Feld, Ph.D.

The Ratio of Free to Total Serum Prostate Specific Antigen and Its Use in Differential Diagnosis of Prostate Carcinoma in Japan
Egawa S, Soh S, Ohori M, et al (Kitasato Univ, Sagamihara, Japan; Hyogo Med Ctr for Adults, Akashi, Japan)
Cancer 79:90–98, 1997   22–14

Background.—Prostate specific antigen (PSA) is useful for diagnosing prostate carcinoma, but its sensitivity and specificity are inadequate. Because the use of PSA assays has increased, there is a need for higher sensitivity and specificity. It is reported that the proportion of free PSA is significantly higher in benign prostatic hyperplasia than in prostate carcinoma. The percentage of free PSA in serum can help differentiate benign histologic conditions from cancer while retaining high sensitivity. The value of this ratio of 2 different molecular forms of PSA in an Asian male population has not been demonstrated; there is less PSA in serum in Japanese men than in white men of the same age.

Methods.—An AIA total PSA assay was developed that equally detects PSA in free or complex form. The value of this ratio was determined using 268 frozen serum samples. The samples were from patients treated for prostate carcinoma or benign prostatic hyperplasia.

Results.—Significantly lower ratios of free to total PSA were detected in patients with prostate carcinoma than in patients with benign prostatic hyperplasia. Total PSA levels were between 2.1 ng/mL and 10 ng/mL; median levels were not significantly different between the 2 groups of patients. There were significant differences in median percentages of free PSA between the 2 groups. The ratio of free to total PSA, but not total PSA, was valuable in identifying prostate carcinoma in palpably benign glands with total PSA of 2.1 ng/mL to 10 ng/mL. Sensitivity was 91.7% and specificity was 72.2% for low total PSA levels between 2.1 ng/mL and 4 ng/mL, with a cutoff value of 17%. In receiver-operating curve analysis, the value of the ratio of free to total PSA and of PSA density were similar.

Discussion.—The ratio of free to total PSA increases the value of total PSA for distinguishing benign histologic conditions from prostate carcinoma. It may be possible to avoid unnecessary biopsies in certain patients. This method can be used in patients with low total PSA. The determination of this ratio may be useful for evaluating older men with benign prostatic hyperplasia before surgical treatment. A larger prospective study is currently being conducted.

▶ There is little doubt that PSA has changed practice patterns. Even though large trials designed to answer the question of whether PSA is actually lengthening life are several years from publication, the number of PSA assays performed increases each year. There is also considerable debate among various medical groups as to whether PSA should be used as a screening tool at all.

Part of the problem with PSA is that minimally elevated levels can be caused by either benign prostatic hyperplasia or cancer. To overcome this shortcoming, various modifications—including age-specific normals, PSA density, and PSA velocity—have been tried to increase specificity. Prostate specific antigen exists in serum in both the free and bound forms. Most bound PSA is complexed to α1–antichymotrypsin. The ratio of free to total PSA is higher in benign prostatic hyperplasia than in cancer, and this measurement has been advocated for increasing specificity and reducing needless biopsies.

Several companies have submitted applications to the Food and Drug Administration for a free PSA assay, but, at the time of this writing, none have been approved. It is almost certain that free PSA will become part of the laboratory menu, but it is less certain that it can still the debate regarding the usefulness of this commonly used screening test.

R. Feld, Ph.D.

Clinical Evaluation of Serial Blood Processing at Point of Care

Estey CA, Felder RA (Univ of Virginia, Charlottesville)
Clin Chem 43:360–362, 1997

22–15

Background.—The clinical performance of the Axial Separation Module, which separates whole blood in Axial Process Containers, was evaluated. The Axial Separation Module was used to serially separate whole blood specimens at point of care to determine turnaround time. It was hypothesized that if blood separation were done at point of care, the turnaround time would be shortened because the specimens would not have to undergo the centrifugation step in the main laboratory, which normally delays processing time.

Methods.—Blood was drawn into an Axial Process Container and separated in the Axial Separation Module at a community-based outpatient clinic laboratory. Blood was also drawn into a Vacutainer Tube and separated in a conventional centrifuge at the main laboratory. Turnaround time for the "chem 17" test was calculated. Turnaround times for both separation systems were calculated and compared.

Results.—The turnaround time was shorter for blood that was serially separated at point of care. The average turnaround time was reduced by 24%. The phlebotomists who drew the blood reported no significant increase in workload with the Axial Separation Module at point of care, and also reported that they could immediately detect hemolysis.

Discussion.—Blood specimen turnaround time at the main laboratory can be reduced by using the Axial Separation Module and Axial Process Container system to serially separate blood at point of care. This procedure may improve the quality of analytical results by allowing immediate blood separation.

▶ The words "laboratory automation" have taken on a whole new meaning. Instead of adapting a manual method to an instrument, we are now talking about robotics and systems that take a tube of blood through the preparation and analytical process untouched by human hands.

Axial separation was developed in Canada when a tube of blood was rolled on a table and wondered what would happen if centrifugation occurred around the long axis. This technology allows a tube of blood to be separated into serum or plasma in 1 minute as opposed to 10 minutes in a conventional centrifuge. In a test of a pre-production model, this paper cites the following advantages for this technology: faster turnaround time, quicker detection of hemolysis and other interferents, and less preanalytical effect on certain analytes. This device might work very well in small laboratories where it could be integrated to the front end of instruments and sample preparation could be continuous rather than batch.

R. Feld, Ph.D.

Serum Alanine Aminotransferase Activity in Obese Children

Tazawa Y, Noguchi H, Nishinomiya F, et al (Akita Univ, Japan)
Acta Paediatr Scand 86:238–141, 1997   22–16

Background.—In adults, simple obesity can be accompanied by hepatic morbidity, termed nonalcoholic steatohepatitis, and is associated with serious hepatic diseases, fatty fibrosis, and fatty cirrhosis. Many children who are obese have persistent hyperaminotransferasemia of unknown origin. These patients may have liver diseases other than fatty liver associated with simple obesity. It is important to determine the incidence and pathogenesis of fatty liver in young children who are obese.

Methods.—Biochemical blood tests were performed in 310 obese school children aged 6–11 years. Tests included aspartate aminotransferase, alanine aminotransferase, and lipids. The children were classified into 3 age groups, as well as 4 groups according to level of obesity, and 3 groups according to length of obesity. Ultrasound was used to examine 77 children with an abnormal alanine aminotransferase test result and 27 children with normal alanine aminotransferase values to identify the liver fatty-fibrotic pattern.

Results.—Of all the children, 24% had an abnormal serum alanine aminotransferase test result. In 64 of the 77 children with abnormal alanine aminotransferase values and in 5 of the 27 children with normal alanine aminotransferase values, the fatty-fibrotic pattern was identified. The sensitivity of the serum alanine aminotransferase test for detecting the fatty-fibrotic pattern proved by US was 92%. The number of individuals with abnormal serum alanine aminotransferase levels increased with length of obesity. In individuals with obesity of short duration, the rate of abnormal results of serum alanine aminotransferase testing did not increase with older age or severity of obesity.

Discussion.—The serum alanine aminotransferase test is useful for screening fatty liver. These findings suggest that in children, fatty liver is associated with severity and length of obesity. Fatty liver or fatty fibrosis may develop in young children with mild obesity or obesity of short duration. Early intervention is needed in these individuals.

▶ Obesity is a serious problem in this country. It is a leading cause of type II diabetes and can affect both quantity and quality of life adversely. Each year reports indicate that more Americans are obese, and as the standard of living in the world increases and animal protein replaces grains, it is thought that this problem will spread.

Obesity is associated with liver disease, specifically, nonalcoholic steatohepatitis or NASH. Nonalcoholic steatohepatitis is caused by fatty infiltration and can lead to fibrosis or cirrhosis. Patients with NASH can exhibit elevated alamine aminotransferase (ALT) values and it is in the differential for the patient with an unexplained elevated ALT.

This Japanese study measured ALT values in obese children divided into groups based on age, duration of obesity, and the extent of obesity. The ALT values were higher in children who had extreme obesity of long duration. Ultrasound evaluations in these patients showed a higher percentage of fatty-fibrotic pattern than in children with lesser obesity. Although weight loss can reverse the pathologic changes in the liver and lower ALT values, it is an extremely difficult task, as anyone who has tried to lose weight can tell you. We can add one more disease that is associated with obesity, and with an increasing rate of obesity in the world, a more common explanation of an unexplained elevated ALT.

R. Feld, Ph.D.

Evaluation of Fasting Plasma Glucose as a Screening Test for Diabetes Mellitus in Singaporean Adults

Lee CH, Fook-Chong S (Toa Payoh Hosp, Singapore; Ministry of Health, Singapore)
Diabetic Med 14:119–122, 1997   22–17

Introduction.—The World Health Organization (WHO) cutoff value for fasting plasma glucose (FPG) is 7.8 mmol L^{-1} for the diagnosis of diabetes mellitus (DM). There is some concern that this level is not adequate for diagnosing often asymptomatic non-insulin-dependent diabetes mellitus. The adequacy and performance of various FPG cutoff values, including the WHO value of 7.8 mmol L^{-1}, were evaluated during screening for DM in a group of Singaporean adults.

Methods.—During a 4 year period, 865 oral glucose tolerance tests were performed on Singaporean outpatients. After an overnight fast, a fasting blood sample was collected. Research subjects took an oral 75 g anhydrous glucose load, and a 2–hour postload plasma glucose blood sample then was obtained. Age range of 502 men and 363 woman was 18 to 67 years. Ethnic origin of the research subjects was as follows: 680 Chinese, 101 Indians, and 84 Malays. Sensitivity and specificity of FPG the diagnosis of DM were calculated.

Results.—Of 865 research subjects, 220 (25.4%) had a 2–hour plasma glucose (2H-PG) level exceeding 11.1 mmol L^{-1}. Of these, 90 had a fasting plasma glucose level of 7.8 mmol L^{-1} or greater; the sensitivity was 40.9%, specificity was 98.8%, and positive predictive value was 92.7%. There was a non-linear relationship between FPG and 2H-PG. Using a cubic equation, the FPG corresponding to a 2H-PG of 11.1 mmol L^{-1} was 5.7 mmol L^{-1}. The predicted 2H-PG corresponding to a FPG of 7.8 mmol L^{-1} was 16.0 mmol L^{-1}. A cutoff FPG of 5.7 mmol L^{-1} produced optimal sensitivity and specificity using the ROCLAB program. When data were reclassified using a FPG cutoff of 5.7 mmol L^{-1}, sensitivity, specificity, and positive predictive values changed to 80.0%, 90.9%, and 74.9%, respectively. When the FPG cutoff was set at 7.0 mmol L^{-1}, there was a satisfactory balance between sensitivity, specificity, and positive predictive value.

Conclusion.—It is suggested that a FPG of 7.0 mmol L^{-1} be adopted because specificity and sensitivity are more appropriate at 98.3% and 56.4%, respectively. The sensitivity of 56.4% is a clinically useful improvement compared with 40.9% according to WHO criteria.

▶ This article examines the sensitivity and specificity of various cutoff values for fasting plasma glucose in the diagnosis of diabetes. The oral glucose tolerance test served as the gold standard. Receiver operating characteristic analysis yielded a "best" cutoff of 103 mg/dL, but this decision level was considered to have too low a specificity (90.9%). When a cutoff value of 126 mg/dL was used, specificity increased to 98.3%.

The American Diabetes Association has recently recommended a decision level of 126 mg/dL for a fasting blood glucose value to diagnose diabetes. The Diabetes Complications and Control Trial (DCCT) has made it clear that tight control greatly reduces the complications of diabetes in patients with type I diabetes. It is expected that similar findings will be demonstrated in type II diabetic patients. It is estimated that this new lower cutoff will cause an additional 2 million new diagnoses of diabetes. The ADA also recommended that people be screened for diabetes with a fasting glucose test starting at age 45 and continuing every 3 years. It is hoped that by identifying diabetes earlier and instituting treatment that diabetic complications can be avoided. The cost of these complications for the nation's 14 million diabetic patients is huge; even though upfront costs may increase to diagnose and treat the new diabetic patients who are identified, overall costs may eventually be reduced. The additional work for laboratories to diagnose and monitor these new diabetic patients will be substantial.

R. Feld, Ph.D.

23 Laboratory Management

A Leadership-Management Training Curriculum for Pathology Residents
Sims KL, Darcy TP (Creighton Univ, Omaha, Neb)
Am J Clin Pathol 108:90–95, 1997   23–1

Introduction.—Leadership and management skills are crucial to the success of a pathologist in and outside of academic centers. A leadership and management curriculum from a combined anatomical and clinical pathology residency program was described.

Leadership-Management Curriculum.—This mentor-based strategy incorporates leadership and management skills throughout the residency, with a dedicated 2-month rotation in the final year of the program. The 2-month rotation is lead by a senior faculty pathologist mentor and incorporates active participation in management activities, small group discussions, reading, and a management process project. Residents who complete this curriculum are followed for outcomes and program evaluations.

Outcome Measures and Results.—Six residents have participated in the 2-month mentor-based leadership and management rotation, and 2 have participated in an abbreviated 1-month rotation. Postrotation participants gave the rotation the highest possible rating on written and verbal evaluations. Three reported that it was their favorite rotation during residency. Of 6 eligible residents who have taken and passed the American Board of Pathology anatomical pathology–clinical pathology certification examinations, 3 reported that their highest relative score was on the management section of the clinical pathology examination. Residents who have completed the program are contacted annually by telephone and written questionnaire. This annual follow-up will continue for at least 5 years for graduates.

Conclusion.—The mentor-based approach to the described leadership-management curriculum is considered productive and has been enthusiastically supported by its graduates. It is suggested that any program of this nature should be led by a senior pathologist with a current leadership role.

▶ Management training is often neglected in pathology residency programs. There are probably several reasons for this. First, there are more than enough clinical material and conferences to fully occupy the resident's time. Second, most laboratory directors have little or no formal management training and are, therefore, reluctant to take on the task of teaching something that they are not comfortable with.

This paper describes a curriculum in leadership and management that was developed at Creighton University. The training occurs throughout the resident's time but culminates in a concentrated 2-month rotation during the senior year. This focused training is mentor-based and relies heavily on small group discussions. In addition, each resident is assigned a "process" project which must be completed by the end of the residency. The projects were assigned according to the current needs of the department.

We have had "management" projects during the chemistry rotation at our institution for many years and find them to be well received and useful. This is a well-reasoned and detailed program which should be copied at institutions that train residents. This type of training will be essential if the pathologist is to be effective in the future health care environment.

R. Feld, Ph.D.

Evaluating Laboratory Usage in the Intensive Care Unit: Patient and Institutional Characteristics That Influence Frequency of Blood Sampling
Zimmerman JE, Seneff MG, Sun X, et al (George Washington Univ, Washington, DC; Univ of Virginia, Charlottesville)
Crit Care Med 25:737–748, 1997   23–2

Introduction.—Overuse of laboratory testing can increase the cost of patient care and result in iatrogenic anemia with the subsequent need for transfusion and its associated risks. Recent economic and federal regulatory developments have mandated re-examination of laboratory use. The number of blood samples drawn for laboratory testing within a large and diverse population of patients admitted to ICUs was evaluated to identify patient and institutional characteristics influencing the frequency of blood drawing.

Methods.—A consecutive sample of 17,440 patients admitted to the ICU was used and 14,043 blood samples obtained for laboratory testing on ICU days 2–7 were evaluated. On ICU day 1, data on patient demographics and physiology were recorded. Information was collected on the type and number of blood samples taken for laboratory testing. Using only data from ICU day 1, the subsequent number of samples drawn on ICU days 2 and 2–7 were predicted.

Results.—In the 42 ICUs analyzed, the mean number of blood samples drawn on ICU days 2–7 was 16.2 per patient. The mean was 23 in teaching ICUs and 9.9 in nonteaching ICUs. The most significant determinants of the number of blood samples drawn on ICU days 2–7 were the ICU day 1 Acute Physiology Score and admission diagnosis. After controlling for patient variables, hospital teaching status, number of beds, and location of hospitals in the East and South were significantly associated with increased blood sampling on ICU days 2 and ICU days 2–7. There was an association between increased blood sampling, more frequent use of arterial cannula, and mechanical ventilation.

Conclusion.—This method of adjusting for patient and institutional variables and being able to predict the number of blood samples drawn for laboratory tests allow ICUs to compare their practices with those of other ICUs. In the present environment of concern regarding cost of medical care, this information can be useful.

▶ The overordering by physicians of laboratory tests and other medical resources has been a continuing problem in American medicine. Efforts to reduce ordering—such as education, Diagnosis-Related Groups, and managed care—have been only partially successful. We will soon institute government-approved profiles in order to attempt to accomplish this end. The problem in the case of the ICU patient is more complicated because of the severity of the illness and the fact that physicians who care for extremely ill patients have easy access to laboratory testing, such as point-of-care instruments and stat laboratories.

This paper tries to predict test ordering on ICU days 2–7, based on data established on day 1. This would allow institutions to compare usage. Severity of illness and admission diagnosis were the primary predictors of test usage. As would be expected, more tests were ordered in teaching hospitals, and there was some geographic influence.

The authors point out all the detriments of test overordering, including blood loss, transfusion risk, and increased cost. This study was not designed to answer the big question, namely, which tests are necessary and how often they should be ordered. Maybe this question will be decided by practice guidelines and market forces. Armed with the data and methods presented in the paper, it should be easier to compare institutions and to track progress in reducing ordering subject to any interventions.

R. Feld, Ph.D.

What Many of Us Are Doing or Should Be Doing in Clinical Pathology: A List of the Activities of the Pathologist in the Clinical Laboratory
Laposata M (Massachusetts Gen Hosp, Boston; Harvard Med School, Boston)
Am J Pathol 106:571–573, 1996   23–3

Background.—Hospital administrators and physicians who are not pathologists are often not aware of the full range of pathologists' activities. This lack of understanding makes clinical pathology activities vulnerable to scrutiny for cost-cutting purposes. A list of the activities of pathologists in the clinical laboratory was presented.

Pathologists' Activities in the Clinical Laboratory.—Clinical activities include providing clinical information. Among other responsibilities, this includes reviewing a sample microscopically at the request of a clinician, interpreting test results, evaluating patients, performing tests not routinely offered or that require a modification of the standard test protocol, explaining a test result that may be confusing to the clinician, discussing the clinical significance of a test, and evaluating a patient's medical history before certain blood samples are collected to ensure accurate test interpretation. Pathologists also control clinical laboratory use. For example, a clinician may ask which test should be done in a particular setting or request an expensive laboratory test only on approval of the pathologist. Pathologists also investigate a laboratory test order that is inapproriate or incomplete and duplicate orders. Pathologists perform quality assurance activities. Management activities in clinical pathology include fiscal and personnel management, negotiation of payment for laboratory services, and revenue enhancement endeavors.

Conclusions.—The list presented may serve as a starting point for a universally accepted group of activities describing modern clinical pathology and will be useful for pathologists who wish to elucidate their significant contributions to administrators and fellow physicians.

▶ Anyone who has had the pleasure of hearing Mike Laposata speak knows that he does not lack enthusiasm. Clinical pathology is like the amnesia victim of many movies searching for an identity. This is compounded by the fact that many payers do not recognize the contributions of the laboratory-based physician.

In this article, Dr. Laposata outlines his thoughts on what laboratory physicians should be doing. The author divides the duties into clinical and management activities. Clinical activities include provision of clinical information, control of laboratory use, and performance of quality assurance activities. He provides several examples in each category. These activities obviously require the establishment of a working relationship between the clinicians and the clinical pathologist. It has been my experience that the laboratory must be proactive in many situations. The laboratory must contact the physician about a problem rather than waiting for the clinician to initiate the interaction.

The last category discussed includes fiscal and personnel management and revenue enhancement endeavors. Although most pathologists are probably already performing most of these tasks, the trick is to get the value-added recognized by others.

R. Feld, Ph.D.

Duplicate Laboratory Orders: A College of American Pathologists Q-Probes Study of Thyrotropin Requests in 502 Institutions

Valenstein P, Schifman RB (St Joseph Mercy Hosp, Ann Arbor, Mich; Tucson VA Med Ctr, Ariz)

Arch Pathol Lab Med 120:917–921, 1996   23–4

Background.—Duplicate laboratory testing is wasteful. A College of American Pathologists Q-probes study of the frequency and cause of duplicate testing for thyrotropin (TSH) at a large number of centers was reported.

Methods.—Five hundred and two centers of various sizes analyzing consecutively processed TSH assays participated in the study. Data on 221,476 TSH orders were reported. Duplicates were defined as 2 or more TSH tests performed within 7 days.

Findings.—A median 1.5% of TSH tests duplicated a TSH order received for the same patient within the previous 7 days. Ten percent of the centers found that 4.5% or more of their TSH tests were duplicates. Higher duplicate rates tended to occur at larger centers. At such centers, duplicate tests were more likely to be ordered by a physician other than the one initially ordering the test. For 19% of these duplicate orders, physicians were not aware that the first test had been ordered. Duplicate assays were ordered to see if a previous result had changed or to check the accuracy of a previous finding. Eleven percent of duplicate TSH assays had apparently never been ordered.

Conclusions.—Many centers are performing duplicate TSH tests that, in most cases, appear to be unnecessary medically. Policies to reduce the opportunity for different physicians to order tests on 1 patient should be considered.

▶ The literature is replete with information concerning the use of laboratory tests in the diagnosis of various diseases, but there is a paucity of information on how often patients should be monitored with laboratory tests once a diagnosis has been established. Hospitalized patients seem to get tests every 24 hours, not because anyone has established this as an effective schedule, but simply because the sun has risen and set.

This paper, one of the Q-probe series by the College of American Pathologists, looks at duplicate ordering of TSH. A duplicate order is defined as 2 TSH values within a 7-day period. The duplicate order rate for more than 500 institutions of varying sizes was 1.9%. Duplicate ordering was more prevalent at larger institutions, which is not surprising given that care for the patient may be shared by several physicians.

In investigating the causes of duplicate orders, the most common explanation was that the physician was unaware of the duplicate order. Fully 11% of the duplicate orders were never ordered and a clerical error was suspected. In many institutions, physicians do not fill in laboratory request slips and the person whose job this is may not know the difference between a TSH and a PSA. Surprisingly, those institutions with computer systems that scanned for duplicate orders did not have a lower duplicate ordering ratio, because these tended to be larger institutions with a higher duplicate rate for other reasons.

There is obviously room for improvement here, both in transmitting orders to the laboratory and in the laboratory's providing decision support to ordering physicians on the proper use of tests.

R. Feld, Ph.D.

Converging Technologies and Their Impact on the Clinical Laboratory
Burtis CA (Oak Ridge Natl Lab, Tenn)
Clin Chem 42:1735–1749, 1996

23–5

Introduction.—Clinical laboratory medicine is changing dramatically. The technological revolution is redefining the ways in which it is organized, staffed, operated, and equipped. These changes are occurring in solid-state physics; material manufacturing; computer, engineering, and laboratory sciences; analytical chemistry; biotechnology; and medicine.

Measurement and Digital Technology.—Measurement technology includes large, multipurpose mainframe chemistry analyzers; immunoassay analyzers; point-of-care analyzers; and portable, single-purpose analyzers for use in the home. Front-end automation has integrated the specimen identification, labeling, preparation, handling, transport, delivery, storage, retrieval, and retesting functions into analytical systems. Miniaturization has dramatically decreased the overall size of the systems. Molecular diagnostics have resulted in clinical methods, such as nuclei acid amplification, that are sensitive and specific. Computer hardware, software, and peripherals are changing the practice of clinical laboratory medicine in statistical processing, word processing, financial management, time and database management, spreadsheets, tracking, and trend analysis. Peripherals include ergonomically designed keyboards, color video terminals, high-capacity hard-disk drives, printers, and modems.

Communications and Transportation Technology.—Computers can be interconnected on a global scale with a network. Telecommunications hardware and media affect the rate at which data are transmitted and received. The Internet provides a wealth of information and allows laboratories to communicate by means of electronic mail, join discussion groups, and generate and distribute relevant information through electronic publishing. Just-in-time manufacturing is a result of transportation technology. This affects clinical laboratories by moving goods from one site to another rapidly, allowing for clinical results to be available within 24 hours.

Conclusion.—The boundaries of time and space are removed by means of the new technologies. A wide repertoire of clinically relevant assays crossing traditional disciplinary boundaries is possible with the new generation of automated chemistry, hematology, immunoassay, coagulation, and microbiology analytical systems now available. A more productive, efficient, and cost-effective operation is possible with the arrival of total automation in the clinical laboratory. Laboratory professionals must engage in continuing education to keep their skills current.

▶ Clinical laboratories have always been heavily influenced by technology. This is especially true in today's environment in which technological change is rapid and market forces are rewarding technological innovation that can also be shown to be cost effective.

The author of this review covers such new technologies as system integration, miniaturization, molecular diagnostics, computers, and communications. System integration has led to total laboratory automation which combines sample introduction, reagent handling, reaction monitoring, and data processing. Molecular diagnostics involves DNA and polymerase chain reaction technology. Computer software and hardware allow for the processing and storage of data that, when combined with communication technology, enable the dissemination of information, including Internet transfer. The author emphasizes the fact that only through the use of these new technologies will the laboratory of the future be able to survive in the changing health care environment.

R. Feld, Ph.D.

Subject Index*

A

Abdominal
  fat aspiration, diagnostic screening of
    systemic amyloidosis by, *98:* 288
AccuProbe
  group B streptococcus test to detect
    group B streptococci in broth
    cultures of vaginal-anorectal
    specimens in pregnancy, *98:* 401
Achondroplasia
  definition by recurrent G380R
    mutations of FGFR3, *96:* 407
Acid
  /EDTA elution method, removal of IgG
    antibodies from intact red cells by,
    98: 386
Acinic
  cell carcinoma of salivary glands,
    well-differentiated, with lymphoid
    stroma, *98:* 184
Acquired immunodeficiency syndrome (*see*
    AIDS)
Acridine
  orange staining of broth blood cultures
    for *Bartonella quintana* detection,
    96: 361
Adenocarcinoma
  bladder, florid cystitis glandularis of
    intestinal type with mucin
    extravasation mimics, *98:* 145
  cervix
    in situ, cone biopsy margins in,
      98: 78
    microinvasive, *98:* 77
  colorectal, lymph node recovery from
    resection specimens removed from,
    98: 203
  cutaneous, CD44 expression in,
    98: 276
  endometrium
    histologic grading with nuclear
      grading system, *96:* 189
    sertoliform, case studies, *98:* 90
  gastric, synchronous with
    mucosa-associated lymphoid tissue
    lymphoma of stomach, *98:* 195
  lung, and atypical alveolar hyperplasia,
    96: 74
  metastatic, immunohistochemical
    identification of tumor markers in,
    98: 357
  pancreas

HER-2/*neu* expression in, *97:* 101
  K-*ras* mutation detection in,
    polymerase chain reaction-based,
    97: 100
  prostate
    androgen ablation therapy in,
      neoadjuvant total, *96:* 150
    with atrophic features, *98:* 149
    intraepithelial tumors as risk factor
      for, *97:* 122
    metastatic, preoperative androgen
      deprivation therapy in, florid
      xanthomatous pelvic lymph node
      reaction to, *97:* 144
    screening, normal range *vs.*
      age-specific prostate-specific antigen
      in, *97:* 306
    single focus of adenocarcinoma in
      prostate biopsy specimen not
      predictive of pathologic stage of
      disease, *98:* 151
    spread within prostatic ducts and
      acini, *98:* 157
    T1-T3/M0, predicting lymph node
      metastases in, *96:* 145
    xanthoma as mimic of, *96:* 154
  sinonasal intestinal type, *97:* 54
  urethral clear cell, *98:* 146
Adenoid
  cystic carcinoma (*see* Carcinoma,
    adenoid cystic)
Adenoma
  bronchial, mucous gland, *97:* 74
  colorectal, papillomavirus DNA in,
    96: 122
  kidney, metanephric, *97:* 115
  nephrogenic, of prostatic urethra,
    96: 138
  pituitary, diagnosis on touch
    preparations by
    immunocytochemistry, *96:* 310
  salivary gland
    basal cell and minimally pleomorphic
      types, cytologic differentiation from
      solid adenoid cystic carcinoma,
      98: 132
    pleomorphic, differentiated from
      adenoid cystic carcinoma on fine
      needle aspiration cytology, *98:* 133
Adenomatoid
  tumor of adrenal gland, *98:* 261
Adenomatous
  hyperplasia

C

Author Index